Hypoxia: Translation in Progress

Hypoxia: Translation in Progress

Editor: Kate Morris

AMERICAN
MEDICAL PUBLISHERS
www.americanmedicalpublishers.com

AMERICAN
MEDICAL PUBLISHERS
www.americanmedicalpublishers.com

Cataloging-in-Publication Data

Hypoxia : translation in progress / edited by Kate Morris.
p. cm.
Includes bibliographical references and index.
ISBN 979-8-88740-585-8
1. Anoxemia. 2. Oxygen in the body. 3. Hypoxia (Water). 4. Diagnosis—Causes and theories of causation.
5. Health. I. Morris, Kate.
RC103.A4 R65 2023
616.989 3--dc23

American Medical Publishers,
41 Flatbush Avenue,
1st Floor, New York,
NY 11217, USA

ISBN 979-8-88740-585-8 (Hardback)

Contents

Preface

Hypoxia refers to a type of condition in which the entire or a part of the body does not receive enough supply of oxygen at the tissue level. Its symptoms include difficulty in breathing, bluish skin, disorientation, a rapid heartbeat and agitation. The underlying illnesses which affect breathing and blood flow, resulting in hypoxia are asthma, emphysema, pneumothorax, sleep apnea, anemia, pulmonary edema and congestive heart failure. There are several ways to diagnose hypoxia, such as arterial blood gas test (ABG), six-minute walk test (6MWT), pulse oximetry, pulmonary function test (PFT), etc. Hypoxic condition can be treated by administering oxygen. It involves various equipments that can be used for inhaling oxygen such as non-rebreather masks, transport ventilators, nasal cannula, bag valve masks and simple oxygen facemasks. This book provides significant information to help develop a good understanding of hypoxia. It aims to understand the clinical perspectives of this medical condition. The readers would gain knowledge that would broaden their perspective in this area of study.

This book unites the global concepts and researches in an organized manner for a comprehensive understanding of the subject. It is a ripe text for all researchers, students, scientists or anyone else who is interested in acquiring a better knowledge of this dynamic field.

I extend my sincere thanks to the contributors for such eloquent research chapters. Finally, I thank my family for being a source of support and help.

Editor

1

Similar Supine Heart Rate Variability Changes during 24-h Exposure to Normobaric vs. Hypobaric Hypoxia

Valérian Tanner[1], Raphael Faiss[2,3], Jonas Saugy[2,3], Nicolas Bourdillon[2], Laurent Schmitt[4] and Grégoire P. Millet[2]*

[1] *Medicine School, Faculty of Biology and Medicine, University of Lausanne, Lausanne, Switzerland,* [2] *Institute of Sport Sciences, University of Lausanne, Lausanne, Switzerland,* [3] *REDs, Research and Expertise in Anti-Doping Sciences, University of Lausanne, Lausanne, Switzerland,* [4] *National Centre of Nordic-Ski, Research and Performance, Prémanon, France*

Correspondence:
Valérian Tanner
valerian.tanner@unil.ch

Purpose: This study aimed to investigate the differences between normobaric (NH) and hypobaric hypoxia (HH) on supine heart rate variability (HRV) during a 24-h exposure. We hypothesized a greater decrease in parasympathetic-related parameters in HH than in NH.

Methods: A pooling of original data from forty-one healthy lowland trained men was analyzed. They were exposed to altitude either in NH (F_IO_2 = 15.7 ± 2.0%; PB = 698 ± 25 mmHg) or HH (F_IO_2 = 20.9%; PB = 534 ± 42 mmHg) in a randomized order. Pulse oximeter oxygen saturation (S_pO_2), heart rate (HR), and supine HRV were measured during a 7-min rest period three times: before (in normobaric normoxia, NN), after 12 (H12), and 24 h (H24) of either NH or HH exposure. HRV parameters were analyzed for time- and frequency-domains.

Results: S_pO_2 was lower in both hypoxic conditions than in NN and was higher in NH than HH at H24. Subjects showed similarly higher HR during both hypoxic conditions than in NN. No difference in HRV parameters was found between NH and HH at any time. The natural logarithm of root mean square of the successive differences (LnRMSSD) and the high frequency spectral power (HF), which reflect parasympathetic activity, decreased similarly in NH and HH when compared to NN.

Conclusion: Despite S_pO_2 differences, changes in supine HRV parameters during 24-h exposure were similar between NH and HH conditions indicating a similar decrease in parasympathetic activity. Therefore, HRV can be analyzed similarly in NH and HH conditions.

Keywords: heart rate variability, arterial oxygen saturation, normobaric normoxia, hypobaric hypoxia, normobaric hypoxia, autonomic nervous system, altitude

INTRODUCTION

Altitude training is an effective method commonly used by elite athletes (Millet and Brocherie, 2020). Prolonged altitude exposure increases erythropoiesis, which is explained by increased plasma erythropoietin concentration (Stray-Gundersen et al., 2001) and leads to an apparent increase in peripheral tissues oxygen delivery. This altitude-related increase in red blood cell mass increases the oxygen-carrying capacity of the blood and improves aerobic power (Hauser et al., 2016). Moreover, skeletal muscle adaptations could improve oxygen extraction during altitude exposition (Brooks et al., 1992).

The two main methods used for hypoxic exposure are hypobaric hypoxia (HH; FIO2 = 20.9%; PB <760 mmHg; real altitude in mountain or hypobaric "decompression" chamber) and normobaric hypoxia (NH; FIO2 <20.9%; PB = 760 mmHg; simulated altitude by using hypoxic facilities). On the one hand, HH has been used for years by endurance athletes during training camps On the other hand, the democratization of NH, accelerated by technical progress, allows the use of the usual lowland infrastructures, and avoids the time and inconvenience of transport to altitude. An updated panorama of all HH and NH hypoxic training methods is available in Girard et al. (2017). Based on the equivalent air altitude equivalent model (Conkin and Wessel, 2008), NH is frequently used as a surrogate to HH. However, recent research suggested that NH and HH are not interchangeable (Fulco et al., 2011; Millet et al., 2012; Saugy et al., 2014, 2016a; Coppel et al., 2015; DiPasquale et al., 2015a; Conkin, 2016) although the differences between HH and NH are still debated (Millet and Debevec, 2020; Richalet, 2020). The following differences were already reported for a matched inspired oxygen pressure (P_IO_2) in HH vs. NH, respectively: (1) lower pulse oximeter oxygen saturation (S_pO_2) (Saugy et al., 2016c; Aebi et al., 2020; Debevec et al., 2020); (2) greater performance impairment (Beidleman et al., 2014; Saugy et al., 2016a), both recently confirmed in a study with perfectly controlled environmental factors (Takezawa et al., 2021); (3) higher oxidative stress (Faiss et al., 2013; Ribon et al., 2016); (4) impaired nitric oxide bioavailability (Faiss et al., 2013); (5) greater fluid retention (Loeppky et al., 2005; Conkin and Wessel, 2008), and (6) sleep structure perturbation (Heinzer et al., 2016; Saugy et al., 2016b). In addition, breathing patterns are affected as well: lower tidal volume, lower minute ventilation, higher physiological dead space, and higher respiratory frequency during HH exposure compared to NH (Savourey et al., 2003; Conkin and Wessel, 2008; Saugy et al., 2014). It was also demonstrated that HH provokes stronger hypoxic pulmonary vasoconstriction, altering the ventilation-perfusion ratio (Loeppky et al., 1997). Moreover, hypocapnia and blood alkalosis are greater in HH than NH (Savourey et al., 2003; Coppel et al., 2015). Despite all these differences, which suggest that exposure in terrestrial altitude (HH) may induce more pronounced stress with larger physiological responses than simulated altitudes (NH), there is still an ongoing debate about their clinical significance. A "point-counterpoint" (Millet et al., 2012; Mounier and Brugniaux, 2012) reported the main arguments on this subject, and a more recent crosstalk (Millet and Debevec, 2020; Richalet, 2020) brought the debate back to the forefront. All protagonists agreed that further studies with a rigorous methodological approach and new perspectives would allow a more comprehensive understanding of the role of barometric pressure *per se* in different hypoxic conditions.

One of the potential perspectives to evaluate the differences between HH and NH could be the heart rate variability (HRV). HRV is the fluctuation in the time intervals between adjacent heartbeats (Malik et al., 1996). There are two main methods for the HRV analyses: time-domain and frequency-domain. Time-domain indices of HRV (LnRMSSD, natural logarithm of root mean square of the successive differences) quantify the amount of variability in measurements of the interbeat interval. Frequency-domain measurements [The low frequency spectral power (LF) and HF, respectively low and high frequency spectral power] estimate the distribution of absolute or relative power into frequency bands. This non-invasive method is used to assess cardiac autonomic control (Buchheit, 2014). It is especially an accurate means of estimating parasympathetic activation by looking specifically at HF with frequency-domain analysis (Malik et al., 1996; Grossman and Taylor, 2007). Moreover, those frequency-domain analyses are known to be more sensitive than time-domain (Schmitt et al., 2015a). In general, acute hypoxia decreases HRV and parasympathetic activity (Wille et al., 2012). Since S_pO_2 is lower in HH, the hypoxic chemoreflex should lead to a greater vagal withdrawal in HH than in NH (Parati et al., 2015) and thus potentially result in differences in the autonomic cardiac control. Moreover, variations in S_pO_2 are related to variations in HRV parameters. Indeed, a decrease in S_pO_2 is related to a decrease in both LnRMSSD (Krejèí et al., 2018) and HF and to an increase in the low-to-high frequency ratio (LF/HF) (Botek et al., 2015). Since ventilation influences cardiac autonomic activity (Brown et al., 1993), the above-mentioned differences in breathing patterns between NH and HH could also generate distinct HRV responses. Considering those physiological mechanisms, one may speculate on different influences of NH vs. HH on HRV.

The effects of NH vs. HH on HRV were studied only during acute exposures ($\leq$ 30 min) (Basualto-Alarcón et al., 2012; Aebi et al., 2020). The LF/HF ratio was slightly higher in HH, but the evidence for a hypobaric effect *per se* on HRV in hypoxia during acute exposures was not strong enough (Aebi et al., 2020). Therefore, the present study aimed to compare the influence of a 24-h exposure in NH vs. HH on supine HRV. Since HH induced a larger desaturation than NH, the hypothesis of a greater decrease in parasympathetic-related HRV parameters (such as LnRMSSD and HF) in HH condition was tested. Furthermore, since breathing patterns are different between HH and NH, greater differences in frequency-domain parameters (especially in HF influenced by respiratory sinus arrhythmia) (Grossman and Taylor, 2007) than in time-domain parameters (i.e., LnRMSSD) were expected.

METHODS

Subjects

Forty-one healthy lowland trained men regularly practicing endurance sports have participated in our study. The main characteristics of all subjects were: age 30 ± 7 years, body height 179 ± 5 cm, body weight 73 ± 7 kg, VO_2max $62 \pm 8\ mL \cdot kg^{-1} \cdot min^{-1}$. Subjects were included only if exposed to the three NN, NH, and HH conditions. They were non-smokers and neither acclimatized nor recently exposed to altitude for at least a month before the experiment. Subjects' characteristics are displayed in **Table 1**.

Study Design

This study brings together original unanalyzed data from three previous studies performed by our laboratory (Faiss et al., 2013; Saugy et al., 2016a,c). All these studies have in common a randomized continuous 24 h exposure in NH and HH for each subject and a comparison with the control condition (NN). The measurements in NN were performed a few hours before each hypoxic exposure, whether in NH or HH. Regarding the washout period that was different between the two hypoxic exposures (see **Table 1**), the minimum duration required has always been respected to avoid potential interactions between hypoxic exposures. Many more methodological details are reported in the already published studies, but their respective main characteristics are also outlined in **Table 1** for the reader's convenience.

TABLE 1 | Data are reported as mean ± standard deviations.

	Faiss et al., 2013	Saugy et al., 2016a	Saugy et al., 2016c
Subjects	12	13	16
Age (years)	35 ± 8	34 ± 9	24 ± 4
Bodyweight (kg)	74 ± 8	76 ± 7	70 ± 5
Height (cm)	179 ± 7	180 ± 4	179 ± 5
VO_2max (mL·kg^{-1}·min^{-1})	61 ± 7	60 ± 10	66 ± 8
Protocol			
Total exposure time (h)	24	26	432
Washout period (days)	23	12	347
Measuring time points used (h)	H0, H8, H12, H20, and H24	H0, H10, and H20	H0, H24
NN			
Altitude (m)	485	485	1150
Barometric pressure (mmHg)	720 ± 1	718 ± 4	665 ± 11
F_IO_2 (%)	20.9	20.9	20.9
P_IO_2 (mmHg)	140.0 ± 1.2	140.5 ± 0.6	140.1 ± 1.0
Temperature (°C)	24 ± 1	23 ± 1	22 ± 2
NH			
"Simulated" altitude (m)	3000	3450	2250
Barometric pressure (mmHg)	720.0 ± 1.0	715.8 ± 3.8	666.6 ± 3.6
F_IO_2 (%)	14.7 ± 0.1	13.6 ± 0.0	18.1 ± 0.0
P_IO_2 (mmHg)	99.0 ± 0.4	91.0 ± 0.6	111.9 ± 0.6
Temperature (°C)	27 ± 2	23 ± 1	22 ± 3
HH			
Altitude (m)	3000	3450	2250
Barometric pressure (mmHg)	530.0 ± 6.0	481.8 ± 4.7	580.2 ± 2.9
F_IO_2 (%)	20.9	20.9	20.9
P_IO_2 (mmHg)	102.0 ± 0.3	90.9 ± 1.0	111.6 ± 0.6
Temperature (°C)	25 ± 2	21 ± 1	20 ± 4

VO2max, maximal oxygen uptake; Washout period, minimum period between the two hypoxic exposures; NN, normobaric normoxia, control condition few hours before each hypoxic exposure; NH, normobaric hypoxia; HH, hypobaric hypoxia; FIO2, fraction of inspired oxygen; PIO2, partial pressure of inspired oxygen.

Since these studies were planned independently and their measurement times do not match exactly, measurement time points were grouped into the following three categories:

- **NN:** H0 (all three studies, control condition before each hypoxic exposition).
- **H12:** H8 and H12 (Faiss et al., 2013); H10 (Saugy et al., 2016a).
- **H24:** H24 (Saugy et al., 2016c); H20 and H24 (Faiss et al., 2013); H20 (Saugy et al., 2016a).

Measurements

Measurements included S_pO_2, heart rate (HR), and supine HRV with identical equipment and measurement protocol between studies. S_pO_2 and HR were recorded continuously using a wrist oximeter connected to a finger sensor (Wristox 3100TM with 8000SM-WO Sensor; Nonin, Plymouth, MN) at each measurement time point during a 7 min supine rest period at 0.25 Hz.

The HRV measurement was performed during the last 5 min of a 7 min supine rest period. Measurement of the interval duration between two R waves of the cardiac electrical activity was performed with an HR monitor. Heartbeats that do not originate from the sino-atrial node have been shown to have drastic effects on the outcome of HRV indexes (Malik et al., 1996). To this end, the RR-intervals were first analyzed to remove ectopic beats from the recordings using automatic and visual inspections of the RR series. Then, time-domain analyses were performed with LnRMSSD, reflecting mainly the activity of the parasympathetic system (Kleiger et al., 2005; Plews et al., 2013). The spectral power was calculated with Fast Fourier Transform and was expressed in ms^2: with HF (0.15–0.40 Hz) reflecting modulation of parasympathetic influence to the heart (Malik et al., 1996; Shaffer et al., 2014) and related to respiratory sinus arrhythmia (Grossman and Taylor, 2007); and LF (0.04–0.15 Hz) reflecting mainly baroreceptor activity during resting conditions (Goldstein et al., 2011; Shaffer et al., 2014; Mccraty and Shaffer, 2015). LF was calculated in absolute spectral power units (ms^2) as described above and in normalized units (nu) with LFnu = LF/(LF + HF). This study does not show HFnu because of its total dependence with LFnu, both in absolute values and statistical analysis. The total spectral power (TP) was calculated by adding LF and HF. The LF/HF ratio was also calculated. All procedures were carried out according to the Task Force recommendations (Malik et al., 1996).

Statistical Analysis

Data are reported as mean ± standard deviation in the text and table, mean ± standard error in graphs. Data were tested for both homogeneity of variance (Fisher-Snedecor *F*-test) and normality (Shapiro–Wilk test). When both conditions were met, a two-way measures analysis of variance (ANOVA) was performed to assess whether physiological variables were differentially affected depending on the condition (NH, HH) and time points (H0, H12, and H24). Tukey's *post hoc* tests were used to localize differences when significant main or interaction effects were found. When either equality of variance or normality were not satisfied, variables were analyzed for each condition using a Friedman test for repeated measures to determine time effects using pairwise multiple comparison procedures (Bonferroni test). Differences between overall exposure mean (H12 and H24 combined) in NH vs. HH were compared using paired t-test. Corrections for multiple comparisons were applied (Bonferroni). Null hypothesis was rejected at $p < 0.05$. The statistical analyses were performed with SPSS 27.0 software (IBM Corp., New York, NY, United States).

RESULTS

The statistical power (calculated with G*Power software, version 3.1.9.7, Heinrich-Heine-Universität Düsseldorf) was satisfying for the four "main" variables in descending order; SpO2 (0.95); LnRMSSD (0.85); HR (0.74); and HF (0.69).

Oxygen Saturation

There were significant main effects on $\mathbf{S_pO_2}$ between exposures ($p = 0.009$) and time points ($p < 0.001$). The interaction was significant ($p = 0.038$). As expected, S_pO_2 decreased in both hypoxic conditions at H12 ($p < 0.001$) and H24 ($p < 0.001$) when compared to NN. S_pO_2 was higher in NH than in HH only at H24 ($p = 0.002$). S_pO_2 was higher at H24 than at H12 in both NH ($p < 0.001$) and HH ($p = 0.021$) (**Figure 1**). The overall exposure mean (H12 and H24 combined) yielded a higher S_pO_2 in NH vs. HH ($p = 0.008$).

Heart Rate

There was a significant main effect on **HR** between time points ($p < 0.001$). HR increased in both exposures at H12 ($p < 0.001$, $p < 0.001$) and H24 ($p < 0.001$, $p < 0.001$) when compared to NN (**Figure 1**). No differences between NH and HH were found either in individual time or overall exposure mean (H12 and H24 combined).

Heart Rate Variability

There were significant main effects between time points on all HRV parameters except LF. **LnRMSSD** was lower in both NH and HH at H12 ($p = 0.044$, $p = 0.022$), but only in HH at H24 ($p = 0.008$), when compared to NN (**Figure 1**). **LF** did not show any significant main effect (**Figure 1**). **HF** decreased in NH and HH at H12 ($p < 0.001$, $p = 0.004$) and H24 ($p = 0.008$, $p < 0.001$) when compared to NN (**Figure 1**). **TP** decreased in both exposures at H12 ($p = 0.041$, $p = 0.041$), but only in HH at H24 ($p = 0.012$) when compared to NN (**Figure 1**). **LFnu** increased in NH and HH at H12 ($p < 0.001$, $p < 0.001$) and H24 ($p < 0.001$, $p = 0.003$) when compared to NN (**Figure 1**). **LF/HF** ratio increased in both exposures at H12 ($p < 0.001$, $p < 0.001$) and H24 ($p < 0.001$, $p < 0.001$) when compared to NN (**Figure 1**). No differences in HRV parameters between NH and HH were found either in individual time or overall exposure mean (H12 and H24 combined).

DISCUSSION

To our knowledge, the present study is the first to compare heart rate variability between normobaric normoxia, normobaric hypoxia, and hypobaric hypoxia during prolonged exposures. The main finding was that NH and HH elicited similar HRV changes during 24-h exposures despite a higher mean S_pO_2 in NH. Indeed, the decrease in parasympathetic-related parameters (LnRMSSD and HF) was similar between NH and HH, contrary to our hypothesis.

To properly interpret the results of this study, it is necessary to mention the main cardiorespiratory adaptations in acute hypoxia: (1) a decrease in S_pO_2 due to reduction in inspired oxygen pressure (P_iO_2) (Maufrais et al., 2017), even at low altitude (Goldberg et al., 2012) and despite the diverse hypoxic-related ventilatory and cardiovascular compensations; (2) an increase in resting heart rate and cardiac output (Duplain et al., 1999; Bärtsch and Gibbs, 2007; Naeije, 2010), due to increased sympathetic activity and vagal withdrawal (Koller et al., 1988, 19) and inversely proportional to the decrease in S_pO_2 to maintain unchanged oxygen delivery to the tissues (Naeije, 2010); and (3) a largely unchanged blood pressure (Wolfel et al., 1994; Parati et al., 2015). The baroreflex and chemoreflex are also of great importance when considering the effects of hypoxia on the autonomic nervous system. On the one hand, the peripheral chemoreceptors in the carotid body respond primarily to hypoxemia and increase sympathetic activity while decreasing parasympathetic activity (Parati et al., 2015). On the other hand, the baroreflex ensures strict blood pressure regulation with stretch-sensitive baroreceptors located in the carotid sinuses and aortic arch. An increased blood pressure activates the baroreceptors, leading to decreased sympathetic activity and greater parasympathetic activation (Pitzalis et al., 1998). Finally, the already well-documented higher S_pO_2 in NH vs. HH can be explained by faster and shallower respiration, which increases dead space ventilation in HH (Faiss et al., 2013). The initial triggers of this S_pO_2 difference between NH and HH are still unclear. However, since chemosensitivity seems not to be changed in altitude (Loeppky et al., 1996), modification in gases density and diffusivity are the main hypotheses (Savourey et al., 2003). Our study confirmed a higher oxygen saturation in NH vs. HH after 24 h of hypoxic exposure. This is already well described for shorter exposition times (Aebi et al., 2020; Debevec et al., 2020) and logically was also already reported in the three support experiments of the present study. However, the latter was still debated for exposures longer than 8 h (Coppel et al., 2015). As expected, HR was higher in hypoxic conditions compared to normoxia in response to the increased sympathetic activity and vagal withdrawal. Several studies have further found lower HR in NH vs. HH (Savourey et al., 2003; DiPasquale et al., 2015b; Heinzer et al., 2016; Ross et al., 2019; Aebi et al., 2020) but only during short exposures. In addition, studies examining longer exposures (>8 h) found no difference in HR (Faiss et al., 2013; Richard et al., 2014). Unsurprisingly, our results hence suggest similar HR between NH and HH.

A decrease in LnRMSSD (Liu et al., 2001; Long et al., 2006) and HF (Bernardi et al., 1998; Sevre et al., 2001) in hypoxia

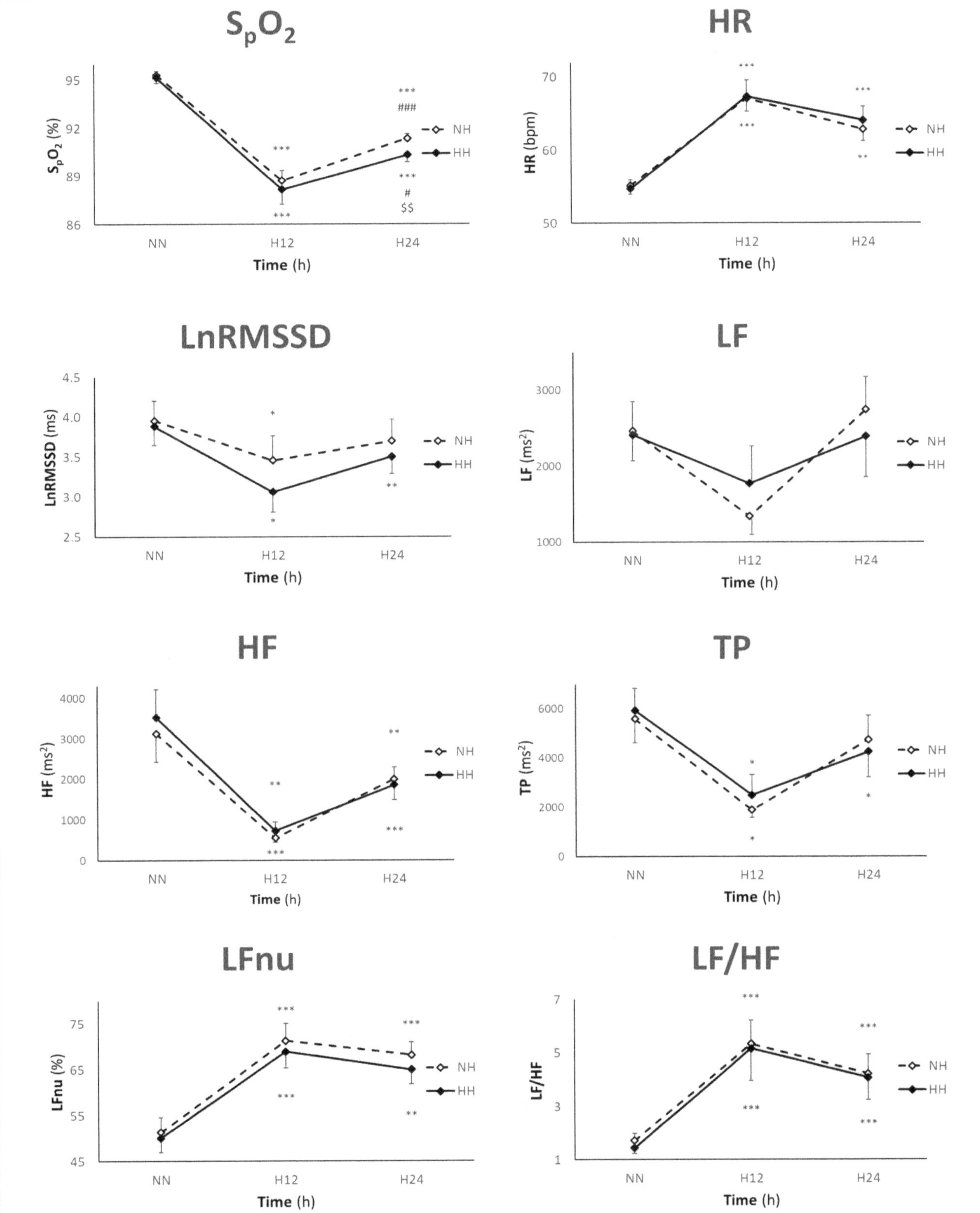

FIGURE 1 | Values are presented as mean ± SE. n = 41, 25, and 41 for NN, H12, and H24, respectively (n = 36, 18, and 37 for S_pO_2). HR, heart rate; LnRMSSD, natural logarithm of the root mean square of the successive differences; LF, low frequency; HF, high frequency; TP, total power; NN, normobaric normoxia; NH, normobaric hypoxia; HH, hypobaric hypoxia; bpm, beat per minute; h, hours; $^{*}p < 0.05$, $^{**}p < 0.01$, and $^{***}p < 0.001$ for difference with NN, $^{\#}p < 0.05$, $^{\#\#\#}p < 0.001$ for difference with H12, $^{\$\$}p < 0.01$ for difference with NH.

is already well described and demonstrates a clear hypoxic-related parasympathetic decrease. Firstly, since LnRMSSD mainly reflects the activity of the parasympathetic system (Kleiger et al., 2005; Plews et al., 2013) and is not very sensitive to respiratory variations (Hill et al., 2009; Buchheit, 2014), its decrease in both hypoxic conditions at H12 was not surprising. When compared to NN, a potentially larger parasympathetic tone reduction might explain that LnRMSSD remained lower in HH but not in NH at H24. However, the difference between NH and HH was not significant ($p = 0.328$). Secondly, since vagal activity is the major contributor to the HF component (Malik et al., 1996; Shaffer et al., 2014), a significant decrease in both hypoxic exposures at H12 and H24 was observed as expected. HF is called the "respiratory band" because it corresponds to the frequency of the respiratory sinus arrhythmia variations (Grossman and Taylor, 2007). Therefore, considering the differences in respiratory patterns between NH and HH mentioned in the introduction, one may expect differences in HF between NH and HH. However, these differences remained non-significant, maybe due to limited breathing differences or other confounding factors (as discussed below in "*Strengths and limitations*"). Thus, considering the LnRMSSD and HF data, it can be concluded that parasympathetic activity is similarly decreased in NH and HH compared to NN.

Hypoxia increases sympathetic activity (Duplain et al., 1999) mainly *via* peripheral chemoreceptor activation (Heistad and Abboud, 1980), as proved by increased plasma and urinary catecholamines (Mazzeo et al., 1991; Bogaard et al., 2002) and skeletal muscle sympathetic activity (Hansen and Sander, 2003). Therefore, the similar increase in HR between NH and HH may be seen as a consequence of similar sympathetic activity between those two hypoxic conditions. However, since there is no well-established marker of sympathetic activity in the HRV parameters measured in this study, it is not possible to make a stronger statement about the sympathetic activity similarities in NH vs. HH here.

LF reflects baroreceptor activity during resting conditions (Goldstein et al., 2011; Shaffer et al., 2014; Mccraty and Shaffer, 2015) which is primarily vagally mediated (Keyl et al., 2001). Therefore, it should not be used as a marker of sympathetic nervous system activity at rest (Eckberg, 1983; Kember et al., 2001; Billman, 2013; Shaffer et al., 2014). Since hypoxia increases sympathetic activity partly through altered baroreceptor function (Hainsworth et al., 2007), and as already reported (Schmitt et al., 2015b, 2018; Aebi et al., 2020), a decrease in LF during hypoxic exposures could theoretically be observed. However, that was not the case in this study since no difference in LF between normoxia and hypoxia was found, thus confirming the challenging interpretation of LF. Two additional precautions should be kept in mind when considering the data presented here. On the one hand, the consequent decrease in HF can alone be the reason behind the significant increase of LFnu in NH and HH exposures, especially considering that both branches of the autonomic nervous system are frequently non-reciprocal (Billman, 2013). On the other hand, it is often assumed that LF/HF ratio reflects the sympathetic-parasympathetic balance (Taylor, 2006). However, it is frequently shifted due to reductions in LF power which do not reflect sympathetic nervous system activity at rest. The LF/HF ratio should thus be interpreted with caution (Shaffer et al., 2014). Moreover, both branches of the autonomic nervous system can be simultaneously active (Berntson and Cacioppo, 1999). Furthermore, the interactions between parasympathetic and sympathetic nervous systems are complex, non-linear, and frequently non-reciprocal (Billman, 2013). Therefore, as LF is not decreased, it can be stated that this increase in LF/HF ratio mainly displays the hypoxic sympathetic-parasympathetic misbalance due mainly to a parasympathetic alteration.

Altogether, despite the greater hypoxemia in HH, which could lead to a potential greater decrease in parasympathetic activity, no differences in HRV between NH and HH were found. When taken as a whole, the above results converge toward lowered parasympathetic activity during hypoxic exposures and confirmed previous findings (Marshall, 1998; Wille et al., 2012), again without differences between NH and HH. However, HRV analyses need to be conducted carefully as many other factors than autonomic tone affects HRV. These are, for instance, the already mentioned regulation loops as baroreflex or respiratory sinus arrhythmia (Aebi et al., 2020).

Perspectives

The present study showed once again that normobaric and hypobaric hypoxia are not interchangeable and elicit different responses on physiological parameters (S_pO_2) but same HRV responses. Because HRV and hypoxic exposures are increasingly used among athletes (Schmitt et al., 2018), this has important implications. Considering our results, HRV can be used independently of the hypoxic methods for monitoring the athletes' adaptations to altitude and training loads. However, further investigations, particularly on standing HRV in NH vs. HH, are required before a possible replication of the diagnosis of fatigue sub-category in hypoxia (Schmitt et al., 2015b). Furthermore, standing HRV provides information about the dynamic adaptations of the autonomic nervous system and orthostatic tolerance (Schmitt et al., 2015b). Moreover, since supine and standing HRV are independent (Schmitt et al., 2015a), one cannot be extrapolated from the other, and hypoxia effects on standing HRV remain to be clarified. Further research could also increase the altitude and lengthen the duration of NH and HH exposures. Further research could also increase the altitude and lengthen the duration of NH and HH exposures.

Strengths and Limitations

On the one hand, this pooling study included more subjects than most other studies in this field, allowing us to reduce the risk of type II errors (false negative). Moreover, the subjects had homogeneous individual characteristics (**Table 1**). As the eight variables in this study are measured only at three different times, and corrections for multiple comparisons were applied, the risk of type I errors (false positive) remained reasonably low as well. Both hypoxic exposures were performed with rigorous protocol ensuring close experimental conditions and thus limiting external confounding factors. This allowed a targeted and specific analysis on the effects of barometric pressure *per se* in hypoxia. Finally, the perfectly matched control conditions between groups allow an appropriate comparison between two close conditions.

On the other hand, despite that the three protocols performed by our laboratory were quite similar (same crossover design, similar subjects, same measuring equipment and protocol, same data analysis, ...), one cannot rule out some potential flaws since the altitude level was different between the three "original" studies. In addition, the present protocols were performed with uncontrolled breathing frequency, known for potentially changing the LF- HF band boundary. However, in our view, this point is not relevant since (1) strictly imposing a breathing frequency may *per se* alter HRV, and (2) this may hide the searched differences in HRV, particularly HF between NH and HH. Moreover, with sensitive variables like HRV, differences in comfort, stress, and environmental conditions such as temperature, humidity, and hypercapnia between exposures may have affected the results (Bernardi et al., 2001).

CONCLUSION

Altitude training (alternating "live high - train high" in HH and "live high - train low" in NH) (Millet et al., 2010) and HRV are increasingly used for enhancing and monitoring the athletes' fatigue and responses to training. In this context, the present study showed that, at least during 24-h hypoxic exposures, the decrease in parasympathetic activity was similar between NH and HH. Therefore, HRV could be analyzed similarly in NH and HH conditions. Furthermore, together with previous results on acute exposures (Aebi et al., 2020), it forms a reliable basis for a similar interpretation of HRV in NH and HH during both acute and long hypoxic exposures.

ETHICS STATEMENT

The studies involving human participants were reviewed and approved by (1) Commission Cantonale Valaisanne d'Ethique Médicale, CCVEM; Agreement 051/09; Sion, Switzerland (2) French National Conference of Research Ethics Committees; NoCPP EST I: 2014/33; Dijon, France. The patients/participants provided their written informed consent to participate in this study.

AUTHOR CONTRIBUTIONS

VT wrote the manuscript. RF, JS, and LS conducted the experiments and collected the data. NB was involved in the data analysis. GM conceived and designed the research, revised the manuscript critically, and gave advice to VT for corrections. All authors reviewed and approved the final manuscript before submission.

ACKNOWLEDGMENTS

We would like to thank all the authors and contributors of the three above-mentioned studies who provided high-quality data. In addition, we acknowledge Michel Amiguet from the Division of Biostatistics, Center for Primary Care and Public Health (Unisanté), University of Lausanne, Switzerland, for his help and valuable advice about statistics and data analysis procedures.

REFERENCES

Aebi, M. R., Bourdillon, N., Bron, D., and Millet, G. P. (2020). Minimal influence of hypobaria on heart rate variability in hypoxia and normoxia. *Front. Physiol.* 11:1072. doi: 10.3389/fphys.2020.01072

Bärtsch, P., and Gibbs, J. S. R. (2007). Effect of altitude on the heart and the lungs. *Circulation* 116, 2191–2202. doi: 10.1161/CIRCULATIONAHA.106.650796

Basualto-Alarcón, C., Rodas, G., Galilea, P. A., Riera, J., Pagés, T., Ricart, A., et al. (2012). Cardiorespiratory parameters during submaximal exercise under acute exposure to normobaric and hypobaric hypoxia. *Apunts Med. Esport* 47, 65–72. doi: 10.1016/j.apunts.2011.11.005

Beidleman, B. A., Fulco, C. S., Staab, J. E., Andrew, S. P., and Muza, S. R. (2014). Cycling performance decrement is greater in hypobaric versus normobaric hypoxia. *Extreme Physiol. Med.* 3:8. doi: 10.1186/2046-7648-3-8

Bernardi, L., Passino, C., Spadacini, G., Calciati, A., Robergs, R., Greene, R., et al. (1998). Cardiovascular autonomic modulation and activity of carotid baroreceptors at altitude. *Clin. Sci.* 95, 565–573. doi: 10.1042/cs0950565

Bernardi, L., Sleight, P., Bandinelli, G., Cencetti, S., Fattorini, L., Wdowczyc-Szulc, J., et al. (2001). Effect of rosary prayer and yoga mantras on autonomic cardiovascular rhythms: comparative study. *BMJ* 323, 1446–1449.

Berntson, G. G., and Cacioppo, J. T. (1999). Heart rate variability: a neuroscientific perspective for further studies. *Card. Electrophysiol. Rev.* 3, 279–282. doi: 10.1023/A:1009920002142

Billman, G. E. (2013). The LF/HF ratio does not accurately measure cardiac sympatho-vagal balance. *Front. Physiol.* 4:26. doi: 10.3389/fphys.2013.00026

Bogaard, H. J., Hopkins, S. R., Yamaya, Y., Niizeki, K., Ziegler, M. G., and Wagner, P. D. (2002). Role of the autonomic nervous system in the reduced maximal cardiac output at altitude. *J. Appl. Physiol. Bethesda Md.* 1985, 271–279. doi: 10.1152/japplphysiol.00323.2001

Botek, M., Krejčí, J., De Smet, S., Gába, A., and McKune, A. J. (2015). Heart rate variability and arterial oxygen saturation response during extreme normobaric hypoxia. *Auton. Neurosci. Basic Clin.* 190, 40–45. doi: 10.1016/j.autneu.2015.04.001

Brooks, G. A., Wolfel, E. E., Groves, B. M., Bender, P. R., Butterfield, G. E., Cymerman, A., et al. (1992). Muscle accounts for glucose disposal but not blood lactate appearance during exercise after acclimatization to 4,300 m. *J. Appl. Physiol.* 72, 2435–2445. doi: 10.1152/jappl.1992.72.6.2435

Brown, T. E., Beightol, L. A., Koh, J., and Eckberg, D. L. (1993). Important influence of respiration on human R-R interval power spectra is largely ignored. *J. Appl. Physiol. Bethesda Md* 1985, 2310–2317. doi: 10.1152/jappl.1993.75.5.2310

Buchheit, M. (2014). Monitoring training status with HR measures: do all roads lead to Rome? *Front. Physiol.* 4:73. doi: 10.3389/fphys.2014.00073

Conkin, J. (2016). Equivalent air altitude and the alveolar gas equation. *Aerosp. Med. Hum. Perform.* 87, 61–64. doi: 10.3357/AMHP.4421.2016

Conkin, J., and Wessel, J. H. (2008). Critique of the equivalent air altitude model. *Aviat. Space Environ. Med.* 79, 975–982. doi: 10.3357/ASEM.2331.2008

Coppel, J., Hennis, P., Gilbert-Kawai, E., and Grocott, M. P. W. (2015). The physiological effects of hypobaric hypoxia versus normobaric hypoxia: a systematic review of crossover trials. *Extreme Physiol. Med.* 4:2. doi: 10.1186/s13728-014-0021-6

Debevec, T., Pialoux, V., Poussel, M., Willis, S. J., Martin, A., Osredkar, D., et al. (2020). Cardio-respiratory, oxidative stress and acute mountain sickness responses to normobaric and hypobaric hypoxia in prematurely born adults. *Eur. J. Appl. Physiol.* 120, 1341–1355. doi: 10.1007/s00421-020-04366-w

DiPasquale, D. M., Strangman, G. E., Harris, N. S., and Muza, S. R. (2015a). Hypoxia, hypobaria, and exercise duration affect acute mountain sickness. *Aerosp. Med. Hum. Perform.* 86, 614–619. doi: 10.3357/AMHP.4266.2015

DiPasquale, D. M., Strangman, Harris, N. S., and Muza, S. R. (2015b). Acute mountain sickness, hypoxia, hypobaria and exercise duration each affect heart rate. *Int. J. Sports Med.* 36, 609–614. doi: 10.1055/s-0034-1398623

Duplain, H., Vollenweider, L., Delabays, A., Nicod, P., Bärtsch, P., and Scherrer, U. (1999). Augmented sympathetic activation during short-term hypoxia and high-altitude exposure in subjects susceptible to high-altitude pulmonary edema. *Circulation* 99, 1713–1718. doi: 10.1161/01.CIR.99.13.1713

Eckberg, D. L. (1983). Human sinus arrhythmia as an index of vagal cardiac outflow. *J. Appl. Physiol.* 54, 961–966. doi: 10.1152/jappl.1983.54.4.961

Faiss, R., Pialoux, V., Sartori, C., Faes, C., Dériaz, O., and Millet, G. P. (2013). Ventilation, oxidative stress, and nitric oxide in hypobaric versus normobaric hypoxia. *Med. Sci. Sports Exerc.* 45, 253–260. doi: 10.1249/MSS.0b013e31826d5aa2

Fulco, C. S., Muza, S. R., Beidleman, B. A., Demes, R., Staab, J. E., Jones, J. E., et al. (2011). Effect of repeated normobaric hypoxia exposures during sleep on acute mountain sickness, exercise performance, and sleep during exposure to terrestrial altitude. *Am. J. Physiol. - Regul. Integr. Comp. Physiol.* 300, R428–R436. doi: 10.1152/ajpregu.00633.2010

Girard, O., Brocherie, F., and Millet, G. P. (2017). Effects of altitude/hypoxia on single- and multiple-sprint performance: a comprehensive review. *Sports Med. Auckl. N. Z.* 47, 1931–1949. doi: 10.1007/s40279-017-0733-z

Goldberg, S., Buhbut, E., Mimouni, F. B., Joseph, L., and Picard, E. (2012). Effect of moderate elevation above sea level on blood oxygen saturation in healthy young adults. *Respiration* 84, 207–211. doi: 10.1159/000336554

Goldstein, D. S., Bentho, O., Park, M.-Y., and Sharabi, Y. (2011). Low-frequency power of heart rate variability is not a measure of cardiac sympathetic tone but may be a measure of modulation of cardiac autonomic outflows by baroreflexes: low-frequency power of heart rate variability. *Exp. Physiol.* 96, 1255–1261. doi: 10.1113/expphysiol.2010.056259

Grossman, P., and Taylor, E. W. (2007). Toward understanding respiratory sinus arrhythmia: relations to cardiac vagal tone, evolution and biobehavioral functions. *Biol. Psychol.* 74, 263–285. doi: 10.1016/j.biopsycho.2005.11.014

Hainsworth, R., Drinkhill, M. J., and Rivera-Chira, M. (2007). The autonomic nervous system at high altitude. *Clin. Auton. Res.* 17, 13–19. doi: 10.1007/s10286-006-0395-7

Hansen, J., and Sander, M. (2003). Sympathetic neural overactivity in healthy humans after prolonged exposure to hypobaric hypoxia. *J. Physiol.* 546, 921–929. doi: 10.1113/jphysiol.2002.031765

Hauser, A., Schmitt, L., Troesch, S., Saugy, J. J., Cejuela-Anta, R., Faiss, R., et al. (2016). Similar hemoglobin mass response in hypobaric and normobaric hypoxia in athletes. *Med. Sci. Sports Exerc.* 48, 734–741. doi: 10.1249/MSS.0000000000000808

Heinzer, R., Saugy, J. J., Rupp, T., Tobback, N., Faiss, R., Bourdillon, N., et al. (2016). Comparison of sleep disorders between real and simulated 3,450-m altitude. *Sleep* 39, 1517–1523. doi: 10.5665/sleep.6010

Heistad, D. D., and Abboud, F. M. (1980). Dickinson W. Richards lecture: circulatory adjustments to hypoxia. *Circulation* 61, 463–470. doi: 10.1161/01.CIR.61.3.463

Hill, L., Siebenbrock, A., Sollers, J., and Thayer, J. (2009). Are all measures created equal? Heart rate variability and respiration. *Biomed. Sci. Instrum.* 45, 71–76.

Kember, G. C., Fenton, G. A., Armour, J. A., and Kalyaniwalla, N. (2001). Competition model for aperiodic stochastic resonance in a Fitzhugh-Nagumo model of cardiac sensory neurons. *Phys. Rev. E* 63:041911. doi: 10.1103/PhysRevE.63.041911

Keyl, C., Schneider, A., Dambacher, M., and Bernardi, L. (2001). Time delay of vagally mediated cardiac baroreflex response varies with autonomic cardiovascular control. *J. Appl. Physiol. Bethesda Md.* 1985, 283–289. doi: 10.1152/jappl.2001.91.1.283

Kleiger, R. E., Stein, P. K., and Bigger, J. T. (2005). Heart rate variability: measurement and clinical utility. *Ann. Noninv. Electrocardiol. Off. J. Int. Soc. Holter Noninvasive Electrocardiol. Inc* 10, 88–101. doi: 10.1111/j.1542-474X.2005.10101.x

Koller, E. A., Drechsel, S., Hess, T., Macherel, P., and Boutellier, U. (1988). Effects of atropine and propranolol on the respiratory, circulatory, and ECG responses to high altitude in man. *Eur. J. Appl. Physiol.* 57, 163–172. doi: 10.1007/BF00640657

Krejèí, J., Botek, M., and McKune, A. J. (2018). Dynamics of the heart rate variability and oxygen saturation response to acute normobaric hypoxia within the first 10 min of exposure. *Clin. Physiol. Funct. Imaging* 38, 56–62. doi: 10.1111/cpf.12381

Liu, X. X., Lu, L. L., Zhong, C. F., Cheng, Z. H., Yuan, Q., and Ren, H. R. (2001). [Analysis of heart rate variability during acute exposure to hypoxia]. *Hang Tian Yi Xue Yu Yi Xue Gong Cheng Space Med. Med. Eng.* 14, 328–331.

Loeppky, J. A., Icenogle, M., Scotto, P., Robergs, R., Hinghofer-Szalkay, H., and Roach, R. C. (1997). Ventilation during simulated altitude, normobaric hypoxia and normoxic hypobaria. *Respir. Physiol.* 107, 231–239. doi: 10.1016/S0034-5687(97)02523-1

Loeppky, J. A., Roach, R. C., Maes, D., Hinghofer-Szalkay, H., Roessler, A., Gates, L., et al. (2005). Role of hypobaria in fluid balance response to hypoxia. *High Alt. Med. Biol.* 6, 60–71. doi: 10.1089/ham.2005.6.60

Loeppky, J. A., Scotto, P., and Roach, R. C. (1996). Acute ventilatory response to simulated altitude, normobaric hypoxia, and hypobaria. *Aviat. Space Environ. Med.* 67, 1019–1022.

Long, M., Qin, J., Huang, L., Tian, K., Yu, S., and Yu, Y. (2006). [Comparison of heart rate variability in healthy young men during exposure to different altitudes]. *Sheng Wu Yi Xue Gong Cheng Xue Za Zhi J. Biomed. Eng. Shengwu Yixue Gongchengxue Zazhi* 23, 1195–1197.

Malik, M., Bigger, J. T., Camm, A. J., Kleiger, R. E., Malliani, A., Moss, A. J., et al. (1996). Heart rate variability: standards of measurement, physiological interpretation, and clinical use. *Eur. Heart J.* 17, 354–381. doi: 10.1093/oxfordjournals.eurheartj.a014868

Marshall, J. M. (1998). Chemoreceptors and cardiovascular control in acute and chronic systemic hypoxia. *Braz. J. Med. Biol. Res. Rev. Bras. Pesqui. Medicas E Biol.* 31, 863–888. doi: 10.1590/s0100-879x1998000700002

Maufrais, C., Rupp, T., Bouzat, P., Doucende, G., Verges, S., Nottin, S., et al. (2017). Heart mechanics at high altitude: 6 days on the top of Europe. *Eur. Heart J. Cardiovasc. Imaging* 18, 1369–1377. doi: 10.1093/ehjci/jew286

Mazzeo, R. S., Bender, P. R., Brooks, G. A., Butterfield, G. E., Groves, B. M., Sutton, J. R., et al. (1991). Arterial catecholamine responses during exercise with acute and chronic high-altitude exposure. *Am. J. Physiol.-Endocrinol. Metab.* 261, E419–E424. doi: 10.1152/ajpendo.1991.261.4.E419

Mccraty, R., and Shaffer, F. (2015). Heart rate variability: new perspectives on physiological mechanisms, assessment of self-regulatory capacity, and health risk. *Glob. Adv. Health Med.* 4, 46–61. doi: 10.7453/gahmj.2014.073

Millet, G. P., and Brocherie, F. (2020). Hypoxic training is beneficial in elite athletes. *Med. Sci. Sports Exerc.* 52, 515–518. doi: 10.1249/MSS.0000000000002142

Millet, G. P., and Debevec, T. (2020). CrossTalk proposal: barometric pressure, independent of PO, is the forgotten parameter in altitude physiology and mountain medicine. *J. Physiol.* 598, 893–896. doi: 10.1113/JP278673

Millet, G. P., Faiss, R., and Pialoux, V. (2012). Point: hypobaric hypoxia induces/does not induce different responses from normobaric hypoxia. *J. Appl. Physiol.* 112, 1783–1784. doi: 10.1152/japplphysiol.00067.2012

Millet, G. P., Roels, B., Schmitt, L., Woorons, X., and Richalet, J. P. (2010). Combining hypoxic methods for peak performance. *Sports Med. Auckl. N. Z.* 40, 1–25. doi: 10.2165/11317920-000000000-00000

Mounier, R., and Brugniaux, J. V. (2012). Counterpoint: Hypobaric hypoxia does not induce different responses from normobaric hypoxia. *J. Appl. Physiol.* 112, 1784–1786. doi: 10.1152/japplphysiol.00067.2012a

Naeije, R. (2010). Physiological adaptation of the cardiovascular system to high altitude. *Prog. Cardiovasc. Dis.* 52, 456–466. doi: 10.1016/j.pcad.2010.03.004

Parati, G., Ochoa, J. E., Torlasco, C., Salvi, P., Lombardi, C., and Bilo, G. (2015). Aging, high altitude, and blood pressure: a complex relationship. *High Alt. Med. Biol.* 16, 97–109. doi: 10.1089/ham.2015.0010

Pitzalis, M. V., Mastropasqua, F., Passantino, A., Massari, F., Ligurgo, L., Forleo, C., et al. (1998). Comparison between noninvasive indices of baroreceptor sensitivity and the phenylephrine method in post-myocardial infarction patients. *Circulation* 97, 1362–1367. doi: 10.1161/01.CIR.97.14.1362

Plews, D. J., Laursen, P. B., Stanley, J., Kilding, A. E., and Buchheit, M. (2013). Training adaptation and heart rate variability in elite endurance athletes: opening the door to effective monitoring. *Sports Med. Auckl. N. Z.* 43, 773–781. doi: 10.1007/s40279-013-0071-8

Ribon, A., Pialoux, V., Saugy, J. J., Rupp, T., Faiss, R., Debevec, T., et al. (2016). Exposure to hypobaric hypoxia results in higher oxidative stress compared to normobaric hypoxia. *Respir. Physiol. Neurobiol.* 223, 23–27. doi: 10.1016/j.resp.2015.12.008

Richalet, J.-P. (2020). CrossTalk opposing view: barometric pressure, independent of, is not the forgotten parameter in altitude physiology and mountain medicine. *J. Physiol.* 598, 897–899. doi: 10.1113/JP279160

Richard, N. A., Sahota, I. S., Widmer, N., Ferguson, S., Sheel, A. W., and Koehle, M. S. (2014). Acute mountain sickness, chemosensitivity, and cardiorespiratory responses in humans exposed to hypobaric and normobaric hypoxia. *J. Appl. Physiol. Bethesda Md.* 1985, 945–952. doi: 10.1152/japplphysiol.00319.2013

Ross, C. I., Shute, R. J., Ruby, B. C., and Slivka, D. R. (2019). Skeletal muscle mRNA response to hypobaric and normobaric hypoxia after normoxic endurance exercise. *High Alt. Med. Biol.* 20, 141–149. doi: 10.1089/ham.2018.0147

Saugy, J. J., Rupp, T., Faiss, R., Lamon, A., Bourdillon, N., and Millet, G. P. (2016a). Cycling time trial is more altered in hypobaric than normobaric hypoxia. *Med. Sci. Sports Exerc.* 48, 680–688. doi: 10.1249/MSS.0000000000000810

Saugy, J. J., Schmitt, L., Hauser, A., Constantin, G., Cejuela, R., Faiss, R., et al. (2016c). Same performance changes after live high-train low in Normobaric vs. Hypobaric hypoxia. *Front. Physiol.* 7:138. doi: 10.3389/fphys.2016.00138

Saugy, J. J., Schmitt, L., Fallet, S., Faiss, R., Vesin, J.-M., Bertschi, M., et al. (2016b). Sleep disordered breathing during live high-train low in normobaric versus hypobaric hypoxia. *High Alt. Med. Biol.* 17, 233–238. doi: 10.1089/ham.2016.0049

Saugy, J. J., Schmitt, L., Cejuela, R., Faiss, R., Hauser, A., Wehrlin, J. P., et al. (2014). Comparison of "Live high-train low" in normobaric versus hypobaric hypoxia. *PLoS One* 9:e114418. doi: 10.1371/journal.pone.0114418

Savourey, G., Launay, J.-C., Besnard, Y., Guinet, A., and Travers, S. (2003). Normo- and hypobaric hypoxia: are there any physiological differences? *Eur. J. Appl. Physiol.* 89, 122–126. doi: 10.1007/s00421-002-0789-8

Schmitt, L., Regnard, J., and Millet, G. P. (2015a). Monitoring fatigue status with HRV measures in elite athletes: an avenue beyond RMSSD? *Front. Physiol.* 6:343. doi: 10.3389/fphys.2015.00343

Schmitt, L., Regnard, J., Parmentier, A., Mauny, F., Mourot, L., Coulmy, N., et al. (2015b). Typology of "Fatigue" by heart rate variability analysis in elite nordic-skiers. *Int. J. Sports Med.* 36, 999–1007. doi: 10.1055/s-0035-1548885

Schmitt, L., Regnard, J., Coulmy, N., and Millet, G. (2018). Influence of training load and altitude on heart rate variability fatigue patterns in elite nordic skiers. *Int. J. Sports Med.* 39, 773–781. doi: 10.1055/a-0577-4429

Sevre, K., Bendz, B., Hankø, E., Nakstad, A. R., Hauge, A., Kåsin, J. I., et al. (2001). Reduced autonomic activity during stepwise exposure to high altitude. *Acta Physiol. Scand.* 173, 409–417. doi: 10.1046/j.1365-201X.2001.00925.x

Shaffer, F., McCraty, R., and Zerr, C. L. (2014). A healthy heart is not a metronome: an integrative review of the heart's anatomy and heart rate variability. *Front. Psychol.* 5:1040. doi: 10.3389/fpsyg.2014.01040

Stray-Gundersen, J., Chapman, R. F., and Levine, B. D. (2001). "Living high-training low" altitude training improves sea level performance in male and female elite runners. *J. Appl. Physiol.* 91, 1113–1120. doi: 10.1152/jappl.2001.91.3.1113

Takezawa, T., Dobashi, S., and Koyama, K. (2021). Cardiorespiratory response and power output during submaximal exercise in normobaric versus hypobaric hypoxia: a pilot study using a specific chamber that controls environmental factors. *High Alt. Med. Biol.* 22, 201–208. doi: 10.1089/ham.2020.0142

Taylor, S. E. (2006). Tend and befriend: biobehavioral bases of affiliation under stress. *Curr. Dir. Psychol. Sci.* 15, 273–277. doi: 10.1111/j.1467-8721.2006.00451.x

Wille, M., Mairer, K., Gatterer, H., Philippe, M., Faulhaber, M., and Burtscher, M. (2012). Changes in cardiac autonomic activity during a passive 8 hour acute exposure to 5 500 m normobaric hypoxia are not related to the development of acute mountain sickness. *Int. J. Sports Med.* 33, 186–191. doi: 10.1055/s-0031-1291325

Wolfel, E. E., Selland, M. A., Mazzeo, R. S., and Reeves, J. T. (1994). Systemic hypertension at 4,300 m is related to sympathoadrenal activity. *J. Appl. Physiol. Bethesda Md.* 1985, 1643–1650. doi: 10.1152/jappl.1994.76.4.1643

2

Mice and Rats Display Different Ventilatory, Hematological and Metabolic Features of Acclimatization to Hypoxia

Christian Arias-Reyes, Jorge Soliz† and Vincent Joseph*†*

Centre de Recherche de l'Institute Universitaire de Cardiologie et de Pneumologie de Québec, Université Laval, Québec, QC, Canada

***Correspondence:**
Jorge Soliz
jorge.soliz@criucpq.ulaval.ca
Vincent Joseph
vincent.joseph@criucpq.ulaval.ca

†These authors have contributed equally to this work and share senior authorship

Phylogeographic studies showed that house mice (*Mus musculus*) originated in the Himalayan region, while common rats (*Rattus rattus* and *Rattus norvegicus*) come from the lowlands of China and India. Accordingly, it has been proposed that its origins gave mice, but not rats, the ability to invade ecological niches at high altitudes (pre-adaptation). This proposal is strongly supported by the fact that house mice are distributed throughout the world, while common rats are practically absent above 2,500 m. Considering that the ability of mammals to colonize high-altitude environments (>2,500 m) is limited by their capability to tolerate reduced oxygen availability, in this work, we hypothesize that divergences in the ventilatory, hematological, and metabolic phenotypes of mice and rats establish during the process of acclimatization to hypoxia (Hx). To test this hypothesis male FVB mice and Sprague-Dawley (SD) rats were exposed to Hx (12% O_2) for 0 h (normoxic controls), 6 h, 1, 7, and 21 days. We assessed changes in ventilatory [minute ventilation (V_E), respiratory frequency (f_R), and tidal volume (V_T)], hematological (hematocrit and hemoglobin concentration), and metabolic [whole-body O_2 consumption (VO_2) and CO_2 production (VCO_2), and liver mitochondrial oxygen consumption rate (OCR) parameters]. Compared to rats, results in mice show increased ventilatory, metabolic, and mitochondrial response. In contrast, rats showed quicker and higher hematological response than mice and only minor ventilatory and metabolic adjustments. Our findings may explain, at least in part, why mice, but not rats, were able to colonize high-altitude habitats.

Keywords: acclimatization to hypoxia, physiology, metabolism, mitochondria, rodents

INTRODUCTION

Animals living at high-altitude present a series of physiological adjustments to prevent an imbalance in the supply and demand of oxygen (Scott et al., 2008; Storz et al., 2010). These adjustments occur along the oxygen cascade, and include a combination of physiological, cellular, molecular, and biochemical modifications that result in either an increased supply, narrowed demand, more efficient use of oxygen, or combinations of those three (Hochachka, 1985; Scott et al., 2008; Storz et al., 2010). Remarkably, such changes may differ in expression and efficiency between species or even between populations of the same species depending on their genetic backgrounds and their phenotypic plasticity (Monge and León-Velarde, 2003; Storz et al., 2010; Storz and Scott, 2021). Such differences appear when comparing house mice (*Mus musculus*), that successfully colonized high-altitude environments, and common rats (*Rattus rattus* and *Rattus norvegicus*), that are rare or absent in natural habitats over 2,500 m above sea level (masl; Jochmans-Lemoine et al., 2015). In previous works, we described the physiological traits of lab mice (FVB) and Sprague-Dawley (SD) rats established at 3,600 masl for more than 20 years and over 30 generations. Compared to rats, mice have a higher metabolic rate, higher tidal volume, increased alveolar surface area and lung volume, lower hematocrit and hemoglobin levels, and reduced right ventricular hypertrophy (a sign of reduced pulmonary hypertension; Jochmans-Lemoine et al., 2015). In following, we were interested in unveiling whether these features had a genetic basis or were the result of phenotypic plasticity, thus, the physiological and molecular responses to acute hypoxia (Hx; 6 h - 12% O_2, roughly equivalent to 4,000 masl) were evaluated at sea level. In comparison to rats, mice had lower metabolic rate, higher minute ventilation, and higher expression of the transcription factor HIF-1α (a master regulator of the hypoxic response) in the brainstem. On the other hand, rats presented increased expressions of glucose transporter 1, indicating an elevated glycolytic metabolism in the brainstem (Jochmans-Lemoine et al., 2016). In summary, these data showed that FVB mice develop a more efficient response than SD rats during the acute phase of exposure to Hx, but it remains unclear whether such differences would persist during acclimatization to chronic hypoxia, a process of gradual changes occurring within few weeks that improves the capture, distribution, and utilization of oxygen (Monge and Leon-Velarde, 1991; Schmitt et al., 1994; Cáceda et al., 2001; Storz et al., 2010; Czerniczyniec et al., 2015; Lukyanova and Kirova, 2015). To answer this question, FVB mice and SD rats were exposed to hypoxia up to 3 weeks to identify the ventilatory, hematological, and metabolic changes occurring at whole-body level as well as in mitochondrial O_2 consumption in the liver (the most metabolically active organ in rodents - accounting for up to 50% of resting O_2 consumption in mice and rats, Wang et al., 2012; Kummitha et al., 2014). We found that mice have a biphasic increase of minute ventilation, peaking after 7 days of exposure to hypoxia and later increased blood hemoglobin content and hematocrit level. Surprisingly, metabolic rate was higher after 7 days of hypoxic exposure, in line with increased mitochondrial O_2 consumption in the liver, mediated by the increased activity of complex II of the electron transport chain (ETC). Contrastingly, apart from an excessive increase in hematological parameters, rats show only minor ventilatory or metabolic adjustments.

MATERIALS AND METHODS

Animals

We used male adult (7 weeks old) FVB-NJ mice (Jackson) and Sprague-Dawley rats (Charles River). Animals were housed at the animal care facility at the "Centre de Recherche de l'Institut Universitaire de Cardiologie et de Pneumologie de Québec" (CRIUCPQ) with food and water ad libitum and exposed to 12:12 h light:dark cycles. All experimental procedures were in concordance with the Canadian Council of animal Care. The animal study was reviewed and approved by the Animal Protection Committee of Université Laval, Québec, Canada.

Exposure to Hypoxia

Animals were exposed to hypoxia (12% O_2) for 6 h ($n_{mice, rats}$ = 15, 13), 1 ($n_{mice, rats}$ = 12, 12), 7 ($n_{mice, rats}$ = 8, 9), or 21 ($n_{mice, rats}$ = 10, 7) days. For the 6 h group, we directly used the plethysmography chambers (see below), while for the other groups, we used plexiglass chambers, controlling oxygen levels with an oxycycler (Biospherix, Redfield, NY). Hypoxic chambers were open once a week during 1 h for changing animals' cages and replacing water and food. Normoxic controls ($n_{mice, rats}$ = 14, 15) were kept in regular room conditions (21% O_2).

Ventilatory and Metabolic Parameters

For the last hours of the exposure protocol, animals were quickly transferred to plethysmography chambers and recordings were made for 3 h (while animals were sleeping) using a whole-body plethysmograph (EMKA Technologies, Paris, France). Mice and rats' plethysmography chambers were constantly supplied with a mix of 12% O_2 balanced in N_2, or room air (21% O_2) for normoxic controls. Inflow was set at 350 ml/min for mice and 1,150 ml/min for rats. A subsampling pump (100 ml/min) was used to control outflow. O_2, CO_2, and water pressure levels were continuously measured using specific gas analyzers (OXZILLA, CA-10, RH-300, Sable Systems, Las Vegas, NV; and CD-3A, AEI Technologies, San Francisco, CA). Levels of O_2, CO_2, and water pressure in the inflowing air were measured at the beginning, after 1 h, and at the end of the recordings to calculate the oxygen consumption (VO_2) and CO_2 production (VCO_2). Animals were weighed after the recordings.

Hematological Parameters

After plethysmography recordings, animals were anesthetized and euthanized. Blood samples were taken to measure the hemoglobin (Hb) concentration and hematocrit (Ht). We used an automated spectroscopic system (HemoCue, Ängelholm, Sweden) to measure the concentration of Hb. The Ht was calculated by conventional methods using a dedicated blood capillaries centrifuge.

Mitochondrial O_2 Consumption

Tissue Sampling

Liver tissue samples (approximately 2 mg) were extracted from rats and mice under normoxia (Nx) or exposed to 1, 7, or 21 days of hypoxia (12% O_2). Samples were immediately transferred to ice-cold respirometry medium MiR05 (0.5 mM EGTA, 3 mM $MgCl_2 * 6H_2O$, 60 mM K-lactobionate, 20 mM taurine, 10 mM KH_2P0_4, 20 mM HEPES, 110 mM sucrose, and 1 g/L bovine serum albumin pH = 7) supplemented with saponin (50 μg/L) for permeabilization of the cell membrane as previously described (Arias-Reyes et al., 2019).

Oxygen Consumption Rates

Quickly after extraction, liver samples were transferred inside the respirometry chambers of the Oxygraph-2k (OROBOROS Instruments – Innsbruck, Austria) filled with the same MiR05 medium supplemented with saponin, and left incubating for 15 min. The mass-specific (pmol $O_2 \cdot s^{-1} \cdot mg\ ww^{-1}$) oxygen consumption rates (OCRs) were measured according to the protocols described below.

In each experiment, the mitochondrial ETC was fueled-up through different electron-transfer pathways by the addition of specific mitochondrial substrates and inhibitors (Gnaiger et al., 2019). The N (NADH electrons through complex I), S ($FADH_2$ electrons through complex II), and F (fatty acids oxidation electrons through ubiquinone) pathways were triggered independently or combined to reach specific mitochondrial activation states namely LEAK and electron transfer (ET). LEAK state results from the proton slippage across the inner mitochondrial membrane toward mitochondrial matrix in presence of mitochondrial metabolic substrates but in absence of ADP. ET state occurs when the electron transfer and oxygen consumption are uncoupled from the adenosine triphosphate (ATP) synthesis by the addition of a protonophore (rapidly returns protons into the mitochondrial matrix independently of the regulation of the ATP synthase) in presence of metabolic mitochondrial substrates (Gnaiger et al., 2019).

LEAK – ET Protocol

After the 15 min incubation, injections of 5 mM pyruvate and 2 mM malate were added consecutively to the respiratory chambers containing the samples to trigger the N pathway and reach LEAK state. In following, 2.5 mM ADP, 10 µM cytochrome C (see rationale below), and 20 µM CCCP (protonophore) were added to uncouple mitochondria and consequently initiate the ET state. Then, timely injections of 10 mM glutamate, 50 mM succinate, 0.5 mM octanoylcarnitine, and 0.5 µM rotenone were made to record OCRs for N, NS, NSF, and S pathways correspondingly (Doerrier et al., 2018). Finally, 2.5 µM antimycin A (inhibitor of complex III) was added to stop mitochondrial respiration and make corrections for non-mitochondrial OCR. Cytochrome C was used to control the integrity of the outer mitochondrial membrane, thus, if OCR increased more than 20% after the addition of cytochrome C the sample was considered damaged and discarded.

ETC Maximum Capacity and Flux Control Ratios

The ETC maximum capacity is defined as the mitochondrial OCR when all the electron-transfer pathways relevant for the analyzed tissue are active during the ET state. In our experiments, the ETC maximum capacity was measured by triggering the NSF pathway. Then, the flux control ratio (FCR) was calculated for each sample by dividing the value of OCR for the electron-transfer pathways N, S, and NS by the value of ETC maximum capacity (NSF pathway). FCR values have the advantages of internal normalization of mitochondrial content (Gnaiger et al., 2019), and of representing the fraction of the ETC maximum capacity covered by each of the N, S, or NS pathways. In this manuscript, FCR is referred as the level of activation of each electron-transfer pathway.

Activity of Cytochrome C Oxidase (Complex IV)

At the end of the experiments of mitochondrial respiration, after antimycin A injections, 2 mM ascorbate (keeps TMPD in reduced state) and 0.5 mM N,N,N′,N′-Tetramethyl-p-phenylenediamine dihydrochloride (TMPD – specific electron donor to complex IV), were added to measure the OCR exclusive to complex IV. Finally, 100 mM sodium azide (inhibitor of complex IV) was added. The activity of cytochrome C oxidase was calculated by subtracting the background chemical oxidation of the medium (after the addition of azide) from the OCR after the injection of TMPD.

Data and Statistical Analysis

Plethysmography recordings were analyzed with the software Spike2 v.7.19 (Cambridge Electronic Design). We used averaged values of three different segments along the recording where the breathing pattern was stable at resting values to obtain respiratory frequency (f_R), minute ventilation (V_E), tidal volume (V_T), the oxygen consumption (VO_2), and CO_2 production (VCO_2) rates. V_T was calculated as described previously (Marcouiller et al., 2014; Ballot et al., 2015; Boukari et al., 2016; Jochmans-Lemoine et al., 2016). VO_2 and VCO_2 were calculated by indirect calorimetry as described in (Boukari et al., 2016). Values of f_R, V_T, VO_2, and VCO_2 were allometrically adjusted to make them comparable between species as described previously (Stahl, 1967; Jochmans-Lemoine et al., 2015).

Ventilatory, metabolic, and hematological data were analyzed by two-way ANOVA tests, followed by *post hoc* analysis (Fisher's Least Significant Difference) using GraphPad Prism 8.3. We used species (mice and rats), and exposure (Nx; 6 h, 1, 7, and 21 days of hypoxia) as factors. Values of V_E, hematocrit, and VO_2, were correlated against each other using Spearman's correlations.

Mitochondrial data were captured using the software DatLab v.7.4.0.4 (OROBOROS Instruments – Innsbruck, Austria). Data was analyzed by two-way RM ANOVA tests using species (mice and rats), and exposure (normoxia; 1, 7, and 21 days of hypoxia) as factors. The combination of mitochondrial respiratory states and active electron-transfer pathways (i.e., LEAK, ET-N, ET-S, ET-NS, and ET-NSF) were the repeated measures. When significant differences in treatments or interactions were found, a *post hoc* Fisher's Least Significant Difference multiple comparison test was performed.

For all the analyses, test significances were set to $p < 0.05$. Data are presented as means ± SD unless stated differently.

RESULTS

Ventilatory Response

Mice Have a Stronger Ventilatory Response Than Rats During the Process of Acclimatization to Hypoxia

A significant effect of the hypoxic exposure on ventilation was observed in both species (Two-way ANOVA $F_{exposure} = 25.17$; d.f. = 4, 105; $p < 0.0001$; $F_{interaction} = 9.05$; d.f. = 4, 105; $p < 0.0001$). In mice, V_E remained unchanged after 6 h of hypoxia in comparison to control levels (Fisher's LSD test $p = 0.0608$). However, significant increases were observed after 1, 7, and 21 days of hypoxia (Fisher's LSD test $p_{1d} = 0.0004$; $p_{7d} < 0.0001$; and $p_{21d} < 0.0001$). A peak of V_E in mice was reached at day 7 (3-fold normoxic control levels) followed by a significant reduction at day 21 (Fisher's LSD test $p_{7d\ vs21d} < 0.0001$; **Figure 1A** – middle panel). In rats, V_E levels increased after 6 h of hypoxia in comparison to control conditions and remained elevated at 1, 7, and 21 days (Fisher's LSD test $p_{6h} = 0.0004$; $p_{1d} = 0.0062$; $p_{7d} = 0.0004$; and $p_{21d} = 0.0035$; **Figure 1A** – left panel). Comparing both species, mice showed significantly higher ventilation levels than rats after 7 days of hypoxia (Fisher's LSD test $p < 0.0001$). However, V_E was not different for mice compared to rats in normoxia, 6 h, 1 and 21 days of hypoxia (Fisher's LSD test $p_{6h} = 0.35$; $p_{1d} = 0.09$; and $p_{21d} = 0.053$; **Figure 1A** – right panel).

Hypoxia affected V_T of mice but not rats (Two-way ANOVA $F_{exposure} = 2.57$; d.f. = 4, 106; $p = 0.068$; $F_{species} = 71.55$; d.f. = 14, 106; $p < 0.0001$; and $F_{interaction} = 2.473$; d.f. = 4, 106; $p = 0.0488$; **Figure 1B** – left and middle panels). Compared to normoxic controls, mice exposed to 6-h hypoxia showed a significant decrease in VT values (Fisher's LSD test $p = 0.0185$). Consistently, mice had higher V_T values in comparison to rats in normoxia and 1-, 7-, and 21-days hypoxia (Fisher's LSD test $p_{Ctrl} < 0.0001$; $p_{1d} < 0.005$; $p_{7d} < 0.0001$; and $p_{21d} < 0.0001$). Such difference was not significant after 6 h-hypoxia (Fisher's LSD test $p = 0.0649$; **Figure 1B** – right panel).

Hypoxia significantly affected the respiratory frequency of mice and rats (Two-way ANOVA $F_{exposure} = 49.50$; d.f. = 4, 107 $p < 0.0001$; $F_{species} = 60.56$; d.f. = 1, 107 $p < 0.0001$; and $F_{interaction} = 2.27$; d.f. = 4, 107 $p = 0.067$). In mice, hypoxia triggered a significant and progressive increase in respiratory frequency after 6 h, reaching peak values after 7 days of exposure (Fisher's LSD test $p_{6h} < 0.0001$; $p_{1d} < 0.0001$; $p_{7d} < 0.0001$; and $p_{21d} < 0.0001$). f_R values dropped by day 21 of hypoxia ($p_{7dvs21d} = 0.0004$). In comparison to control levels, rats showed an augmentation in f_R after 6 h of hypoxia (Fisher's LSD test $p < 0.0001$) and maintained elevated values until 21 days of hypoxic exposure

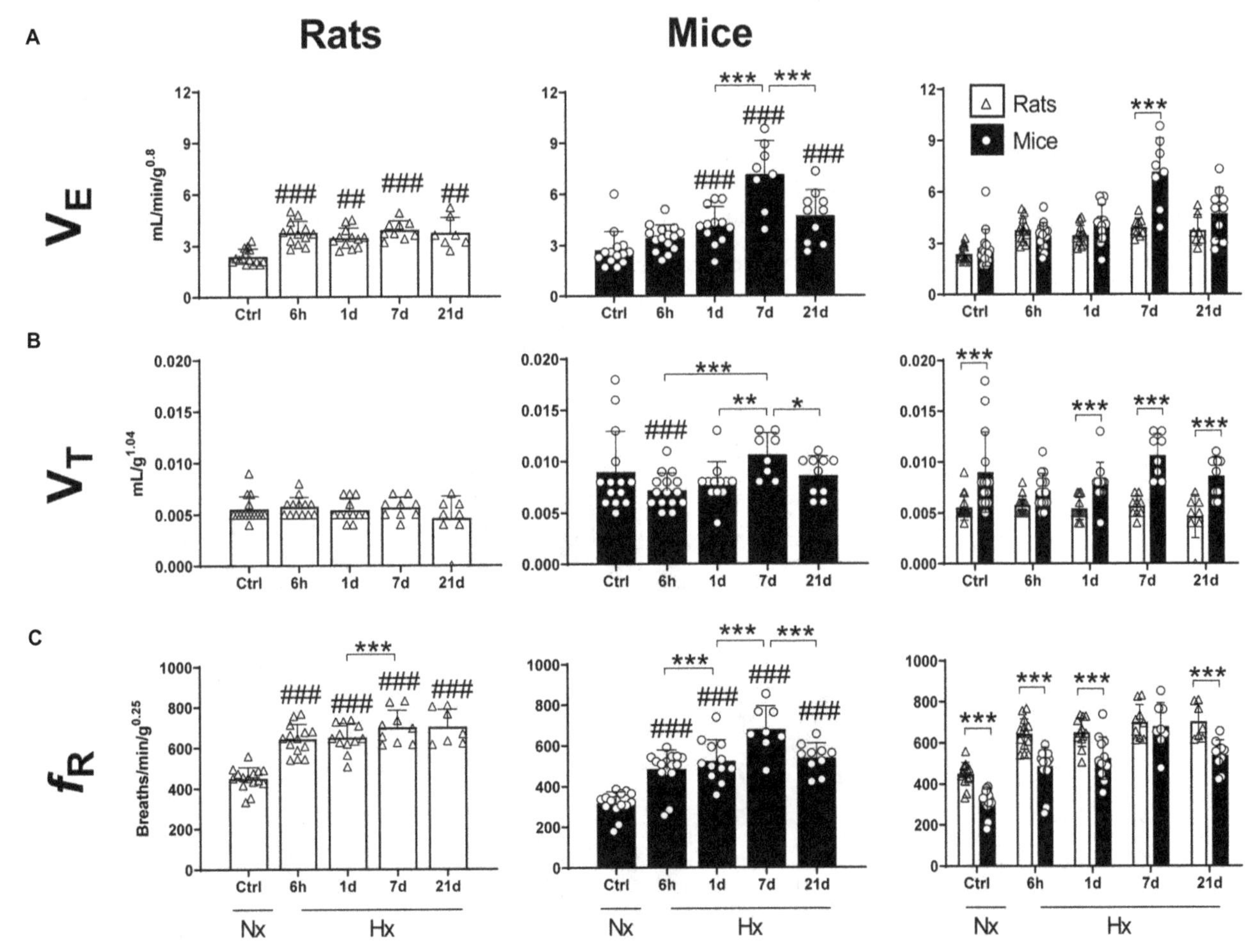

FIGURE 1 | Mass-corrected ventilatory parameters of adult rats and mice in normoxia (Nx) or exposed to 6 h, 1, 7, or 21 days of hypoxia (Hx). Mice show a stronger ventilatory response in hypoxic conditions than rats. **(A)** Mass-corrected ventilation (V_E), **(B)** mass-corrected tidal volume (V_T), and **(C)** mass-corrected respiratory frequency (f_R). *$p < 0.05$; **$p < 0.01$; and ***$p < 0.001$; ##$p < 0.01$ and ###$p < 0.001$ vs. the control. $n = 7–15$.

inclusively. f_R values in mice were significantly lower than in rats in either normoxic conditions ($p < 0.0001$), or after 6 h, 1 and 21 days of hypoxia (Fisher's LSD test $p_{6h} < 0.0001$; $p_{1d} < 0.0001$; $p_{21d} < 0.0001$). Such difference disappears transiently after 7 days of hypoxia (Fisher's LSD test $p = 0.574$; **Figure 1C**).

Hematological Response

Mice Have a Late Hematological Response Compared to Rats During the Process of Acclimatization to Hypoxia

Hypoxia significantly affected the hematocrit (Two-way ANOVA $F_{interaction} = 3.828$; d.f. = 4, 75; $p = 0.0069$) and hemoglobin concentration (Two-way ANOVA $F_{interaction} = 3.208$; d.f. = 4, 82; $p = 0.017$) of mice and rats. The Ht of mice significantly increased in comparison to controls after 21-days hypoxia (Fisher's LSD test $p < 0.0001$; **Figure 2A** – center panel). In rats, a progressive augmentation of Ht was observed early after 1 day of hypoxia (Fisher's LSD test $p = 0.0046$; **Figure 2A** – left panel). When comparing both species, no differences were observed in normoxic conditions, 6 h, 1 and 21 days of hypoxia. At day 7 of hypoxia, however, mice showed significantly lower Ht levels than rats (Fisher's LSD test $p = 0.0003$; **Figure 2A** – right panel).

While the concentration of hemoglobin was significantly increased in mice only after 21 days of hypoxia (Fisher's LSD test $p = 0.0046$; **Figure 2B** – center panel), in rats we observed a progressive augmentation after 1 day of hypoxic exposure, reaching maximum values at day 21 (Fisher's LSD test vs. control: $p_{1d} = 0.013$; $p_{7d} < 0.0001$; $p_{21d} < 0.0001$; $p_{1dvs7d} = 0.018$; and $p_{7dvs21d} = 0.004$; **Figure 2B** – left panel). In normoxic conditions mice showed significantly higher Hb than rats (Two-way ANOVA $F = 7.286$; d.f. = 1, 82; $p = 0.008$), however, when exposed to hypoxia, no differences between species were observed after 6 h, 7 and 21 days. Moreover, in animals exposed to hypoxia for 1 day, Hb was higher in mice than in rats (Fisher's LSD test $p = 0.028$; **Figure 2B** – right panel).

Metabolic Response

Mice and Rats Have a Transitory Drop in Body Temperature During the Process of Acclimatization to Hypoxia

Hypoxia had a significant effect on body temperature (BT) in mice and rats (Two-way ANOVA $F_{exposure} = 2.712$; d.f. = 4, 117; $p = 0.033$; $F_{species} = 3.466$; d.f. = 1, 117; $p = 0.065$; and $F_{interaction} = 2.517$; d.f. = 4, 117; $p = 0.045$). In mice, a significant drop occurred after 1-day hypoxia (Fisher's LSD test $p = 0.014$), however, after 7 days, control levels were restored. Rats showed an early decline of BT after 6 h of hypoxia (Fisher's LSD test $p = 0.01$), moreover, control levels were re-established after 7 days. Both species showed similar body temperatures in normoxic conditions, 6-h and 21-days hypoxia. At days 1 and 7 of hypoxic exposure, mice had significantly lower values of BT than rats (Fisher's LSD test $p_{1d} = 0.029$; $p_{7d} = 0.016$; **Table 1**).

Mice but Not Rats Increase Their Whole-Body O_2 Consumption and CO_2 Production During the Process of Acclimatization to Hypoxia

A significant effect of hypoxia on the oxygen consumption (VO_2) was observed in mice but not in rats (Two-way ANOVA

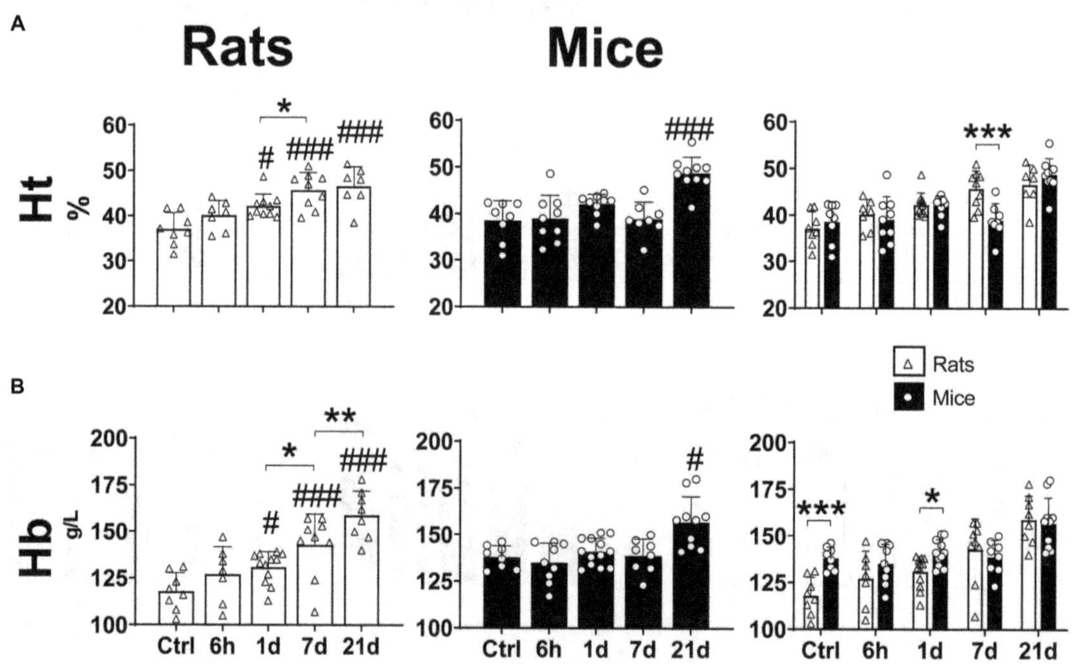

FIGURE 2 | Hematological parameters (hematocrit – **A** and hemoglobin concentration – **B**) of adult rats and mice in normoxia (Nx) or exposed to 6 h, 1, 7 or 21 days of hypoxia (Hx). The hematological response to chronic hypoxia is delayed in mice compared to rats. *$p < 0.05$; **$p < 0.01$; and ***$p < 0.001$; #$p < 0.05$ and ###$p < 0.001$ vs. the control. n = 7–15.

TABLE 1 | Ventilatory, hematological, and metabolic parameters in rats and mice during the process of acclimatization to hypoxia at sea-level and at high-altitude.

	Sea level					High altitude*
Rats	**Normoxia**	**Hypoxia 6 h**	**1 day**	**7 days**	**21 days**	**3,600 masl**
Body mass (g)	309.7 ± 88.2	279.8 ± 47.3	242.7 ± 19.7	317.5 ± 31.1	372.6 ± 83.9	232 ± 9
Body temp. (°C)	34.5 ± 1	33.6 ± 1.1	34.3 ± 0.8	34.8 ± 0.7	34.1 ± 0.8	35.2 ± 0.2
V_E (ml/min/100 g)	73.3 ± 11.9	115.6 ± 19.7	109.4 ± 19	116.9 ± 16.4	106.3 ± 25.1	153 ± 97
V_T (ml/100 g)	0.675 ± 0.153	0.723 ± 0.101	0.665 ± 0.13	0.708 ± 0.099	0.677 ± 0.114	0.79 ± 0.34
f_R (bpm)	110.2 ± 13.5	157.9 ± 19.5	165.7 ± 16.8	166.3 ± 20.5	155.6 ± 18	186 ± 38
Hematocrit (%)	37.1 ± 3.6	40.1 ± 3.2	42.2 ± 2.6	45.7 ± 3.9	46.6 ± 4.3	60.5 ± 1.1
Hemoglobin (g/L)	117.9 ± 9.9	127 ± 14.8	130.8 ± 8.3	142.8 ± 16.7	158.9 ± 12.9	204 ± 3
VO_2 (ml/min/100 g)	1.72 ± 0.44	1.59 ± 0.71	2.04 ± 0.69	1.51 ± 0.36	1.54 ± 0.33	1.7 ± 0.26
VCO_2 (ml/min/100 g)	1.63 ± 0.32	1.17 ± 0.26	1.74 ± 0.33	1.58 ± 0.18	1.25 ± 0.3	1.98 ± 0.41
RER (VCO_2/VO_2)	0.95 ± 0.22	0.84 ± 0.35	0.94 ± 0.3	1.1 ± 0.3	0.81 ± 0.09	1.128 ± 0.105
V_E/VO_2	46.13 ± 17.18	65.82 ± 25.43	56.98 ± 12.49	80.8 ± 18.82	70.33 ± 17.27	87.7 ± 47.6
O_2 extraction	12.56 ± 3.63	17.24 ± 8.51	17.61 ± 3.72	12.92 ± 3.28	14.85 ± 3.44	6.7 ± 2.8
Mice	**Normoxia**	**Hypoxia 6 h**	**1 day**	**7 days**	**21 days**	**3,600 masl**
Body mass (g)	25.9 ± 2.6	25.1 ± 3.4	24.7 ± 1.1	16 ± 11.9	24.8 ± 1.5	13.7 ± 0.9
Body temp. (°C)	34.3 ± 1.2	33.9 ± 0.9	33.4 ± 0.5	33.7 ± 1.1	34.4 ± 1.1	35.2 ± 0.2
V_E (ml/min/100 g)	138.5 ± 54.7	174.3 ± 36.8	211 ± 56.9	367.3 ± 102.2	238.8 ± 77.2	461.4 ± 199.5
V_T (ml/100 g)	1.014 ± 0.451	0.824 ± 0.192	0.904 ± 0.219	1.186 ± 0.24	0.978 ± 0.221	1.49 ± 0.67
f_R (bpm)	141.1 ± 23.7	216.1 ± 37	235.4 ± 46.1	306.6 ± 49.1	240.5 ± 32.9	320.9 ± 75.8
Hematocrit (%)	38.5 ± 4.3	39 ± 5	42.1 ± 2.1	39 ± 3.7	48.8 ± 3.5	47.0 ± 1.7
Hemoglobin (g/L)	137.9 ± 6.1	135 ± 10.6	140.8 ± 7.3	138.8 ± 8.9	156.9 ± 13.8	116 ± 10
VO_2 (ml/min/100 g)	4.11 ± 1.3	3.56 ± 1.13	3.87 ± 0.98	4.99 ± 0.91	4.85 ± 1.11	5.85 ± 0.96
VCO_2 (ml/min/100 g)	3.16 ± 0.9	3 ± 0.54	3.18 ± 0.56	4.54 ± 0.9	3.89 ± 1.22	4.95 ± 0.92
RER (VCO_2/VO_2)	0.78 ± 0.09	0.93 ± 0.38	0.86 ± 0.23	0.91 ± 0.04	0.8 ± 0.12	0.859 ± 0.169
V_E/VO_2	36.22 ± 17.37	52.49 ± 15.9	58.62 ± 24.39	73.34 ± 15.2	50.4 ± 14.33	79.8 ± 31.6
O_2 extraction	17.62 ± 7.21	18.62 ± 4.55	18.02 ± 7.25	13.12 ± 3.28	18.61 ± 6.14	7.1 ± 3.2

*Values are means ± SD. Data for normoxia (Nx) and sea level hypoxia (6 h, 1, 7, and 21 days) is presented in this study. *High altitude values were published by Jochmans-Lemoine et al. (2015).*

$F_{exposure}$ = 2.222 d.f. = 4, 103; p = 0.072; $F_{species}$ = 36.27 d.f. = 1, 103; p < 0.0001; and $F_{interaction}$ = 2.865 d.f. = 4, 103; p = 0.027). In comparison to normoxic controls, mice exposed to hypoxia for 7 and 21 days showed an increase of 10 and 25% in VO_2, respectively (Fisher's LSD test p_{7d} = 0.017; p_{21d} = 0.016; **Figure 3A** – center panel). No changes were observed in rats (**Figure 3A** – left panel). Compared to rats, VO_2 in mice resulted significantly higher in normoxia and after 7 and 21 days of hypoxia (Fisher's LSD test p_{7d} < 0.0001; p_{21d} < 0.0001; **Figure 3A** – right panel).

CO_2 production was significantly affected by hypoxic exposure in mice and rats (Two-way ANOVA $F_{exposure}$ = 8.375; d.f. = 4, 104; p < 0.0001; $F_{species}$ = 45.29; d.f. = 1, 104; p < 0.0001; and $F_{interaction}$ = 5.836; d.f. = 4, 104; p = 0.0003). Mice showed an augmentation in VCO_2 starting after 7 days of hypoxia (Fisher's LSD test p_{7d} < 0.0001; p_{21d} < 0.004; **Figure 3B** – center panel). In rats, a transient reduction of VCO_2 after 6 h of hypoxia was observed (Fisher's LSD test p < 0.001), however, in rats exposed to hypoxia for 1, 7, and 21 days, VCO_2 values were not different from normoxic controls (**Figure 3B** – left panel). When both species were compared, mice showed higher VCO_2 values than rats after 7 and 21 days of hypoxia (Fisher's LSD test p_{7d} < 0.0001; p_{21d} < 0.0001; **Figure 3B** – right panel).

The respiratory exchange ratio (RER) is calculated as the ratio of VCO_2 divided by VO_2. The RER is associated with the favored metabolic fuel (carbohydrates, proteins, or fatty acids). A value close to 1 represents a predominant glycolytic metabolism, while a value closer to 0.7 implies a metabolism more dependent on the oxidation of fatty acids (Deuster and Heled, 2008). In mice, we calculated values of RER between 0.778 and 0.929, while for rats between 0.813 and 1.096, however, no significant effects of hypoxia or species were found (**Figure 3C**; $F_{exposure}$ = 0.25; d.f. = 4, 103; p = 0.248; $F_{species}$ = 2.256; d.f. = 1, 103; p = 0.136; and $F_{interaction}$ = 1.212; d.f. = 4, 103; p = 0.3104).

Plasticity in the S (Complex II-Linked) and NS (Complex I&II-Linked) Pathways Upregulates the ETC Maximum Capacity During Acclimatization to Hypoxia in Liver Mitochondria of Mice but Not in Rats

We tested the effect of hypoxia on the oxidative machinery in the ETC of liver mitochondria of mice and rats during LEAK and ET states. Furthermore, we calculated the FCR as a measurement of the fraction of the ETC maximum capacity covered by the activation of N, S, or NS electron-transfer pathways. No changes were observed for LEAK state in any species either in normoxia or hypoxia (**Figures 4A,C**). Regarding ET state, in mice, while the N pathway (complex I-linked) remained unaltered in normoxia and hypoxia, after 21-days hypoxia the S (complex II-linked), NS (complexes I&II-linked), and NSF (complexes I&II&FAO-linked) pathways increased significantly in comparison to normoxic control levels (RM ANOVA Fisher's LSD test p_S = 0.0002; p_{NS} < 0.0001; p_{NSF} < 0.0001; **Figure 4C**). Accordingly, the activation of NS pathway was upregulated by 30% after 21 days of hypoxia (RM ANOVA Fisher's LSD test p < 0.0001). The activation of S pathway was seemingly increased as well (+12%) after 21-days

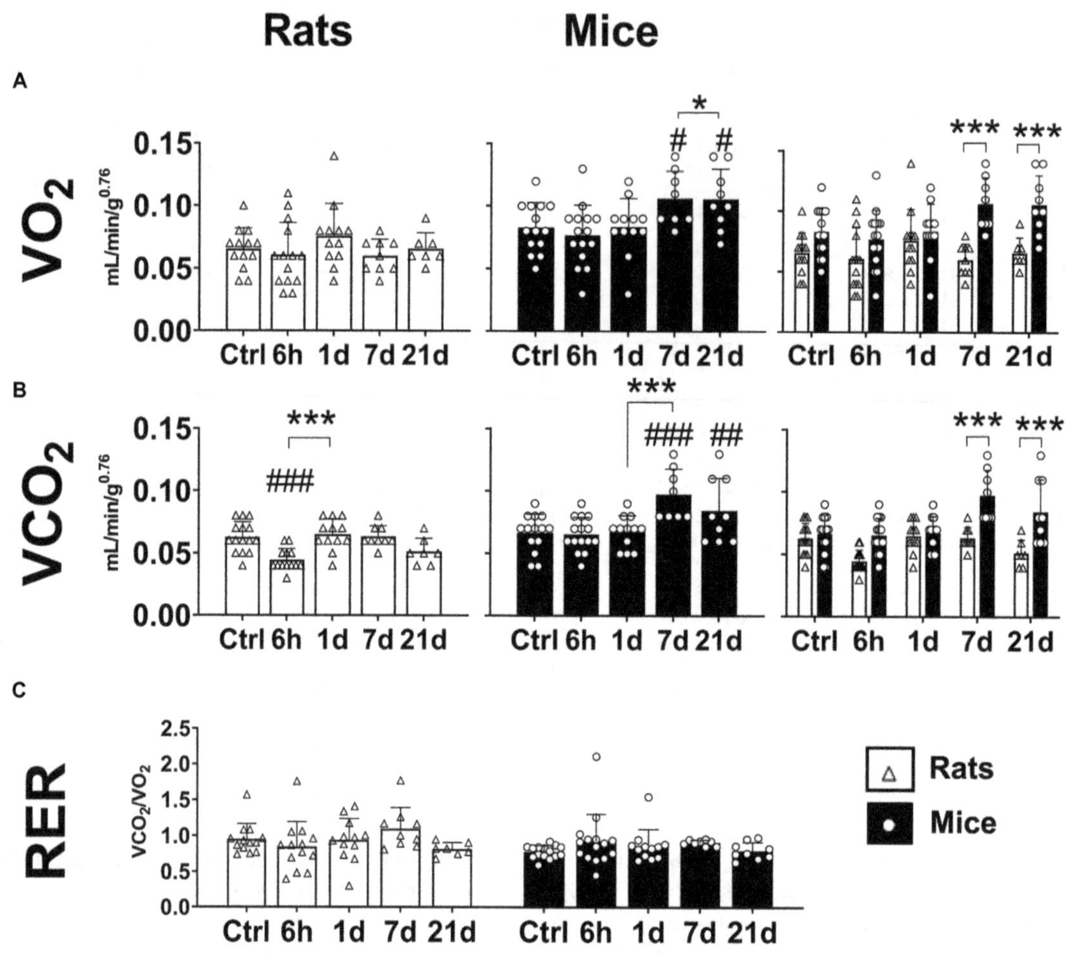

FIGURE 3 | Metabolic parameters of adult rats and mice in normoxia (Nx) or exposed to 6 h, 1, 7, or 21 days of hypoxia (Hx). Mice, but not rats, have an increase in metabolic rate during the process of acclimatization to hypoxia. Mice show increased values of mass-corrected oxygen consumption (VO_2; **A**) and mass-corrected CO_2 production **(B)** under hypoxia. The respiratory exchange ratio (RER) remains unchanged in mice and rats **(C)**. $^*p < 0.05$ and $^{***}p < 0.001$; $^{\#}p < 0.05$; $^{\#\#}p < 0.01$; and $^{\#\#\#}p < 0.001$ vs. the control. $n = 7–15$.

hypoxia, and while the difference with the normoxic controls was not statistically significant (RM ANOVA Fisher's LSD test $p = 0.0548$), the improved activation was significant in comparison to 1 and 7-days hypoxia levels (RM ANOVA Fisher's LSD test $p_{1d} < 0.0005$; $p_{7d} < 0.0259$; **Figure 4D**). Rats showed no alterations in oxygen consumption nor in the activation of electron-transfer pathways during ET state (**Figures 4A,B**). When both species were compared, mice showed higher OCRs during ET state than rats in both normoxic and hypoxic conditions (RM ANOVA $F_{species\_x\_exposure} = 10.42$; d.f. = 7, 39; $p < 0.0001$), independently of the activation of S (Fisher's LSD test $p_{ctrl} = 0.023$; $p_{1d} = 0.0018$; $p_{7d} = 0.0023$; and $p_{21d} < 0.0001$), NS (Fisher's LSD test $p_{ctrl} = 0.027$; $p_{1d} < 0.001$; $p_{7d} < 0.001$; and $p_{21d} < 0.0001$), or NSF (Fisher's LSD test $p_{ctrl} < 0.0001$; $p_{1d} < 0.0001$; $p_{7d} < 0.0001$; and $p_{21d} < 0.0001$) pathways. The same occurred when only the N pathway was active after 1 and 21 days of hypoxia, however, no differences were evidenced in normoxic control conditions and after 7-days hypoxia (Fisher's LSD test $p_{ctrl} = 0.2216$; $p_{1d} = 0.0486$; $p_{7d} = 0.1649$; and $p_{21d} = 0.0253$; **Figure 4E**). Rats and mice showed similar levels of activation (FCR) of the N pathway in normoxic and hypoxic conditions, however, the S pathway was significantly less active in mice than in rats when exposed to normoxia, 1 and 7-days hypoxia ($p_{1d} < 0.0001$; $p_{7d} < 0.001$). This difference disappears after 21 days of hypoxia ($p = 0.438$). Similarly, the activation of NS pathway was weaker in mice compared to rats in normoxic conditions and after 1 day of hypoxia ($p_{ctrl} < 0.0001$; $p_{1d} = 0.002$). Differences disappear after 7 and 21 days of hypoxia ($p_{7d} = 0.303$; $p_{21d} = 0.315$; **Figure 4F**). Finally, we measured the activity of complex IV, the final enzyme in the oxidation of oxygen, because it is known to be structurally modified upon exposure to hypoxia. In this regard, mice and rats were not different in normoxic conditions, however, when under hypoxia, mice reached higher values independently of the time of exposure (Fisher's LSD test $p_{ctrl} = 0.005$; $p_{1d} < 0.0001$; $p_{7d} < 0.0001$; and $p_{21d} < 0.0001$). Mice significantly increased the activity of complex IV after 1 and 21 days-hypoxia in comparison to the normoxic group and showed

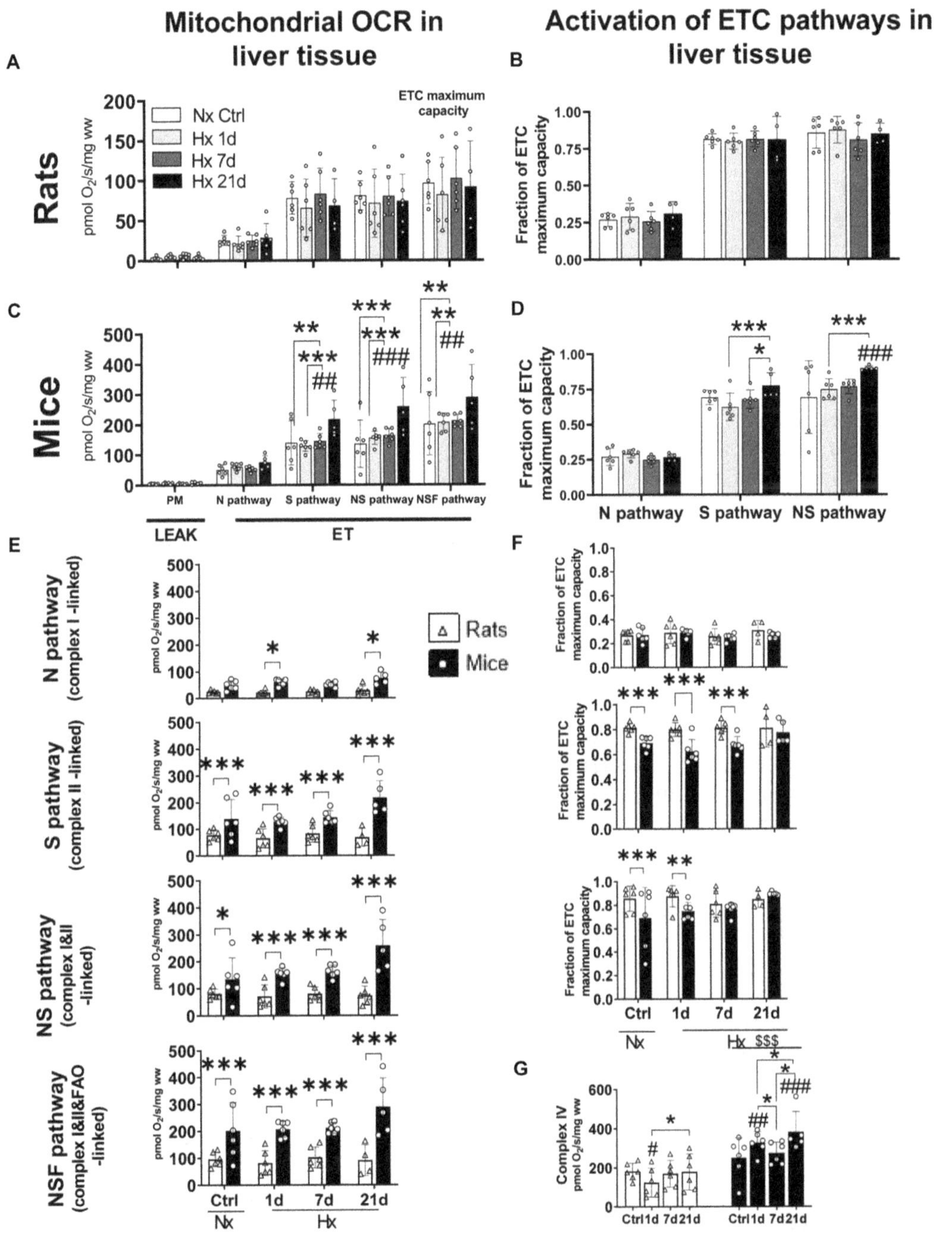

FIGURE 4 | Oxygen consumption rates (OCR) and activation of mitochondrial electron transport chain (ETC) pathways in liver tissue of adult rats and mice exposed to normoxia (Nx) or 1, 7, or 21 days of hypoxia (Hx). The OCR was measured during inactive adenosine triphosphate (ATP) production (LEAK) or uncoupled electron transfer (ET) fueled with substrates for the N (complex I), S (complex II), NS (complexes I&II), or NSF (complexes I&II and fatty acids oxidation) pathways. Activation values represent the fraction of the ETC maximum capacity covered by the activation of N (complex I-linked), S (complex II-linked), or NS (complexes I&II) pathways. OCR in rats' liver-mitochondria is not affected by hypoxia **(A)**. Likewise, rats showed no changes in the activation of N, S, or NS pathways in normoxic nor hypoxic conditions **(B)**. Mice increased its OCR (+44%) after 21-days hypoxia due to an overactivation of S pathway (complex II). Additionally, the maximum ETC capacity (NSF pathway) was 70% increased after 21 days of hypoxia **(C)**. A non-significant overactivation (+11%) of S pathway occurred in mice after 21 days of hypoxia together with the increased activation of NS pathway (+20%; **D**). Mice have higher OCR levels than rats in normoxic and hypoxic conditions. This occurs mainly because of higher S pathway (complex II) activities. The ETC maximum capacity in mice is higher in normoxia (+52%) and hypoxia (up to +69% at day 21) than in rats **(E)**. Rats show a higher activation of N, S, and NS mitochondrial pathways compared to mice during acclimatization to hypoxia prior 7 days of hypoxia. The overactivation of S pathway in mice compensates for these differences after 21-days hypoxia **(F)**. The overactivation of complex IV triggered by hypoxia hints to an improved efficiency in oxygen use in mice but not in rats **(G)**. $^{*}p < 0.05$; $^{**}p < 0.01$; and $^{***}p < 0.001$; $^{\#}p < 0.05$; $^{\#\#}p < 0.01$; and $^{\#\#\#}p < 0.001$ vs. the control. n = 4–6.

control-like values at day 7 (Fisher's LSD test $p_{1d} = 0.002$; $p_{7d} = 0.329$; and $p_{21d} < 0.0001$). In contrast, rats had a transient decline at day 1, then re-establishing normoxic control levels (Fisher's LSD test $p_{1d} = 0.0194$; $p_{7d} = 0.636$; and $p_{21d} = 0.9161$; **Figure 4G**).

DISCUSSION

Our data show that mice and rats have divergent profiles of ventilatory, hematological, metabolic, and mitochondrial acclimatization to hypoxia. At ventilatory level, mice have an early and progressive augmentation in respiratory frequency and minute ventilation, while this response is limited in rats. On the other hand, the increase of hematocrit and hemoglobin occurs only after 3 weeks of hypoxic exposure in mice. Rats on the contrary, increased both hematological parameters during the first day of hypoxia. Furthermore, while there is an elevation of whole-body oxygen consumption and CO_2 production in mice, metabolism in rats remains unaffected. These changes correspond well with the increased activity of the electron-transfer pathways involving complex II (S pathway) in liver mitochondria of mice, which is absent in rats.

Ventilatory Adjustments in Mice Are More Beneficial Than in Rats

We observed in FVB mice and SD rats, a rapid increase (after 6-h and 1-day hypoxia correspondingly) in respiratory frequency and ventilation, in agreement with previous observations in our laboratory (Jochmans-Lemoine et al., 2016). This response is well-known to occur in mammals and birds (Storz et al., 2010) since hyperventilation contributes to limit the decrease in alveolar oxygen partial pressure, thus supports oxygen diffusion toward blood. In mice, such increase continued for 7 days, reaching values of V_E 2.6-fold and f_R 2.1-fold control levels. Similar sustained increasing trends in ventilation after different times of exposure to hypoxia have been observed in other species like the deer mice, pekin duck, and bar-headed goose (Black and Tenney, 1980; Powell, 2007; Ivy and Scott, 2017). After 21 days of hypoxia, however, mice presented an attenuation in V_E and f_R, a change hypothesized to be advantageous for species living permanently under chronic hypoxia (i.e., high altitude) by reducing the oxygen cost of breathing when other adaptations are present (Powell, 2007). At this point, both parameters were only 1.7 control levels and were about 30% lower than the values reported for FVB mice born and grown at 3,600 m of altitude (Jochmans-Lemoine et al., 2015). In rats, V_E and f_R values were sustained around 1.6-fold control levels starting after 6 h and remained unchanged even at 21 days of hypoxia. Interestingly, the values of mass-corrected V_E, we observed in rats after 6-h, 1-, 7-, and 21-days hypoxia ($V_{E6h} = 3.4 \pm 0.8$; $V_{E1d} = 3.4 \pm 0.6$; $V_{E7d} = 3.9 \pm 0.5$; and $V_{E21d} = 3.7 \pm 0.9$ ml/min/g$^{0.8}$), were only 15–20% lower than those reported by Jochmans-Lemoine et al. (2015) in adult (2–3 months old) laboratory rats raised at high-altitude (4.5 ± 2.7 ml/min/g$^{0.8}$), suggesting that the process of ventilatory acclimatization to hypoxia in rats is somehow limited to the acute phase of exposure (6 h). This divergent ventilatory response between mice and rats may be explained by the higher protein level of HIF-1α, in the brainstem (the region of the brain that contains the respiratory control network) after 6 h of hypoxic exposure (O_2 12%) observed in mice but not in rats (Jochmans-Lemoine et al., 2016). Contrary to our findings, Schmitt et al. (1994) reported a continuous increase in V_E until day 14 of hypoxic exposure in male SD rats, although, animals were kept under lower (10%) oxygen concentration, and it is well known that this affects the magnitude of the hypoxic ventilatory response (Powell et al., 1998). Finally, despite the changes observed in V_E and f_R, V_T were only slightly affected by hypoxia in mice and not affected at all in rats. Moreover, V_T in mice was significantly higher than in rats in normoxia and hypoxia, as we reported previously (Jochmans-Lemoine et al., 2015). Overall, these results show that mice have a more plastic respiratory control system than rats.

Hematological Acclimatization Is Stronger and Quicker in Rats Than Mice

Increases in hematocrit and hemoglobin concentration are common hematological responses to hypoxic exposure in lowland individuals (Bullard, 1972; Monge and Whittembury, 1976; Monge and León-Velarde, 2003), helping to ensure the oxygen availability to supply tissues and organs. In this study, we found significantly increased hematocrit and hemoglobin levels after 21 days of hypoxia (12% O_2) in comparison to normoxic controls in mice (Ht = +26%, Hb = +14%) and rats (Ht = +26%, Hb = +35%). Interestingly, in mice, values of Ht observed after 21 days of hypoxia were identical to those reported previously for adult mice from high-altitude colonies (cf. **Table 1**). However, Hb levels in mice were higher than those reported at high altitude (Jochmans-Lemoine et al., 2015). It has been argued that the increase in Hb levels is classical in lowland native species because mammals native to high altitude shows unchanged Hb levels upon hypoxic exposure (Monge and Leon-Velarde, 1991). Furthermore, genetic studies in "wild" South American *Mus musculus* collected at sea level and high altitude found no signs of natural selection in the locus coding for subunits alpha and beta of hemoglobin, in fact, both South American populations coincided genetically with European haplotypes, leading to the conclusion that high altitude residency did not affect hemoglobin affinity for oxygen as an adaptive trait in this species (Storz et al., 2007). These observations suggest that the hematological mechanisms of acclimatization to hypoxia in mice are triggered late and are constrained to the first 21 days of hypoxic exposure. On the other hand, rats showed lower values of Ht and Hb in this study than those reported for high-altitude animals (**Table 1**) hinting that the hematological acclimatization in this species extends longer than 3 weeks. Another possibility is that the phenotype shown by adult rats in high-altitude colonies is also affected by changes during gestation or development. The later was shown to be true in adult SD rats (3 months-old) exposed to postnatal hypoxia (12% O_2 for 10 days) as newborns. These animals developed identical levels of Ht and Hb concentration to those observed in adult rats grown in high-altitude lab colonies (Lumbroso and Joseph, 2009; Jochmans-Lemoine et al., 2015). A limitation of our study is that we did not evaluate the change in cardiovascular parameters such as heart rate and arterial oxygen saturation (SaO_2) along the process of acclimatization to hypoxia. It is known that cardiovascular features interact with respiratory and hematological adjustments to counterbalance the diminished oxygen availability. Indeed, the heart rate of SD rats living permanently at high altitude (3,600 masl) is seemingly increased compared to sea level animals. This does not occur in FVB mice (Jochmans-Lemoine et al., 2015).

Elevated Metabolic Rates in Mice Are Supported by Coordinated Ventilatory and Hematological Adjustments That Are Disjointed in Rats

The metabolism of animals exposed to hypoxia has been classically pointed to be reduced as a strategy to save energy in conditions of limited oxygen availability (Scott et al., 2008; Storz et al., 2010). However, cumulative evidence shows that upon chronic hypoxic exposure metabolic rates can increase in vertebrate species adapted to hypoxic conditions such as the deer mice and the bar-headed geese (Ward et al., 2002; Scott et al., 2008, 2018; Scott and Milsom, 2009; Ivy and Scott, 2017). We found that in rats, hypoxia had no effect on the O_2 consumption and CO_2 production rates, while these values increase in mice suggesting an increased metabolic expenditure linked with the mechanisms underlying hypoxia-acclimatization. The values of VO_2, we found in our experiments after 21 days of hypoxia were about 20% lower than those observed in mice born and grown in high-altitude colonies (see **Table 1**), suggesting further margins to increase metabolic rates during permanent residency at high altitude. However, body weights after 21 days-hypoxia are higher than in high-altitude animals (see **Table 1**), such difference may be due to the effects of hypoxia during gestation and growth similar to those we described for SD rats (Lumbroso and Joseph, 2009). Such metabolic upsurge may also be interpreted as a compensatory mechanism to restore the body temperature independently of the hypoxic exposure. However, the metabolic rate (VO_2) in mice was augmented after day 7 and remained this way until day 21 of hypoxia, while the rectal temperature was significantly lower only at day 1. Interestingly, the VO_2 values we observed after 21 days of hypoxic exposure in rats are much closer (less than 10%) to those reported for high-altitude born and grown SD rats than they are for the FVB mice (**Table 1**), suggesting wider margins for plasticity of metabolic systems in mice compared to rats. Moreover, after the rise in oxygen consumption occurring at day 7 of hypoxia, VO_2 was significantly higher in mice than rats, similarly to what happens in high-altitude acclimatized animals (Hochachka et al., 1983; Ivy and Scott, 2017).

Notably, the forementioned ventilatory and hematological systems normally act in coordination to compensate any imbalance in the relation of oxygen demand and supply (d_{O2}/q_{O2}) produced by hypoxia. Indeed, we observed increased levels of Ht and Hb in mice only after 21 days of hypoxia, while these changes occurred much earlier in rats. This suggests that in mice the ventilatory compensations are sufficient to supply enough O_2 during the first 3 weeks. In rats, however, the restricted ventilatory response accompanied by an early and persistent hematological modulation hint to an improper compensation of the imbalanced ratio d_{O2}/q_{O2}. Consequently, we explored the relations among the response patterns of V_E, Ht, and VO_2 by plotting these features against each other. We noticed distinct interactions between ventilatory, hematological, and metabolic parameters in mice and rats. In mice, an initially large ventilatory response is withdrawn after the day 7 of hypoxia in synchrony with the activation of hematological adjustments (**Figure 5B**). Hematological tuning during acclimatization to hypoxia is classically thought to be triggered slightly later than respiratory modulations, and is considered energetically more efficient than ventilatory and cardiovascular modifications (Monge and León-Velarde, 2003). Moreover, the enhanced ventilation accompanies the increased oxygen consumption up to a steady state reached at day 7 of hypoxic exposure (**Figure 5D**). The latter is further supported by augmented levels of hematocrit (**Figure 5F**), suggesting that ventilatory mechanisms act early during the process of acclimatization of mice and are coordinately backed by subsequent hematological adjustments to ensure an enhanced oxygen supply. Rats, however, have limited ventilatory adjustments, hence require stronger hematological compensations to cope with hypoxic conditions. This is well illustrated by a clear threshold in ventilation right after 6 h of hypoxic exposure while (red dashed line in **Figure 5**), in contrast, continuously rising hematological adjustments are present for over 3 weeks (**Figure 5A**). Likewise, although no significant statistical correlation was found, negative correlation coefficients indicate that VO_2 is not further increased either by ventilatory or hematological modifications following the acute response occurring in the first day of hypoxia (**Figures 5C,E**). The fact, we observed a concurrent acute initiation of ventilatory and hematological mechanisms in rats further supports the hypothesis that blood-level modifications play a more significant role compared to ventilation in the acclimatization of rats.

Plasticity in Liver Mitochondria of Mice, but Not Rats, Permits a More Efficient Use of Subcellular Oxygen in Hypoxic Conditions

We used liver tissue to study the role of mitochondria in the metabolic response to chronic hypoxia since this organ accounts for around 50% of the whole-body energy expenditure in mice and rats (Wang et al., 2012; Kummitha et al., 2014). We quantified the maximum capacity of the ETC by measuring the OCR uncoupled from the ATP synthesis (Gnaiger et al., 2019). We did not find significant alterations in the mitochondrial oxygen consumption in the liver of rats. Concurring with our observations, Costa et al. (1988) found no changes in the respiration of isolated liver-mitochondria after 9-months hypoxia (equivalent to 4,400 masl) in Wistar rats. Contrastingly, Pickett et al. (1979) observed a slight initial reduction in the

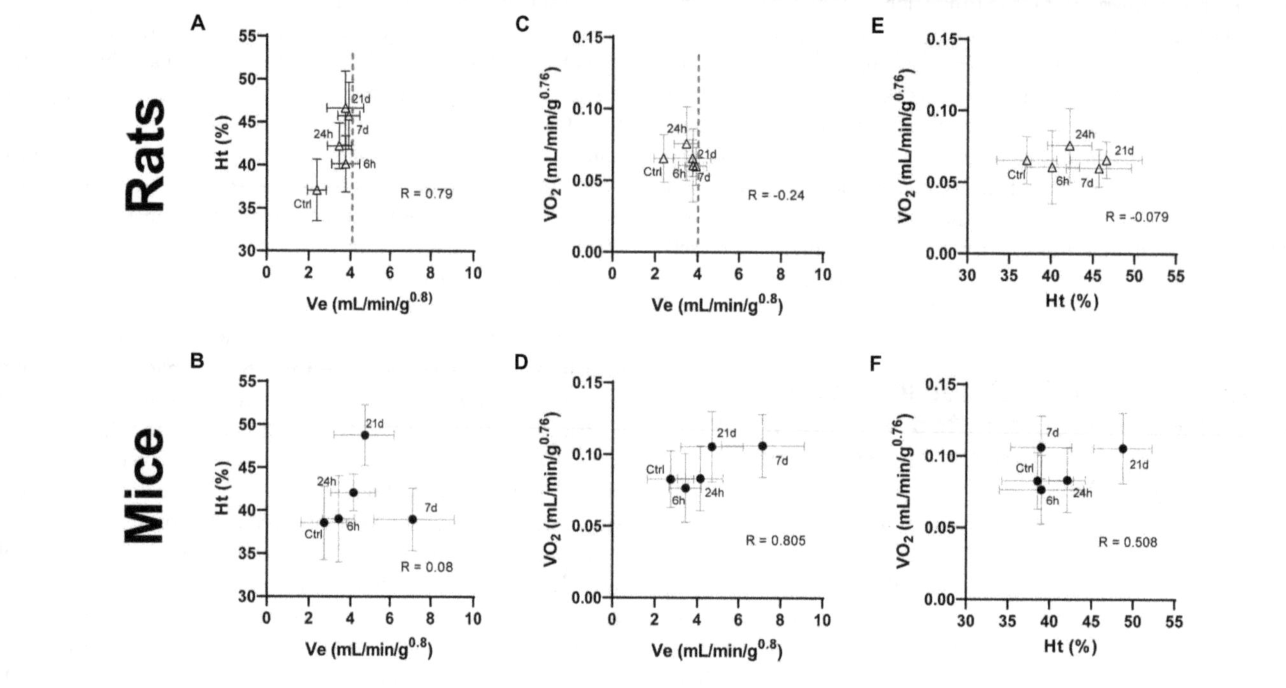

FIGURE 5 | Interaction between ventilatory and hematological parameters **(A,B)** and the effect of ventilatory **(C,D)** and hematological **(E,F)** parameters on the whole-body oxygen consumption in adult rats and mice exposed to normoxia (Ctrl) or 1, 7, or 21 days of hypoxia. A metabolic increase (oxygen consumption – VO_2) in response to chronic hypoxia in mice is supported by cooperative changes in ventilatory and hematological systems. This outcome in rats is impaired due to a limited ventilatory response evident after 6 h of hypoxia (dashed line), thus, requiring excessive hematological compensations to cope with hypoxic conditions.

activity of complex II during the first 2 weeks of hypoxia with an outburst over normoxic levels around the third week of normobaric hypoxia in SD rats. Of note, the levels of oxygen used in this work were much lower than those we applied to our animals (equivalent to 6,600 vs. 4,000 masl respectively), under these circumstances, the lack of response we found suggests that liver mitochondria in rats may only respond to extreme oxygen limitation.

Interestingly, we did see patterns in the liver mitochondrial respiration of mice that coincide with features of species adapted to high-altitude hypoxia. Deer mice show augmented mitochondrial respiratory capacities in the diaphragm muscle after exposure to hypoxia (equivalent to 4,300 masl for 6–8 weeks; Dawson et al., 2018; Scott et al., 2018). As well, in the gastrocnemius muscle, this species have elevated expression levels and activity of enzymes involved in fatty acid β-oxidation and oxidative phosphorylation (Cheviron et al., 2012), and a higher density of subsarcolemmal mitochondria (Mahalingam et al., 2017). HA native deer mice can maintain high metabolic rates during acclimatization to hypoxia (Cheviron et al., 2012; Ivy and Scott, 2017). This occurs either in field conditions at HA (Hayes, 1989) or in response to cold exposure (Cheviron et al., 2012). These biochemical changes are supported by high capillarity and oxidative fiber density (Lui et al., 2015), and result in elevated mitochondrial respiratory capacities (Mahalingam et al., 2017). In our mice, liver mitochondria show an increased ETC maximum capacity (NSF pathway) after 3-week hypoxia propelled by an increased activity of complex II, while complex I remains unchanged. Similar enhancement of complex II activity in ETC under hypoxic exposure has been reported in brain cortex of mice and hypoxia-resistant rats (Lukyanova, 1997; Cáceda et al., 2001; Lukyanova et al., 2008; Lukyanova and Kirova, 2015). Contrary to complex I, which is sensitive to drops in intracellular oxygen concentration, the activity of complex II is only dependent on the availability of its substrate: succinate (Hawkins et al., 2010). Remarkably, in mammals, succinate is accumulated in mitochondria during hypoxia (Hohl et al., 1987; Cáceda et al., 1997; Lukyanova et al., 2018) and acts as a stabilizer of HIF-1α by attenuating the activity of the polyhydroxylases (PHDs; which mark HIF1-α for denaturation in normoxic conditions), thus supporting acclimatization to hypoxia (Fuhrmann and Brüne, 2017). Also, succinate is involved with auxiliar (albeit less efficient) avenues to produce ATP by (1) substrate phosphorylation (produces GTP) catalyzed by succinate thiokinase and (2) the reduction of oxalacetate to succinate that is coupled with the reverse reaction of malate dehydrogenase and the concomitant electron transfer to the ETC *via* complex I (Cáceda et al., 2001). Complex II (succinate dehydrogenase) participates in the second mechanism. Moreover, complex II is also the gateway for cytosolic NADH to enter mitochondria *via* the glycerophosphate shuttle and for the reduced equivalents from fatty acids oxidation, that way having a great participation in ATP production. Accordingly, the fatty acids metabolism has been suggested to be augmented in high-altitude conditions (León-Velarde and Arregui, 1994). Overall, this supports the notion that an increased CII activity as reported here would promote a more efficient O_2 utilization by liver mitochondria in mice. Indeed, the increased activity of complex II is regarded as an "*evolutionarily formed, urgent, protective, regulatory, and compensatory mechanism*" occurring in most tissues upon hypoxic exposure and during acclimatization (Lukyanova and Kirova, 2015). Contrastingly, Leon-Velarde et al. (1986) reported no changes in the respiration of isolated liver mitochondria in Swiss mice exposed to hypobaric hypoxia (equivalent to 4,400 masl) for 90–120 days concluding that isolated mitochondria are not suitable to perform experiments on the effects of hypoxia. However, the exposure period they tested is long enough to allow mitochondrial ETC to recover levels of respiratory complexes activity seen in normoxic animals (Lukyanova and Kirova, 2015). Finally, we learned that liver mitochondria in mice consume more oxygen than their counterparts in rats regardless of the availability of oxygen and the active electron-transfer pathways. This may explain, at least in part, the higher whole-body O_2 consumption in mice compared to rats. Interestingly, during normoxia and the first day of hypoxic exposure, the activation of S and NS pathways is lower in mice than in rats, however, by day 7 of hypoxia such difference in activation disappears hinting to the existence of a "spare capacity" in the liver mitochondrial ETC, a feature observed in other tissues in high-altitude-adapted species (Storz et al., 2010; Lukyanova and Kirova, 2015). Overall, the higher plasticity during acclimatization to hypoxia in mice supports our hypothesis of a genetic background supporting the ability of mice to cope with hypoxia, which is limited or absent in rats.

Why Mice Respond Better to Chronic Hypoxia Than Rats?

Whereas cellular mechanisms work generally at maximum efficiency, especially in the context of energy generation and expenditure, there are cases when "spare" room for further improved efficiency remains as genetical vestiges from ancient more demanding circumstances. This confers populations the capacity to invade new ecological niches thanks to previously acquired appropriate structural and/or functional changes, with the concomitant emergence of multiple "adaptive peaks" (Griffiths et al., 2000), a process called "pre-adaptation" (Monge and León-Velarde, 2003). Indeed, the acclimatizing mitochondrial traits, we observed in mice have been previously posed as well-adaptive or as distinctive from high-altitude adapted species (Lukyanova, 1997; Lukyanova and Dudchenko, 1999; Cáceda et al., 2001; Czerniczyniec et al., 2015; Lukyanova and Kirova, 2015). On the other hand, acclimatizing changes at systemic level in rats are almost exclusively reliant on hematological adjustments, a strategy that has been tagged as disadvantageous due to its limitations to compensate for the reduced levels of oxygen delivery, and instead causing stress to the cardiovascular system (Lumbroso and Joseph, 2009; Storz et al., 2010; Lumbroso et al., 2012) on top of the inadequate or inexistent ventilatory, metabolic, and mitochondrial responses.

Mice (*Mus musculus*) and rats (*Rattus rattus* and *Rattus norvegicus*) are species with very different natural and phylogeographical histories, this can perfectly justify the physiological differences found in their mechanisms of acclimatization to hypoxia. The phylogeographic origin of *M. musculus* lies in the Irani-, Iraqi-, and Pakistani-Himalayan region, from where they initially colonized European and Asian lands by successfully overcoming migrations across mountain chains facing high-altitude challenges and certainly undergoing processes of natural selection (Bonhomme and Searle, 2012). On the contrary, *R. rattus* originated in India and South-Asia, and dispersed towards lowlands evading the northern mountain passes (Aplin et al., 2011). Even more contrastingly, *R. norvegicus* are original from the lowlands of central China and their expansion occurred almost strictly linked to human migration in recent historic times (Song et al., 2014; Puckett et al., 2016). Together with our present and past (Lumbroso and Joseph, 2009; Lumbroso et al., 2012; Jochmans-Lemoine et al., 2015, 2016, 2018; Jochmans-Lemoine and Joseph, 2018) results, this phylogeographic pattern strongly supports the hypothesis of mice being pre-adapted to high-altitude hypoxia.

We conclude that FVB mice and SD rats develop divergent physiological and mitochondrial mechanisms of acclimatization to hypoxia. Mice have an adaptive response with adjustments in oxygen capture, distribution, and utilization that allow them to maintain an unaltered or even increased whole-body and liver-mitochondrial metabolism. On the contrary, rats deploy an excessive and detrimental alteration in oxygen transport systems in blood and fail to trigger adjuvant ventilatory, metabolic, and subcellular procedures, therefore, presenting a deficient acclimatizing response. The adaptive adjustments during the process of acclimatization of mice may explain, at least in part, their ability to colonize high-altitude habitats in contrast to rats and further supports the hypothesis that mice are pre-adapted to high-altitude hypoxia.

ETHICS STATEMENT

The animal study was reviewed and approved by Animal Protection Committee of Université Laval, Québec, Canada.

AUTHOR CONTRIBUTIONS

CA-R performed all the experiments and data analyses. CA-R, JS, and VJ wrote and approved the manuscript. All authors contributed to the article and approved the submitted version.
Ph. D. scholarships from the "Reseau de Santé Respiratoire du Québec" and the "Fonds de Recherche du Québec- Santé" (292950). JS is supported by the "Fonds de recherché du Quebec-Santé" (FRQ-S; FQ121919). VJ is supported by NSERC. JS and VJ are members of the "Physiological breathing disorders" axis of the Quebec Respiratory Health Network.

REFERENCES

Aplin, K. P., Suzuki, H., Chinen, A. A., Chesser, R. T., Have, J. T., Donnellan, S. C., et al. (2011). Multiple geographic origins of commensalism and complex dispersal history of black rats. *PLoS One* 6:e26357. doi: 10.1371/journal.pone.0026357

Arias-Reyes, C., Losantos-Ramos, K., Gonzales, M., Furrer, D., and Soliz, J. (2019). NADH-linked mitochondrial respiration in the developing mouse brain is sex-, age- and tissue-dependent. *Respir. Physiol. Neurobiol.* 266, 156–162. doi: 10.1016/j.resp.2019.05.011

Ballot, O., Joseph, V., and Soliz, J. (2015). Endogenous brain erythropoietin is a potent sex-specific respiratory stimulant in adult and newborn mice. *J. Appl. Physiol.* 118, 1386–1395. doi: 10.1152/japplphysiol.00143.2015

Black, C. P., and Tenney, S. M. (1980). Oxygen transport during progressive hypoxia in high-altitude and sea-level waterfowl. *Respir. Physiol.* 39, 217–239. doi: 10.1016/0034-5687(80)90046-8

Bonhomme, F., and Searle, J. B. (2012). "House mouse phylogeography" in *Evolution of the house mouse. Vol. 3.* eds. M. Macholán, S. J. E. Baird, P. Munclinger and J. Piálek (Cambridge, UK: Cambridge University Press), 278.

Boukari, R., Rossignol, O., Baldy, C., Marcouiller, F., Bairam, A., and Joseph, V. (2016). Membrane progesterone receptor-β, but not-α, in dorsal brain stem establishes sex-specific chemoreflex responses and reduces apnea frequency in adult mice. *J. Appl. Physiol.* 121, 781–791. doi: 10.1152/japplphysiol.00397.2016

Bullard, R. (1972). "Vertebrates at altitude" in *Physiological adaptations: Desert and mountain.* eds. M. K. Yousef, S. M. Horvath and R. W. Bullard (New York, USA: Academic Press), 210–225.

Cáceda, R., Boero, J., and Arregui, A. (1997). Increase in succinate dehydrogenase activity in mice brain during chronic hypoxia. *Acta Andin* 6, 142–144.

Cáceda, R., Gamboa, J. L., Boero, J. A., Monge-C, C., and Arregui, A. (2001). Energetic metabolism in mouse cerebral cortex during chronic hypoxia. *Neurosci. Lett.* 301, 171–174. doi: 10.1016/S0304-3940(01)01630-5

Cheviron, Z. A., Bachman, G. C., Connaty, A. D., McClelland, G. B., and Storz, J. F. (2012). Regulatory changes contribute to the adaptive enhancement of thermogenic capacity in high-altitude deer mice. *Proc. Natl. Acad. Sci. U. S. A.* 109, 8635–8640. doi: 10.1073/pnas.1120523109

Costa, L. E., Boveris, A., Koch, O. R., and Taquini, A. C. (1988). Liver and heart mitochondria in rats submitted to chronic hypobaric hypoxia. *Am. J. Physiol* 255, C123–C129. doi: 10.1152/ajpcell.1988.255.1.C123

Czerniczyniec, A., La Padula, P., Bustamante, J., Karadayian, A., Lores-Arnaiz, S., and Costa, L. (2015). Mitochondrial function in rat cerebral cortex and hippocampus after short-and long-term hypobaric hypoxia. *Brain Res.* 1598, 66–75. doi: 10.1016/j.brainres.2014.12.018

Dawson, N. J., Lyons, S. A., Henry, D. A., and Scott, G. R. (2018). Effects of chronic hypoxia on diaphragm function in deer mice native to high altitude. *Acta Physiol.* 223:e13030. doi: 10.1111/apha.13030

Deuster, P. A., and Heled, Y. (2008). "Chapter 41-testing for maximal aerobic power" in *The sports medicine resource manual.* eds. P. H. Seidenberg and A. I. Beutler (Philadelphia: W.B. Saunders), 520–528.

Doerrier, C., Garcia-Souza, L. F., Krumschnabel, G., Wohlfarter, Y., Mészáros, A. T., and Gnaiger, E. (2018). "High-resolution fluorespirometry and OXPHOS protocols for human cells, permeabilized fibers from small biopsies of muscle, and isolated mitochondria" in *Mitochondrial bioenergetics.* eds. C. M. Palmeira and A. J. Moreno (Springer), 31–70.

Fuhrmann, D. C., and Brüne, B. (2017). Mitochondrial composition and function under the control of hypoxia. *Redox Biol.* 12, 208–215. doi: 10.1016/j.redox.2017.02.012

Gnaiger, E., Åsander Frostner, E., Abdul Karim, N., Abumrad, N., Acuna-Castroviejo, D., Adiele, R., et al. (2019). "Mitochondrial respiratory states and rate". MitoEAGLE task group, COST action CA15203 MitoEAGLE.

Griffiths, A. J., Miller, J. H., Suzuki, D. T., Lewontin, R. C., and Gelbart, W. M. (2000). "Multiple adaptive peaks" in *An introduction to genetic analysis. 7th Edn.* ed. W. H. Freeman.

Hawkins, B. J., Levin, M. D., Doonan, P. J., Petrenko, N. B., Davis, C. W., Patel, V. V., et al. (2010). Mitochondrial complex II prevents hypoxic but not calcium-and proapoptotic Bcl-2 protein-induced mitochondrial membrane potential loss. *J. Biol. Chem.* 285, 26494–26505. doi: 10.1074/jbc.M110.143164

Hayes, J. P. (1989). Altitudinal and seasonal effects on aerobic metabolism of deer mice. *J. Comp. Physiol. B.* 159, 453–459. doi: 10.1007/BF00692417

Hochachka, P. W. (1985). *Exercise limitations at high altitude: The metabolic problem and search for its solution.* Springer Berlin Heidelberg, 240–249.

Hochachka, P. W., Stanley, C., Merkt, J., and Sumar-Kalinowski, J. (1983). Metabolic meaning of elevated levels of oxidative enzymes in high altitude adapted animals: an interpretive hypothesis. *Respir. Physiol.* 52, 303–313. doi: 10.1016/0034-5687(83)90087-7

Hohl, C., Oestreich, R., Rösen, P., Wiesner, R., and Grieshaber, M. (1987). Evidence for succinate production by reduction of fumarate during hypoxia in isolated adult rat heart cells. *Arch. Biochem. Biophys.* 259, 527–535. doi: 10.1016/0003-9861(87)90519-4

Ivy, C. M., and Scott, G. R. (2017). Control of breathing and ventilatory acclimatization to hypoxia in deer mice native to high altitudes. *Acta Physiol.* 221, 266–282. doi: 10.1111/apha.12912

Jochmans-Lemoine, A., and Joseph, V. (2018). "Case study: developmental physiology at high altitude" in *Development and environment.* eds. W. Burggren and B. Dubansky (Cham: Springer International Publishing), 435–457.

Jochmans-Lemoine, A., Revollo, S., Villalpando, G., Valverde, I., Gonzales, M., and Laouafa, S., et al. (2018). Divergent mitochondrial antioxidant activities and lung alveolar architecture in the lungs of rats and mice at high altitude. *Front. Physiol.* 9:311. doi: 10.3389/fphys.2018.00311

Jochmans-Lemoine, A., Shahare, M., Soliz, J., and Joseph, V. (2016). HIF1α and physiological responses to hypoxia are correlated in mice but not in rats. *J. Exp. Biol.* 219, 3952–3961. doi: 10.1242/jeb.142869

Jochmans-Lemoine, A., Villalpando, G., Gonzales, M., Valverde, I., Soria, R., and Joseph, V. (2015). Divergent physiological responses in laboratory rats and mice raised at high altitude. *J. Exp. Biol.* 218, 1035–1043. doi: 10.1242/jeb.112862

Kummitha, C. M., Kalhan, S. C., Saidel, G. M., and Lai, N. (2014). Relating tissue/organ energy expenditure to metabolic fluxes in mouse and human: experimental data integrated with mathematical modeling. *Phys. Rep.* 2:e12159. doi: 10.14814/phy2.12159

León-Velarde, F., and Arregui, A. (1994). *Desadaptación a la vida en las grandes alturas.* Lima, Peru: Universidad Privada Cayetano Heredia, 145.

Leon-Velarde, F., Whittembury, J., and Monge, C. (1986). Oxidative phosphorylation of liver mitochondria from mice acclimatized to hypobaric hypoxia. *Int. J. Biometeorol.* 30, 283–289. doi: 10.1007/BF02189472

Lui, M. A., Mahalingam, S., Patel, P., Connaty, A. D., Ivy, C. M., and Cheviron, Z. A., et al. (2015). High-altitude ancestry and hypoxia acclimation have distinct effects on exercise capacity and muscle phenotype in deer mice. *Am. J. Phys. Regul. Integr. Comp. Phys.* 308, R779–R791. doi: 10.1152/ajpregu.00362.2014

Lukyanova, L. (1997). Bioenergy hypoxia: concept, mechanisms, correction. *Bull. Exp. Biol. Med.* 124, 244–254.

Lukyanova, L., and Dudchenko, A. (1999). "Regulatory role of the adenylate pool in the formation of hepatocyte resistance to hypoxia" in *The adaptation biology and medicine.* eds. K. B. Pandolf, N. Takeda, and P. K. Singal (New Delhi: Narosa Publishing House), 139–150.

Lukyanova, L., Dudchenko, A., Tzybina, T., and Germanova, E. (2008). "Mitochondrial signaling in adaptation to hypoxia" in *Adaptation biology and medicine. Vol. 5.* eds. L. Lukyanova, N. Takeda and P. K. Singai (New Delhi, India: Narosa Publishing house), 245.

Lukyanova, L. D., and Kirova, Y. I. (2015). Mitochondria-controlled signaling mechanisms of brain protection in hypoxia. *Front. Neurosci.* 9:320. doi: 10.3389/fnins.2015.00320

Lukyanova, L. D., Kirova, Y. I., and Germanova, E. L. (2018). The role of succinate in regulation of immediate HIF-1α expression in hypoxia. *Bull. Exp. Biol. Med.* 164, 298–303. doi: 10.1007/s10517-018-3976-2

Lumbroso, D., and Joseph, V. (2009). Impaired acclimatization to chronic hypoxia in adult male and female rats following neonatal hypoxia. *Am. J. Phys. Regul. Integr. Comp. Phys.* 297, R421–R427. doi: 10.1152/ajpregu.00068.2009

Lumbroso, D., Lemoine, A., Gonzales, M., Villalpando, G., Seaborn, T., and Joseph, V. (2012). Life-long consequences of postnatal normoxia exposure in rats raised at high altitude. *J. Appl. Physiol.* 112, 33–41. doi: 10.1152/japplphysiol.01043.2011

Mahalingam, S., McClelland, G. B., and Scott, G. R. (2017). Evolved changes in the intracellular distribution and physiology of muscle mitochondria in high-altitude native deer mice. *J. Physiol.* 595, 4785–4801. doi: 10.1113/JP274130

Marcouiller, F., Boukari, R., Laouafa, S., Lavoie, R., and Joseph, V. (2014). The nuclear progesterone receptor reduces post-sigh apneas during sleep and increases the ventilatory response to hypercapnia in adult female mice. *PLoS One* 9:e100421. doi: 10.1371/journal.pone.0100421

Monge, C., and Leon-Velarde, F. (1991). Physiological adaptation to high altitude: oxygen transport in mammals and birds. *Physiol. Rev.* 71, 1135–1172. doi: 10.1152/physrev.1991.71.4.1135

Monge, C. C., and León-Velarde, F. (2003). *El reto fisiológico de vivir en los Andes*: Travaux de l'I. F. E. A.

Monge, C., and Whittembury, J. (1976). "High altitude adaptations in the whole animal" in *Environmental physiology of animals*. eds. J. Bligh, A. G. MacDonald and J. L. Cloudsley-Thompson (New York, USA: Blackwell Sc. Publications).

Pickett, C. B., Cascarano, J., and Wilson, M. A. (1979). Acute and chronic hypoxia in rats. 1. Effect on organismic respiration, mitochondrial protein mass in liver and succinic dehydrogenase activity in liver, kidney and heart. *J. Exp. Zool.* 210, 49–57. doi: 10.1002/jez.1402100106

Powell, F. L. (2007). The influence of chronic hypoxia upon chemoreception. *Respir. Physiol. Neurobiol.* 157, 154–161. doi: 10.1016/j.resp.2007.01.009

Powell, F. L., Milsom, W. K., and Mitchell, G. S. (1998). Time domains of the hypoxic ventilatory response. *Respir. Physiol.* 112, 123–134. doi: 10.1016/S0034-5687(98)00026-7

Puckett, E. E., Park, J., Combs, M., Blum, M. J., Bryant, J. E., Caccone, A., et al. (2016). Global population divergence and admixture of the brown rat (*Rattus norvegicus*). *Proc. Biol. Sci.* 283:20161762. doi: 10.1098/rspb.2016.1762

Schmitt, P., Soulier, V., Péquignot, J. M., Pujol, J. F., and Denavit-Saubié, M. (1994). Ventilatory acclimatization to chronic hypoxia: relationship to noradrenaline metabolism in the rat solitary complex. *J. Physiol.* 477, 331–337. doi: 10.1113/jphysiol.1994.sp020194

Scott, G. R., Cadena, V., Tattersall, G. J., and Milsom, W. K. (2008). Body temperature depression and peripheral heat loss accompany the metabolic and ventilatory responses to hypoxia in low and high altitude birds. *J. Exp. Biol.* 211, 1326–1335. doi: 10.1242/jeb.015958

Scott, G. R., Guo, K. H., and Dawson, N. J. (2018). The mitochondrial basis for adaptive variation in aerobic performance in high-altitude deer mice. *Integr. Comp. Biol.* 58, 506–518. doi: 10.1093/icb/icy056

Scott, G. R., and Milsom, W. K. (2009). "Control of breathing in birds: implications for high-altitude flight" in *Cardio-respiratory control in vertebrates: Comparative and evolutionary aspects*. eds. M. L. Glass and S. C. Wood (Berlin, Heidelberg: Springer Berlin Heidelberg), 429–448.

Song, Y., Lan, Z., and Kohn, M. H. (2014). Mitochondrial DNA phylogeography of the Norway rat. *PLoS One* 9:e88425. doi: 10.1371/journal.pone.0116455

Stahl, W. R. (1967). Scaling of respiratory variables in mammals. *J. Appl. Physiol.* 22, 453–460. doi: 10.1152/jappl.1967.22.3.453

Storz, J. F., Baze, M., Waite, J. L., Hoffmann, F. G., Opazo, J. C., and Hayes, J. P. (2007). Complex signatures of selection and gene conversion in the duplicated globin genes of house mice. *Genetics* 177, 481–500. doi: 10.1534/genetics.107.078550

Storz, J. F., and Scott, G. R. (2021). Phenotypic plasticity, genetic assimilation, and genetic compensation in hypoxia adaptation of high-altitude vertebrates. *Comp. Biochem. Physiol. A Mol. Integr. Physiol.* 253:110865. doi: 10.1016/j.cbpa.2020.110865

Storz, J. F., Scott, G. R., and Cheviron, Z. A. (2010). Phenotypic plasticity and genetic adaptation to high-altitude hypoxia in vertebrates. *J. Exp. Biol.* 213, 4125–4136. doi: 10.1242/jeb.048181

Wang, Z., Zhang, J., Ying, Z., and Heymsfield, S. B. (2012). Organ-tissue level model of resting energy expenditure across mammals: new insights into kleiber's law. *ISRN Zool.* 2012, 1–9. doi: 10.5402/2012/673050

Ward, S., Bishop, C. M., Woakes, A. J., and Butler, P. J. (2002). Heart rate and the rate of oxygen consumption of flying and walking barnacle geese (*Branta leucopsis*) and bar-headed geese (*Anser indicus*). *J. Exp. Biol.* 205, 3347–3356.

3

Histone Deacetylase 5 is an Early Epigenetic Regulator of Intermittent Hypoxia Induced Sympathetic Nerve Activation and Blood Pressure

*Ning Wang, Ying-Jie Peng, Xiaoyu Su, Nanduri R. Prabhakar and Jayasri Nanduri**

Institute for Integrative Physiology, Center for Systems Biology of O_2 Sensing, The University of Chicago, Chicago, IL, United States

***Correspondence:**
Jayasri Nanduri
jnanduri@uchicago.edu

Intermittent hypoxia (IH) is a hallmark manifestation of obstructive sleep apnea (OSA). Long term IH (LT-IH) triggers epigenetic reprogramming of the redox state involving DNA hypermethylation in the carotid body chemo reflex pathway resulting in persistent sympathetic activation and hypertension. Present study examined whether IH also activates epigenetic mechanism(s) other than DNA methylation. Histone modification by lysine acetylation is another major epigenetic mechanism associated with gene regulation. Equilibrium between the activities of histone acetyltransferases (HATs) and histone deacetylases (HDACs) determine the level of lysine acetylation. Here we report that exposure of rat pheochromocytoma (PC)-12 cells to IH *in vitro* exhibited reduced HDAC enzyme activity due to proteasomal degradation of HDAC3 and HDAC5 proteins. Mechanistic investigations showed that IH-evoked decrease in HDAC activity increases lysine acetylation of α subunit of hypoxia inducible factor (HIF)-1α as well as Histone (H3) protein resulting in increased HIF-1 transcriptional activity. Trichostatin A (TSA), an inhibitor of HDACs, mimicked the effects of IH. Studies on rats treated with 10 days of IH or TSA showed reduced HDAC activity, HDAC5 protein, and increased HIF-1 dependent NADPH oxidase (NOX)-4 transcription in adrenal medullae (AM) resulting in elevated plasma catecholamines and blood pressure. Likewise, heme oxygenase (HO)-2 null mice, which exhibit IH because of high incidence of spontaneous apneas (apnea index 72 ± 1.2 apnea/h), also showed decreased HDAC activity and HDAC5 protein in the AM along with elevated circulating norepinephrine levels. These findings demonstrate that lysine acetylation of histone and non-histone proteins is an early epigenetic mechanism associated with sympathetic nerve activation and hypertension in rodent models of IH.

Keywords: intermittent hypoxia, obstructive sleep apnea, lysine deacetylase, HDAC5, histone 3, HIF-1, hypertension

INTRODUCTION

Obstructive sleep apnea (OSA) is a widespread breathing disorder affecting 10–15% of adult population (Peppard et al., 2013). OSA is defined as periodic disruption of air flow during sleep either due to complete (apneas) or partial collapse (hypopnea) of the upper airway. Population based studies showed high prevalence of essential hypertension with strong correlation to severity of OSA (Morrell et al., 2000; Nieto et al., 2000).

Intermittent hypoxia (IH), a hallmark manifestation of OSA, is a major contributing factor to hypertension (reviewed in Prabhakar et al., 2020). Rats treated with long-term-IH (30 days; LT-IH) exhibit hypertension and heightened sympathetic nerve activity persisting even after a 30-day recovery in room air (Nanduri et al., 2017). The long-lasting blood pressure elevation evoked by LT-IH is reminiscent of treatment-resistant hypertension reported in a subset of OSA patients. LT-IH evoked long-lasting hypertension was due to persistent elevation of ROS caused by epigenetic suppression of anti-oxidant enzyme genes by DNA methylation (Nanduri et al., 2017).

Lysine acetylation of histones (H2A, H2B, H3, and H4) is another important epigenetic mechanism which regulates gene transcription by altering chromatin structure. Hyper-acetylation activates, while hypo-acetylation represses transcriptional activation (Grunstein, 1997; Audia and Campbell, 2016). Lysine acetylation is a dynamic process involving opposing activities of histone/lysine acetyl transferases (HAT) and histone deacetylases (HDAC's) (Yang and Seto, 2007). A recent study reported that chronic stress decreases HDAC activity, leading to increased histone acetylation and transcriptional activation of target genes (Renthal et al., 2007). Given that IH is a form of chronic stress, whether lysine acetylation resulting from reduced HDAC activity participate in gene activation by IH has not been investigated.

In addition to histones, lysine acetylation of non-histone proteins like transcription factors also control gene transcription (Park et al., 2015). Hypoxia inducible factor (HIF-1) is a master regulator for gene transcription during hypoxia (Semenza et al., 1998). Studies on tumor cell lines showed that HDAC1 and HDAC3 positively regulate HIF-1α stability while HDAC4 and HDAC5 increase HIF-1-dependent transcriptional activation (Kim et al., 2007; Seo et al., 2009; Geng et al., 2011). Our earlier studies showed that mice partially deficient in HIF-1α, the O_2 regulated subunit of the HIF-1 complex, exhibit remarkable absence of IH-evoked elevation of ROS, sympathetic activation and hypertension (Peng et al., 2006). Moreover, HIF-1 is a potent activator of pro-oxidant enzyme genes including NADPH oxidases (NOX) (Yuan et al., 2011; Wang et al., 2020). Given that HDACs regulate the stability of HIF-1α as well as HIF-1 activity (Qian et al., 2006; Kim et al., 2007; Seo et al., 2009), we hypothesized that IH reduces HDAC activity and stabilizes HIF-1α through lysine acetylation leading to HIF-1-dependent transcriptional activation involving lysine acetylation of histone proteins. These possibilities were first tested in rat pheochromocytoma (PC)-12 cells and then further validated in two rodent models of OSA, namely rats treated with IH and OSA-exhibiting hemeoxygenase (HO)-2 null mice (Peng et al., 2018).

MATERIALS AND METHODS

Experimental protocols were approved by the Institutional Animal Care and Use Committee (IACUC) of the University of Chicago and were performed on adult Sprague Dawley rats (SD; 2–4 months age, approved protocol #71811), age and gender matched wild-type (WT; C57BL6) and HO-2 null mice (6–8 months age, approved protocol #71810).

Exposure of Rats to Intermittent Hypoxia (IH)

The protocols for exposing rats to IH were essentially the same as described previously (Peng et al., 2006). Briefly, conscious rats were placed in a specialized chamber and exposed to alternating cycles of hypoxia (15 s of ~5% O_2 at nadir followed by 5 min of room air, 8 h/day) for 10 days. Parallel experiments were performed on rats exposed to alternating cycles of room air (control) in an identical chamber. The duration of the gas flow was regulated by timer-controlled solenoid valves. Ambient O_2 and CO_2 levels in the chamber were continuously monitored and the CO_2 levels were maintained at ~0.1%.

Exposure of Rat Pheochromocytoma (PC)-12 Cells to IH

PC12 cells (original clone from Dr. Lloyd A. Greene, Columbia University, NY, United States) (Greene and Tischler, 1976) were cultured in Dulbecco's modified Eagle's medium (DMEM) supplemented with 5% fetal bovine serum (FBS), 10% horse serum under 10% CO_2 and 90% room air (20% O_2) at 37°C (Yuan et al., 2005). Experiments were performed on cells serum-starved overnight in DMEM medium. Cells were exposed to *in vitro* IH (alternating cycles of 1.5% O_2 for 30 s followed by 20% O_2 for 5 min at 37°C) as described (Yuan et al., 2004). Ambient O_2 levels in the IH chamber were monitored by an O_2 analyzer (Alpha Omega Instruments, Huston, TX). In the experiments involving treatment with drugs, cells were pre-incubated for 30 min prior to and during IH exposure with either drug or vehicle.

Measurement of Blood Pressure (BP) and Plasma Norepinephrine

BP was measured in conscious rats between 09.00 and 11.00 a.m. by tail-cuff method using a non-invasive BP system (IITC Life Science Inc., CA, United States). Blood samples were collected in heparinized vials (30 IU/ml) from rats/mice anesthetized with urethane (1.2 g/kg, IP). Plasma was separated by centrifugation and stored at −80°C. Plasma norepinephrine (NE) levels were determined by high pressure liquid chromatography (HPLC) combined with electrochemical detection using dihydroxybenzylamine hydrobromide (DHBA; Sigma-Aldrich) as an internal standard. The NE levels were corrected for recovery loss and expressed as nanograms per milliliter of plasma calculated from an NE standard curve (Peng et al., 2006).

Measurement of Breathing

Breathing was monitored by whole-body plethysmography in conscious mice at ambient temperature of 25 ± 1°C as described (Peng et al., 2018). Apneas were scored by two individuals who were blinded to genotype. Number of apneas (defined as cessation of breathing for more than the duration of three breaths) per hour was analyzed and presented as the apnea index. Sighs, sniffs and movement-induced changes in breathing were excluded in the analysis.

Measurement of HDAC, SIRT, and NOX Activity

HDAC and Sirtuin (SIRT) activities were measured in nuclear lysates using colorimetric Epigenase HDAC activity and SIRT activity kit, respectively (Epigentek, Farmington, NY, United States). Briefly, 5 μg of nuclear extract (from two rat adrenal medullae (AM) and 4 mice AM) were added to a plate coated with acetylated histone HDAC or SIRT substrate. Active HDAC or SIRT binds and deacetylates H3 which is recognized with a specific antibody and measured by reading the absorbance at 450 nm. The activity is directly proportional to the OD intensity measured and expressed as ng/min/mg protein. NADPH oxidase activity in the membrane-enriched protein fractions (50 μg: two rat AM and 4 mice AM) were measured by superoxide dismutase-inhabitable rate of cytochrome c reduction, and reading the absorbance at 550 nm. NADPH oxidase activity was calculated based on the extinction coefficient [21 mmol/(L)] per cm, and is expressed as nmol/min/mg protein (Khan et al., 2011).

Immunoblot and Immunoprecipitation Assays

Nuclear extracts of PC12 cells were prepared using nuclear extraction kit (Active Motif, Carlsbad, CA, United States). Briefly, cells (1×10^6) were homogenized in 200 μl of hypotonic buffer provided in the kit and centrifuged at 850 *g* for 10 min at 4°C. The pellet was re-suspended in 200 μl of hypotonic buffer and a small sample was checked under the microscope to verify cells were efficiently lysed and nuclei were released. The suspension was centrifuged at 14,000 *g* for 30 s. The nuclear pellet was re-suspended in 40 μl of complete lysis buffer provided and fractionated by polyacrylamide-SDS gel electrophoresis. Immunoblots were probed with either HIF-1α (1/1,000 dilution; #NB100-479, Novus Biologicals, Centennial, CO), HDAC1-5 (1/2000; #5356, #5113, #3949, #7628, and #20458, respectively) and H3 (1/4,000; #4499) (Cell signaling, Danvers, MA), TBP (1/1,000; Tata binding protein; #ab51841, Abcam) or tubulin (1/10,000; #T6199, Sigma, St. Louis, MO, United States) antibodies followed by corresponding HRP-conjugated secondary antibody detected by Clarity Western ECL substrate kit (Bio-Rad, Hercules, CA, United States). Immunoblots were scanned and quantified using an Odyssey Fc imaging system (LI-COR, Lincoln, NE, United States). For analysis of HIF-1α acetylation, PC12 cells transfected with FLAG-tagged HIF-1α plasmid were exposed to IH. Cell lysates were immunoprecipitated with anti-FLAG antibody (#1804, Sigma, St. Louis, MO, United States) and the immunoprecipitates were analyzed by acetylated lysine (1/500, #SC-32268, Santa Cruz, Dallas, TX, United States) antibody as described above. Rat/mice adrenal medulla cell extracts were prepared in RIPA buffer (phosphate buffer, pH 7.4 containing 150 mM NaCl, 1% triton X-100, 1% sodium deoxycholate, 0.1% SDS, 5 mM EDTA, and protease inhibitor cocktail) and analyzed using automated capillary electrophoresis size-based separation followed by immunoassay using the WES System from Protein Simple according to the manufacturer's instructions. Data were analyzed with Compass software (Protein Simple). Primary antibodies against the following proteins were used at a dilution of 1/50 for immunoblot assays: HIF-1α (#NB100-123, Novus Biologicals, Centennial, CO). HDAC5 (#ab20458, Cell Signaling Danvers, MA, United States). Sample loading variability was normalized to tubulin (#T6199, Sigma, St. Louis, MO, United States) antibody. Acetylated H3 and NOX4 protein expression was analyzed in AM cell lysates by polyacrylamide-SDS gel electrophoresis and immunoblots were probed with acetylated lysine antibody (1/500, #SC-32268, Santa Cruz, Dallas, TX, United States) or NOX4 antibody (1/1,000; NB110-58851, Novus Biologicals, Centennial, CO, United States).

qRT-PCR (Quantitative Reverse Transcription -PCR)

Total RNA was isolated with TRIZOL (Invitrogen), and cDNA was synthesized using the iScript cDNA synthesis kit (Bio-Rad). qRT- PCR was performed using SsoFast EvaGreen (Bio-RAD) as a fluorogenic binding dye. Housekeeping genes 18S RNA and β-actin were included as quantitation controls. Changes in target mRNA expression was calculated based on the Δ(ΔCt) method as described previously (Nanduri et al., 2009). Primer sequences used for real-time PCR amplification were: Rat NOX4; (NM_053524.1): Forward; CGGGTGGCTTGTTGAAGTAT; Reverse; TGGAACTTGGGTTCTTCCAG, Mouse NOX4; (NM_015760.5): Forward: TGTTGGGCCTAGGATTGTGTT; Reverse: AGGGACCTTCTGTGATCCTCG, 18S (NR_003278): Forward; CGCCGCTAGAGGTGAAATTC; Reverse; CGAACCTCCGACTTTCGTTCT. β-actin (NM_031144.3): Forward; AGG CCC AGA GCA AGA GAG G; Reverse; TAC ATG GCT GGG GTG TTG AA.

Transient Transfections and HRE Reporter Gene Assay

PC12 cells were transiently transfected with overexpression plasmids pHDAC5 and pHDAC3 (addgene) or with control vector plasmid pcDNA using TransIT-2020 (Mirus) transfection reagent. Briefly, cells were plated in 60 mm tissue culture plates at a density of 2×10^6 cells/plate in serum containing growth medium. After 24 h, DNA-TransIT reagent in the ratio of 1:3 was added. After 36 h, serum starved cells were exposed to IH. To analyze HIF-1 transcriptional activity, cells were co-transfected with two reporter plasmids: p2.1, which contains firefly luciferase coding sequences downstream of a basal SV40 promoter and a 68 bp hypoxia response element (HRE) from the human *EPO1* gene (Semenza et al., 1996) and *Renilla* Luciferase Control Reporter Vector (pRL). The Bright-Glo™ Luciferase Assay System (Promega, Madison, WI, United States) was used to measure luciferase activity in nuclear cell lysates and normalized to protein content measured by Bio-Rad protein assay kit (Bio-Rad, Richmond, CA, United States).

Data Analysis

Data is expressed as mean ± SEM from mice (8–12 animals per group) and 3–5 independent cell culture experiments. Statistical analysis was performed by analysis of variance (one-way ANOVA with *post-hoc* Turkey HSD test) and Mann-Whitney test. $p < 0.05$ were considered significant.

RESULTS

IH Decreases HDAC Enzyme Activity

Pheochromocytoma (PC) 12 cells cultures were chosen because experiments require transient transfection protocols for reporter gene assays and ectopic expression of proteins can be best performed in cell cultures rather than tissues from rats (Prabhakar et al., 2012). HDACs comprise of four classes of proteins (Haberland et al., 2009), including Class I (HDACs 1, 2, 3, and 8), Class II (HDACs 4, 5, 6, 7, 9, and 10), Class III (NAD^+-dependent sirtuins) and Class IV (HDAC11). The enzyme activities of HDAC and Sirtuins (SIRT) were determined in cells treated with 60 cycles of IH (IH_{60}) or alternating cycles of room air (N) which served as controls. Cells treated with IH_{60} showed reduced HDAC activity, whereas SIRT activity was unaltered (**Figures 1A,B**). Treating cells with 50 nM Trichostatin A (TSA), which is an inhibitor of HDACs but not SIRTs (Finnin et al., 1999; Bertrand, 2010), mimicked the effects of IH by markedly reducing HDAC activity compared to vehicle treated controls (**Figure 1C**).

IH Reduces HDAC5 and HDAC3 Proteins

We next determined whether reduced expression of HDAC protein(s) account for the decreased HDAC activity by IH. To this end, HDAC1-5 protein abundances were determined in nuclear extracts of IH treated cells by immunoblot assay. IH treated cells showed decreased levels of HDAC3 and HDAC5 proteins, whereas the levels of HDAC1, HDAC2, and HDAC4 proteins were unaltered (**Figures 2A,B**).

IH had no effect on HDAC3 or HDAC5 mRNA expression (**Figure 2C**), suggesting that reduced HDAC3 and HDAC5 proteins by IH are not due to decreased transcription. HDACs can undergo post-translational modifications leading to ubiquitin-mediated proteasomal degradation (Adenuga et al., 2009). To determine whether the effects of IH are due to increased proteasomal degradation, cells were treated with MG-132 (5 μM), a proteasomal inhibitor. As shown in **Figure 2D**, cells treated with MG-132 showed absence of IH-induced reduction in HDAC3 and HDAC5 proteins compared to vehicle treated cells. These data suggest that proteasomal degradation of HDAC3 and HDAC5 contribute to decreased HDAC activity in PC12 cells exposed to IH_{60}.

Reduced HDACs Contributes to HIF-1α Stability by IH Through Lysine Acetylation

IH stabilizes HIF-1α protein and activates HIF-1-dependent transcription in PC12 cells (Yuan et al., 2005, 2011). Given that HDACs can affect HIF-1α stability (Qian et al., 2006; Kim et al., 2007; Seo et al., 2009), we hypothesized that reduced HDAC activity by IH contributes to HIF-1α stabilization through lysine acetylation. This possibility was tested by first monitoring HIF-1α proteins in nuclear extracts of PC12 cells treated with either IH_{60} or 50 nM TSA (positive control). Decreased HDAC3 and HDAC5 protein expressions were associated with elevated HIF-1α protein in IH as well as in TSA-treated cells (**Figure 3A**).

We next determined whether IH or TSA-induced HIF-1α protein accumulation is associated with increased lysine acetylation of HIF-1α. Assessing endogenous HIF-1α lysine acetylation in PC12 cells was technically challenging. To circumvent this limitation, PC12 cells were transfected with a FLAG-tagged HIF-1α expressing plasmid and then treated with either IH_{60} or TSA (50 nM for 7 h). HIF-1α was immunoprecipitated with FLAG-antibody in nuclear extracts and lysine acetylation was determined using anti-acetylated lysine antibody. Cells treated with IH_{60} as well as TSA showed increased abundance of lysine acetylated HIF-1α protein compared to room air (N) or vehicle treated controls (**Figures 3B,C**).

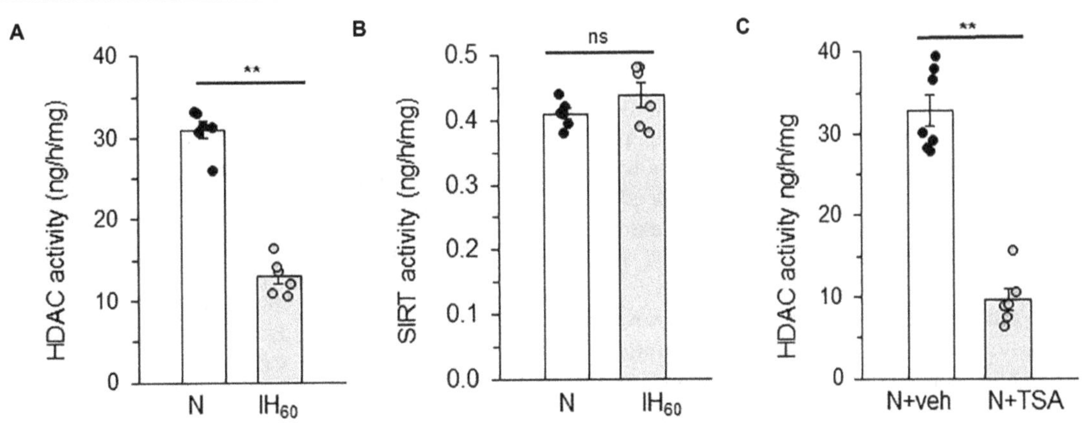

FIGURE 1 | Effect of IH on HDAC and SIRT activity in PC12 cells treated with 60 cycles of IH (IH_{60}) or HDAC inhibitor Trichostatin A (TSA). **(A,B)** HDAC and SIRT activity in nuclear lysates from room air (N) and IH-exposed (IH_{60}) PC12 cells. **(C)** HDAC activity in nuclear lysates from PC12 cells treated with TSA (HDAC inhibitor; 50 nM) for 7 h in room air (N) (mean ± SEM; n = 4–6). $^{**}p \leq 0.05$; ns = not significant ($p > 0.05$) as determined by Mann-Whitney test.

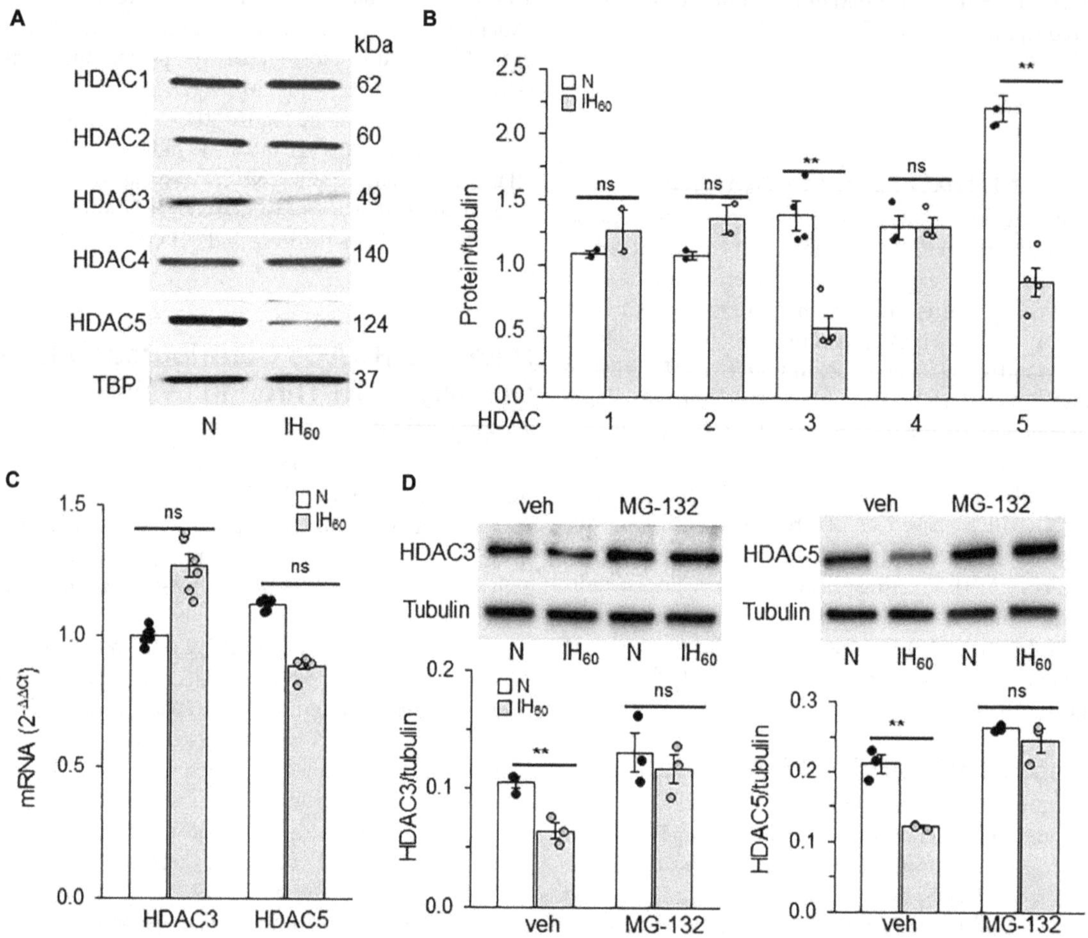

FIGURE 2 | Effect of IH on HDAC proteins and mRNA expression. **(A)** Representative example of an immunoblot showing HDAC1-5 protein expression and Tata binding protein (TBP) as a loading control in nuclear lysates from room air (N) and IH-exposed PC12 cells. **(B)** Quantitative analysis of the blots by ImageJ. **(C)** HDAC3 and HDAC5 mRNA expression by qRT-PCR. **(D)** *Top panel:* HDAC3 and HDAC5 protein expression in cells treated with vehicle or MG132 (proteasomal inhibitor; 5 μM) and exposed to IH. *bottom panel:* Quantitative analysis of the blots (mean ± SEM; n = 3–4) by Image Studio by Odyssey Fc imaging system. $^{**}p \leq 0.05$; ns = not significant ($p > 0.05$) as determined by One-way ANOVA with *post-hoc* Turkey HSD test.

HDACs Regulate IH-Induced HIF-1 Transcription Through Histone Lysine Acetylation

We then asked whether HIF-1α stabilization by lysine acetylation accompanies HIF-1 transcriptional activation by IH. To this end, cells were transfected with a plasmid containing a hypoxia response element (HRE) upstream of luciferase coding sequences. Increased luciferase activity was monitored as an index of HIF transcriptional activity. Cells treated with IH_{60} as well as TSA showed robust HIF-1 dependent transcriptional activation as evidenced by marked increase in luciferase activity (**Figure 4A**).

Lysine acetylation of histones regulate transcription by facilitating binding of transcription factors to promoter regions of target genes through altering chromatin structure (Yang and Seto, 2003; Seto and Yoshida, 2014). We assessed whether reduced HDAC activity contributes to HIF-1 transcriptional activation by IH through increased histone lysine acetylation. This possibility was tested first by determining which histones were acetylated in PC12 cells with IH or TSA. Immunoblot assay with a pan acetylated lysine antibody detected a band around 17 kDa in IH and TSA treated cell lysates. This molecular mass corresponds to histone 3 (H3) rather than histone 4 (~11 kD) (**Figure 4B**). To confirm that IH increases H3 lysine acetylation, H3 was immunoprecipitated from nuclear extracts with anti-H3 antibody and the immunoprecipitates were probed for lysine acetylation with acetylated lysine antibody. Abundance of lysine acetylated H3 protein increased in IH as well as in TSA treated cells with no change in the total H3 protein expression (**Figures 4B,C**). These observations establish that decreased HDAC activity increase lysine acetylation of H3 protein, which accompanies HIF-1 transcriptional activation by IH.

HDAC5 but Not HDAC3 Regulates HIF-1 Activation by IH

HDACs function as multimeric protein complexes with homo- and/or heterodimer structure (Yang and Seto, 2003). Given

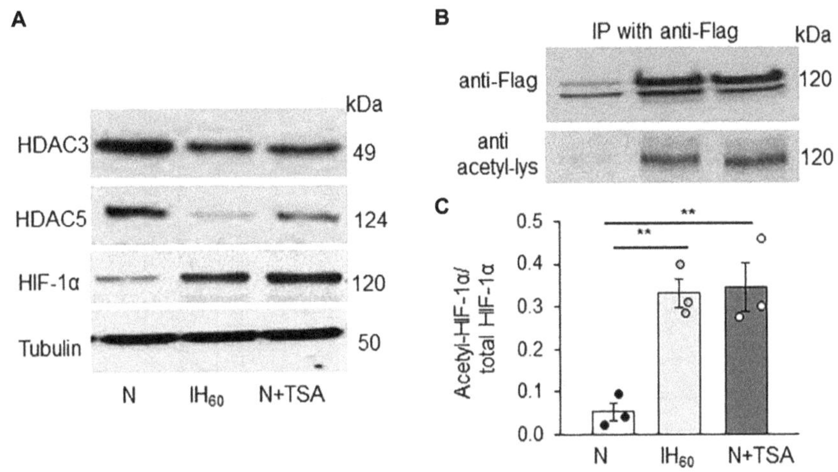

FIGURE 3 | Effect of IH_{60} and TSA on HIF-1α protein and HIF-1α acetylation in PC12 cells. **(A)** HDAC3, HDAC5 and HIF-1 protein expression with tubulin as a loading control in nuclear lysates from room air (N), IH-exposed and TSA (50 nM for 7 h) treated PC12 cells; **(B)** PC12 cells transiently transfected with FLAG-tagged HIF-1 overexpression plasmids were treated with either IH_{60} or TSA and HIF-1α was immunoprecipitated with anti-FLAG antibody from nuclear extracts. Acetylation of HIF-1α was analyzed in the immunoprecipitations by immunoblots using anti-acetylated lysine antibody. HIF-1 protein was analyzed by anti-Flag antibody. **(C)** Quantitative analysis of the blots expressed as ratio of acetylated HIF-1α to total HIF-1α protein (mean ± SEM; $n = 3$). $^{**}p \leq 0.05$ as determined by One-way ANOVA with *post-hoc* Turkey HSD test.

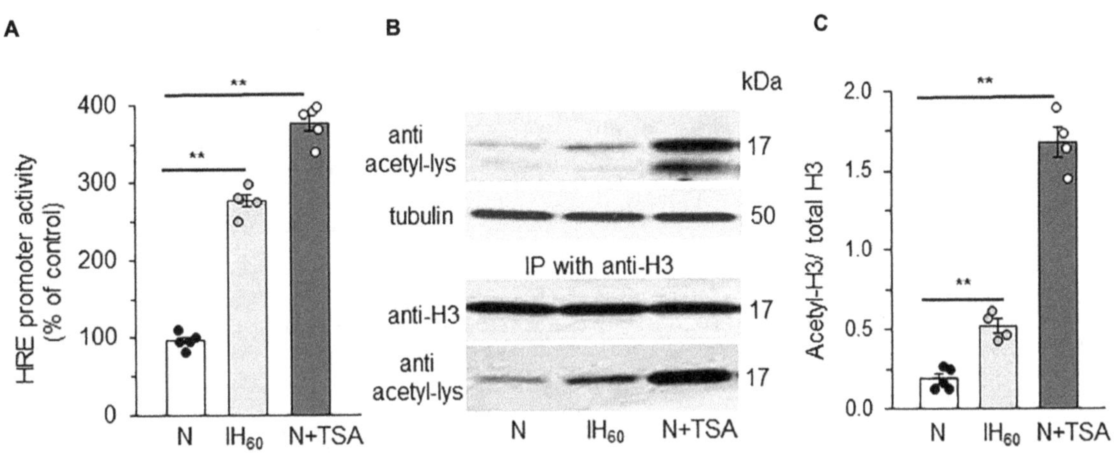

FIGURE 4 | Effect of IH_{60} and TSA on HIF-1 transcriptional activity and Histone (H3) acetylation in PC12 cells. **(A)** HRE transcriptional activity in nuclear lysates of cells co-transfected with a plasmid p2.1 containing HRE upstream of SV40 promoter and luciferase coding sequence and Renilla luciferase control vector and exposed to room air (N), IH and TSA treated. **(B)** Acetylation of Histone 3 (H3) as analyzed by immunoblots with anti-acetyl lysine antibody. Acetylation of H3 was confirmed by immunoprecipitating with anti H3 antibody and the immunoprecipitations probed with anti-H3 antibody and anti-acetyl lysine antibody. **(C)** Quantitative analysis of the blots expressed as ratio of acetylated H3 to total H3 protein (mean ± SEM; $n = 3$–4). $^{**}p \leq 0.05$ as determined by One-way ANOVA with *post-hoc* Turkey HSD test.

that IH decreases both HDAC3 and HDAC5 proteins, we examined the relative contribution of HDAC3 and HDAC5 to IH-evoked HIF-1 transcriptional activation. To this end, cells were transfected with over expression plasmids encoding either HDAC3 or HDAC5, and then exposed to IH_{60} or normoxia (control). Over expression of HDAC5 blocked the reduced HDAC5 expression as well as HIF-1α protein accumulation characteristic to IH (**Figure 5A**) with no significant effect on HDAC3 protein. On the other hand, overexpression of HDAC3 blocked IH-induced decrease in HDAC3 expression but had no effect on either IH-induced HIF-1α or HDAC 5 protein expression (**Figure 5A**). Furthermore, IH-evoked HRE transcriptional activity was absent in cells with ectopic expression of HDAC5 but not HDAC3 (**Figure 5B**). The effects of IH on HDAC5 and HIF-1α protein were reversed within 16 h after recovery of cells in room air (**Figures 5C,D**). These findings demonstrate that reduced HDAC5 but not HDAC3 contribute to HIF-1α stability and HIF-1 transcriptional activation by IH and that the effects of IH on the HDAC5 protein are reversible.

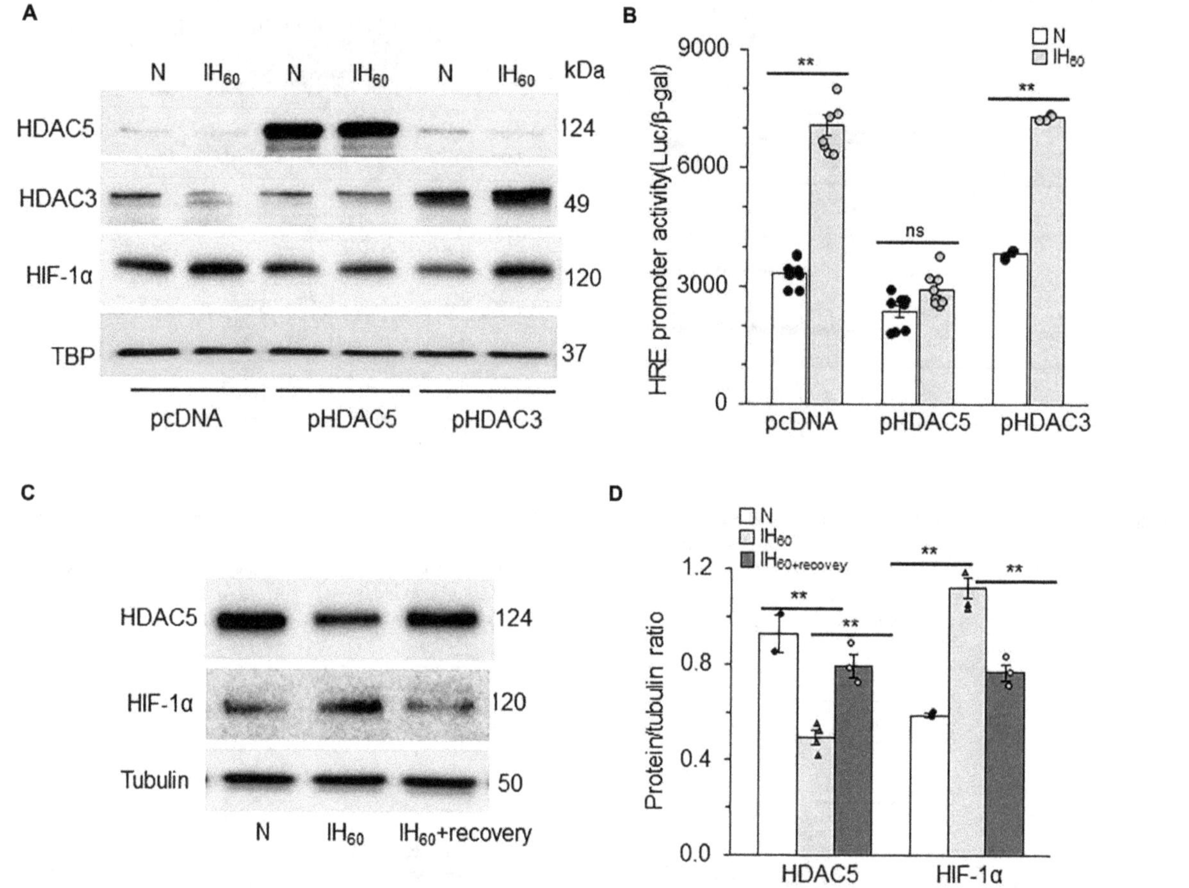

FIGURE 5 | HDAC5 but not HDAC3 contributes to IH-augmented HIF-1 transcriptional activity. **(A)** Representative example of an immunoblot showing HDAC5, HDAC3, and HIF-1α protein expression with Tata binding protein (TBP) as a loading control in nuclear lysates from room air (N) and IH-exposed PC12 cells transfected with overexpression plasmids encoding either HDAC3, HDAC5, or control vector pcDNA (mean ± SEM; $n = 3$). **(B)** HRE transcriptional activity in nuclear lysates from control (N) and IH-exposed PC12 cells overexpressing HDAC3, or HDAC5 protein (mean ± SEM; $n = 6$). $^{**}p \leq 0.05$; ns = not significant ($p > 0.05$) as determined by Mann-Whitney test. **(C)** Immunoblot showing HDAC5, HIF-1α protein and acetyl-H3 protein expression with tubulin as a loading control in cell lysates from room air (N) IH-exposed (IH_{60}) and IH-exposed cells after room air recovery for 16 h ($IH_{60+recovery}$). **(D)** Quantitative analysis of the blots. $^{**}p \leq 0.05$ as determined by One-way ANOVA with *post-hoc* Turkey HSD test.

HDAC Regulation of HIF-1 Activity in Rodent Models of OSA

To validate the observations in cell culture studies, the following experiments were performed on rodents. Two rodent models of IH were studied: (1) rats treated with 10 days of IH patterned after blood O_2 profiles during OSA; and (2) mice deficient in hemeoxygenase (HO)-2, which experience IH because of high incidence of spontaneous apneas (Peng et al., 2017).

Rats Treated With IH

Adult rats were treated with IH or TSA (10 mg/kg; I.P), an inhibitor of HDAC, for 10 days, the latter as a positive control for HDACs. Rats treated with alternating cycles of room air served as controls. HDAC activity, HDAC5, and HIF-1α protein as well as H3 acetylation were determined in adrenal medulla (AM) harvested from anesthetized rats. The AM tissue was chosen for two reasons: (1) PC12 cells, which were used in the above cell culture studies are of adrenal medullary chromaffin cell origin (Greene and Tischler, 1976); and (2) AM plays a critical role in IH-induced hypertension (Bao et al., 1997; Prabhakar et al., 2012). Technical limitations precluded measurements of lysine acetylation of HIF-1α protein in these experiments. HDAC activity and HDAC5 protein expressions were reduced in AM of rats treated with IH as well as TSA (**Figures 6A,B**). These effects were associated with increased H3 lysine acetylation, increased HIF-1α protein and elevated NOX4 mRNA, a HIF-1 target gene (**Figures 6B,C**). The elevated NOX4 mRNA was accompanied with increased NOX enzyme activity as compared to room air treated controls (**Figure 6D**).

Studies on HO-2 Null Mice

Mice deficient in the enzyme hemeoxygenase-2 (HO-2), exhibit sleep apnea (Peng et al., 2017). Apnea index (AI = number of apneas/h) was analyzed by recording breathing by plethysmography for 5 h in un-sedated WT and HO-2 null mice. Examples of breathing in WT and HO-2 null mice are

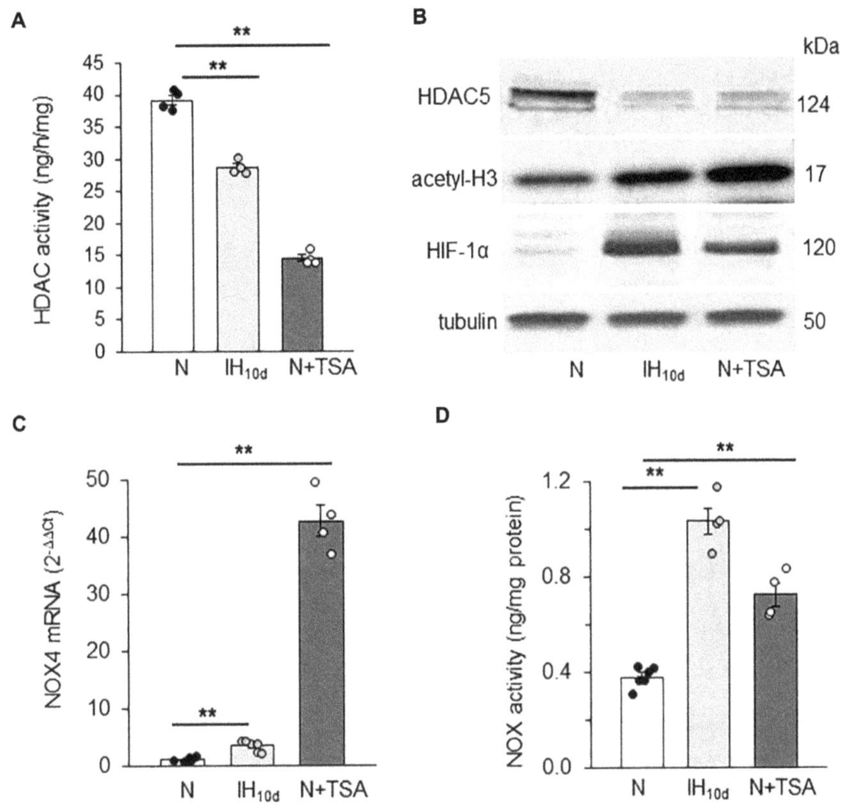

FIGURE 6 | Effect of IH or TSA treatment on HDAC activity, HDAC5, HIF-1α and H3 protein, NOX 4 mRNA and NOX activity in AM of SD rats. Adult rats were either exposed to IH (IH_{10d}) or treated with TSA (10 mg/Kg; IP) for 10 days. Control experiments were performed on rats exposed to room air (N). Cell lysates prepared from AM were analyzed for **(A)** HDAC activity, **(B)** HDAC5, acetyl-H3, HIF-1α protein expression with tubulin as loading control by immunoblots, **(C)** NOX4 mRNA expression by qRT-PCR and **(D)** NOX activity, which was analyzed in membrane protein fractions (2 a.m. from each rat pooled) as described in methods. Data are mean ± SEM from 8 rats per group. $^{**}p \leq 0.05$ as determined by One-way ANOVA with *post-hoc* Turkey HSD test.

shown in **Figure 7A**. WT mouse displayed stable breathing with an apnea index (AI) of 10 ± 7 apneas/hr. HO-2 null mice showed irregular breathing with a high incidence of apneas, with an AI of 75 ± 16 apneas/h (**Figures 7A,B**). AM from HO-2 null mice showed reduced HDAC activity and HDAC5 protein compared to WT AM (**Figures 7C,D**). In addition, HO-2 null AM showed higher abundance of HIF-1α protein and increased H3 acetylation with concomitant increase in NOX4 mRNA (target gene of HIF-1α), NOX4 protein and NOX activity compared to WT AM (**Figures 7D–F**).

Reduced HDAC Expression Elevates Blood Pressure and Plasma NE Levels

IH treated rodents exhibit elevated sympathetic nerve activity and hypertension and these responses are associated with HIF-1-dependent transcriptional activation of NOX (Prabhakar et al., 2015). Given that reduced HDAC activity by IH leads to HIF-1-dependent NOX activation, we hypothesized that these responses will be accompanied with activation of the sympathetic nervous system and elevated BP. To assess whether the systemic effects are linked to reduced HDAC activity, BP and plasma NE levels (a marker of sympathetic nerve activation) were monitored in rats treated with IH or TSA (10 mg/kg/day; 10 days; I.P). TSA treated rats exhibited elevated BP and plasma NE levels similar to IH treated rats (**Figures 8A,B**). Likewise, HO-2 null mice, which showed higher AI and decreased HDAC activity also showed elevated BP and plasma NE levels compared to WT mice (**Figures 8C,D**).

DISCUSSION

The present study examined the role of HDACs in HIF-1 transcriptional activation by IH. Cell culture studies showed that: (1) IH decreases HDAC activity, which was due to reduced HDAC5 and HDAC3 protein expression; (2) reduced HDAC activity stabilizes HIF-1α through lysine acetylation of the HIF-1 protein and (3) activates HIF-1-mediated transcriptional activity via histone (H)-3 lysine acetylation. Similar to PC12 cells, AM tissue from rats treated with IH and from HO-2 null mice, which exhibited a high incidence of spontaneous apneas, also showed reduced HDAC5 protein and enzyme activity while simultaneously exhibiting elevated plasma NE levels and BP. Treating control rats with TSA, a pan HDAC inhibitor, in room air mimicked the effects of IH. These findings demonstrate a

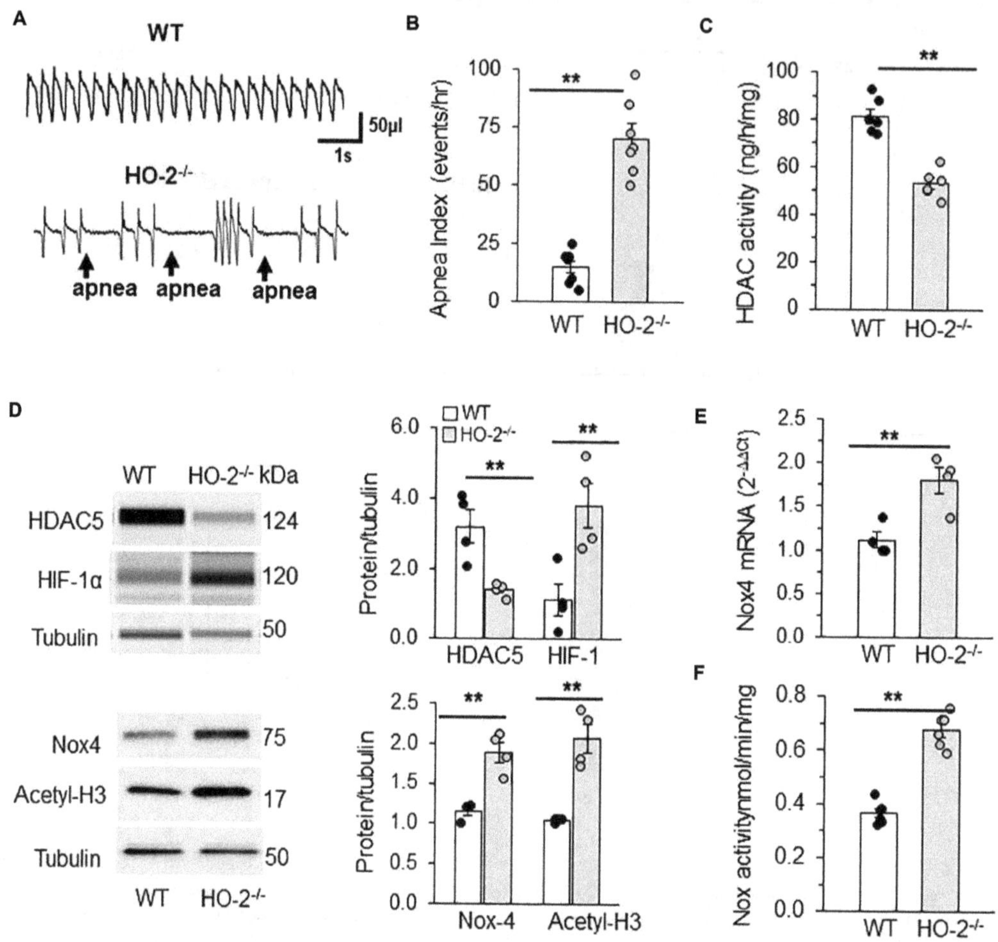

FIGURE 7 | HDAC regulation of HIF-1 in rodent model of OSA. **(A)** Representative tracing of breathing in age matched (6 months) C57BL6 mice (WT) and HO-2 null mice (*HO-2*$^{-/-}$) mice as measured by plethysmography. **(B)** Number of apneas (cessation of breathing for more than three breaths) measured per hour represented as apnea index. **(C)** HDAC activity in nuclear extracts (pooled 4 a.m. for single measurement). **(D)** Top panel: Representative immunoblot of HDAC5, HIF-1α and tubulin (loading control) protein expression as determined by the WES system from Protein simple; Nox4, Acetyl H3 and tubulin (loading control) proteins determined by SDS-PAGE gel electrophoresis. Bottom panel: Quantitative analysis of HDAC5 and HIF-1 proteins using Compass software (Protein Simple). NOX4 and acetyl H3 data was analyzed by ImageJ. $^{**}p \leq 0.05$ determined by One-way ANOVA with *post-hoc* Turkey HSD test. **(E)** Nox4 mRNA expression by qRT-PCR and **(F)** NOX activity in the membrane lysates of AM (pooled 4 a.m. for single measurement) of C57BL6 mice (WT) and *HO-2*$^{-/-}$ mice. Data are mean ± SEM from 12 mice per group. $^{**}p \leq 0.05$ as determined by Mann-Whitney test.

hitherto uncharacterized role for HDACs in HIF-1 activation by IH leading to autonomic morbidities in rodent models of OSA.

Although both HDACs and SIRTs function as histone deacetylases (Lim et al., 2010; Geng et al., 2011), IH decreased HDAC but not SIRT enzyme activity. Furthermore, TSA, a selective inhibitor of HDACs but not SIRTs, mimicked the effects of IH in both cell culture and in rodent models of OSA. The role of SIRT in IH evoked HIF-1 activity, if any, remains to be investigated.

Reduced HDAC activity leads to hyperacetylation, which is known to activate gene transcription (Grunstein, 1997). Consistent with this possibility, decreased HDAC activity by IH was associated with increased HIF-1-dependent gene activation, a major molecular mechanism implicated in autonomic morbidity caused by IH (Prabhakar et al., 2020). Activation by HIF-1-mediated transcription of target genes requires two steps: (1) Stabilization of HIF-1α, the O_2 regulated subunit; and (2) transactivation of the target gene. Inhibition of prolyl hydroxylases (PHDs) is generally thought to stabilize HIF-1α in response to continuous hypoxia (Semenza, 2001). However, PHDs appear to play a less prominent role in IH-induced HIF-1α stabilization (Yuan et al., 2008). Emerging evidence suggests that additional mechanisms including acetylation-deacetylation of HIF-1α protein also contribute to HIF-1α stability (Jeong et al., 2002; Lim et al., 2010). Co-immunoprecipitation studies with nuclear extracts from IH or TSA treated PC12 cells demonstrated increased lysine acetylation of HIF-1α protein, consistent with the notion that HDACs can regulate acetylation of non-histone proteins (Park et al., 2015). Multiple acetylation sites have been identified within the HIF-1α protein, which can contribute to stabilization of the HIF-1α protein (Jeong et al., 2002; Lim et al., 2010; Geng et al., 2011; Seo et al., 2015).

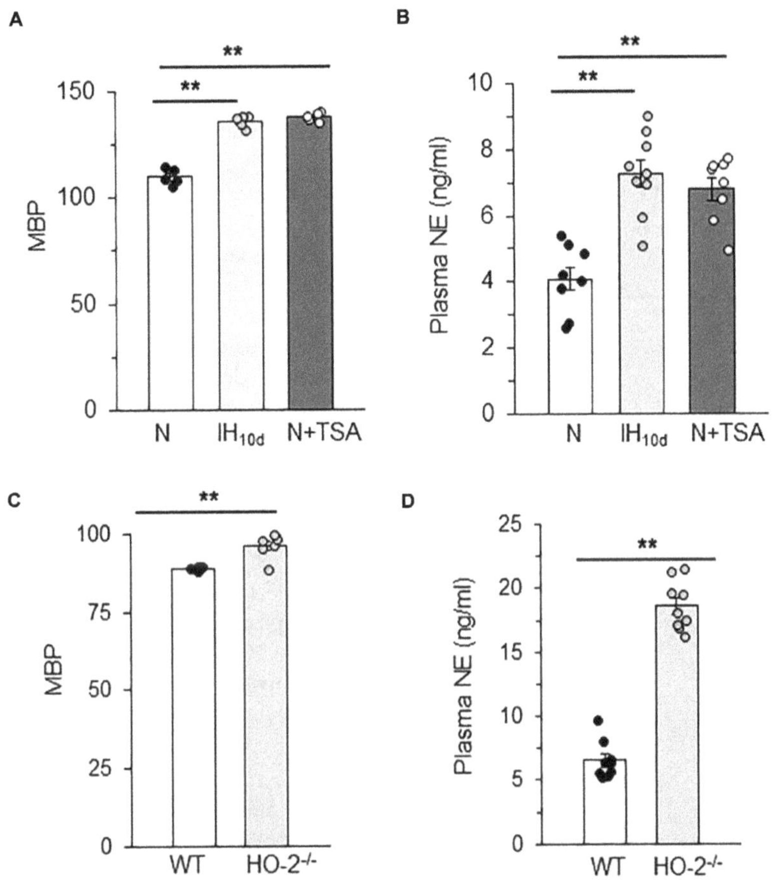

FIGURE 8 | Plasma norepinephrine and BP in TSA treated rats and HO-2 null mice **(A)** Mean blood pressures (MBP) measured after 15 h of terminating IH or TSA treatment. **(B)** Plasma norepinephrine (NE) levels in rats treated with IH with or TSA. Data are mean ± SEM from 8 rats per group. $^{**}p \leq 0.05$ as determined by One-way ANOVA test. **(C)** Mean blood pressures and **(D)** plasma NE levels in age matched (6 months) C57BL6 (WT) and *HO-2*$^{-/-}$mice. Data are mean ± SEM from eight mice per group. $^{**}p \leq 0.05$ as determined by Mann-Whitney test.

Lysine acetylation was shown to inhibit ubiquitination dependent proteasome-mediated degradation (Caron et al., 2005). It is therefore likely that under normoxia, HDACs keep HIF-1α in a deacetylated state, making it susceptible to proteasome degradation. During IH, decreased HDAC activity leads to increased lysine acetylation of HIF-1α, thereby enhancing the protein stability (**Figure 9**).

IH activated HIF-1 transcription in cell cultures as well as tissues from rodents. The increased HIF-1 transcription was accompanied with increased lysine acetylation of H3 (**Figure 4B**). Given that lysine acetylation of histone opens up the chromatin thereby facilitating binding of transcription factors (Seto and Yoshida, 2014), it is conceivable that H3 acetylation contributes to transcriptional activation of HIF-1 by facilitating the accessibility of HIF-1 to the promoter region of target genes such as NOX4, a possibility that requires additional studies and is beyond the scope of the current investigation.

The reduced HDAC activity by IH was accompanied with decreased HDAC5 (class II) and HDAC3 (class I) protein abundance. Because HDACs function as multimeric protein complexes (Seto and Yoshida, 2014), we anticipated that coordinated reduction of HDAC5 and HDAC3 is necessary for HIF-1 activation by IH. Contrary to our expectation, overexpression of HDAC5 alone was sufficient to block IH-induced HIF-1α protein accumulation as well as transcriptional activation. On the other hand, overexpression of HDAC3 was ineffective in altering HIF-1 activation by IH. These findings suggest that individual HDACs have distinct functions in the context of IH. However, further studies are necessary to delineate the role, if any, of HDAC3 in IH-induced physiological changes.

The reduced HDAC3 and HDAC5 protein expressions by IH were not due to reduced transcription but to increased proteasomal degradation (**Figures 2A,B**). HDACs can undergo post-translational modification by phosphorylation, leading to ubiquitination and proteasomal degradation (Adenuga et al., 2009). HDAC5 is known to shuttle between the nucleus and cytoplasm in a calcium- and phosphorylation-dependent manner in response to stimuli (Chawla et al., 2003; Renthal et al., 2007). It is likely that post-translational modifications involving phosphorylation play a role in reduced HDAC5 protein by IH. We have previously shown that IH increases reactive oxygen species (ROS) levels in several tissues (Peng and Prabhakar, 2003)

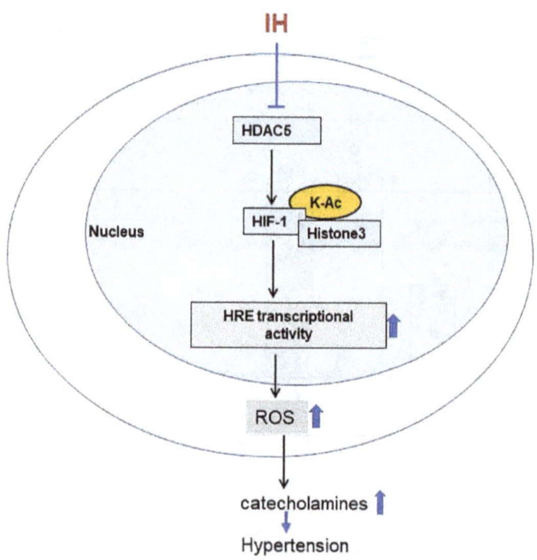

FIGURE 9 | Schematic representation for the role of HDAC5 in IH induced sympathetic activation. IH-decreased HDAC activity leads to increased acetylation of HIF-1 and H3 resulting in augmented HIF-transcriptional activity of pro-oxidant enzyme NADPH oxidases. This effect is associated with elevated ROS levels leading to increased plasma catecholamines, a marker of heightened sympathetic activation, and hypertension.

which are known to regulate protein kinases and phosphatases (Yuan et al., 2008; Corcoran and Cotter, 2013). Whether the decreased HDAC3 and HDAC5 proteins by IH involve ROS-dependent post-translational phosphorylation modifications remains to be studied.

The current study provides important insights linking HDAC alterations, sympathetic nerve activation, and elevated BP in rodent models of OSA. How might augmented HIF-1 transcriptional activity by HDACs contribute to heightened sympathetic nerve activation and BP elevation by IH? HIF-1–dependent transcriptional activation of pro-oxidant enzyme genes such as NOX and the ensuing ROS signaling have been identified as an important molecular mechanisms underlying IH-induced sympathetic activation and BP elevation (Prabhakar et al., 2020). HIF-1-dependent NOX activation augments CA release from AM and elevates BP in IH treated rats as reported previously (Kumar et al., 2006; Kuri et al., 2007; Peng et al., 2014). Whether HDAC-dependent HIF-1 activation in addition to NOX also affects CA secretion from the AM through one or more components of the exocytosis mechanisms of adrenal medullary chromaffin cells remains to be investigated. Despite these limitations, our findings establish a pathogenic mechanism linking HDACs, HIF-1, ROS generation and cardiovascular pathology associated with IH/OSA (**Figure 9**).

The present study demonstrates that IH activates lysine acetylation of H3 and HIF-1α, an epigenetic mechanism that alters chromatin, thereby affecting the accessibility of DNA for transcription factors without changes in the coding sequence of DNA *per se.* We previously reported that IH triggers epigenetic re-programming of the redox state involving DNA hypermethylation (Nanduri et al., 2017). However, there are important differences between the DNA methylation and lysine acetylation by HDAC, the two epigenetic mechanisms activated by IH. These include: (1) DNA methylation is activated by long-term IH, whereas lysine acetylation resulting from reduced HDAC is initiated even with short-term IH treatment; (2) DNA methylation is linked primarily to anti-oxidant enzyme genes, whereas lysine acetylation is linked to NOX activation, which is a pro-oxidant gene; and (3) DNA methylation is linked to long lasting elevation of BP and plasma NE responses which were not reversed even after 30 days recovery in room air, whereas the systemic responses associated with lysine acetylation and reduced HDAC5 are reversed by a few hours of recovery in room air as shown in the present study (**Figures 5C,D**) and as reported previously (Nanduri et al., 2017). Epigenetic mechanisms involving histone post-translational modifications and DNA methylation are interrelated mechanisms. It is therefore possible that early epigenetic changes involving lysine acetylation of histone and non-histone proteins due to decreased HDAC activity may trigger DNA methylation seen with LT-IH which remains to be established.

HDACs function as transcriptional repressors or activators in health and disease (Haberland et al., 2009). For example, certain types of cancers are associated with increased expression of HDACs. Consequently, HDAC inhibitors are currently considered novel potential therapeutic interventions for alleviating cancers. On the other hand, HDACs are known to have a protective role in patients with inflammatory lung disease Adcock et al., 2005) as well as cardiac damage (Chang et al., 2004). The current results indicate an additional unexplored role for HDACs in contributing to autonomic morbidities associated with OSA, a wide-spread breathing disorder.

ETHICS STATEMENT

The animal study was reviewed and approved by the Institutional Animal Care and Use Committee (IACUC) of the University of Chicago.

AUTHOR CONTRIBUTIONS

JN conceived, designed the experiments, and wrote the manuscript. NW, XS, and Y-JP performed the experiments and analyzed the data. NP edited the manuscript. All authors contributed to the article and approved the submitted version.

REFERENCES

Adcock, I. M., Ito, K., and Barnes, P. J. (2005). Histone deacetylation: an important mechanism in inflammatory lung diseases. *COPD* 2, 445–455. doi: 10.1080/15412550500346683

Adenuga, D., Yao, H., March, T. H., Seagrave, J., and Rahman, I. (2009). Histone deacetylase 2 is phosphorylated, ubiquitinated, and degraded by cigarette smoke. *Am. J. Respir. Cell Mol. Biol.* 40, 464–473. doi: 10.1165/rcmb.2008-0255oc

Audia, J. E., and Campbell, R. M. (2016). Histone modifications and cancer. *Cold Spring Harb. Perspect. Biol.* 8:a019521.

Bao, G., Metreveli, N., Li, R., Taylor, A., and Fletcher, E. C. (1997). Blood pressure response to chronic episodic hypoxia: role of the sympathetic nervous system. *J. Appl. Physiol.* 83, 95–101. doi: 10.1152/jappl.1997.83.1.95

Bertrand, P. (2010). Inside HDAC with HDAC inhibitors. *Eur. J. Med. Chem.* 45, 2095–2116. doi: 10.1016/j.ejmech.2010.02.030

Caron, C., Boyault, C., and Khochbin, S. (2005). Regulatory cross-talk between lysine acetylation and ubiquitination: role in the control of protein stability. *Bioessays* 27, 408–415. doi: 10.1002/bies.20210

Chang, S., McKinsey, T. A., Zhang, C. L., Richardson, J. A., Hill, J. A., and Olson, E. N. (2004). Histone deacetylases 5 and 9 govern responsiveness of the heart to a subset of stress signals and play redundant roles in heart development. *Mol. Cell Biol.* 24, 8467–8476. doi: 10.1128/mcb.24.19.8467-8476.2004

Chawla, S., Vanhoutte, P., Arnold, F. J., Huang, C. L., and Bading, H. (2003). Neuronal activity-dependent nucleocytoplasmic shuttling of HDAC4 and HDAC5. *J. Neurochem.* 85, 151–159. doi: 10.1046/j.1471-4159.2003.01648.x

Corcoran, A., and Cotter, T. G. (2013). Redox regulation of protein kinases. *FEBS J.* 280, 1944–1965. doi: 10.1111/febs.12224

Finnin, M. S., Donigian, J. R., Cohen, A., Richon, V. M., Rifkind, R. A., Marks, P. A., et al. (1999). Structures of a histone deacetylase homologue bound to the TSA and SAHA inhibitors. *Nature* 401, 188–193. doi: 10.1038/43710

Geng, H., Harvey, C. T., Pittsenbarger, J., Liu, Q., Beer, T. M., Xue, C., et al. (2011). HDAC4 protein regulates HIF1α protein lysine acetylation and cancer cell response to hypoxia. *J. Biol. Chem.* 286, 38095–38102. doi: 10.1074/jbc.m111.257055

Greene, L. A., and Tischler, A. S. (1976). Establishment of a noradrenergic clonal line of rat adrenal pheochromocytoma cells which respond to nerve growth factor. *Proc. Natl. Acad. Sci. U.S.A.* 73, 2424–2428. doi: 10.1073/pnas.73.7.2424

Grunstein, M. (1997). Histone acetylation in chromatin structure and transcription. *Nature* 389, 349–352. doi: 10.1038/38664

Haberland, M., Montgomery, R. L., and Olson, E. N. (2009). The many roles of histone deacetylases in development and physiology: implications for disease and therapy. *Nat. Rev. Genet.* 10, 32–42. doi: 10.1038/nrg2485

Jeong, J. W., Bae, M. K., Ahn, M. Y., Kim, S. H., Sohn, T. K., Bae, M. H., et al. (2002). Regulation and destabilization of HIF-1alpha by ARD1-mediated acetylation. *Cell* 111, 709–720. doi: 10.1016/s0092-8674(02)01085-1

Khan, S. A., Nanduri, J., Yuan, G., Kinsman, B., Kumar, G. K., Joseph, J., et al. (2011). NADPH oxidase 2 mediates intermittent hypoxia-induced mitochondrial complex I inhibition: relevance to blood pressure changes in rats. *Antioxid. Redox Signal.* 14, 533–542. doi: 10.1089/ars.2010.3213

Kim, S. H., Jeong, J. W., Park, J. A., Lee, J. W., Seo, J. H., Jung, B. K., et al. (2007). Regulation of the HIF-1alpha stability by histone deacetylases. *Oncol. Rep.* 17, 647–651.

Kumar, G. K., Rai, V., Sharma, S. D., Ramakrishnan, D. P., Peng, Y. J., Souvannakitti, D., et al. (2006). Chronic intermittent hypoxia induces hypoxia-evoked catecholamine efflux in adult rat adrenal medulla via oxidative stress. *J. Physiol.* 575, 229–239. doi: 10.1113/jphysiol.2006.112524

Kuri, B. A., Khan, S. A., Chan, S. A., Prabhakar, N. R., and Smith, C. B. (2007). Increased secretory capacity of mouse adrenal chromaffin cells by chronic intermittent hypoxia: involvement of protein kinase C. *J. Physiol.* 584, 313–319. doi: 10.1113/jphysiol.2007.140624

Lim, J. H., Lee, Y. M., Chun, Y. S., Chen, J., Kim, J. E., and Park, J. W. (2010). Sirtuin 1 modulates cellular responses to hypoxia by deacetylating hypoxia-inducible factor 1alpha. *Mol. Cell* 38, 864–878. doi: 10.1016/j.molcel.2010.05.023

Morrell, M. J., Finn, L., Kim, H., Peppard, P. E., Badr, M. S., and Young, T. (2000). Sleep fragmentation, awake blood pressure, and sleep-disordered breathing in a population-based study. *Am. J. Respir. Crit. Care Med.* 162, 2091–2096. doi: 10.1164/ajrccm.162.6.9904008

Nanduri, J., Peng, Y. J., Wang, N., Khan, S. A., Semenza, G. L., Kumar, G. K., et al. (2017). Epigenetic regulation of redox state mediates persistent cardiorespiratory abnormalities after long-term intermittent hypoxia. *J. Physiol.* 595, 63–77. doi: 10.1113/jp272346

Nanduri, J., Wang, N., Yuan, G., Khan, S. A., Souvannakitti, D., Peng, Y. J., et al. (2009). Intermittent hypoxia degrades HIF-2alpha via calpains resulting in oxidative stress: implications for recurrent apnea-induced morbidities. *Proc. Natl. Acad. Sci. U.S.A.* 106, 1199–1204. doi: 10.1073/pnas.0811018106

Nieto, F. J., Young, T. B., Lind, B. K., Shahar, E., Samet, J. M., Redline, S., et al. (2000). Association of sleep-disordered breathing, sleep apnea, and hypertension in a large community-based study. sleep heart health study. *JAMA* 283, 1829–1836. doi: 10.1001/jama.283.14.1829

Park, J. M., Jo, S. H., Kim, M. Y., Kim, T. H., and Ahn, Y. H. (2015). Role of transcription factor acetylation in the regulation of metabolic homeostasis. *Protein Cell* 6, 804–813. doi: 10.1007/s13238-015-0204-y

Peng, Y. J., and Prabhakar, N. R. (2003). Reactive oxygen species in the plasticity of respiratory behavior elicited by chronic intermittent hypoxia. *J. Appl. Physiol.* 94, 2342–2349. doi: 10.1152/japplphysiol.00613.2002

Peng, Y. J., Yuan, G., Khan, S., Nanduri, J., Makarenko, V. V., Reddy, V. D., et al. (2014). Regulation of hypoxia-inducible factor-α isoforms and redox state by carotid body neural activity in rats. *J. Physiol.* 592, 3841–3858. doi: 10.1113/jphysiol.2014.273789

Peng, Y. J., Yuan, G., Ramakrishnan, D., Sharma, S. D., Bosch-Marce, M., Kumar, G. K., et al. (2006). Heterozygous HIF-1alpha deficiency impairs carotid body-mediated systemic responses and reactive oxygen species generation in mice exposed to intermittent hypoxia. *J. Physiol.* 577, 705–716. doi: 10.1113/jphysiol.2006.114033

Peng, Y. J., Zhang, X., Gridina, A., Chupikova, I., McCormick, D. L., Thomas, R. J., et al. (2017). Complementary roles of gasotransmitters CO and H2S in sleep apnea. *Proc. Natl. Acad. Sci. U.S.A.* 114, 1413–1418. doi: 10.1073/pnas.1620717114

Peng, Y. J., Zhang, X., Nanduri, J., and Prabhakar, N. R. (2018). Therapeutic targeting of the carotid body for treating sleep apnea in a pre-clinical mouse model. *Adv. Exp. Med. Biol.* 1071, 109–114. doi: 10.1007/978-3-319-91137-3_14

Peppard, P. E., Young, T., Barnet, J. H., Palta, M., Hagen, E. W., and Hla, K. M. (2013). Increased prevalence of sleep-disordered breathing in adults. *Am. J. Epidemiol.* 177, 1006–1014.

Prabhakar, N. R., Kumar, G. K., and Peng, Y. J. (2012). Sympatho-adrenal activation by chronic intermittent hypoxia. *J Appl Physiol.* 113, 1304–1310. doi: 10.1152/japplphysiol.00444.2012

Prabhakar, N. R., Peng, Y. J., and Nanduri, J. (2020). Hypoxia-inducible factors and obstructive sleep apnea. *J. Clin. Invest.* 130, 5042–5051. doi: 10.1172/jci137560

Prabhakar, N. R., Peng, Y. J., Kumar, G. K., and Nanduri, J. (2015). Peripheral chemoreception and arterial pressure responses to intermittent hypoxia. *Compr. Physiol.* 5, 561–577. doi: 10.1002/cphy.c140039

Qian, D. Z., Kachhap, S. K., Collis, S. J., Verheul, H. M., Carducci, M. A., Atadja, P., et al. (2006). Class II histone deacetylases are associated with VHL-independent regulation of hypoxia-inducible factor 1 alpha. *Cancer Res.* 66, 8814–8821. doi: 10.1158/0008-5472.can-05-4598

Renthal, W., Maze, I., Krishnan, V., Covington, H. E., Xiao, G., Kumar, A., et al. (2007). Histone deacetylase 5 epigenetically controls behavioral adaptations to chronic emotional stimuli. *Neuron* 56, 517–529. doi: 10.1016/j.neuron.2007.09.032

Semenza, G. L. (2001). HIF-1, O(2), and the 3 PHDs: how animal cells signal hypoxia to the nucleus. *Cell* 107, 1–3. doi: 10.1016/s0092-8674(01)00518-9

Semenza, G. L., Agani, F., Iyer, N., Jiang, B. H., Leung, S., Wiener, C., et al. (1998). Hypoxia-inducible factor 1: from molecular biology to cardiopulmonary physiology. *Chest* 114, 40S–45S.

Semenza, G. L., Jiang, B. H., Leung, S. W., Passantino, R., Concordet, J. P., Maire, P., et al. (1996). Hypoxia response elements in the aldolase A, enolase 1, and lactate dehydrogenase A gene promoters contain essential binding sites for hypoxia-inducible factor 1. *J. Biol. Chem.* 271, 32529–32537. doi: 10.1074/jbc.271.51.32529

Seo, H. W., Kim, E. J., Na, H., and Lee, M. O. (2009). Transcriptional activation of hypoxia-inducible factor-1alpha by HDAC4 and HDAC5 involves differential recruitment of p300 and FIH-1. *FEBS Lett.* 583, 55–60. doi: 10.1016/j.febslet.2008.11.044

Seo, K. S., Park, J. H., Heo, J. Y., Jing, K., Han, J., Min, K. N., et al. (2015). SIRT2 regulates tumour hypoxia response by promoting HIF-1α hydroxylation. *Oncogene* 34, 1354–1362. doi: 10.1038/onc.2014.76

Seto, E., and Yoshida, M. (2014). Erasers of histone acetylation: the histone deacetylase enzymes. *Cold Spring Harb. Perspect. Biol.* 6:a018713. doi: 10.1101/cshperspect.a018713

Wang, N., Shi, X. F., Khan, S. A., Wang, B., Semenza, G. L., Prabhakar, N. R., et al. (2020). Hypoxia-inducible factor-1 mediates pancreatic β-cell dysfunction by intermittent hypoxia. *Am. J. Physiol. Cell Physiol.* 11, C922–C932.

Yang, X. J., and Seto, E. (2003). Collaborative spirit of histone deacetylases in regulating chromatin structure and gene expression. *Curr. Opin. Genet. Dev.* 13, 143–153. doi: 10.1016/s0959-437x(03)00015-7

Yang, X. J., and Seto, E. (2007). HATs and HDACs: from structure, function and regulation to novel strategies for therapy and prevention. *Oncogene* 26, 5310–5318. doi: 10.1038/sj.onc.1210599

Yuan, G., Adhikary, G., McCormick, A. A., Holcroft, J. J., Kumar, G. K., and Prabhakar, N. R. (2004). Role of oxidative stress in intermittent hypoxia-induced immediate early gene activation in rat PC12 cells. *J. Physiol.* 557, 773–783. doi: 10.1113/jphysiol.2003.058503

Yuan, G., Khan, S. A., Luo, W., Nanduri, J., Semenza, G. L., and Prabhakar, N. R. (2011). Hypoxia-inducible factor 1 mediates increased expression of NADPH oxidase-2 in response to intermittent hypoxia. *J. Cell Physiol.* 226, 2925–2933. doi: 10.1002/jcp.22640

Yuan, G., Nanduri, J., Bhasker, C. R., Semenza, G. L., and Prabhakar, N. R. (2005). Ca2+/calmodulin kinase-dependent activation of hypoxia inducible factor 1 transcriptional activity in cells subjected to intermittent hypoxia. *J. Biol. Chem.* 280, 4321–4328. doi: 10.1074/jbc.m407706200

Yuan, G., Nanduri, J., Khan, S., Semenza, G. L., and Prabhakar, N. R. (2008). Induction of HIF-1alpha expression by intermittent hypoxia: involvement of NADPH oxidase, Ca2+ signaling, prolyl hydroxylases, and mTOR. *J. Cell Physiol.* 217, 674–685. doi: 10.1002/jcp.21537

4

Ethnic Differences on Cardiac Rhythms and Autonomic Nervous System Responses during a High-Altitude Trek: A Pilot Study Comparing Italian Trekkers to Nepalese Porters

Vittore Verratti[1*†], *Alessandro Tonacci*[2†], *Danilo Bondi*[3], *Annalisa Chiavaroli*[4], *Claudio Ferrante*[4], *Luigi Brunetti*[4], *Antonio Crisafulli*[5] and *Paolo Cerretelli*[6]

[1] *Department of Psychological, Health and Territorial Sciences, University "G. d'Annunzio" of Chieti-Pescara, Chieti, Italy,* [2] *Institute of Clinical Physiology, National Research Council of Italy, Pisa, Italy,* [3] *Department of Neuroscience, Imaging and Clinical Sciences, University "G. d'Annunzio" of Chieti-Pescara, Chieti, Italy,* [4] *Department of Pharmacy, University "G. d'Annunzio" of Chieti-Pescara, Chieti, Italy,* [5] *Department of Medical Science and Public Health, University of Cagliari, Cagliari, Italy,* [6] *Institute of Bioimaging and Molecular Physiology, National Research Council of Italy, Segrate, Italy*

***Correspondence:**
Vittore Verratti
vittore.verratti@unich.it

† *These authors have contributed equally to this work and share first authorship*

Altitude hypoxia exposure results in increased sympathetic activity and heart rate due to several mechanisms. Recent studies have contested the validity of heart rate variability (HRV) analysis on sympathetic activity measurement. But the plethora of HRV metrics may provide meaningful insights, particularly if linked with cardiovascular and autonomic nervous system parameters. However, the population-specific nature of HRV and cardiorespiratory response to altitude hypoxia are still missing. Six Italian trekkers and six Nepalese porters completed 300 km of a Himalayan trek. The ECG analysis was conducted at baseline, and before (*bBC*) and after (*aBC*) the high-altitude (HA) circuit. Urine was collected before and after the expedition in Italians, for assessing catecholamines. Heart rate increased with altitude significantly ($p < 0.001$) in the Italian group; systolic ($p = 0.030$) and diastolic ($p = 0.012$) blood pressure, and mean arterial pressure ($p = 0.004$) increased with altitude. Instead, pulse pressure did not change, although the Nepalese group showed lower baseline values than the Italians. As expected, peripheral oxygen saturation decreased with altitude ($p < 0.001$), independently of the ethnic groups. Nepalese had a higher respiratory rate ($p = 0.007$), independent of altitude. The cardiac vagal index increased at altitude, from baseline to *bBC* ($p = 0.008$). Higuchi fractal dimension (HFD) showed higher basal values in the Nepalese group ($p = 0.041$), and a tendency for the highest values at *bBC*. Regarding the urinary catecholamine response, exposure to HA increased urinary levels, particularly of norepinephrine ($p = 0.005$, $d = 1.623$). Our findings suggest a better cardiovascular resilience of the Nepalese group when compared with Italians, which might be due to an intrinsic adaptation to HA, resulting from their job.

Keywords: heart rate variability, urinary catecholamines, himalayas, altitude hypoxia, adaptiveness, blood pressure

INTRODUCTION

The occurrence of hypobaric hypoxia at high altitude (HA) challenges human homeostasis, providing an ecological model for measuring the physiological responses to such environmental stressors (Cerretelli, 2013; West, 2016; Moore, 2017), both in the short- and long-term (Beall, 2003; Mulliri et al., 2019). The cardiorespiratory system is massively affected by altitude exposure since low partial pressure of oxygen in arterial blood induces acute and chronic hemodynamic changes (West, 2016; Verratti et al., 2020a). Hyperventilation occurs as an essential step of acclimatization (San et al., 2013), with a hypoxia-related switch to rapid and shallow breaths, rather than an increase in tidal volume (Brinkman et al., 2020). Concerning blood pressure (BP), the acute response in lowlanders is typically increased during ascent, especially at the beginning of exposure (Calbet and Lundby, 2009). The BP increment occurs early even after exposure to moderate altitude (Torlasco et al., 2020) and persists after acclimatization (Parati et al., 2015). BP also increases as a chronic response, despite the fact that systemic O_2 delivery improves with acclimatization (Calbet, 2003).

The higher the altitude, the higher the heart rate, both at rest and at a standardized workload (Gamboa et al., 2003; Princi et al., 2008). What subsequently generates a chronic acclimatization process is the maintenance of cardiac output, while heart rate may continue to be high and stroke volume decreases, probably due to a reduction in plasma volume (Reeves et al., 1987; Stembridge et al., 2019). The major extrinsic factor for heart rhythmicity is the autonomic nervous system (ANS), which regulates heart rate by modulating sympathetic and parasympathetic tone (Mangoni and Nargeot, 2008). In humans, during acute exposure to altitude hypoxia, a significant increase in sympathetic activity and heart rate occurs due to the carotid body and brain stem chemoreceptors activation (Marshall, 1994; Solomon, 2000).

The sympathetic branch of ANS acts on the cardiovascular system by stimulating all the four hemodynamic effectors: inotropism, chronotropism, cardiac preload, and afterload (Furnival et al., 1971; Schümann, 1983; Takahashi et al., 1993; Ullian, 1999). Plasmatic and urinary catecholamines levels increases in response to HA exposure in subjects staying for more than 1 week (Rostrup, 1998). However, combining pharmacological inhibition of sympathetic and/or parasympathetic control of the heart, Siebenmann et al. demonstrated reduced cardiac parasympathetic activity as the main mechanisms underlying the increase of resting heart rate in response to middle-term exposure to altitude hypoxia (Siebenmann et al., 2017). The same evidence was reported in rats, with a parasympathetic withdrawal after 24 h of exposure to 3,270 m above sea level (Beltrán et al., 2020). A few evidence exists about ethnic differences in the autonomic control of the cardiovascular response to altitude hypoxia; e.g., altered muscle sympathetic nerve activity and beneficial lower sympathetic vasoconstrictor activity have been suggested as beneficial hypoxic adaptations in Sherpas (Simpson et al., 2019). Cardioprotective phenotypes in Sherpas prevent them from developing apnea-induced bradyarrhythmias at altitude (Busch et al., 2018).

Despite broad historical use of HRV as a convenient surrogate of other measures to evaluate ANS activity, strong reservations have been recently claimed, especially regarding the sympathetic influence on HRV (Thomas et al., 2019). Moreover, in HRV analysis, the contextual measurement importance of the factors has been stressed along with the accurate interpretation of the diverse parameters, which can be clustered in time-domain, frequency-domain, and non-linear indexes (Shaffer and Ginsberg, 2017). Indeed, the recent development of non-linear metrics allowed to extend the methodological rationale of HRV, e.g., Gomes and colleagues (Gomes et al., 2017) reported physical exercise to acutely reduce the chaotic behavior of heart rate dynamics, through the complex Higuchi Fractal Dimension (HFD) analysis. Indeed, alternative approaches to the typical HRV investigation may add novel interpretation levels to the non-uniform alterations in the several HRV domains observed in response to altitude exposure (Verratti et al., 2019). Dhar et al. (2018) reported higher mean RR, LF (low frequency) power ms^2, LF (normalized units: nu), and LF/HF ratio values, with lower RMSSD (root mean square of successive RR interval differences), NN50, pNN50 (percentage of successive RR intervals that differ by more than 50 ms), SD1 (Poincaré plot standard deviation perpendicular the line of identity), HF (high frequency) power ms^2 and HF (nu) values, in acclimatized lowlanders (15–18 months residence at >3,500 m asl) compared to HAs native and sea-level residents never exposed to HAs. However, to our knowledge, no study investigated the differential response of non-habitual altitude trekkers, compared with the altitude porters, both lowland natives. Studying the possible differences in Westerner trekkers vs. Himalayan porters could be of great interest to identify, if any, the advantages of lowland native Nepalese porters in cardiac rhythms adaptations, for providing novel insights on the occupational adaptation to HA, and for defining extended models of physiology and pathophysiology related for current expeditioners.

In the broad and extensive background of cardiovascular responses to hypoxia, population-specificity of HRV, BP, and breathing response to middle-term altitude hypoxia remains to be elucidated. The present study aimed to explore the cardiorespiratory adaptive response during a Himalayan trek, comparing Westerners and Easterners using an ecological field study design. In particular, the present work aimed to focus on the physiological meaning of the several responses as a function of altitude and/or ethnicity, as depicted by the different metrics.

METHODS

Study Design and Participants

This study was part of the "Kanchenjunga Exploration & Physiology" project, a subset of the broad project entitled "Environmentally-modulated metabolic adaptation to hypoxia in altitude natives and sea-level dwellers: from integrative to molecular (proteomics, epigenetics, and ROS) level," approved by the Ethics Review Board of the Nepal Health Research Council (NHRC)—ref. no. 458. All study procedures were performed under the ethical standards of the 1964 Declaration of Helsinki and all its amendments (World Medical Association, 2013).

All participants provided their written, informed consent to participate in the study.

The participants completed a combined circuit of 300 km distance (south and north base camps of Kanchenjunga), covering a daily average of about 6 h walk for about 110 h. They were exposed throughout the trek to low (500–2,000 m), moderate (2,000–3,000 m) and high (3,000–5,500 m) altitudes (Schommer and Bärtsch, 2011), along a demanding route with ascent and descent tracts covering totally over 16,000 m in altitude, in the Himalayan mountain range of eastern Nepal (**Figure 1**).

This research project investigated adaptive cardiovascular responses to HA exposure stressors in two experimental groups composed of six healthy Italian trekkers and six healthy Nepalese porters, both lowland dwellers. Characteristics of the two studied groups were as follows: Italians, five men, and one woman, aged 44 ± 15 years, body mass index (BMI) of 25.81 ± 3.25 Kg/m^2; Nepalese, all men, aged 30 ± 8 years, BMI of 24.36 ± 4.70 kg/m^2. The Italian trekkers usually live at low altitudes, and some of them reported previous HA experiences, although not in the last 3 years. The Nepalese trekkers habitually live at low altitudes and reported frequent exposure to HAs, with a working experience of 2-to-5 similar expeditions per year in the last 3 years.

The expedition was continuously supervised by an expert medical doctor. None of the participants suffered from AMS during the trek, neither did they report any cardiovascular nor respiratory disease. The Caucasian participants only took one acetazolamide pill of 250 mg daily, at 6 p.m. during the 2 days between the acclimatization day and the stay at the highest altitude point of the expedition. However, two out of three measurements were conducted before the use, and the last measurement was conducted largely after the drug washout. No drugs were used by participants that may have affected uptake transporter proteins, metabolizing enzymes, or clearance of catecholamines. The technical requirements of the devices concerning transport, storage, and operating temperature were all met. Even though distance and difference in altitude were identical among groups, the workload was different, reflecting the typical situation in modern Himalayan expeditions: while Italian trekkers carried light loads, Nepalese porters carried heavier loads (10–30 kg), throughout the whole route. All participants underwent ECG recording, before the trek (*Pre*), at 3,427 m of altitude before the North base camp (5,143 m of altitude) circuit (*bBC*), and after that circuit (*aBC*). BP and SpO_2 assessments were conducted eight times during the trek. From urine samples collected before (*Pre*) and after the expedition (*Post*), catecholamines concentration was assessed. Urine samples were obtained only by Italians, before and 10 days after the expedition. Unfortunately, the logistics of the current study did not allow to sample and store adequately the urine samples of the Nepalese.

Procedures and Data Analysis

Peripheral oxygen saturation (SpO_2) was measured using a pulse oximeter (APN-100, Contec Medical Systems Co. Ltd, China); values allowing several seconds to detect a pulse and waiting for a stable value were considered. The device measured in the range of 70–100% with an accuracy of 2%. A rubber finger SpO_2 probe was attached over a clean and dry skin (WHO, 2011), in the morning before breakfast. All the SpO_2 tests were performed in duplicate.

Systolic blood pressure (SBP) and diastolic blood pressure (DBP) were measured using an oscillometric device (ABPM50, Contec Medical Systems Co. Ltd, China). The devices measured in a range of 40–270 mmHg with an accuracy of 3 mmHg. SBP and DBP data were taken in a sitting position at rest, with the cuff at heart level (Whelton et al., 2018), in the morning before breakfast. Pulse pressure (PP) was calculated as a diastolic–systolic difference and mean arterial pressure (MAP) was calculated as (SBP + 2DBP) ÷ 3 (Giles and Sander, 2013). All the BP tests were performed in duplicate.

The ECG signal was captured with the individual lying in a supine position through a single-lead Shimmer2ECG sensor (Shimmer Sensing, Dublin, Ireland) with a sampling frequency of 500 Hz to allow the estimation of the relevant HRV features according to the guidelines (Malik, 1996) and taking advantage of the Einthoven I derivative. From 5 min-ECG recording at rest, we extracted the tachogram by the Pan-Tompkins algorithm (Pan and Tompkins, 1985) and we evaluated HRV by the mean of time-domain (SDNN and pNN50), frequency-domain (absolute LF and HF power, and the normalized counterparts, computed taking into account the whole Power Spectral Density) and non-linear parameters (CSI, CVI, and HFD). Spectral calculations (see **Figure 2**) were computed according to the Welch model (Welch, 1967) using 64 samples in the window, 32 to overlap, and 512 points in the frequency axis. As for frequency bands, we employed the bands 0.04–0.15 Hz for LF and 0.15–0.4 Hz for HF, according to the literature (Shaffer and Ginsberg, 2017), which was also used as a reference to extrapolate considerations about short-term HRV applicability.

The sensor was attached to the body of the volunteer through a fitness-like chest strap (Polar Electro Oy, Kempele, Finland), avoiding discomfort for the individuals tested.

Catecholamines Dosage

The obtained first-voided urinary samples were immediately stored and transferred in ice (−20°C) and subsequently analyzed frozen in liquid nitrogen for transport until analyses were carried out in Italy in the Department of Pharmacy Laboratory, University "G. d'Annunzio" of Chieti. One milliliter urine samples were stirred for 1 min using a vortex mixer, centrifuged at 13,000 *g* for 10 min to remove sediments, and finally filtered through Millipore 0.25 μm nylon filters. This was followed by HPLC-EC assay of NE and E and HPLC-UV assessment of creatinine. The detailed protocols are described below. Urinary creatinine levels were determined as previously reported (Verratti et al., 2020a,b). The HPLC apparatus consisted of a Jasco (Tokyo, Japan) PU-2080 chromatographic pump and a Jasco MD-2010 Plus absorbance detector. Integration was performed by Jasco Borwin Chromatography software, version 1.5. The chromatographic separation was performed by isocratic elution on the GraceSmart reverse phase column (C18, 150 mm × 4.6 mm i.d., 5 μm). The mobile phase was (1:99, v/v) acetonitrile and 25 mM pH 5.00 phosphate buffer containing octanesulfonic acid 10 mM and triethylamine 0.03%, v/v. The flow rate was 1.0 ml/min, and the samples were

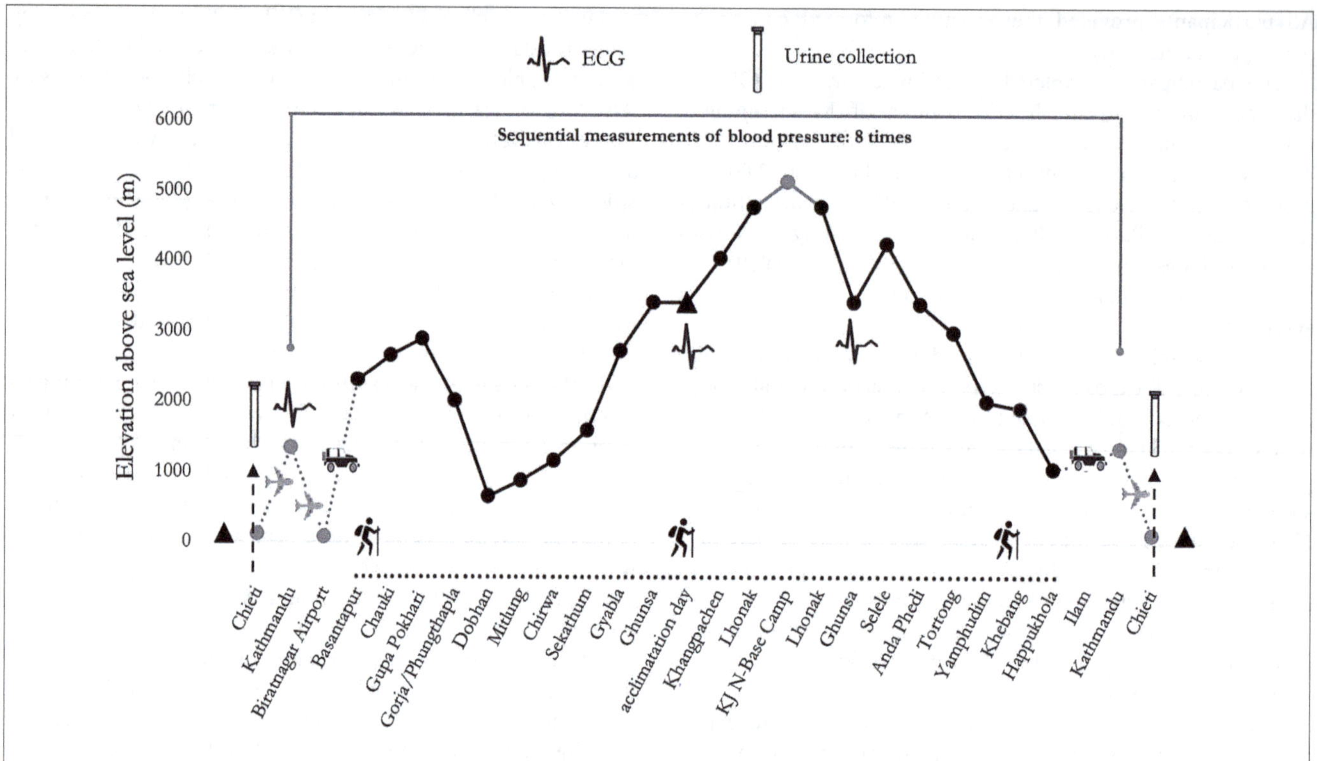

FIGURE 1 | Altimetric plan and measurement time of psychological tests of "Kanchenjunga Exploration and Physiology" project.

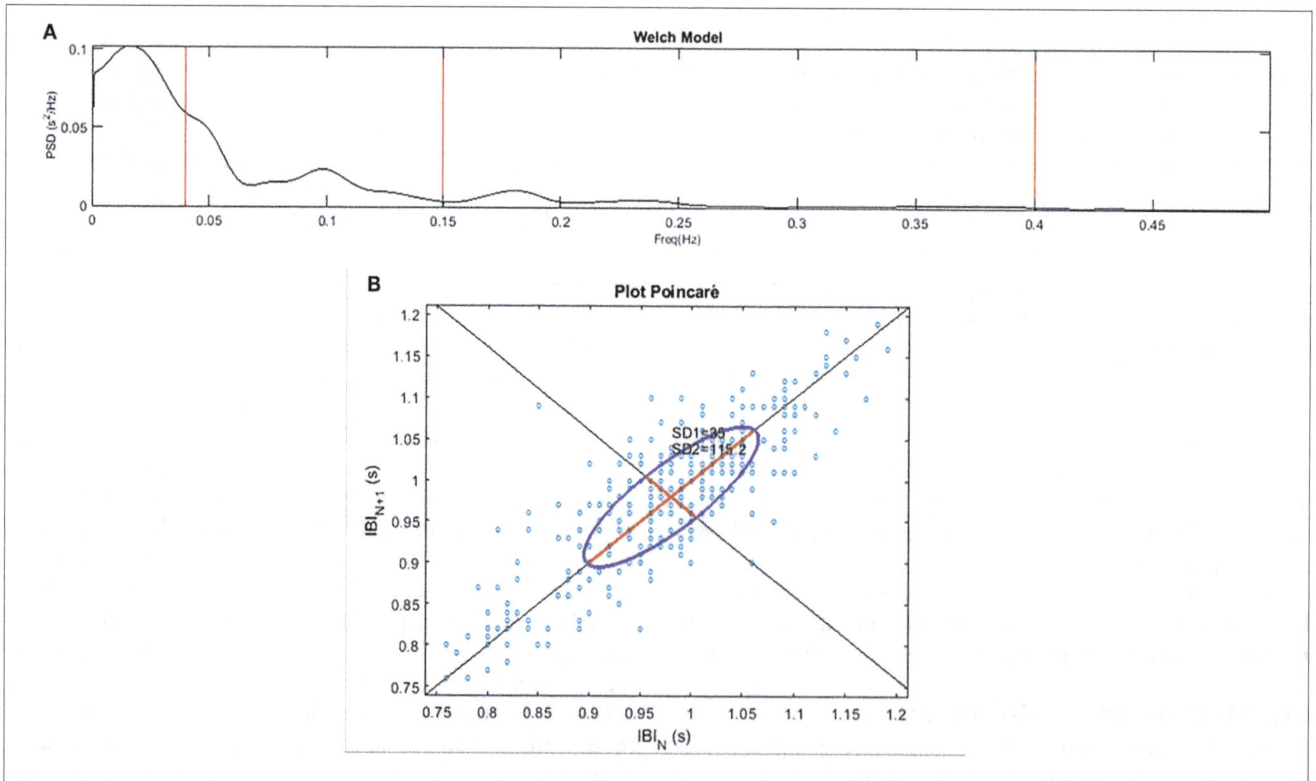

FIGURE 2 | An example of the frequency spectra **(A)** and of the Poincaré plot **(B)** for a sample individual enrolled in the study.

manually injected through a 20 µl loop. Creatinine analyses were performed by two hundred-fold diluting urinary samples before injection and monitoring absorbance at 235 nm. Creatinine peaks were identified by comparison with pure standard retention time, while their concentrations in the urinary samples were calculated by linear regression curve (y = bx + m) obtained with the standard. The standard stock solution of the solution of creatinine (2 mg/ml) was purchased from Alexis Biochemicals, San Diego, CA, USA. The stock solution was stored at 4°C. Work solutions (20–200 µg/ml) were daily obtained, progressively diluting stock solutions in the mobile phase. NE and E levels were analyzed through an HPLC apparatus consisting of a Jasco (Tokyo, Japan) PU-2080 chromatographic pump and an ESA (Chelmsford, MA, USA) Coulochem III coulometric detector, equipped with a microdialysis cell (ESA-5014b) porous graphite working electrode and a solid-state palladium reference electrode. The experimental conditions for biogenic amine identification and quantification were selected as follows. The analytical cell was set at −0.150 V for detector 1 and at +0.300 V for detector 2, with a range of 100 nA. The chromatograms were monitored at the analytical detector 2. Integration was performed by Jasco Borwin Chromatography software version 1.5. The chromatographic separation was performed by isocratic elution on a Phenomenex Kinetex reverse phase column (C18, 150 × 4.6 mm i.d., 2.6 µm). Regarding the separation of NE and E, the mobile phase was (10:90, v/v) acetonitrile and 75 mM pH 3.00 phosphate buffer containing octanesulfonic acid 1.8 mM, EDTA 30 µM, and triethylamine 0.015%, v/v. The flow rate was 0.6 ml/min, and the samples were manually injected through a 20 µl loop. Neurotransmitter peaks were identified by comparison with the retention time of pure standard. Neurotransmitter concentrations in the samples were calculated by linear regression curve ($y = bx + m$) obtained with the standard. The standard stock solutions of NE and E at 2 mg/ml were prepared in bidistilled water containing 0.004% EDTA and 0.010% sodium bisulfite. The stock solutions were stored at 4°C. Work solutions (1.25–20.00 ng/ml) were obtained daily by progressively diluting the stock solutions in the mobile phase.

Statistics

The statistical analysis of HR, BP, SpO_2, and breathing rate was carried out using the R-based open-source software Jamovi Version 1.2.27.0 (retrieved from https://www.jamovi.org). Graphs were created using the GraphPad Prism Version 5.01 (GraphPad Software, La Jolla, USA). The assumption check was based on Shapiro–Wilk's test for normality, Levene's tests for homoscedasticity and Q–Q plots. General linear mixed model (GLMM) was used to test altitude × ethnicity comparison, with residual maximum likelihood (REML) estimator, AIC and BIC as model fit measures, the Satterthwaite method for degrees of freedom, and participants as a random variable; the random effect was tested by likelihood ratio test (LRT). Marginal R^2 and conditional R^2 were reported, and partial eta squared (η_p^2) and partial omega squared (ω_p^2) were calculated as measures of effect size (Fritz et al., 2012). Experimental data of urine NE and E were analyzed through paired sample Student's *t*-test; considering the small sample size, Cohen's *d* was adjusted to unbiased Cohen's *d* (d_{unb}) (Fritz et al., 2012).

Concerning the ECG signal, a normality test (Shapiro–Wilk's test) was conducted prior to the overall analysis. Given the results obtained with this investigation (significant deviation from the normality), we performed non-parametric tests for the various features, including Friedman's Test with Wilcoxon *post-hoc* correction for the comparison between the different phases within the same group, or Mann–Whitney's test for comparing the data between the two different cohorts included in the investigation.

RESULTS

Heart rate increased with altitude; this trend was particularly evident for Italians, who also had lower overall values than Nepalese; SBP and DBP increased with altitude, as well as MAP, without significant differences by ethnicity. Instead, PP did not change, but Nepalese had lower overall values than Italians. SpO_2 decreased with altitude, without differences in the ethnic comparison. Surprisingly, breath frequency was overall lower in Nepalese, and statistical analysis failed to demonstrate a significant response to HA exposure (see **Table 1**). Among the several measurements, SpO_2 represented the best parameter to identify the response to HA, considering the greatest effect size (see **Supplementary Materials**) and the lowest model fit measures (AIC and BIC). In all the models, individuality played a significant role in response to HA, particularly for BP parameters.

Results of HRV are summarized in **Table 2**. Splitting the whole population based on nationality, Italian volunteers have displayed the same trends as the whole group concerning pNN50—a trend also reported among Nepalese participants, with no difference by altitude. In contrast, significance was found in CSI decrease at mid-point, further increase at the final evaluation, and in HFD, displaying the opposite trend. The baseline comparison between Italian and Nepalese individuals displayed higher values for Nepalese volunteers concerning HFD (1.601 ± 0.036 vs. 1.553 ± 0.026, $p = 0.041$). The total power of frequency bands was significantly higher before the trek started, compared with the midpoint; therefore, the absolute power of both VLF, LF, and HF bands followed the same trend. No other features were found to be significantly different between the two ethnicities.

As depicted in **Figure 3**, the exposure to HA increased the urinary levels of epinephrine and norepinephrine, expressed as µg/mg of creatinine. This difference was significant for NE, with $t_{(5)} = 4.719$, $p = 0.005$, and $d_{unb} = 1.623$ whereas there was a strong tendency for *E*, with $t_{(5)} = 2.382$, $p = 0.063$, and $d_{unb} = 0.819$.

DISCUSSION

A recent massive increase in activities at HA, such as touristic sojourn, hiking, mountaineering, and sports training, raises the call for the evaluation of adaptive health consequences. In this regard, monitoring the cardiorespiratory variables emerges as a

TABLE 1 | Cardiorespiratory results, clustered by altitude, and ethnic group.

Altitude	Group	HR (bpm)	SpO_2 (%)	BR (bpm)	SBP (mmHg)	DBP (mmHg)	PP (mmHg)	MAP (mmHg)
1450m	*Ita*	58 ± 8	98 ± 1	12 ± 4	129 ± 8	77 ± 8	52 ± 6	95 ± 8
	Nep	76 ± 6	96 ± 1	16 ± 4	129 ± 10	86 ± 12	43 ± 7	100 ± 11
2316m	*Ita*	59 ± 5	95 ± 2	12 ± 3	137 ± 13	87 ± 7	50 ± 8	103 ± 9
	Nep	70 ± 11	95 ± 2	18 ± 3	132 ± 18	87 ± 14	45 ± 10	102 ± 15
2895m	*Ita*	67 ± 8	94 ± 3	13 ± 5	131 ± 7	83 ± 9	48 ± 9	99 ± 7
	Nep	77 ± 12	95 ± 3	18 ± 8	137 ± 15	94 ± 13	43 ± 8	108 ± 14
1173m	*Ita*	62 ± 9	98 ± 1	13 ± 1	125 ± 3	81 ± 7	43 ± 5	96 ± 5
	Nep	76 ± 15	97 ± 2	17 ± 4	129 ± 9	86 ± 9	43 ± 6	100 ± 9
3400m	*Ita*	67 ± 11	92 ± 3	15 ± 2	132 ± 9	84 ± 6	48 ± 9	100 ± 6
	Nep	71 ± 8	92 ± 1	17 ± 4	127 ± 13	89 ± 15	38 ± 8	102 ± 14
4750m	*Ita*	74 ± 9	86 ± 4	15 ± 6	136 ± 10	87 v 7	49 ± 7	103 ± 8
	Nep	80 ± 7	85 ± 3	18 ± 5	130 ± 17	90 ± 15	40 ± 5	103 ± 16
3000m	*Ita*	59 ± 4	95 ± 2	13 ± 2	130 ± 12	82 v 5	48 ± 7	98 ± 7
	Nep	68 ± 11	95 ± 2	21 ± 3	131 ± 10	87 ± 12	44 ± 6	101 ± 11
1747m	*Ita*	60 ± 6	97 ± 1	13 ± 3	129 ± 9	80 ± 4	49 ± 11	96 ± 3
	Nep	71 ± 10	96 ± 2	18 ± 3	126 ± 12	82 ± 13	44 ± 9	97 ± 12

Ita, Italians; Nep, Nepalese; HR, heart rate; SpO_2, peripheral oxygen saturation; BR, breathing rate; SBP, systolic blood pressure; DBP, diastolic blood pressure; PP, pulse pressure; MAP, mean arterial pressure; bpm, beats (or breaths) per minute.

TABLE 2 | Data extracted from the ECG signal for the whole study population.

	Pre	bBC	aBC	Pre vs. bBC	bBC vs. aBC
HR (bpm)	66.1 ± 8.7	59.9 ± 8.7	59.4 ± 6.6	n.s.	n.s.
SDNN (ms)	47.8 ± 24.0	74.6 ± 37.6	65.9 ± 31.5	0.010	n.s.
pNN50 (%)	11.6 ± 14.0	33.1 ± 26.4	27.8 ± 23.2	0.003	n.s.
CSI	2.72 ± 0.86	2.26 ± 1.15	2.35 ± 0.96	n.s.	n.s.
CVI	3.08 ± 0.40	3.51 ± 0.52	3.42 ± 0.38	0.008	n.s.
Total power (ms^2)	2.27 ± 2.56	6.37 ± 5.68	3.92 ± 4.47	0.008	n.s.
VLF power (ms^2)	1.06 ± 1.18	2.49 ± 2.79	1.44 ± 1.25	n.s.	n.s.
LF power (ms^2)	0.66 ± 0.91	1.68 ± 1.87	1.04 ± 1.54	0.034	n.s.
HF power (ms^2)	0.55 ± 0.64	2.20 ± 2.31	1.44 ± 2.13	0.010	n.s.
nLF (n.u.)	0.56 ± 0.16	0.45 ± 0.18	0.45 ± 0.20	n.s.	n.s.
nHF (n.u.)	0.44 ± 0.16	0.55 ± 0.18	0.55 ± 0.20	n.s.	n.s.
LF/HF	1.57 ± 0.90	1.03 ± 0.75	1.24 ± 1.31	n.s.	n.s.
Peak (VLF) (Hz)	0.010 ± 0.012	0.010 ± 0.008	0.008 ± 0.009	n.s.	n.s.
Peak (LF) (Hz)	0.088 ± 0.029	0.105 ± 0.025	0.085 ± 0.024	n.s.	n.s.
Peak (HF) (Hz)	0.236 ± 0.076	0.228 ± 0.051	0.247 ± 0.067	n.s.	n.s.
HFD	1.577 ± 0.039	1.597 ± 0.029	1.576 ± 0.032	n.s.	n.s.

Pre, before the trek; bBC, before the base camp circuit; aBC, after the base camp circuit; HR, heart rate; SDNN, standard deviation of the normal R-to-R intervals; pNN50, percentage of normal R-to-R intervals >50 ms; CSI, cardiac sympathetic index; CVI, cardiac vagal index; LF, low-frequency spectral band; HF, high-frequency spectral band; n.u., normalized units; VLF, very low frequency; HFD, Higuchi fractal dimension; n.s., non-significant.

cornerstone and raises the need to use devices with adequate characteristics, i.e., compact and portable enough to perform in this harsh environment (Ridolfi et al., 2010).

Of particular importance is the assessment of a vast amount of information using simplified, low-cost, lightweight instruments, like the ECG sensor interfaced with a fitness-like chest strap. This kind of device can be carried on without a significant increase in the efforts of the carriers, but at the same time providing useful information about the ANS activation, as previously demonstrated (Billeci et al., 2019; Tonacci et al., 2019). It is worth noting that HRV metrics have been claimed as measures of ANS response, particularly regarding the sympathetic influence on heart rate and the autonomic reactivity (Thomas et al., 2019). However, logistics sometimes impairs the possibility to obtain direct measures of ANS functioning during field studies in extreme conditions. In the current work, no direct measures

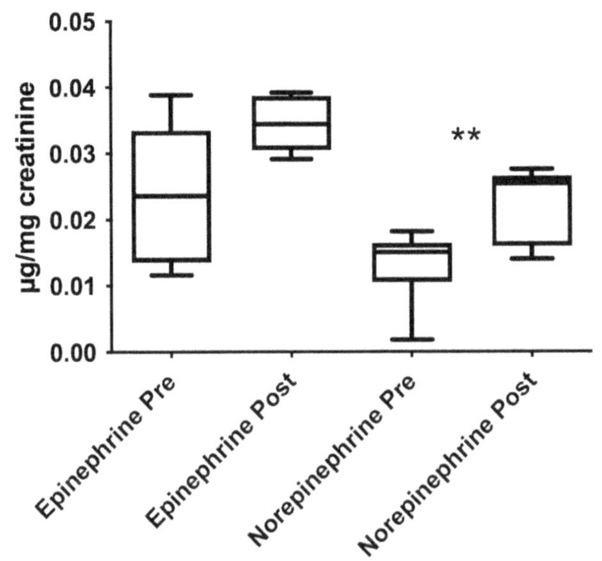

FIGURE 3 | Stimulating effects induced by HA trek on urinary norepinephrine and epinephrine levels, expressed as µg/mg of creatinine and shown as boxplots. Urine samples were collected in Italians only. Data were analyzed through paired samples Student's *t*-test; $^{**}p < 0.01$.

of ANS were conducted, but a wide set of metrics related to the cardiorespiratory system were assessed. According to the results obtained from the ECG analysis, all participants displayed likely ANS response at *bBC*. This was likely due to the higher altitude reached in this stage. This response remained sustained even at *aBC*, albeit the absolute value of SDNN did not reach the lower values displayed at the *Pre* point.

This overall trend can be affected by the higher vagal activation described by the pNN50, which could drive the overall ANS reactivity toward higher values at *bBC*. As a confirmation for this trend on the overall population, the CVI was also increased at *bBC* with respect to the Pre, with a further decrease at *aBC*, thus confirming a parasympathetic activation that occurred at the second assessment with respect to the baseline and to the third evaluation point. Conversely, limitedly to the Italian trekkers, CSI followed the opposite trend, with lower values reported at *bBC*. The higher values found for both absolute LF and HF power bands at *bBC* compared with baseline followed the higher values of total power. However, it may be misleading to use absolute power values *per se*, rather than relative values of power bands and/or integrating time-domain and non-linear values. Indeed, absolute values are greatly sensitive to artifacts and to the computational model used (Miranda Dantas et al., 2012; Stapelberg et al., 2018).

Taken together, these results might indicate a counter-intuitive autonomic behavior at HA, since several investigations have clearly demonstrated a significant sympathetic activation with the hypoxic conditions experienced at altitude (Hainsworth et al., 2007). However, it is worth noting that, in the present protocol, the *Pre* test was performed at 3,427 m, which could have driven basal measurements. Indeed, despite the response preceding the protocol start, the effects of hypoxia on the sympathetic activation within the autonomic nervous system might already appear as low as 3,000 m, especially in non-natives (Hainsworth et al., 2007).

Such effects are more likely to occur at higher altitudes. However, the concentration required to prepare the trekking might have challenged the sympathetic tone before the expedition, eventually experienced toward a higher parasympathetic activation at *bBC* with respect to the previous measurement. After the trek, the effect of physical activity on the delay of parasympathetic response, already demonstrated by others investigators (Al Haddad et al., 2012), could have determined a lack of variation with respect to the *bBC* measurement. Indeed, it can be supposed that, before the trek started, participants had greater arousal and stress with respect to *bBC*. After the base camp circuit, albeit participants were tested at the same altitude as *bBC*, the hypobaric hypoxia exposure, along with the physical conditioning, posed a high stressor on participants, determining a chronic sympathetic activation and parasympathetic de-activation, as previously reported (Siebenmann et al., 2017; Beltrán et al., 2020). Considering reduced cardiac parasympathetic activity as the main mechanisms underlying the increase of resting heart rate in response to middle-term exposure to altitude hypoxia (Siebenmann et al., 2017), and that HRV metrics could be considered more adequate in estimate parasympathetic, rather than sympathetic, dynamics (Fontolliet et al., 2018; Thomas et al., 2019), all in all, HRV can be considered effective in monitoring altitude effects on autonomic control of cardiac rhythms, when direct or more effective measures (such as microneurography) are harsh to implement.

Urinary catecholamines have been highlighted as an effective assessment of ANS role in regulating blood pressure (Missouris et al., 2016). The urinary catecholamines findings of Italians revealed the likely summatory and chronic response of the sympathetic system due to the HA trek. Indeed, consistent with our recent findings, we found an increase in urinary levels of catecholamines, thus suggesting the activation of the sympathetic nervous system following exposure to HA (Verratti et al., 2020b). Although structurally similar, catecholamines have different affinities for specific adrenergic receptors, inducing a wide range of physiological effects (Eisenhofer and Lenders, 2018). Physiologically, epinephrine produces a prolonged increase in resting energy expenditure, with increased carbohydrate oxidation (Ratheiser et al., 1998).

It has been suggested that the lipolytic activity of the skeletal muscle is increased by endogenous catecholamines *in vivo* and appears to be more responsive to epinephrine than norepinephrine stimulation (Qvisth et al., 2006). For its part, norepinephrine significantly affects blood pressure, primarily acting on alpha-adrenoreceptors in the blood vessels. In particular, urinary norepinephrine is linked with chronic alterations of blood pressure, as the higher BP, the higher urinary

NE excretion (Missouris et al., 2016). Thus, a more marked increase of norepinephrine in our study indicates that BP increase after hypobaric hypoxia exposure may be due to a large extent by vasoconstriction.

Short-term exposure to hypobaric hypoxia does not increase plasma catecholamines; to be noted that, although these findings are biased by increased clearance, reduced synthesis of catecholamines during short-term hypoxia has been demonstrated (Rostrup, 1998). The time course of HRV parameters in our study, together with the chronic increase in urinary catecholamines, is in line with these findings. Therefore, we support the notion that middle (>1 week) and long-term hypobaric hypoxia exposure increases sympathetic activity (Rostrup, 1998) and consequently, blood pressure. Among the mechanisms shown to drive the cardiovascular responses to altitude hypoxia, muscle sympathetic nerve activity, sympathetic vasoconstrictor activity (Simpson et al., 2019), pulmonary arterial baroreceptors (Simpson et al., 2020), asymmetric dimethylarginine activity (Verratti et al., 2020b) have been recently pointed out.

Finally, the comparison between Italians and Nepalese individuals showed no significant differences at baseline, except for a slightly increased value for HFD in the latter. This result could demonstrate a better cardiovascular resilience (He et al., 2019) for Nepalese trekkers with respect to the Italian colleagues, possibly due to a wider experience, and consequent habit, to HAs. This phenomenon appears to be challenging in being demonstrated by "ordinary" HRV features, but non-linear, fractal measures could help retrieve possibly hidden information related to such physiological processes (Di Rienzo et al., 2010). Therefore, we suggest using non-linear measures, such as HFD (Gomolka et al., 2018), in addition to the most common ones in HRV, to evaluate hypoxia-related responses.

The result of a higher breathing rate of Nepalese porters, compared with Italian trekkers, add a novel finding to the results of Dhar and colleagues (2018), who reported a higher respiration rate of HAs native and acclimatize lowlanders (15–18 months residence at >3,500 m asl) compared with sea-level residents never exposed to HAs. As breathing rate is regulated by the brain, brainstem, respiratory muscles, lungs, airways, and blood vessels (Chourpiliadis and Bhardwaj, 2020), the ethnic difference in this summary physiological outcome, related to acute or chronic altitude exposure, may unveil novel insights on cardiorespiratory responses and adaptations.

In BP regulation at altitude, ion channels should deserve to be focused on, as they are sensitive to oxygen deprivation and play a major role in cardiac contractility and control of vasomotor tone (Shimoda and Polak, 2011). A worth investigating topic also lies on nitric oxide (NO) system, as it plays a fundamental role in cardiovascular homeostasis; NO synthases enzymes and oral nitrate-reducing bacteria supply bioactive NO (Pignatelli et al., 2020). Thus, the interplay of NOS activity, nutrition, and oral health may unveil novel insights on altitude-related hypertension. Finally, HRV has been interpreted as a global measure of the network of an organism interconnectedness and complexity, reflecting biologic rhythm variability and adaptability of the human organism (Sturmberg et al., 2015). In this vein, unveiling the different responses of HRV indexes, particularly the novel ones of non-linear analysis, will provide insights into a novel interpretation of human responses to acute and chronic environmental and physical stressors.

This study did not come without limitations, particularly related to the baseline differences between tourists and porters, and to the difference in the load carried throughout the trek. However, the ecological nature of this study did not allow to control for the baseline variables to adhere to the homogeneity of groups. These differences that may have biased the results are likely to occur in similar field studies aiming to detect the response of different populations. Therefore, further evidence is needed to extend and ameliorate the original findings herein discussed.

Considering our results, further studies may focus on the starting point of the expedition, evaluating the mood state of expeditioners, that may experience feelings such as enjoyment and emotional stresses, that are strongly linked to HRV parameters, as a sign of the well-known mind-cardiorespiratory system connection (Bernardi et al., 2001). This starting state is possibly different between the diverse groups of expeditioners (tourists, mountaineers, porters, medical doctors, and guides).

ETHICS STATEMENT

The studies involving human participants were reviewed and approved by Ethics Review Board of the Nepal Health Research Council (NHRC). The patients/participants provided their written informed consent to participate in this study.

AUTHOR CONTRIBUTIONS

VV, AT, and DB contributed to the conception and design of the study and wrote the first draft of the manuscript. VV and DB performed the acquisition of data and samples. AT, ACh, CF, and LB performed the analyses. AT and DB performed the statistical analysis. VV, AT, DB, ACh, CF, LB, ACr, and PC wrote sections of the manuscript. All authors contributed to manuscript revision, read, and approved the submitted version.

ACKNOWLEDGMENTS

The authors thank the Mission Nepal Holidays Pvt. Ltd. (Kathmandu, Nepal), and all the Italian trekkers and Nepalese porters involved in this project.

REFERENCES

Al Haddad, H., Mendez-Villanueva, A., Bourdon, P. C., and Buchheit, M. (2012). Effect of acute hypoxia on post-exercise parasympathetic reactivation in healthy Men. *Front. Physiol.* 3. doi: 10.3389/fphys.2012.00289

Beall, C. M. (2003). High-altitude adaptations. *Lancet Lond. Engl.* 362 (Suppl), s14–15. doi: 10.1016/S0140-6736(03)15058-1

Beltrán, A. R., Arce-Álvarez, A., Ramirez-Campillo, R., Vásquez-Muñoz, M., von Igel, M., Ramírez, M. A., et al. (2020). Baroreflex modulation during acute high-altitude exposure in rats. *Front. Physiol.* 11:1049. doi: 10.3389/fphys.2020.01049

Bernardi, L., Sleight, P., Bandinelli, G., Cencetti, S., Fattorini, L., Wdowczyc-Szulc, J., et al. (2001). Effect of rosary prayer and yoga mantras on autonomic cardiovascular rhythms: comparative study. *BMJ* 323, 1446–1449. doi: 10.1136/bmj.323.7327.1446

Billeci, L., Tonacci, A., Brunori, E., Raso, R., Calderoni, S., Maestro, S., et al. (2019). Autonomic nervous system response during light physical activity in adolescents with anorexia nervosa measured by wearable devices. *Sensors* 19:19122820. doi: 10.3390/s19122820

Brinkman, J. E., Toro, F., and Sharma, S. (2020). *Physiology, Respiratory Drive. StatPearls Publishing* Available online at: https://www.ncbi.nlm.nih.gov/books/NBK482414/ (accessed October 14, 2020).

Busch, S. A., Davies, H., van Diepen, S., Simpson, L. L., Sobierajski, F., Riske, L., et al. (2018). Chemoreflex mediated arrhythmia during apnea at 5,050 m in low- but not high-altitude natives. *J. Appl. Physiol.* 124, 930–937. doi: 10.1152/japplphysiol.00774.2017

Calbet, J. A. L. (2003). Chronic hypoxia increases blood pressure and noradrenaline spillover in healthy humans. *J. Physiol.* 551, 379–386. doi: 10.1113/jphysiol.2003.045112

Calbet, J. A. L., and Lundby, C. (2009). Air to muscle O2 delivery during exercise at altitude. *High Alt. Med. Biol.* 10, 123–134. doi: 10.1089/ham.2008.1099

Cerretelli, P. (2013). Career perspective: paolo cerretelli. *Extreme Physiol. Med.* 2:13. doi: 10.1186/2046-7648-2-13

Chourpiliadis, C., and Bhardwaj, A. (2020). "Physiology, Respiratory Rate," in *StatPearls* (Treasure Island (FL): StatPearls Publishing). Available online at: http://www.ncbi.nlm.nih.gov/books/NBK537306/ (accessed April 27, 2020).

Dhar, P., Sharma, V. K., Das, S. K., Barhwal, K., Hota, S. K., and Singh, S. B. (2018). Differential responses of autonomic function in sea level residents, acclimatized lowlanders at >3500 m and Himalayan high altitude natives at >3500 m: a cross-sectional study. *Respir. Physiol. Neurobiol.* 254, 40–48. doi: 10.1016/j.resp.2018.04.002

Di Rienzo, M., Castiglioni, P., Rizzo, F., Faini, A., Mazzoleni, P., Lombardi, C., et al. (2010). Linear and fractal heart rate dynamics during sleep at high altitude. investigation with textile technology. *Methods Inf. Med.* 49, 521–525. doi: 10.3414/ME09-02-0053

Eisenhofer, G., and Lenders, J. W. M. (2018). "Catecholamines," in *Encyclopedia of Endocrine Diseases* (Cambridge, TN: Academic Press).

Fontolliet, T., Pichot, V., Bringard, A., Fagoni, N., Adami, A., Tam, E., et al. (2018). Testing the vagal withdrawal hypothesis during light exercise under autonomic blockade: a heart rate variability study. *J. Appl. Physiol. Bethesda Md* 125, 1804–1811. doi: 10.1152/japplphysiol.00619.2018

Fritz, C. O., Morris, P. E., and Richler, J. J. (2012). Effect size estimates: current use, calculations, and interpretation. *J. Exp. Psychol. Gen.* 141, 2–18. doi: 10.1037/a0024338

Furnival, C. M., Linden, R. J., and Snow, H. M. (1971). The inotropic and chronotropic effects of catecholamines on the dog heart. *J. Physiol.* 214, 15–28. doi: 10.1113/jphysiol.1971.sp009416

Gamboa, A., León-Velarde, F., Rivera-Ch, M., Palacios, J.-A., Pragnell, T. R., O'Connor, D. F., et al. (2003). Selected contribution: acute and sustained ventilatory responses to hypoxia in high-altitude natives living at sea level. *J. Appl. Physiol.* 94, 1255–1262. doi: 10.1152/japplphysiol.00856.2002

Giles, T. D., and Sander, G. E. (2013). Diastolic blood pressure and hypertension phenotypes: The US food and drug administration has it right. *J. Clin. Hypertens.* 15, 145–146. doi: 10.1111/jch.12053

Gomes, R. L., Vanderlei, L. C. M., Garner, D. M., Vanderlei, F. M., and Valenti, V. E. (2017). Higuchi fractal analysis of heart rate variability is sensitive during recovery from exercise in physically active men. *Med. Express* 4, 1–8. doi: 10.5935/MedicalExpress.2017.02.03

Gomolka, R. S., Kampusch, S., Kaniusas, E., Thürk, F., Széles, J. C., and Klonowski, W. (2018). Higuchi fractal dimension of heart rate variability during percutaneous auricular vagus nerve stimulation in healthy and diabetic subjects. *Front. Physiol.* 9:1162. doi: 10.3389/fphys.2018.01162

Hainsworth, R., Drinkhill, M. J., and Rivera-Chira, M. (2007). The autonomic nervous system at high altitude. *Clin. Auton. Res. Off. J. Clin. Auton. Res. Soc.* 17, 13–19. doi: 10.1007/s10286-006-0395-7

He, L., Wang, J., Zhang, L., Zhang, X., Dong, W., and Yang, H. (2019). Decreased fractal dimension of heart rate variability is associated with early neurological deterioration and recurrent ischemic stroke after acute ischemic stroke. *J. Neurol. Sci.* 396, 42–47. doi: 10.1016/j.jns.2018.11.006

Malik, M. (1996). Heart Rate Variability. *Ann. Noninvasive Electrocardiol.* 1, 151–181. doi: 10.1111/j.1542-474X.1996.tb00275.x

Mangoni, M. E., and Nargeot, J. (2008). Genesis and regulation of the heart automaticity. *Physiol. Rev.* 88, 919–982. doi: 10.1152/physrev.00018.2007

Marshall, J. M. (1994). Peripheral chemoreceptors and cardiovascular regulation. *Physiol. Rev.* 74, 543–594. doi: 10.1152/physrev.1994.74.3.543

Miranda Dantas, E., Lima Sant'Anna, M., Varejão Andreão, R., Pereira Gonçalves, C., Aguiar Morra, E., Perim Baldo, M., et al. (2012). Spectral analysis of heart rate variability with the autoregressive method: What model order to choose? *Comput. Biol. Med.* 42, 164–170. doi: 10.1016/j.compbiomed.2011.11.004

Missouris, C. G., Markandu, N. D., He, F. J., Papavasileiou, M. V., Sever, P., and MacGregor, G. A. (2016). Urinary catecholamines and the relationship with blood pressure and pharmacological therapy. *J. Hypertens.* 34, 704–709. doi: 10.1097/HJH.0000000000000843

Moore, L. G. (2017). Measuring high-altitude adaptation. *J. Appl. Physiol. Bethesda Md* 123, 1371–1385. doi: 10.1152/japplphysiol.00321.2017

Mulliri, G., Sainas, G., Magnani, S., Roberto, S., Ghiani, G., Mannoni, M., et al. (2019). Effects of exercise in normobaric hypoxia on hemodynamics during muscle metaboreflex activation in normoxia. *Eur. J. Appl. Physiol.* 119, 1137–1148. doi: 10.1007/s00421-019-04103-y

Pan, J., and Tompkins, W. J. (1985). A Real-Time QRS Detection Algorithm. *IEEE Trans. Biomed. Eng.* BME-32, 230–236. doi: 10.1109/TBME.1985.325532

Parati, G., Ochoa, J. E., Torlasco, C., Salvi, P., Lombardi, C., and Bilo, G. (2015). Aging, high altitude, and blood pressure: a complex relationship. *High Alt. Med. Biol.* 16, 97–109. doi: 10.1089/ham.2015.0010

Pignatelli, P., Fabietti, G., Ricci, A., Piattelli, A., and Curia, M. C. (2020). How periodontal disease and presence of nitric oxide reducing oral bacteria can affect blood pressure. *Int. J. Mol. Sci.* 21:7538. doi: 10.3390/ijms21207538

Princi, T., Zupet, P., Finderle, Z., and Accardo, A. (2008). Linear and nonlinear assessment of heart rate variability in nonacclimatized middleaged subjects at different hypoxic levels. *Biomed. Sci. Instrum.* 44, 380–385.

Qvisth, V., Hagström-Toft, E., Enoksson, S., Moberg, E., Arner, P., and Bolinder, J. (2006). Human skeletal muscle lipolysis is more responsive to epinephrine than to norepinephrine stimulation in vivo. *J. Clin. Endocrinol. Metab.* 91, 665–670. doi: 10.1210/jc.2005-0859

Ratheiser, K. M., Brillon, D. J., Campbell, R. G., and Matthews, D. E. (1998). Epinephrine produces a prolonged elevation in metabolic rate in humans. *Am. J. Clin. Nutr.* 68, 1046–1052. doi: 10.1093/ajcn/68.5.1046

Reeves, J. T., Groves, B. M., Sutton, J. R., Wagner, P. D., Cymerman, A., Malconian, M. K., et al. (1987). Operation Everest II: preservation of cardiac function at extreme altitude. *J. Appl. Physiol. Bethesda Md* 63, 531–539. doi: 10.1152/jappl.1987.63.2.531

Ridolfi, A., Vetter, R., Sol,à, J., and Sartori, C. (2010). Physiological monitoring system for high altitude sports. *Procedia Eng.* 2, 2889–2894. doi: 10.1016/j.proeng.2010.04.083

Rostrup, M. (1998). Catecholamines, hypoxia and high altitude. *Acta Physiol. Scand.* 162, 389–399. doi: 10.1046/j.1365-201X.1998.00335.x

San, T., Polat, S., Cingi, C., Eskiizmir, G., Oghan, F., and Cakir, B. (2013). Effects of high altitude on sleep and respiratory system and theirs adaptations. *Sci. World J.* 2013. doi: 10.1155/2013/241569

Schommer, K., and Bärtsch, P. (2011). Basic Medical Advice for Travelers to High Altitudes. *Dtsch. Ärztebl. Int.* 108, 839. doi: 10.3238/arztebl.2011.0839

Schümann, H. J. (1983). What role do alpha- and beta-adrenoceptors play in the regulation of the heart? *Eur. Heart J.* 4 (Suppl A), 55–60. doi: 10.1093/eurheartj/4.suppl_A.55

Shaffer, F., and Ginsberg, J. P. (2017). An overview of heart rate variability metrics and norms. *Front. Public Health* 5:258. doi: 10.3389/fpubh.2017.00258

Shimoda, L. A., and Polak, J. (2011). Hypoxia. 4. Hypoxia and ion channel function.

Am. J. Physiol. Cell Physiol. 300, C951-967. doi: 10.1152/ajpcell.00512.2010

Siebenmann, C., Rasmussen, P., Hug, M., Keiser, S., Flück, D., Fisher, J. P., et al. (2017). Parasympathetic withdrawal increases heart rate after 2 weeks at 3454 m altitude. *J. Physiol.* 595, 1619–1626. doi: 10.1113/JP273726

Simpson, L. L., Busch, S. A., Oliver, S. J., Ainslie, P. N., Stembridge, M., Steinback, C. D., et al. (2019). Baroreflex control of sympathetic vasomotor activity and resting arterial pressure at high altitude: insight from Lowlanders and Sherpa. *J. Physiol.* 597, 2379–2390. doi: 10.1113/JP277663

Simpson, L. L., Meah, V. L., Steele, A., Thapamagar, S., Gasho, C., Anholm, J. D., et al. (2020). Evidence for a physiological role of pulmonary arterial baroreceptors in sympathetic neural activation in healthy humans. *J. Physiol.* 598, 955–965. doi: 10.1113/JP278731

Solomon, I. C. (2000). Excitation of phrenic and sympathetic output during acute hypoxia: contribution of medullary oxygen detectors. *Respir. Physiol.* 121, 101–117. doi: 10.1016/S0034-5687(00)00122-5

Stapelberg, N. J. C., Neumann, D. L., Shum, D. H. K., McConnell, H., and Hamilton-Craig, I. (2018). The sensitivity of 38 heart rate variability measures to the addition of artifact in human and artificial 24-hr cardiac recordings. *Ann. Noninvasive Electrocardiol.* 23:e12483. doi: 10.1111/anec.12483

Stembridge, M., Ainslie, P. N., Boulet, L. M., Anholm, J., Subedi, P., Tymko, M. M., et al. (2019). The independent effects of hypovolaemia and pulmonary vasoconstriction on ventricular function and exercise capacity during acclimatisation to 3800 m. *J. Physiol.* 597, 1059–1072. doi: 10.1113/JP275278

Sturmberg, J. P., Bennett, J. M., Picard, M., and Seely, A. J. E. (2015). The trajectory of life. Decreasing physiological network complexity through changing fractal patterns. *Front. Physiol.* 6:169. doi: 10.3389/fphys.2015.00169

Takahashi, M., Yamada, T., and Kinoshita, M. (1993). [Catecholamines and beta-blockers for the treatment of heart failure]. *Nihon Rinsho Jpn. J. Clin. Med.* 51, 1268–1275.

Thomas, B. L., Claassen, N., Becker, P., and Viljoen, M. (2019). Validity of commonly used heart rate variability markers of autonomic nervous system function. *Neuropsychobiology*, 1–13. doi: 10.1159/000495519

Tonacci, A., Billeci, L., Sansone, F., Masci, A., Pala, A. P., Domenici, C., et al. (2019). An Innovative, Unobtrusive approach to investigate smartphone interaction in nonaddicted subjects based on wearable sensors: a pilot study. *Med. Kaunas Lith.* 55:37. doi: 10.3390/medicina55020037

Torlasco, C., Bilo, G., Giuliano, A., Soranna, D., Ravaro, S., Oliverio, G., et al. (2020). Effects of acute exposure to moderate altitude on blood pressure and sleep breathing patterns. *Int. J. Cardiol.* 301, 173–179. doi: 10.1016/j.ijcard.2019.09.034

Ullian, M. E. (1999). The role of corticosteroids in the regulation of vascular tone. *Cardiovasc. Res.* 41, 55–64. doi: 10.1016/S0008-6363(98)00230-2

Verratti, V., Bondi, D., Mulliri, G., Ghiani, G., Crisafulli, A., Pietrangelo, T., et al. (2020a). Muscle oxygen delivery in the forearm and in the vastus lateralis muscles in response to resistance exercise: a comparison between Nepalese porters and Italian trekkers. *Front. Physiol.* 11:7616. doi: 10.3389/fphys.2020.607616

Verratti, V., Ferrante, C., Soranna, D., Zambon, A., Bhandari, S., Orlando, G., et al. (2020b). Effect of high-altitude trekking on blood pressure and on asymmetric dimethylarginine and isoprostane production: Results from a Mount Ararat expedition. *J. Clin. Hypertens.* 22, 1494–1503. doi: 10.1111/jch.13961

Verratti, V., Mrakic-Sposta, S., Moriggi, M., Tonacci, A., Bhandari, S., Migliorelli, D., et al. (2019). Urinary physiology and hypoxia: a pilot study of moderate-altitude trekking effects on urodynamic indexes. *Am. J. Physiol. Renal Physiol.* 317, F1081–F1086. doi: 10.1152/ajprenal.00333.2019

Welch, P. (1967). The use of fast Fourier transform for the estimation of power spectra: A method based on time averaging over short, modified periodograms. *IEEE Trans. Audio Electro.* 15, 70–73. doi: 10.1109/TAU.1967.1161901

West, J. B. (2016). Early history of high-altitude physiology. *Ann. N. Y. Acad. Sci.* 1365, 33–42. doi: 10.1111/nyas.12719

Whelton, P. K., Carey, R. M., Aronow, W. S., Casey, D. E., Collins, K. J., Dennison Himmelfarb, C., et al. (2018). 2017 ACC/AHA/AAPA/ABC/ACPM/AGS/APhA/ASH/ASPC/NMA/PCNA Guideline for the Prevention, Detection, Evaluation, and Management of High Blood Pressure in Adults. *J. Am. Coll. Cardiol.* 71, e127–e248. doi: 10.1016/j.jacc.2017.11.006

WHO (2011). *Pulse Oximetry Training Manual.* Available online at: https://www.who.int/patientsafety/safesurgery/pulse_oximetry/who_ps_pulse_oxymetry_training_manual_en.pdf?ua=1.

World Medical Association (2013). World Medical Association Declaration of Helsinki: Ethical Principles for Medical Research Involving Human Subjects. *JAMA* 310:2191. doi: 10.1001/jama.2013.281053

5

Right Ventricular Response to Acute Hypoxia Exposure

*Argen Mamazhakypov[1], Meerim Sartmyrzaeva[2,3], Nadira Kushubakova[2,3], Melis Duishobaev[2,3], Abdirashit Maripov[2,3], Akylbek Sydykov[1,2] and Akpay Sarybaev[2,3]**

[1] Department of Internal Medicine, Excellence Cluster Cardio-Pulmonary Institute (CPI), Member of the German Center for Lung Research (DZL), Justus Liebig University of Giessen, Giessen, Germany, [2] Department of Mountain and Sleep Medicine and Pulmonary Hypertension, National Center of Cardiology and Internal Medicine, Bishkek, Kyrgyzstan, [3] Kyrgyz Indian Mountain Biomedical Research Center, Bishkek, Kyrgyzstan

***Correspondence:**
Akpay Sarybaev
ak_sar777@mail.ru

Background: Acute hypoxia exposure is associated with an elevation of pulmonary artery pressure (PAP), resulting in an increased hemodynamic load on the right ventricle (RV). In addition, hypoxia may exert direct effects on the RV. However, the RV responses to such challenges are not fully characterized. The aim of this systematic review was to describe the effects of acute hypoxia on the RV in healthy lowland adults.

Methods: We systematically reviewed PubMed and Web of Science and article references from 2005 until May 2021 for prospective studies evaluating echocardiographic RV function and morphology in healthy lowland adults at sea level and upon exposure to simulated altitude or high-altitude.

Results: We included 37 studies in this systematic review, 12 of which used simulated altitude and 25 were conducted in high-altitude field conditions. Eligible studies reported at least one of the RV variables, which were all based on transthoracic echocardiography assessing RV systolic and diastolic function and RV morphology. The design of these studies significantly differed in terms of mode of ascent to high-altitude, altitude level, duration of high-altitude stay, and timing of measurements. In the majority of the studies, echocardiographic examinations were performed within the first 10 days of high-altitude induction. Studies also differed widely by selectively reporting only a part of multiple RV parameters. Despite consistent increase in PAP documented in all studies, reports on the changes of RV function and morphology greatly differed between studies.

Conclusion: This systematic review revealed that the study reports on the effects of acute hypoxia on the RV are controversial and inconclusive. This may be the result of significantly different study designs, non-compliance with international guidelines on RV function assessment and limited statistical power due to small sample sizes. Moreover, the potential impact of other factors such as gender, age, ethnicity, physical activity, mode of ascent and environmental factors such as temperature and humidity on RV responses to hypoxia remained unexplored. Thus, this comprehensive overview will promote reproducible research with improved study designs and methods for the future large-scale prospective studies, which eventually may provide important insights into the RV response to acute hypoxia exposure.

Keywords: acute hypoxia, high-altitude, right ventricle, pulmonary hypertension, echocardiography

INTRODUCTION

With increasing altitude, the partial pressure of oxygen in the atmosphere falls along with the barometric pressure, leading to a gradually decreasing oxygen availability. Consequently, exposure to high-altitude results in diminished arterial blood oxygen content and initiates acclimatization processes consisting in a series of physiological responses of various organs and systems to maintain an adequate oxygen delivery to the tissues. Particularly, major changes occur in the cardiovascular system. While, the systemic vascular resistance may increase only up to 20%, there is more significant elevation of pulmonary artery pressure (PAP) and pulmonary vascular resistance (PVR) due to hypoxic pulmonary vasoconstriction (HPV), against which the right ventricle (RV) should maintain its contractility (Baggish et al., 2014). HPV is a remarkable cardiovascular response to high-altitude hypoxia exposure (Sydykov et al., 2021). Although, the main purpose of the HPV is to maintain local ventilation-perfusion matching and improve blood oxygenation, in the setting of global lung hypoxia during high-altitude exposure, diffuse HPV results in PAP and PVR increase (Swenson, 2013). The degree of the PAP elevation is usually mild-to-moderate and is not associated with serious adverse health consequences (Sydykov et al., 2021). If exposure to hypoxia persists, PAP may remain elevated (Hilty et al., 2016; Gaur et al., 2021) or become partially attenuated over the course of 2–3 weeks (Ghofrani et al., 2004; Baggish et al., 2010). However, a certain proportion of the population displays an exaggerated HPV (B?rtsch and Gibbs, 2007), which may predispose to high altitude pulmonary edema (HAPE), a potentially life-threatening condition that typically occurs in otherwise healthy individuals after rapid ascent to high-altitude (Sydykov et al., 2021). Importantly, alleviation of HPV by an immediate descent leads to a full recovery from HAPE.

A fall in arterial blood oxygen content initiates cardiac responses, including cardiac output increase, in order to maintain adequate oxygen delivery to the tissues (Naeije, 2010). The cardiac output enhancement observed upon high-altitude exposure is explained mainly by increased heart rate with maintained or decreased stroke volume (Naeije, 2010). In high-altitude hypoxia conditions with decreased oxygen availability, augmented cardiac output along with the enhanced load to the RV due to elevated PVR increases myocardial oxygen demand, thus predisposing the RV to myocardial dysfunction. In addition, cardiac performance may be hampered by various factors associated with the high-altitude exposure, such as increased blood viscosity, sympathetic nervous system activation and hypovolemia (Naeije, 2010). Thus, the RV not only should maintain or couple its contractility to increased afterload but also withstand other adverse challenges associated with high-altitude. All these factors together require RV functional and geometrical adaptation to maintain cardiac function and oxygen delivery to the tissues.

Available studies that evaluated the effects of acute high-altitude exposure on the RV produced conflicting results (Naeije and Dedobbeleer, 2013; Richalet and Pichon, 2014). While some studies demonstrated an augmented RV function in response to acute hypoxia-induced afterload increase (Berger et al., 2018; Sareban et al., 2020), others found no change (Huez et al., 2005) or even an impaired RV function (Reichenberger et al., 2007; Hanaoka et al., 2011; Page et al., 2013). Furthermore, there is anecdotal evidence of acute RV failure due to increased RV pressure overload in a healthy individual upon high-altitude exposure (Huez et al., 2007). These discrepancies in the existing literature are poorly understood but might be related to the considerable differences in methods and research designs between the studies and lack of compliance with the guidelines for the assessment of the RV function and morphology (Rudski et al., 2010). In addition, gender (Boos et al., 2016), age (Stewart et al., 2020), ethnicity (Gaur et al., 2021), individual susceptibility (Huez et al., 2007) and some other factors can impact RV performance upon high-altitude hypoxia exposure. Further, at high altitude, RV might be subjected to hemodynamic load of variable severity in different individuals due to great inter-individual variability in the HPV.

In lowlanders, prolonged high-altitude stay is associated with sustained HPV and pulmonary vascular remodeling (Groves et al., 1987; Maggiorini et al., 2001; Luks et al., 2017). Depending on their severity, these changes can cause persistent elevation of PAP and PVR resulting in increased RV afterload, which may lead to RV remodeling and dysfunction (Yang et al., 2015). During prolonged stay at extreme high-altitudes (5800-6700 m), some healthy lowlanders might develop severe RV failure with peripheral congestion syndrome, which is fully reversible upon returning to low altitude (Anand et al., 1990). However, it remains unknown whether acute RV dysfunction affects subsequent development of RV remodeling and failure with prolonged stay at high-altitude.

Although right heart catheterization is the gold standard method for the assessment of pulmonary hemodynamics and RV function, its application in healthy humans in high-altitude settings is challenging due to logistics (remote area) and its invasive nature. Alternatively, echocardiography has become a widely available and reliable method to study cardiovascular physiology (Soria et al., 2016, 2019). It has been proven to be a valuable tool to characterize RV function and morphology in various cardiovascular conditions (Taleb et al., 2013; Greiner et al., 2014). Importantly, echocardiography allows measuring cardiac function serially over the specified time periods and altitude levels (Galie et al., 2016). Consequently, echocardiography has become a widely available and reliable method to study cardiovascular physiology in high-altitude research (Fagenholz et al., 2012; Feletti et al., 2018).

Recently emerged state-of-the-art echocardiography imaging modalities such as speckle-tracking and 3D echocardiography have significantly improved our understanding of the left ventricular (LV) physiology in lowlanders acutely exposed to high-altitude and in permanent high-altitude residents (Stembridge et al., 2015, 2016, 2019). However, these techniques remain underutilized for the in-depth characterization of the RV function and morphology in high-altitude settings. Understanding the physiology of the RV responses to acute hypoxia is of significant importance for gaining insights into mechanisms underlying acute RV dysfunction and failure in various cardiopulmonary diseases. Thus, this systematic review

TABLE 1 | Summary of the studies evaluating right ventricular function and morphology upon acute simulated altitude exposure.

Study	Sample size (M/F)	Age (mean ± SD or mean (range) years)	Health status	Type of hypoxia exposure	Baseline altitude (m)	FiO_2 (%) or altitude level (m)	Rate of exposure	Hypoxic duration	Pulmonary hemodynamics parameters	RV diastolic functional parameters	RV systolic functional parameters	RV morphology parameters
Huez et al., 2005	25 (14/11)	32 ± 8	Healthy	Hypoxic breathing	Brussels (13)	FiO_2–12% (≈4,500)	NA	90 min	TRG, PAAT/ET	RV E/A, RV E′, RV A′, RV E′/A′	TAPSE, RV-S′	RV-EDA
Kjaergaard et al., 2007	14 (13/1)	33 (21–55)	Healthy	Hypoxic breathing	NA	FiO_2–12.5%	NA	1 h	sPAP, PAAT, PVR	RV-E′, RV-A′	TAPSE, RV-MPI, RV-S′, RV-FAC	RV-EDA
Reichenberger et al., 2007	14 (12/2)	37 (23–55)	Healthy	Hypoxia breathing	Giessen (171)	FiO_2–10% (≈5,500)	NA	2 h	sPAP, PAAT/ET		TAPSE, RV-MPI	
(HAPE-s) (Hanaoka et al., 2011)	11 (11/0)	50.9 ± 13.2	Healthy	Hypoxic breathing	Matsumoto (610)	4,000	NA	30 min	sPAP		RV-MPI	
(HAPE-r) (Hanaoka et al., 2011)	9 (9/9)	53.1 ± 13.4	Healthy	Hypoxic breathing	Matsumoto (610)	4,000	NA	40–45 min	sPAP		RV-MPI	
Pavelescu and Naeije, 2012	10 (7/3)	24 ± 3	Healthy	Hypoxic breathing	NA	FiO_2–12%	NA	2 h	sPAP, TRG, PAAT/ET, PVR	RV-E/A, RV-E′, RV-A′, RV-E′/A′	TAPSE, RV-S′, RV-FAC	RV-EDA
Goebel et al., 2013	14 (12/2)	NA (25–41)	Healthy	Normobaric hypoxia chamber	NA	FiO_2–9.9%	2h → 4,000 m (4 h) → 5,500	2 h	TRG, PVR	RV-E/A	TAPSE, RV-GLS	
Boos et al., 2013	14 (14/0)	30.5 ± 4.3	Healthy	Hypobaric hypoxia chamber	Henlow (40)	4,800	1,219 m per min	>150 min	sPAP, PAAT,	RV-E, RV-A, RV-E/A, RV-E′, RV-A′	TAPSE, RV-MPI, RV-S′	
(Women) (Boos et al., 2016)	7 (0/7)	25.9 ± 3.2	Healthy	Normobaric hypoxia chamber	Leeds (113)	FiO_2–11.4% (≈4,800)	NA	>150 min	sPAP, PAAT, PVR		TAPSE	
(Men) (Boos et al., 2016)	7 (7/0)	27.3 ± 4.4	Healthy	Normobaric hypoxia chamber	Leeds (113)	FiO_2–11.4%	NA	>150 min	PAAT, sPAP, PVR		TAPSE	
Seccombe et al., 2017	7 (4/3)	51 ± 15	Healthy	Hypoxic breathing		FiO_2–15%	NA	20 min	sPAP		TAPSE, RV-MPI, RV-FAC	RV-ESA
Netzer et al., 2017	35 (24/11)	NA	Healthy	Normobaric hypoxia chamber	Bad Aibling (492)	FiO_2–11%	NA	30, 60, 100, 150 min	sPAP, PAAT	RV-E′, RV-A′	TAPSE, RV-MPI, RV-S′	RV-EDA, RVD1, RVD2, RVD3
Pezzuto et al., 2018	17 (10/7)	24 ± 6	Healthy	Hypoxic breathing	NA	FiO_2–12%	NA	15, 30, 45, 60 min	mPAP, PVR		TAPSE, RV-S′, RV-FAC	RV-EDA
Ewalts et al., 2021	15 (12/3)	25 ± 4	Healthy	Hypoxic breathing	Cardiff (17)	FiO_2–12%	NA	30 min	sPAP, mPAP, PVR		RV-FAC, RV-GLS	RV-EDA, RV-ESA

TRG, tricuspid regurgitation gradient; sPAP, systolic pulmonary artery pressure; mPAP, mean pulmonary artery pressure; PAAT, pulmonary artery acceleration time; PAAT/ET, pulmonary acceleration time to ejection time ratio; PVR, pulmonary vascular resistance; RV-E, tricuspid inflow early diastolic velocity; RV-A, tricuspid inflow late diastolic velocity; RV-E/A, tricuspid inflow early diastolic velocity to late diastolic velocity; RV-E′, tricuspid annulus early diastolic velocity by tissue Doppler imaging; RV-A′, tricuspid annulus late diastolic velocity by tissue Doppler imaging; RV-E′/A′, tissue Doppler early and late diastolic tricuspid velocities ratio; RV-S′, peak systolic velocity with tissue Doppler imaging at the tricuspid annulus; TAPSE, tricuspid annular plane systolic excursion, RV-MPI, right ventricular myocardial performance index; RV-FAC, right ventricular fractional area change; RV-EDA, right ventricular end-diastolic area; RV-ESA, right ventricular end-systolic area; RVD1, right ventricular end-diastolic basal cavity dimension; RVD2, right ventricular end-diastolic mid cavity dimension; RVD3, right ventricular end-diastolic longitudinal dimension; RV-GLS, right ventricular global longitudinal strain.

TABLE 2 | Summary of the studies evaluating right ventricular function and morphology upon acute high-altitude exposure.

Study	Sample size (M/F)	Age (mean ± SD or mean (range) years)	Health status	Baseline altitude (m)	High altitude location (altitude in m)	Ascent mode/duration of ascent	High altitude measurement timepoints	Pulmonary hemodynamics parameters	RV diastolic functional parameters	RV systolic functional parameters	RV structural parameters
Huez et al., 2009	15 (7/8)	36 ± 12	Healthy	Brussels (13)	La Paz (3,750), Huayna Potosi (4,850 m)	Direct/24 h	1st day (3,750 m), 10th day (4,850 m)	TRG, PAAT, mPAP	RV-E, RV-A, RV-E′, RV-A′, RV-E′/A′	TAPSE, RV-S′, RV-MPI	
de Vries et al., 2010	7 (4/3)	41 ± 16	Healthy	Zwolle (4)	Aconcagua (4,200)	Staged/10-day trip	10th day		RV-E′	TAPSE	
Pratali et al., 2010	18 (10/8)	45 ± 10	Healthy	Aosta (583)	Namche Bazaar (3,440), Gokyo (4,790), Gorak shep (5,130)	Staged/6 days	6th day (3,440 m), 10th day (4,790 m), 14th day (5,130 m)	sPAP		TAPSE	
Page et al., 2013	14 (8/6)	46 ± 12.4	Healthy	Montreal (30)	Namche Bazar (3,450), Chukkung (4,730)	Staged/4 day	4th and 7th days	sPAP, PVR	RV-E/A	TAPSE, RV-S′, RV-MPI, RV-GLS, RV-FWLS	
Boos et al., 2014	19 (10/9)	35.4 ± 8.3	Healthy	NA (1,300)	Namche Bazar (3,440), Pheriche (4,270), Gorak Shep (5,150)	Staged/2 days	2nd day (3,440 m), 6th day (4,270 m), 9th day (5,150 m)	sPAP	RV-E, RV-E′	RV-S′	
Stembridge et al., 2014	9 (9/0)	34 ± 7	Healthy	Kelowna (344)	Lobuche (5,050)	Staged/10-day trip	10th day	sPAP	RV-E′, RV-A′	TAPSE, RV-S′	RV-EDA, RV-ESA
Dedobbeleer et al., 2015	25 (13/12)	31 ± 13	Healthy	Brussels (13)	Cerro de Pasco (4,350)	Staged/4 days	4th day	TRG, mPAP, PVR		TAPSE, RV-S′, RV-FAC, RV-MPI	
Hilty et al., 2016	7 (7/0)	26.6 ± 1.4	Healthy	Zurich (488)	Jungfraujoch (3,454)	Direct/24 h (train)	2nd, 10th, 18th, and 26th days	sPAP, PVR, PAAT		TAPSE, RV-FAC, RV-MPI	RV-EDA
De Boeck et al., 2018	23 (15/8)	43 ± 9	Healthy	Zurich (450)	Margherita hut (4,559)	(car, climb) (1 night at 3,647 m)	2nd, 3rd, and 4th days	TRG		TAPSE, RV-S′, RV-FAC	RV-EDA, RV-ESA
Maufrais et al., 2017	11 (11/0)	28 ± 8	Healthy	Grenoble (212)	Mont Blanc (4,350)	Direct/3 ± 2 h (helicopter)	0.5th, 2nd, 4th, and 6th days	sPAP, TRG, PVR	RV-E, RV-A, RV-E/A, RV-E′, RV-A′	TAPSE, RV-S′, RV-FAC, RV-FWLS	RV-EDA, RV-ESA

(Continued)

TABLE 2 | Continued

Study	Sample size (M/F)	Age (mean ± SD or mean (range) years)	Health status	Baseline altitude (m)	High altitude location (altitude in m)	Ascent mode/duration of ascent	High altitude measurement timepoints	Pulmonary hemodynamics parameters	RV diastolic functional parameters	RV systolic functional parameters	RV structural parameters
Qiu et al., 2017	123 (123/0)	23.77 ± 4.5	Healthy	Chengdu (500)	Lhasa (3,700)	Direct/2 h (airplane)	1st day	mPAP		RV-MPI	
Berger et al., 2018	17 (11/6)	36 ± 12	Healthy	Salzburg (423)	Monte Rosa (4,559)	20 h (car, climb), 1 night at 3,611 m	7th, 20th, 32nd, 44th h	sPAP		TAPSE, RV-S′, RV-FAC, RV-MPI	
Hilty et al., 2019	41 (22/19)	45.8 ± 11.9	Healthy	Bern (553)	C2 (6,022 m), C3 (7,042)	Staged/1 week (by foot)	8th (n = 36), and 15th (n = 15) days	TRG		TAPSE	
Maufrais et al., 2019	20 (29/0)	39 ± 16	Healthy	Bangor (65)	Larkyu (5,085)	Staged/10-day trip	10th day	sPAP	RV-E, RV-A, RV-E/A, RV-E‘, RV-A′	TAPSE, RV-S′, RV-FAC	
Stembridge et al., 2019	12 (12/0)	27 ± 6	Healthy	Kelowna (344)	Barcroft Laboratory (3,800)	Direct (9–10 h in motor vehicle)	5–10th days	sPAP, PVR	RV-E, RV-A, RV-E/A	RV-FAC, RV-GLS	RV-EDA, RV-ESA
(Young) (Stewart et al., 2020)	14 (8/6)	32 ± 5	Healthy	Moshi (880)	Shira (3,100), Barafu (4,800)	Staged/3 days	3rd (3,100 m), and 8th (4,800 m) days	RVSP, mPAP, PVR	RV-E′, RV-A′, RV-E′/A′,	TAPSE, RV-S′, RV-FAC	RV-EDA, RV-ESA
(Old) (Stewart et al., 2020)	13 (8/5)	59 ± 5	Healthy	Moshi (880)	Shira (3,100), Barafu (4,800)	Staged/3 days	3rd (3,100 m), 8th (4,800 m) days	RVSP, mPAP, PVR	RV-E′, RV-A′, RV-E′/A′,	TAPSE, RV-S′, RV-FAC	RV-EDA, RV-ESA
Tian et al., 2020	240 (240/0)		Healthy	Chongqing (500)	Litang (4,100)	Staged/7 days (bus)	5th day	sPAP, mPAP, PAAT/ET	RV-E, RV-A, RV-E/A, RV-E′	RV-S′, RV-FAC, RV-MPI	RV-EDAI, RV-ESAI
Yang et al., 2020b	121 (121/0)	20 (19, 21)	Healthy	Chongqing (400)	Litang (4,100)	Staged/7 days (bus)	1st day	sPAP, mPAP, PAWP, PVR	RV-E/A, RV-E′	RV-S′, RV-FAC	RV-EDA, RV-ESA
Yang et al., 2020a	108 (108/0)	20 (19, 22)	Healthy	Chongqing (400)	Litang (4,100)	Staged/7 days (bus)	1st day	sPAP, PAAT, PAAT/ET, mPAP	RV-E/A, RV-E‘,	TAPSE, RV-S′, RV-FAC, RV-GLS	RV-EDA, RV-ESA,
Ewalts et al., 2021	10 (10/0)	27 ± 6	Healthy	Kelowna (344)	Barcroft Laboratory (3,800)	Direct (9–10 h in motor vehicle)	5–10th days	TRV, sPAP, mPAP, PVR		RV-FAC, RV-GLS	RV-EDA, RV-ESA,
Sareban et al., 2020	50 (50/0)	36 ± 11	Healthy	Sulzburg (424)	Monte Rosa (4,559)	20 h (car, climb) (1 night at 3,611 m)	7th, 20th, 44th h	sPAP		TAPSE, RV-S′, RV-FAC, RV-MPI, RV-GLS	RV-EDA, RV-ESA, RVD1, RVD2, RVD3
(Indians) (Gaur et al., 2021)	10 (10/0)	23.8 ± 2.1	Healthy	Bishkek (800)	Sook Pass (4,111)	Direct/3 h (car)	3rd, 7th, 14th, 21st days	PVR, TRG	RV-E, RV-A, RV-E/A, RV-E′, RV-A′, RV-E′/A′	TAPSE, RV-S′, RV-MPI	RVD1, RVD2, RVD3
(Kyrgyz) (Gaur et al., 2021)	20 (20/0)	22.6 ± 2.1	Healthy	Bishkek (800)	Sook Pass (4,111)	Direct/3 h (car)	3rd, 7th, 14th, 21st days	PVR, TRG	RV-E, RV-A, RV-E/A, RV-E′, RV-A′, RV-E′/A′	TAPSE, RV-S′, RV-MPI	RVD1, RVD2, RVD3

(Continued)

TABLE 2 | Continued

Study	Sample size (M/F)	Age (mean ± SD or mean (range) years)	Health status	Baseline altitude (m)	High altitude location (altitude in m)	Ascent mode/duration of ascent	High altitude measurement timepoints	Pulmonary hemodynamics parameters	RV diastolic functional parameters	RV systolic functional parameters	RV structural parameters
He et al., 2021	82 (82/0)	20 (19–21)	Healthy	Anggongqiao (400)	Litang (4,100)	Direct/Staged/7-day trip	5 ± 2 h	sPAP, TRG	RV-E, RV-A, RV-E/A, RV-E′, RV-A′, RV-E′/A′		RV-EDAI, RV-ESAI
Lichtblau et al., 2021	21 (8/13)	25 (21–28)	Healthy	Chile (520)	ALMA (5,050)	Staged/Car, walk, 1 night at 2,900 m	4–8 h	sPAP, TRG, PVR		TAPSE, RV-FAC	
Yuan et al., 2021	99 (69/30)	25 (21.3, 29)	Healthy	Chengdu (500)	Litang (4,100)	Staged/2 days (bus)	1st day	sPAP, mPAP, PAAT, PAAT/ET, PVR, PAWP	RV-E, RV-A, RV-E/A, RV-E′	TAPSE, RV-S′, RV-FAC, RV-GLS	RV-EDA, RV-ESA, RVD1, RVD2

TRG, tricuspid regurgitation gradient; sPAP, systolic pulmonary artery pressure; mPAP, mean pulmonary artery pressure; PAAT, pulmonary artery acceleration time; PAAT/ET, pulmonary acceleration time to ejection time ratio; PAWP, pulmonary artery wedge pressure; PVR, pulmonary vascular resistance; RV-E, tricuspid inflow early diastolic velocity; RV-A, tricuspid inflow late diastolic velocity; RV-E/A, tricuspid inflow early diastolic velocity to late diastolic velocity; RV-E′, tricuspid annulus early diastolic velocity by tissue Doppler imaging; RV-A′, tricuspid annulus late diastolic velocity by tissue Doppler imaging; RV-E′/A′, tissue Doppler early and late diastolic tricuspid velocities ratio; RV-S′, peak systolic velocity with tissue Doppler imaging at the tricuspid annulus; TAPSE, tricuspid annular plane systolic excursion, RV-MPI, right ventricular myocardial performance index; RV-FAC, right ventricular fractional area change; RV-EDA, right ventricular end-diastolic area; RV-ESA, right ventricular end-systolic area; RV-EDAI, right ventricular end-diastolic area index; RV-ESAI, right ventricular end-systolic area index; RVD1, right ventricular end-diastolic basal cavity dimension; RVD2, right ventricular end-diastolic mid cavity dimension; RVD3, right ventricular end-diastolic longitudinal dimension; RV-GLS, right ventricular global longitudinal strain.

aims to evaluate the RV responses to acute simulated altitude exposure and high-altitude ascent in healthy lowland individuals.

METHODS

Data Sources and Search Strategy

A comprehensive literature search for the relevant articles was performed between January 2005 and May 2021 using online databases PubMed and Web of Science. The aim was to identify studies investigating the effects of acute simulated altitude or high-altitude exposure on RV systolic and diastolic function and morphologic parameters in healthy lowland adults. The search strategy was implemented using the following Boolean operators (AND/OR) and terms: "right ventricular function" OR "right ventricular dysfunction" OR "cardiac function" AND healthy subjects OR healthy individuals OR humans AND "echocardiography" OR "ultrasound imaging" AND hypoxia exposure OR "high altitude" OR hypoxia chamber OR hypoxia room. The search was refined by applying the limits "Humans" and "All adult: +19 years" in PubMed and searching within the subject areas of physiology, respiratory system, cardiovascular system and cardiology in the Web of Science. The exact search terms and Boolean operators used in PubMed and Web of Science are provided in the **Supplementary Material**. Additionally, manual searches were conducted using Google Scholar and reference lists of the eligible articles to retrieve further articles.

Inclusion and Exclusion Criteria

The inclusion criteria for the relevant studies were: (1) involving healthy lowland subjects aged ≥19 years that had not been exposed to altitudes over 2,500 m in the last 3 weeks before study inclusion; (2) simulated altitude or high-altitude field studies at elevations of 2,500 m and over; (3) reporting at least one of the echocardiographic parameters of the RV systolic or diastolic function or its morphology with numerical values or plots with indicated statistical changes; (4) measurements were performed at baseline (see level with normoxia breathing) and after hypoxia exposure for 15 min up to 1 month; (5) full-text in English; and (6) human subjects. Exclusion criteria were: (1) not reporting measurement results at baseline or after hypoxia exposure; (2) studies with unclear design; (3) case reports, reviews, abstracts, and editorials.

Study Selection and Data Extraction

Two authors (Argen Mamazhakypov and Meerim Sartmyrzaeva) independently screened the retrieved articles by titles and abstracts according to the inclusion and exclusion criteria. Then, the full-texts of the relevant articles were obtained, and the same two authors independently screened the full-text of the articles. Disagreements were resolved by discussions between all the authors.

Two authors (Argen Mamazhakypov and Meerim Sartmyrzaeva) independently extracted the following data (**Tables 1, 2**): publication details (authors, publication year), sample characteristics (sample size, gender, age), hypoxia exposure profile (simulated altitude or high-altitude field

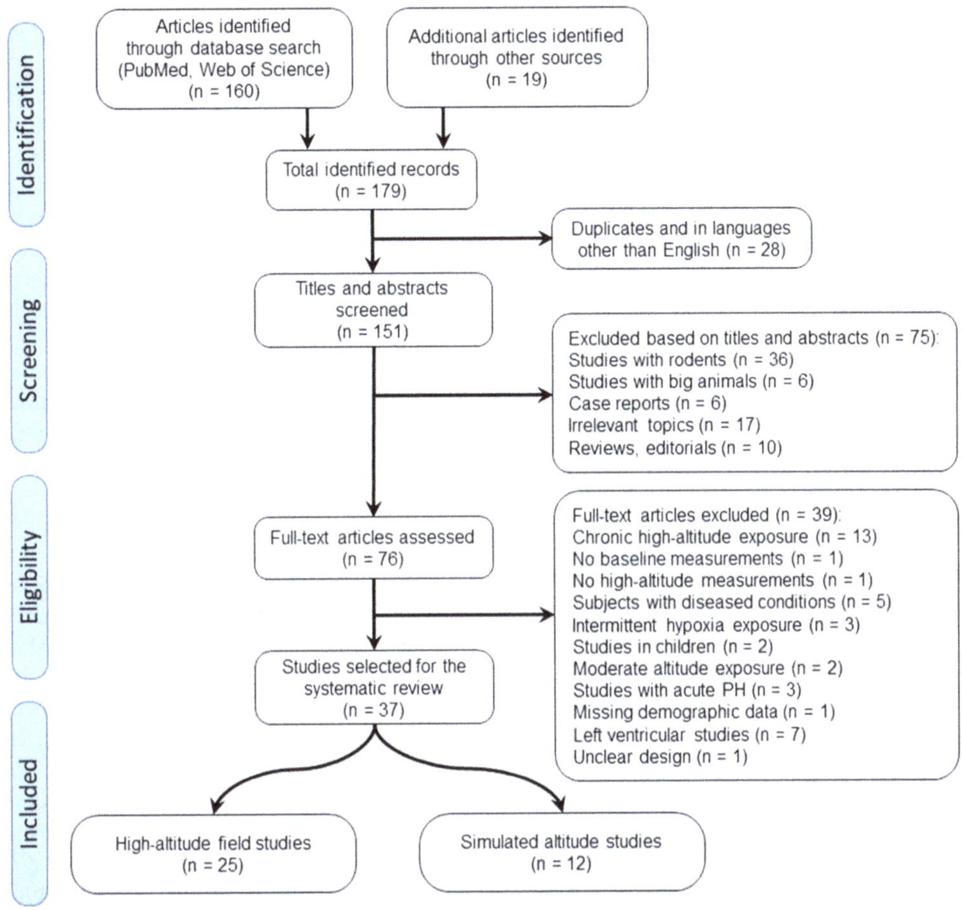

FIGURE 1 | Flow chart representation of literature search.

study, hypoxia exposure duration, altitude elevation), mode of ascent (staged acclimatization or without pre-acclimatization), and summarized the outcome measures (RV function and morphology parameters) and the changes in RV parameters upon simulated altitude or high-altitude exposure (**Tables 4, 6**).

RESULTS

Study Selection

Using electronic searches of the databases PubMed and Web of Science, the initial search retrieved 160 records. Additional 19 articles were identified through other sources. After excluding duplicates and articles in languages other than English, we screened the remaining 151 articles by their title and abstract and excluded animal experiments, case reports, review articles, editorials, conference abstracts and articles on irrelevant topics. The remaining 76 records were evaluated for eligibility by full-text assessment, of which 37 studies fulfilled the inclusion criteria and thus were selected for systematic review. The selection process is shown in the PRISMA flow diagram in **Figure 1**.

Study Characteristics

The characteristics of the selected 37 studies are summarized in **Tables 1, 2**. The studies differed in their design (e.g., mode of ascent, altitude level, and measurement time-points at high-altitude), simulated altitude characteristics (e.g., hypoxia breathing, normobaric or hypobaric hypoxia chamber exposure), reported RV parameters, and subject characteristics (number, gender, and age). The marked methodological heterogeneity across these studies and the small number of papers prevented meta-analysis. Hence, we provide a descriptive analysis of the results.

According to the mode of hypoxia exposure the selected studies were divided into simulated altitude and high-altitude field studies. Twelve studies exploited simulated altitude using normobaric or hypobaric hypoxia chambers or hypoxia breathing, and 25 studies were conducted in high-altitude field conditions.

Effects of Simulated Altitude on the Right Ventricle

Twelve studies explored effects of simulated altitude and included a total of 199 healthy adults (Huez et al., 2005; Kjaergaard

TABLE 3 | Echocardiographic parameters assessed in acute simulated altitude studies.

Studies	Diastolic function						Systolic function					Morphology				
	RV-E	RV-A	RV-E/A	RV-E′	RV-A′	RV- E′/A′	RV-S′	TAPSE	RV-FAC	RV-MPI	RV-GLS	RVD1	RVD2	RVD3	RV-EDA	RV-ESA
Huez et al., 2005			✓	✓	✓	✓	✓	✓							✓	
Kjaergaard et al., 2007				✓	✓		✓	✓	✓	✓					✓	
Reichenberger et al., 2007								✓		✓						
Hanaoka et al., 2011										✓						
Pavelescu and Naeije, 2012			✓	✓	✓	✓	✓	✓	✓							
Goebel et al., 2013			✓					✓								
Boos et al., 2013	✓	✓	✓	✓			✓	✓		✓						
Boos et al., 2016								✓								
Seccombe et al., 2017								✓	✓	✓						
Netzer et al., 2017				✓	✓		✓	✓		✓		✓	✓	✓	✓	
Pezzuto et al., 2018							✓	✓	✓						✓	
Ewalts et al., 2021									✓		✓				✓	✓

✓ Indicates that the echocardiographic parameter was provided in the corresponding studies; empty cell indicate that the echocardiographic parameter is not provided in the corresponding studies.

et al., 2007; Reichenberger et al., 2007; Hanaoka et al., 2011; Pavelescu and Naeije, 2012; Boos et al., 2013, 2016; Goebel et al., 2013; Netzer et al., 2017; Seccombe et al., 2017; Pezzuto et al., 2018; Ewalts et al., 2021). Study participants were exposed to various degrees of hypoxia from 9.9 to 12.5% fraction of inspired oxygen (FiO_2), which correspond to altitude levels ranging from 4,000 to 5,500 m. Altitude was simulated by either hypobaric or normobaric hypoxic chamber exposure or hypoxia breathing. Duration of the hypoxia exposure varied from 15 to 150 min. In the majority of the studies, a single echocardiography investigation was performed at high altitude, but in few of them, serial investigations were done. Echocardiographic parameters assessed systolic and diastolic RV function and RV morphology. The summary of the assessed RV parameters is presented in **Table 3** and the changes of the parameters upon hypoxia exposure are summarized in **Table 4**.

Right Ventricular Systolic Function

In all of the studies, at least one of the following RV systolic function parameters was reported: tricuspid annular plane systolic excursion (TAPSE), RV fractional area change (RV-FAC), tissue Doppler-derived peak tricuspid annulus systolic velocity (RV-S′), RV myocardial performance index (RV-MPI) and RV global longitudinal strain (RV-GLS). The most frequently measured RV systolic parameter was TAPSE, which was evaluated in 10 studies (Huez et al., 2005; Kjaergaard et al., 2007; Reichenberger et al., 2007; Pavelescu and Naeije, 2012; Boos et al., 2013, 2016; Goebel et al., 2013; Netzer et al., 2017; Seccombe et al., 2017; Pezzuto et al., 2018). In 7 of these studies, TAPSE values remained unchanged upon exposure to acute hypoxia (Huez et al., 2005; Pavelescu and Naeije, 2012; Boos et al., 2013, 2016; Goebel et al., 2013; Seccombe et al., 2017; Pezzuto et al., 2018). One study reported significant elevation of TAPSE following 1 h of hypoxia breathing ($FiO_2 = 12.5\%$) suggesting augmented RV function (Kjaergaard et al., 2007). Significantly decreased TAPSE values upon hypoxia breathing ($FiO_2 = 10\%$), suggesting RV systolic dysfunction, were observed in one study (Reichenberger et al., 2007). One more study evaluating TAPSE at several time points over the course of 150 min hypoxia showed that TAPSE decreased after 1 h of hypoxia breathing (Netzer et al., 2017).

Other frequently reported RV systolic function parameters included RV-MPI (Kjaergaard et al., 2007; Reichenberger et al., 2007; Hanaoka et al., 2011; Boos et al., 2013; Netzer et al., 2017; Seccombe et al., 2017) and RV-S′ (Huez et al., 2005; Kjaergaard et al., 2007; Pavelescu and Naeije, 2012; Boos et al., 2013; Netzer et al., 2017; Pezzuto et al., 2018), which were evaluated in 6 studies each. RV-MPI was not changed in 3 studies (Kjaergaard et al., 2007; Boos et al., 2013; Seccombe et al., 2017), while its values were significantly increased in one study (Reichenberger et al., 2007). In addition, RV-MPI values increased in subjects susceptible to HAPE (Hanaoka et al., 2011) and in those who were exposed to hypoxia for more than 100 min (Netzer et al., 2017). RV-S′ values remained unchanged in 4 studies (Huez et al., 2005; Kjaergaard et al., 2007; Pavelescu and Naeije, 2012; Pezzuto et al., 2018) and were increased in one study (Boos et al., 2013) or decreased in another study after 1 h hypoxia exposure (Netzer

TABLE 4 | Summary of the studies evaluating the impact of simulated altitude exposure on the right ventricle.

Study	Subjects (n)	Measurement points (minutes or hours)	FiO_2 (%)	Equivalent altitude (m)	Systolic function parameters	Diastolic function parameters	Morphology parameters
Huez et al., 2005	25	90 min	12	4,500	↔ RV-FS, ↔ TAPSE, ↔ RV-S′	↓ RV-E/A, ↔ RV-E′, ↑ RV-A′, ↓ RV-E′/A′	↔ RV-EDA,
Kjaergaard et al., 2007	14	1 h	12.5	4,200	↑ TAPSE, ↔ RV-FAC, ↔ RV-S′, ↔ RV-MPI	↔ RV-E′, ↔ RV-A′	↔ RV-EDA,
Reichenberger et al., 2007	14	2 h	10	4,500	↑ RV-MPI, ↓ TAPSE		
(HAPE-s) (Hanaoka et al., 2011)	11	30 min	NA	4,000	↑ RV-MPI		
(HAPE-r) (Hanaoka et al., 2011)	9	30 min	NA	4,000	↔ RV-MPI		
Pavelescu and Naeije, 2012	10	2 h	12	4,500	↔ RV-FAC, ↔ TAPSE, ↔ RV-S′	↓ RV-E/A, ↔ RV-E′, ↑ RV-A′, ↓RV-E′/A′	↔ RV-EDA
Goebel et al., 2013	14	2 h	9.9	5,500	↔ TAPSE, ↑ RV-strain		
Boos et al., 2013	14	≥150 min	11.4	4,800	↔ TAPSE, ↑ RV-S′, ↔ RV-MPI	↔ RV-E, ↔ RV-A, ↔ RV-E/A, ↔ RV-E′, ↑ RV-A′	
(Females) (Boos et al., 2016)	7	≥150 min	11.4	4,800	↔ TAPSE		
(Males) (Boos et al., 2016)	7	≥150 min	11.4	4,800	↔ TAPSE		
Seccombe et al., 2017	7	20 min	15	2,500	↔ RV-FAC, ↔ RV-MPI, ↔ TAPSE		↔ RV-EDA, ↔ RV-ESA
Netzer et al., 2017	35	30 min	10	4,500	↔ RV-MPI, ↔ TAPSE, ↔ RV-S′	↔ RV-E′, ↔ RV-A′	↑ RVD1, ↑ RVD2, ↑ RVD3, ↑ RV-EDA
		60 min	10	4,500	↔ RV-MPI, ↓ TAPSE, ↓ RV-S′	↔ RV-E′, ↔ RV-A′	↑ RVD1, ↑ RVD2, ↑ RVD3, ↑ RV-EDA
		100 min	10	4,500	↑ RV-MPI, ↓ TAPSE, ↓ RV-S′	↔ RV-E′, ↔ RV-A′	↑ RVD1, ↑ RVD2, ↑ RVD3, ↑ RV-EDA
		150 min	10	4,500	↑ RV-MPI, ↓ TAPSE, ↓ RV-S′	↔ RV-E′, ↔ RV-A′	↑ RVD1, ↑ RVD2, ↑ RVD3, ↑ RV-EDA
Pezzuto et al., 2018	17	15 min	12	4,500	↔ TAPSE, ↔ RV-S′, ↔ RV-FAC,		↔ RV-EDA
		30 min	12	4,500	↔ TAPSE, ↔ RV-S′, ↔ RV-FAC,		↔ RV-EDA
		45 min	12	4,500	↔ TAPSE, ↔ RV-S′, ↔ RV-FAC,		↔ RV-EDA
		60 min	12	4,500	↔ TAPSE, ↔ RV-S′, ↔ RV-FAC,		↔ RV-EDA
Ewalts et al., 2021	15	30 min	12	45,00	↔ RV-FAC, ↔ RV-SV, ↔ RV-GLS, ↔ RV-GLSR		↔ RV-EDA, ↔ RV-ESA

↑, *high-altitude values of the measured parameters are significantly increased compared to baseline values;* ↓, *high-altitude values of measured parameters are significantly decreased compared to baseline values;* ↔ *high-altitude values of measured parameters are not changed significantly compared to baseline values.*

TABLE 5 | Echocardiographic parameters assessed in acute high-altitude exposure studies.

Studies	Diastolic function						Systolic function					Morphology				
	RV-E	RV-A	RV-E/A	RV-E′	RV-A′	RV-E′/A′	RV-S′	TAPSE	RV-FAC	RV-MPI	RV-GLS	RVD1	RVD2	RVD3	RV-EDA	RV-ESA
Huez et al., 2009	✓	✓		✓	✓	✓	✓	✓		✓						
de Vries et al., 2010				✓				✓								
Pratali et al., 2010								✓								
Page et al., 2013			✓				✓	✓		✓	✓					
Boos et al., 2014	✓			✓			✓									
Stembridge et al., 2014				✓	✓		✓	✓			✓				✓	✓
Dedobbeleer et al., 2015							✓	✓	✓	✓						
Hilty et al., 2016								✓	✓	✓					✓	✓
De Boeck et al., 2018							✓	✓							✓	✓
Qiu et al., 2017										✓						
Maufrais et al., 2017	✓	✓	✓	✓	✓		✓	✓	✓		✓				✓	✓
Berger et al., 2018							✓	✓	✓	✓						
Hilty et al., 2019								✓								
Stembridge et al., 2019	✓	✓	✓						✓		✓				✓	✓
Maufrais et al., 2019	✓	✓	✓	✓	✓		✓	✓	✓							
Sareban et al., 2020							✓	✓	✓	✓	✓	✓	✓	✓	✓	✓
Stewart et al., 2020				✓	✓	✓	✓	✓	✓						✓	✓
Yang et al., 2020b			✓	✓			✓		✓						✓	✓
Yang et al., 2020a			✓	✓			✓	✓	✓		✓				✓	
Tian et al., 2020	✓	✓	✓	✓			✓		✓	✓					✓	✓
Ewalts et al., 2021									✓		✓				✓	✓
Gaur et al., 2021	✓	✓	✓	✓	✓	✓	✓	✓		✓		✓	✓	✓		
Yuan et al., 2021	✓	✓	✓	✓			✓	✓	✓		✓	✓	✓		✓	✓
He et al., 2021	✓	✓	✓	✓	✓	✓	✓		✓						✓	✓
Lichtblau et al., 2021								✓	✓							

✓Indicates that the echocardiographic parameter was provided in the corresponding studies; empty cell indicate that the echocardiographic parameter is not provided in the corresponding studies.

TABLE 6 | Summary of the studies evaluating the impact of high-altitude exposure on the right ventricle.

Study	Measurement timepoints (hours or days)	Altitude (m)	Systolic function parameters	Diastolic function parameters	Morphology parameters
Huez et al., 2009	1 day	3,750	↔ RV-S′, ↔ TAPSE, ↑ RV-MPI	↓ RV-E, ↔ RV-A, ↓ RV-E/A, ↔ RV-E′, ↔ RV-A′, ↔ RV-E′/A′	
	10 days	4,850	↔ RV-S′, ↔TAPSE, ↑ RV-MPI	↓ RV-E, ↔ RV-A, ↓ RV-E/A, ↔ RV-E′, ↔ RV-A′, ↔ RV-E′/A′	
de Vries et al., 2010	10 days	4,200	↓ TAPSE	↔RV-E′	
Pratali et al., 2010	6 days	3,440	↔ TAPSE		
	15 days	5,130	↔ TAPSE		
Page et al., 2013	4 days	3,450	↔ RV-S′, ↔ TAPSE, ↑ RV-MPI, ↔ RV-GLS	↓ RV-E/A	
	7 days	4,730	↔ RV-S′, ↔ TAPSE, ↑ RV-MPI, ↔ RV-GLS	↓ RV-E/A	
Boos et al., 2014	2 days	3,440	↔ RV-S′	↔ RV-E, ↔RV-E′	
	6 days	4,270	↔ RV-S′	↔ RV-E, ↔RV-E′	
	9 days	5,150	↔ RV-S′	↔ RV-E, ↔RV-E′	
Stembridge et al., 2014	10 days	5,050	↓ TAPSE, ↔ RV-S′, ↓ RV-GLS	↔ RV-E′, ↔ RV-A′	↔ RV-EDA, ↔ RV-ESA
Dedobbeleer et al., 2015	4 days	4,350	↔ RV-S′, ↓ TAPSE, ↑ RV-MPI, ↔ RV-FAC		
Hilty et al., 2016	2–3 days	3,454	↔ TAPSE, ↔ RV-FAC, ↑ RV-MPI		↔ RV-EDA
	8–10 days	3,454	↔ TAPSE, ↔ RV-FAC, ↑ RV-MPI		↔ RV-EDA
	17–18 days	3,454	↔ TAPSE, ↔ RV-FAC, ↑ RV-MPI		↔ RV-EDA
	26–27 days	3,454	↔ TAPSE, ↔ RV-FAC, ↑ RV-MPI		↔ RV-EDA
De Boeck et al., 2018	3 days	4,559	↔ RV-FAC, ↔ RV-S′, ↔ TAPSE		↑ RV-EDA, ↑ RV-ESA
	4 days	4,559	↔ RV-FAC, ↑ RV-S′, ↔ TAPSE		↔ RV-EDA, ↔ RV-ESA
Qiu et al., 2017	1 day	3,700	↑ RV-MPI		
Maufrais et al., 2017	0.5 days	4,350	↔ RV-FAC, ↔ TAPSE, ↔ RV-S′, ↔ RV-GLS	↔ RV-E, ↑RV-A, ↓ RV-E/A, ↑ RV-E′, ↑ RV-A′	↔ RV-EDA, ↔ RV-ESA
	2 days	4,350	↔ RV-FAC, ↔ TAPSE, ↔ RV-S′, ↔ RV-GLS	↔ RV-E, ↔RV-A, ↓ RV-E/A, ↔RV-E′, ↑ RV-A′	↔ RV-EDA, ↔ RV-ESA
	4 days	4,350	↔ RV-FAC, ↔ TAPSE, ↔ RV-S′, ↔ RV-GLS	↔ RV-E, ↔RV-A, ↓ RV-E/A, ↔RV-E′, ↔RV-A′,	↔ RV-EDA, ↔ RV-ESA
	6 days	4,350	↔ RV-FAC, ↔ TAPSE, ↔ RV-S′, ↔ RV-GLS	↔ RV-E, ↔RV-A, ↓ RV-E/A, ↔RV-E′, ↔RV-A′	↔ RV-EDA, ↔ RV-ESA

(Continued)

TABLE 6 | Continued

Study	Measurement timepoints (hours or days)	Altitude (m)	Systolic function parameters	Diastolic function parameters	Morphology parameters
Berger et al., 2018	7 h	4,559	↑ TAPSE, ↔ RV-MPI, ↑ RV-S′, ↔ RV-FAC		
	20 h	4,559	↑ TAPSE, ↔ RV-MPI ↑ RV-S′, ↔ RV-FAC		
	44 h	4,559	↑ TAPSE, ↔ RV-MPI ↑ RV-S′, ↔ RV-FAC		
Stembridge et al., 2019	5–10 days	3,800	↔ RV-FAC, ↔ RV-GLS	↔ RV-E, ↔RV-A, ↔ RV-E/A	↔ RV-EDA, ↔ RV-ESA
Maufrais et al., 2019	10 days	5,058	↔ RV-FAC, ↔ TAPSE, ↑ RV-S′, ↔ RV-GLS	↔ RV-E, ↑ RV-A, ↓ RV-E/A, ↔ RV-A′, ↔RV-E′,↔ RV-E′/A′	
Hilty et al., 2019	8 days	6,022	↓ TAPSE		
	15 days	7,042	↔ TAPSE		
Ewalts et al., 2021	5–10 days	3,800	↔ RV-FAC, ↔ RV-SV, ↔ RV-GLS		↔ RV-EDA, ↔ RV-ESA
Tian et al., 2020	5 days	4,100	↓ RV-FAC, ↔ RV-S′, ↑ RV-MPI	↓ RV-E, ↓ RV-A, ↓ RV-E/A, ↔ RV-E′	↓ RV-EDAI, ↔ RV-ESAI
Yang et al., 2020b	1 day	4,100	↓ RV-FAC, ↔ RV-S′,	↓ RV-E/A, ↔RV-E′	↔ RV-EDA, ↔ RV-ESA
Yang et al., 2020a	1 day	4,100	↓ RV-FAC, ↓ TAPSE, ↔ RV-S′, ↓ RV-GLS,	↓ RV-E/A, ↔RV-E′,	↓ RV-EDA, ↔ RV-ESA
(Young) (Stewart et al., 2020)	3 days	3,100	↓ RV-FAC, ↔ RV-S′, ↓TAPSE	↔ RV-A′, ↔RV-E′, ↔ RV-E′/A′	↑ RV-EDA, ↑ RV-ESA
	8 days	4,800	↓ RV-FAC, ↑ RV-S′, ↓TAPSE	↑ RV-A′, ↔RV-E′, ↓ RV-E′/A′	↑ RV-EDA, ↑ RV-ESA
(Old) (Stewart et al., 2020)	3 days	3,00	↓ RV-FAC, ↑ RV-S′, ↓TAPSE	↑ RV-A′, ↔RV-E′, ↓ RV-E′/A′	↑ RV-EDA, ↑ RV-ESA
	8 days	4,800	↓ RV-FAC, ↑ RV-S′, ↓TAPSE	↑ RV-A′, ↔RV-E′, ↓ RV-E′/A′	↑ RV-EDA, ↑ RV-ESA
Sareban et al., 2020	7 h	4,559	↔ TAPSE, ↔ RV-FAC, ↑ RV-S′, ↔ RV-MPI, ↔ RV-GLS		↔ RVD1, ↔ RVD2, ↔ RVD3, ↔ RV-EDA, ↔ RV-ESA
	20 h	4,559	↑ TAPSE, ↔ RV-FAC, ↑ RV-S′, ↔ RV-MPI, ↔ RV-GLS		↔ RVD1, ↔ RVD2, ↔ RVD3, ↔ RV-EDA, ↔ RV-ESA
	44 h	4,559	↔ TAPSE, ↔ RV-FAC, ↑ RV-S′, ↔ RV-MPI, ↔ RV-GLS		↔ RVD1, ↔ RVD2, ↔ RVD3, ↔ RV-EDA, ↔ RV-ESA
(Kyrgyz) (Gaur et al., 2021)	3 days	4,111	↔ TAPSE, ↔ RV-S′, ↔ RV-MPI	↔ RV-A, ↔ RV-E, ↔ RV-E/A, ↔ RV-E′, ↔ RV-A′, ↔ RV-E′/A′	↔ RVD1, ↔ RVD2, ↔ RVD3
	7 days	4,111	↔ TAPSE, ↔ RV-S′, ↔ RV-MPI	↔ RV-A, ↔ RV-E, ↔ RV-E/A, ↔ RV-E′, ↔ RV-A′, ↔ RV-E′/A′	↔ RVD1, ↔ RVD2, ↔ RVD3
	14 days	411	↔ TAPSE, ↔ RV-S′, ↔ RV-MPI	↔ RV-A, ↔ RV-E, ↔ RV-E/A, ↔ RV-E′, ↓ RV-A′, ↔ RV-E′/A′	↔ RVD1, ↔ RVD2, ↔ RVD3
	21 days	4,111	↓ TAPSE, ↔ RV-S′, ↔ RV-MPI	↔ RV-A, ↔ RV-E, ↔ RV-E/A, ↓ RV-E′, ↓ RV-A′, ↔ RV-E′/A′	↔ RVD1, ↔ RVD2, ↔ RVD3

(Continued)

TABLE 6 | Continued

Study	Measurement timepoints (hours or days)	Altitude (m)	Systolic function parameters	Diastolic function parameters	Morphology parameters
(Indians) (Gaur et al., 2021)	3 days	4,111	↔ TAPSE, ↔ RV-S′, ↔ RV-MPI	↔ RV-A, ↔ RV-E, ↔ RV-E/A, ↔ RV-E′, ↔ RV-A′, ↔ RV-E′/A′	↔ RVD1, ↔ RVD2, ↔ RVD3
	7 days	4,111	↔ TAPSE, ↔ RV-S′, ↔ RV-MPI	↔ RV-A, ↔ RV-E, ↔ RV-E/A, ↓ RV-E′, ↔ RV-A′, ↔ RV-E′/A′	↔ RVD1, ↔ RVD2, ↔ RVD3
	14 days	4,111	↓ TAPSE, ↔ RV-S′, ↔ RV-MPI	↔ RV-A, ↓ RV-E, ↔ RV-E/A, ↓ RV-E′,↔ RV-A′, ↔ RV-E′/A′	↔ RVD1, ↔ RVD2, ↔ RVD3
	21 days	4,111	↔ TAPSE, ↔ RV-S′, ↔ RV-MPI	↔ RV-A, ↔ RV-E, ↔ RV-E/A, ↓ RV-E′, ↔ RV-A′, ↔ RV-E′/A′	↔ RVD1, ↔ RVD2, ↔ RVD3
He et al., 2021	5–2 h	4,100	↓ RV-FAC, ↔ RV-S′	↓ RV-E, ↓ RV-A, ↓ RV-E/A, ↔RV-E′, ↓ RV-A′	↓ RV-EDAI, ↔ RV-ESAI
Lichtblau et al., 2021	4–8 h	5,050	↔ TAPSE, ↔ RV-FAC		
Yuan et al., 2021	15 ± 3 h	4,100	↓ TAPSE, ↓ RV-FAC, ↑ RV-S′, ↓ RV-GLS	↓ RV-E, ↑ RV-A, ↓ RV-E/A, ↔ RV-E′	↔ RVD1, ↑ RVD2, ↔ RV-EDA, ↔ RV-EDA

↑, high-altitude values are significantly increased compared to baseline values; ↓, high-altitude values are significantly decreased compared to baseline values; ↔ high-altitude values are not changed significantly compared to baseline values.

et al., 2017). RV-GLS was evaluated in 2 studies and showed opposite results (Goebel et al., 2013; Ewalts et al., 2021).

Right Ventricular Diastolic Function

In 6 studies, at least one of the following RV diastolic function parameters was reported: early diastolic tricuspid inflow velocity (RV-E), late diastolic tricuspid inflow velocity (RV-A), early-to-late diastolic tricuspid inflow velocities ratio (RV-E/A), tissue Doppler-derived early diastolic tricuspid annular velocity (RV-E′), tissue Doppler-derived late diastolic tricuspid annular velocity (RV-A′), tissue Doppler-derived early-to-late diastolic tricuspid annular velocities ratio (RV-E′/A′) (Huez et al., 2005; Kjaergaard et al., 2007; Pavelescu and Naeije, 2012; Boos et al., 2013; Goebel et al., 2013; Netzer et al., 2017). The RV diastolic parameters RV-E′ and RV-A′ were assessed in 5 (Huez et al., 2005; Kjaergaard et al., 2007; Pavelescu and Naeije, 2012; Boos et al., 2013; Netzer et al., 2017) and 4 studies (Huez et al., 2005; Kjaergaard et al., 2007; Pavelescu and Naeije, 2012; Netzer et al., 2017), respectively. In all these studies, RV-E′ remained unchanged upon exposure to acute hypoxia. In 3 studies, RV-A′ values increased upon hypoxia exposure suggesting increased right atrial (RA) contribution to the RV filling (Huez et al., 2005; Pavelescu and Naeije, 2012; Boos et al., 2013). Consequently, two studies reported decreased RV-E′/A′ values upon acute hypoxia exposure (Huez et al., 2005; Pavelescu and Naeije, 2012).

Right Ventricular Morphology

Seven of the studies reported at least one of the following RV morphology parameters: RV end diastolic area (RV-EDA), RV end systolic area (RV-ESA), RV basal diameter (RVD1), RV mid diameter (RVD2), RV longitudinal size (RVD3) (Huez et al., 2005; Kjaergaard et al., 2007; Pavelescu and Naeije, 2012; Netzer et al., 2017; Seccombe et al., 2017; Pezzuto et al., 2018; Ewalts et al., 2021). The most frequently evaluated RV morphology parameter RV-EDA was reported in 7 studies (Huez et al., 2005; Kjaergaard et al., 2007; Pavelescu and Naeije, 2012; Netzer et al., 2017; Seccombe et al., 2017; Pezzuto et al., 2018; Ewalts et al., 2021). None of the studies revealed changes in the RV morphology following simulated altitude exposure (Huez et al., 2005; Kjaergaard et al., 2007; Pavelescu and Naeije, 2012; Seccombe et al., 2017; Pezzuto et al., 2018; Ewalts et al., 2021), except one study, which showed RV dilation after 10% oxygen breathing (Netzer et al., 2017).

Effects of High-Altitude Exposure on the Right Ventricle

Twenty-five studies were conducted in high-altitude field conditions and included 1144 healthy adults exposed to altitudes of 3100 to 7042 m (Huez et al., 2009; de Vries et al., 2010; Pratali et al., 2010; Page et al., 2013; Boos et al., 2014; Stembridge et al., 2014, 2019; Dedobbeleer et al., 2015; Hilty et al., 2016, 2019; Maufrais et al., 2017, 2019; Qiu et al., 2017; Berger et al., 2018; De Boeck et al., 2018; Sareban et al., 2020; Stewart et al., 2020; Tian et al., 2020; Yang et al., 2020a,b; Ewalts et al., 2021; Gaur et al., 2021; He et al., 2021; Lichtblau et al., 2021; Yuan et al., 2021). At high-altitude, echocardiographic examinations were conducted at various time points of the sojourn ranging from a few hours to

26 days. In some studies, serial echocardiographic investigations were performed over the course of several days of high-altitude stay (Huez et al., 2009; Page et al., 2013; Boos et al., 2014; Hilty et al., 2016, 2019; Maufrais et al., 2017; Berger et al., 2018; De Boeck et al., 2018; Sareban et al., 2020; Stewart et al., 2020; Gaur et al., 2021). In 3 of them, measurements were taken serially over a progressive altitude increment (Huez et al., 2009; Boos et al., 2014; Stewart et al., 2020). In 12 studies, both male and female subjects were included (Huez et al., 2009; de Vries et al., 2010; Pratali et al., 2010; Page et al., 2013; Boos et al., 2014; Dedobbeleer et al., 2015; Berger et al., 2018; De Boeck et al., 2018; Hilty et al., 2019; Stewart et al., 2020; Lichtblau et al., 2021; Yuan et al., 2021), while in 13 studies participants consisted of male subjects only (Stembridge et al., 2014, 2019; Hilty et al., 2016; Maufrais et al., 2017, 2019; Qiu et al., 2017; Sareban et al., 2020; Tian et al., 2020; Yang et al., 2020a,b; Ewalts et al., 2021; Gaur et al., 2021; He et al., 2021). Mode of ascent also differed significantly between the studies ranging from a rapid transportation to high-altitude by airplanes to a staged acclimatization with spending nights at intermediate altitudes. Echocardiographic examination included assessment of RV systolic and diastolic function and morphology. The summary of the assessed RV parameters is presented in **Table 5** and the changes of the parameters following high-altitude exposure are summarized in **Table 6**.

Right Ventricular Systolic Function

In all studies, at least one of the following RV systolic function parameters was reported: TAPSE, RV-S′, RV-FAC or RV-MPI. In addition, RV free wall or global strain were assessed in 8 studies (Page et al., 2013; Stembridge et al., 2014, 2019; Maufrais et al., 2017; Sareban et al., 2020; Yang et al., 2020a,b; Ewalts et al., 2021). The most frequently reported RV systolic function parameter TAPSE was assessed in 18 studies (Huez et al., 2009; de Vries et al., 2010; Pratali et al., 2010; Page et al., 2013; Stembridge et al., 2014; Dedobbeleer et al., 2015; Hilty et al., 2016, 2019; Maufrais et al., 2017, 2019; Berger et al., 2018; De Boeck et al., 2018; Sareban et al., 2020; Stewart et al., 2020; Yang et al., 2020a; Gaur et al., 2021; Lichtblau et al., 2021; Yuan et al., 2021). In 6 of these studies (de Vries et al., 2010; Stembridge et al., 2014; Dedobbeleer et al., 2015; Maufrais et al., 2019; Lichtblau et al., 2021; Yuan et al., 2021), TAPSE was evaluated once while in others it was measured at two (Huez et al., 2009; Pratali et al., 2010; Page et al., 2013; De Boeck et al., 2018; Hilty et al., 2019; Stewart et al., 2020), or 3 (Berger et al., 2018; Sareban et al., 2020) or 4 (Hilty et al., 2016; Maufrais et al., 2017; Sareban et al., 2020; Gaur et al., 2021) time-points over the course of high altitude acclimatization. Regardless of measured time-points in 8 studies out of 18, TAPSE values were maintained during high-altitude stay suggesting preserved RV systolic function (Huez et al., 2009; Pratali et al., 2010; Page et al., 2013; Hilty et al., 2016; Maufrais et al., 2017, 2019; De Boeck et al., 2018; Lichtblau et al., 2021). Only one study reported increased TAPSE values upon high-altitude exposure (Berger et al., 2018). However, other six studies reported reduced TAPSE values at high-altitude on days 3, 4, 8, 10, 12, and 14 suggesting RV systolic dysfunction (de Vries et al., 2010; Stembridge et al., 2014; Dedobbeleer et al., 2015; Stewart et al., 2020; Yang et al., 2020a; Yuan et al., 2021). In addition, three studies reported inconsistent changes in TAPSE values over the course of high-altitude acclimatization (Hilty et al., 2019; Sareban et al., 2020; Gaur et al., 2021).

Another frequently evaluated RV systolic function parameter RV-S′ was reported in 17 studies (Huez et al., 2009; Page et al., 2013; Boos et al., 2014; Stembridge et al., 2014; Dedobbeleer et al., 2015; Maufrais et al., 2017, 2019; Berger et al., 2018; De Boeck et al., 2018; Sareban et al., 2020; Stewart et al., 2020; Tian et al., 2020; Yang et al., 2020a,b; Gaur et al., 2021; He et al., 2021; Yuan et al., 2021). In 11 studies, RV-S′ values were maintained up to 21 days of high-altitude sojourn suggesting preserved RV systolic function (Huez et al., 2009; Page et al., 2013; Boos et al., 2014; Stembridge et al., 2014; Dedobbeleer et al., 2015; Maufrais et al., 2017; Tian et al., 2020; Yang et al., 2020a,b; Gaur et al., 2021; He et al., 2021). Moreover, in 5 studies, RV-S′ values were significantly increased on days 3, 8, and 10 of high-altitude stay, suggesting enhanced RV performance (Berger et al., 2018; De Boeck et al., 2018; Sareban et al., 2020; Stewart et al., 2020; Yang et al., 2020a; Yuan et al., 2021).

Similarly, no changes in RV-FAC were revealed in 9 studies out of 15 (Dedobbeleer et al., 2015; Hilty et al., 2016; Maufrais et al., 2017; Berger et al., 2018; De Boeck et al., 2018; Stembridge et al., 2019; Sareban et al., 2020; Ewalts et al., 2021; Lichtblau et al., 2021). In contrast, in other 6 studies, decreased RV-FAC upon acute high-altitude induction suggested reduced RV systolic function (Stewart et al., 2020; Tian et al., 2020; Yang et al., 2020a,b; He et al., 2021; Yuan et al., 2021). Maintained RV-MPI over the course of high-altitude stay was reported in 3 studies out of 9 (Berger et al., 2018; Sareban et al., 2020; Gaur et al., 2021). In other 6 studies, elevated RV-MPI values suggested compromised RV function (Huez et al., 2009; Page et al., 2013; Dedobbeleer et al., 2015; Hilty et al., 2016; Qiu et al., 2017; Tian et al., 2020). Unchanged RV-GLS was revealed in 6 studies out of 8 suggesting preserved RV function (Page et al., 2013; Maufrais et al., 2017, 2019; Stembridge et al., 2019; Sareban et al., 2020; Ewalts et al., 2021). Reduced RV-GLS values were reported in other 3 studies (Stembridge et al., 2014; Yang et al., 2020a; Yuan et al., 2021).

Right Ventricular Diastolic Function

Fifteen studies reported at least one of the following RV diastolic function parameters upon high-altitude exposure: RV-E, RV-A, RV-E/A, RV-E′, RV-A′, or RV-E′/A′(Huez et al., 2009; de Vries et al., 2010; Page et al., 2013; Boos et al., 2014; Stembridge et al., 2014, 2019; Maufrais et al., 2017, 2019; Stewart et al., 2020; Tian et al., 2020; Yang et al., 2020a,b; Gaur et al., 2021; He et al., 2021; Yuan et al., 2021). The most frequently evaluated parameter was RV-E′ (Huez et al., 2009; de Vries et al., 2010; Boos et al., 2014; Stembridge et al., 2014; Maufrais et al., 2017, 2019; Stewart et al., 2020; Tian et al., 2020; Yang et al., 2020a,b; Gaur et al., 2021; He et al., 2021; Yuan et al., 2021). In 11 studies out of 13, no changes in RV-E′ values were revealed at various time-points and altitude levels (Huez et al., 2009; de Vries et al., 2010; Boos et al., 2014; Stembridge et al., 2014; Maufrais et al., 2019; Stewart et al., 2020; Tian et al., 2020; Yang et al., 2020a,b; He et al., 2021; Yuan et al., 2021). In one study, RV-E′ values increased at an early time point of high-altitude acclimatization and subsequently returned to baseline values at later stages (Maufrais et al., 2017), while they decreased after 3 weeks of high-altitude stay in another study (Gaur et al., 2021).

Another frequently evaluated diastolic parameter RV-E/A was reported in 11 studies (Huez et al., 2009; Page et al., 2013; Maufrais et al., 2017, 2019; Stembridge et al., 2019; Tian et al., 2020; Yang et al., 2020a,b; Gaur et al., 2021; He et al., 2021; Yuan et al., 2021). RV-E/A was decreased in 9 studies (Huez et al., 2009; Page et al., 2013; Maufrais et al., 2017, 2019; Tian et al., 2020; Yang et al., 2020a,b; He et al., 2021; Yuan et al., 2021) and it was unchanged in two studies (Stembridge et al., 2019; Gaur et al., 2021). In 5 studies out of 9, RV-E values remained unaffected at high-altitude (Boos et al., 2014; Maufrais et al., 2017, 2019; Stembridge et al., 2019; Gaur et al., 2021), and they were significantly reduced in 4 studies (Huez et al., 2009; Tian et al., 2020; He et al., 2021; Yuan et al., 2021). RV-A values were not affected upon high altitude exposure in 3 studies out of 8 (Huez et al., 2009; Stembridge et al., 2019; Gaur et al., 2021) and were reduced in 2 studies (Tian et al., 2020; He et al., 2021). Three studies reported significantly increased RV-A values at high-altitude (Maufrais et al., 2017, 2019; Yuan et al., 2021). RV-E′/A′ was reported in 4 studies, which showed preserved values in 2 studies (Huez et al., 2009; Maufrais et al., 2019) and reduced values in one study (Stewart et al., 2020; Gaur et al., 2021).

Right Ventricular Morphology

Fourteen studies reported at least one of the following RV morphology parameters: RV-EDA, RV-ESA, RVD1, RVD2, or RVD3 (Stembridge et al., 2014, 2019; Hilty et al., 2016; Maufrais et al., 2017; De Boeck et al., 2018; Sareban et al., 2020; Stewart et al., 2020; Tian et al., 2020; Yang et al., 2020a,b; Ewalts et al., 2021; Gaur et al., 2021; He et al., 2021; Yuan et al., 2021). The most frequently reported RV morphology parameters were RV-EDA and RV-ESA (Stembridge et al., 2014, 2019; Hilty et al., 2016; Maufrais et al., 2017; De Boeck et al., 2018; Sareban et al., 2020; Stewart et al., 2020; Tian et al., 2020; Yang et al., 2020a,b; Ewalts et al., 2021; He et al., 2021; Yuan et al., 2021). In some studies, RV-EDA and RV-ESA values were indexed to body surface area (Tian et al., 2020; He et al., 2021). In 8 studies out of 13, RV-EDA values remained unchanged upon high-altitude exposure (Stembridge et al., 2014, 2019; Hilty et al., 2016; Maufrais et al., 2017; Sareban et al., 2020; Yang et al., 2020b; Ewalts et al., 2021; Yuan et al., 2021), while they were increased in 2 (De Boeck et al., 2018; Stewart et al., 2020) and decreased in 3 studies (Tian et al., 2020; Yang et al., 2020a; He et al., 2021). Similarly, high-altitude induction did not alter RV-ESA values in 10 studies (Stembridge et al., 2014, 2019; Maufrais et al., 2017; Sareban et al., 2020; Tian et al., 2020; Yang et al., 2020a,b; Ewalts et al., 2021; He et al., 2021; Yuan et al., 2021) and was associated with increased RV-ESA values in 2 studies (De Boeck et al., 2018; Stewart et al., 2020).

Three studies reported unaltered RVD1 and RVD2 values upon high-altitude exposure (Sareban et al., 2020; Gaur et al., 2021; Yuan et al., 2021). Similarly, RVD3 values remained unchanged at high-altitude in 2 studies (Sareban et al., 2020; Gaur et al., 2021).

DISCUSSION

The present systematic review aimed to analyze the effects of acute altitude simulation and high-altitude exposure on the echocardiography-based RV systolic and diastolic function as well as RV morphology parameters in healthy lowland individuals. Both, simulated altitude and high-altitude field conditions have been used to study the effects of reduced arterial partial oxygen pressure on the RV function and morphology. Literature search identified 37 eligible articles that assessed at least one of the RV echocardiography parameters at sea level and at various time points after hypoxia exposure. Of these, 12 studies were conducted using simulated altitude (Huez et al., 2005; Kjaergaard et al., 2007; Reichenberger et al., 2007; Hanaoka et al., 2011; Pavelescu and Naeije, 2012; Boos et al., 2013, 2016; Goebel et al., 2013; Netzer et al., 2017; Seccombe et al., 2017; Pezzuto et al., 2018; Ewalts et al., 2021) and 25 studies were performed in high-altitude field conditions (Huez et al., 2009; de Vries et al., 2010; Pratali et al., 2010; Page et al., 2013; Boos et al., 2014; Stembridge et al., 2014, 2019; Dedobbeleer et al., 2015; Hilty et al., 2016, 2019; Maufrais et al., 2017, 2019; Qiu et al., 2017; Berger et al., 2018; De Boeck et al., 2018; Sareban et al., 2020; Stewart et al., 2020; Tian et al., 2020; Yang et al., 2020a,b; Ewalts et al., 2021; Gaur et al., 2021; He et al., 2021; Lichtblau et al., 2021; Yuan et al., 2021). The simulated altitude studies have exploited either hypoxic breathing (Huez et al., 2005; Kjaergaard et al., 2007; Hanaoka et al., 2011; Pezzuto et al., 2018; Ewalts et al., 2021) or normobaric hypoxia (Goebel et al., 2013; Boos et al., 2016; Netzer et al., 2017) or hypobaric hypoxia chambers (Boos et al., 2013; Goebel et al., 2013).

Right Ventricular Systolic Function

Only a few studies followed the international guidelines and assessed multiple parameters for the comprehensive RV evaluation (Pavelescu and Naeije, 2012; Boos et al., 2013; Maufrais et al., 2017; Netzer et al., 2017; Stewart et al., 2020; Tian et al., 2020; Yang et al., 2020a; Gaur et al., 2021; Yuan et al., 2021). Most of the studies have evaluated only one or 2 or 3 of the following RV systolic function parameters: TAPSE, RV-S′, RV-FAC, RV-MPI or RV-GLS.

Assessment of multiple parameters revealed inconsistent changes in RV systolic function parameters at different time-points and altitude levels. More specifically, TAPSE and RV-S′ remained unchanged upon exposure to high-altitude in the majority of the studies (Huez et al., 2009; Page et al., 2013; Hilty et al., 2016; Maufrais et al., 2017; Gaur et al., 2021). However, in a few studies, RV function assessed by TAPSE was augmented at earlier time-points of exposure (with 24 h) (Berger et al., 2018; Sareban et al., 2020) and then decreased at later stages of high-altitude stay (Stewart et al., 2020; Gaur et al., 2021). Similarly, RV-S′ values were increased at certain time-points of high-altitude exposure in several studies (Berger et al., 2018; De Boeck et al., 2018; Sareban et al., 2020; Stewart et al., 2020; Yang et al., 2020a). Notably, assessment of RV-FAC and RV-MPI revealed augmented RV systolic function in none of the studies (Huez et al., 2009; Page et al., 2013; Dedobbeleer et al., 2015; Maufrais et al., 2017; Berger et al., 2018; De Boeck et al., 2018; Stembridge et al., 2019; Sareban et al., 2020; Stewart et al., 2020; Tian et al., 2020; Yang et al., 2020a; Ewalts et al., 2021; He et al., 2021; Lichtblau et al., 2021; Yuan et al., 2021). In fact, in several studies, the changes of RV-FAC and RV-MPI values indicated diminished RV systolic function (Huez et al., 2009; Page et al., 2013; Dedobbeleer et al., 2015; Hilty et al., 2016; Qiu et al., 2017; Stewart et al., 2020; Tian et al., 2020; Yang et al., 2020a; He et al., 2021; Yuan et al., 2021). Moreover, serial assessment of the RV systolic function parameters within the same study showed inconsistent changes over the course of high-altitude acclimatization (Sareban et al., 2020; Stewart et al., 2020; Gaur et al., 2021). Taken together, in the majority of the studies conventional echocardiography demonstrated maintained RV systolic function upon acute high-altitude exposure, although with variations in the directions of changes in RV systolic parameters and measurement points over the course of high-altitude acclimatization.

Recently, the advent of speckle-tracking echocardiography and its utilization to assess myocardial strain allowed less angle-dependent and load-independent insights into intrinsic myocardial function (Salvo et al., 2015). Speckle-tracking echocardiography has been shown to be a reliable technique in the analysis of RV myocardial mechanics (Kossaify, 2015). In addition, it enables assessment of additional alterations of myocardial mechanics such as contraction dyssynchrony (Badagliacca et al., 2015). Using this technique, RV dyssynchrony was shown in various cardiopulmonary conditions associated with an increased RV pressure overload (Kalogeropoulos et al., 2008; Badagliacca et al., 2017; Pezzuto et al., 2018). Speckle-tracking echocardiography was utilized to evaluate RV-GLS in two simulated altitude studies (Goebel et al., 2013; Ewalts et al., 2021) and in several high-altitude studies (Page et al., 2013; Maufrais et al., 2017; Stembridge et al., 2019; Sareban et al., 2020; Yang et al., 2020a; Ewalts et al., 2021; Yuan et al., 2021). Although, the RV-GLS values remained unchanged upon hypoxia exposure in most of the studies (Page et al., 2013; Maufrais et al., 2017, 2019; Stembridge et al., 2019; Sareban et al., 2020; Ewalts et al., 2021), three studies demonstrated RV dyssynchrony in healthy adults upon exposure to acute simulated altitude and high-altitude (Pezzuto et al., 2018; Ewalts et al., 2021; Yuan et al., 2021).

Augmented RV afterload predisposes the RV to myocardial dysfunction. Although, there is significant amount of information on the pressure overload-induced RV dysfunction, hypoxia itself induces activation of several molecular pathways that could contribute to RV remodeling and dysfunction (Pena et al., 2020). In addition, preclinical studies have demonstrated that hypoxia can directly exert negative inotropic effects in intact animal preparations (Tucker et al., 1976) and in isolated cardiomyocytes (Silverman et al., 1997). The depressive effects of hypoxia on embryonic mouse cardiomyocytes may be related to hypoxia-inducible factor-1 mediated sarcoplasmic reticulum Ca^{2+}-ATPase downregulation (Ronkainen et al., 2011). Direct negative inotropic effects of hypoxia were corroborated in a recent study that demonstrated preservation of the RV contractile function by improved oxygen delivery to the hypoxic myocardium in lambs exposed to acute hypoxia (Boehme et al., 2018).

Besides the direct effects of hypoxia on the myocardium, reduced venous return due to plasma volume contraction might also be responsible for the RV dyssynchrony as increasing venous return to the right heart alleviates it (Ewalts et al., 2021). In addition, in a recent study, high-altitude-induced RV dyssynchrony was associated with a lower degree of oxygen saturation and higher PAP (Yang et al., 2020a) suggesting its relationship with hypoxemia and increased RV afterload. Interestingly, there were no differences in the conventional echocardiography systolic function parameters between subjects with RV dyssynchrony and those without (Yang et al., 2020a). Taken together, while conventional echocardiography-derived parameters suggest maintained RV systolic function upon exposure to hypoxia, subtle changes can be revealed by speckle-tracking echocardiography. Interestingly, the findings derived by the latter suggested that these changes might be driven not only by increased afterload but also by other factors such as decreased preload and direct effects of hypoxia.

High-altitude exposure causes major changes in various functions of the cardiovascular system (Naeije, 2010). In addition to HPV and an associated increase in PAP and PVR, other initial cardiovascular responses include an increase in cardiac output along with tachycardia (Naeije, 2010). Of note, non-cardiovascular factors might contribute to the cardiovascular responses at high-altitude. For example, previous studies demonstrated plasma volume contraction upon high-altitude exposure (Singh et al., 1990), which can remain below sea level values even for up to 4–6 months above 4,000 m (Pugh, 1964). Reduced plasma volume causes, in turn, alterations in the LV function (Stembridge et al., 2019). These findings are supported by recent studies with plasma volume expansion (Stembridge et al., 2019). In healthy lowlanders, plasma volume expansion during acclimatization to 3,800 m restored LV end-diastolic volume, mitral inflow velocities and stroke volume (Stembridge et al., 2019).

Differences in ethnicity (Gaur et al., 2021), age (Stewart et al., 2020), gender (Boos et al., 2016) and exposure duration (Gaur et al., 2021) and physical activity might account for the discrepancies between the study results. The magnitude of the RV response to high-altitude exposure might also be related to the susceptibility to HAPE. For example, exposure to normobaric hypoxia was associated with RV dysfunction in Japanese HAPE-susceptible subjects, while HAPE-resistant subjects displayed maintained RV function (Hanaoka et al., 2011). In line with these findings, in healthy subjects at high-altitude, the degree of RV dysfunction was associated with subclinical pulmonary edema (Page et al., 2013). Importantly, HAPE-susceptible individuals exhibit an exaggerated HPV and display higher PAP values at high-altitude compared to HAPE-resistant subjects (Hanaoka et al., 2011). There is anecdotal evidence of severe acute hypoxic PH with RV dilatation in a previously healthy lowlander upon arrival to 3,700 m within 24 h (Huez et al., 2007). All these findings suggest that lowland apparently healthy HAPE-susceptible subjects are also prone to develop RV dysfunction, most probably due to an augmented HPV. However, direct effects of the gene-variants associated with HAPE susceptibility on the RV cannot be ruled out yet.

Right Ventricular Diastolic Function

It should be noted that only a few studies followed the international guidelines to evaluate multiple parameters for full characterization of the RV diastolic function. Most of the studies provided only a few RV diastolic function parameters. Thus, 7 out of 12 simulated altitude and 15 out of 24 high-altitude exposure studies reported at least one of the following RV diastolic function parameters: RV-E, RV-A, RV-E/A, RV-E′, RV-A′, and RV-E′/A′.

The most consistent change upon high-altitude exposure was the decrease in RV-E/A (Huez et al., 2009; Page et al., 2013; Maufrais et al., 2017, 2019; Tian et al., 2020; Yang et al., 2020a; He et al., 2021; Yuan et al., 2021). However, in a few studies, RV-E/A values remained unchanged (Stembridge et al., 2019; Gaur et al., 2021). Interestingly, the values of RV-E and RV-A were unaffected in the majority of the studies (Boos et al., 2014; Stembridge et al., 2014, 2019; Maufrais et al., 2017, 2019; Gaur et al., 2021). In contrast to the conventional Doppler echocardiography, only a few studies reported changes of RV-E′, RV-A′, RV-E′/A′ in the TDI-derived RV filling parameters (Huez et al., 2009; de Vries et al., 2010; Boos et al., 2014; Stembridge et al., 2014; Maufrais et al., 2019; Stewart et al., 2020; Tian et al., 2020; Yang et al., 2020a; He et al., 2021; Yuan et al., 2021).

Hypoxia has been shown to alter myocardial relaxation (Tucker et al., 1976; Gibbs, 2007). However, LV and RV intrinsic relaxation estimated by TDI echocardiography derived E′ remained unchanged upon acute exposure to high-altitude suggesting that ventricular early filling may be unaffected by hypoxia (He et al., 2021). Interventricular interaction between the RV and LV may impair LV filling through the septal shift toward the LV due to RV pressure overload (B?rtsch and Gibbs, 2007). Alterations in the traditional LV diastolic function markers such as E/A ratio at high-altitude may not be associated with an impairment in myocardial relaxation but might rather reflect lower LV filling pressure (Holloway et al., 2011). Impairment of the LV relaxation seems less likely because pulmonary capillary wedge pressure, which is considered as a surrogate marker of left atrial pressure, is not elevated upon exposure to high-altitude (Reeves et al., 1987). Moreover, increased LV untwist velocity upon acute high-altitude exposure despite attenuated LV filling (Dedobbeleer et al., 2015; Stembridge et al., 2015; Osculati et al., 2016), suggests preserved or even augmented LV relaxation. Increased sympathetic activation may contribute to the enhanced LV untwisting (Rademakers et al., 1992). Likewise, changes in RV diastolic filling patterns upon hypoxia exposure may develop due to increased RV afterload and sympathetic nervous system activation but not due to altered RV relaxation (Huez et al., 2005, 2009; Naeije, 2010).

Atrial contraction is the final component of the ventricular diastole and contributes ∼15–20% of stroke volume (He et al., 2021), and thus is intricately related to cardiac performance. As atria actively participate in the ventricular filling, atrial function is considered as a part of ventricular diastolic function. Atrial function can be affected by a number of factors such as decreased energy supply and preload, increased afterload, and altered ventricular mechanics observed upon exposure to high-altitude (Yang et al., 2020a; Ewalts et al., 2021; He et al., 2021). However, despite its importance, literature on atrial function at high-altitude remains scarce. Only a few studies evaluated atrial function upon exposure to high-altitude using speckle-tracking echocardiography (Sareban et al., 2020; He et al., 2021). Thus, unchanged left atrial and enhanced RA contractile function was reported a few hours following an ascent to 4,559 m (Sareban et al., 2019, 2020). In contrast, a more recent study revealed a slightly impaired left atrial function and a prominent RA dysfunction at high-altitude (He et al., 2021). More specifically, acute high-altitude exposure led to a decrease of the reservoir and conduit functions of both atria and reduced RA contractility (He et al., 2021). Notably, atrial dyssynchrony occurred only to the RA and was associated with worse RV performance (He et al., 2021). Taken together, in addition to conventional RV diastolic indices, evaluating RA function by means of speckle-tracking echocardiography can provide additional insights into the RV diastolic function in response to high-altitude exposure. However, exploitation of such methods remains underutilized.

Clinical Implication of Acute Hypoxia Induced Right Ventricular Dysfunction

Understanding the physiology of the RV responses to acute hypoxia is important for gaining insights into mechanisms underlying acute RV dysfunction and failure in some diseases encountered at low-altitude. For example, acute RV dysfunction associated with HPV is common during exacerbation of respiratory diseases such as chronic obstructive pulmonary disease and diffuse fibrotic lung diseases (Weitzenblum, 1994; Judge et al., 2012; Swenson, 2013). Further, episodes of transient hypoxemia accompany sleep-disordered breathing. The most common type of sleep-disordered breathing is obstructive sleep apnea. HPV contributes to transient increases in PAP during sleep in obstructive sleep apnea patients (Kholdani et al., 2015). Taken together, acute hemodynamic load exerted on the RV due to HPV is common during exacerbation in diverse cardiopulmonary conditions and understanding of its pathophysiology may lead to the development of better management strategies.

Therapeutic approaches that could potentially improve RV performance upon acute high-altitude exposure should either reduce RV afterload or improve RV oxygenation. Decreased aerobic exercise capacity observed upon exposure to high-altitude is ascribed to both a decrease in arterial oxygen content and a limitation in maximal cardiac output (Fulco et al., 1998). Combined effects of several factors such as decreased blood volume, hypocapnia, increased blood viscosity, alterations of autonomic nervous system have been shown to limit maximal cardiac output (Wagner, 2000). A limitation in RV flow output due to HPV has also been shown to contribute to reduced maximal cardiac output and exercise capacity (Naeije et al., 2010). Indeed, several vasodilators such as sildenafil (Ghofrani et al.,

2004; Richalet et al., 2005), bosentan (Faoro et al., 2009) and sitaxsentan (Naeije et al., 2010) have been shown to improve maximal exercise capacity along with decreasing PAP in humans upon acute high-altitude exposure. Sitaxsentan (Naeije et al., 2010), sildenafil (Reichenberger et al., 2007) and epoprostenol (Pavelescu and Naeije, 2012) also improved RV function in healthy volunteers upon acute high-altitude exposure or hypoxic breathing. Although, their direct impact on the RV cannot be excluded, these beneficial effects on the RV were probably due to lowering PAP and PVR. Taken together, vasodilators can improve RV function and exercise capacity at least in part due to reduction of RV afterload.

Another strategy to improve RV function is to improve RV oxygenation. Artificial oxygen carriers initially developed as "blood substitutes" are now considered also for other therapeutic concepts as "oxygen therapeutics" (Spahn, 2018). Recently, a beneficial effect of a novel cross-linked hemoglobin-based oxygen carrier was demonstrated in an experimental model of acute mountain sickness in rabbits and goats (Zhang et al., 2021). Application of a carbon monoxide-saturated hemoglobin-based oxygen carrier significantly improved cardiac performance in mice exposed to high-altitude (Wang et al., 2017). Furthermore, in lambs exposed to acute hypoxia, administration of a novel oxygen delivery biotherapeutic Omniox-cardiovascular was associated with preserved RV contractile function despite elevated PVR (Boehme et al., 2018). Thus, artificial oxygen carriers might be useful in improving RV function in conditions of acute hypoxia exposure. Similarly, agents improving cardiomyocyte tolerance to hypoxia may also help to maintain cardiac function and exercise capacity at high-altitude. For example, trimetazidine has been shown to prevent cardiorespiratory fitness impairment and improve left ventricular systolic function in healthy volunteers during acute high-altitude exposure (Yang et al., 2019). However, it remains unknown whether trimetazidine can improve RV function upon acute exposure to high-altitude.

LIMITATIONS

Our systematic review has several limitations. As with any systematic review, publication bias and the possibility of missing potentially relevant articles cannot be excluded. However, we attempted to minimize such issues by using a robust search strategy including checking bibliography of original and review articles on the relevant topics.

In general, heterogeneity and small sample size limit the conclusions that can be drawn from the systematic analysis of the studies. Our systematic review identified considerable heterogeneity between study results. In the majority of the studies, RV function and morphology parameters were under-reported. Studies also differed significantly in terms of mode of altitude ascent. In studies with a staged acclimatization, participants spent nights at intermediate altitudes, while in other studies, subjects were brought to high-altitude by vehicles within a short time. In addition, results of acute altitude simulation studies cannot be fully extrapolated to the high-altitude field conditions. For example, reduction of total blood volume that occurs at high-altitude is not observed during acute simulated altitude (Stembridge et al., 2016). Moreover, the debate about the potential differences in modalities of hypoxia challenge remains unresolved (Savourey et al., 2003; Mounier and Brugniaux, 2012). Furthermore, echocardiography examinations were performed at different time-points of exposure to hypoxia. All these factors might have influenced the changes in the RV function parameters at a target altitude. Moreover, only very few studies considered other factors potentially influencing the RV response to acute hypoxia such as gender (Boos et al., 2016), age (Stewart et al., 2020) and ethnicity (Gaur et al., 2021).

With the advent of speckle-tracking echocardiography, detection of subtle cardiac abnormalities might have been improved. However, only in a few of the included studies such a sensitive technique was employed. In addition, in most of the studies, participants were middle-aged males; thus, our results probably are not applicable to other groups such as females and other age groups. Since we considered studies only on healthy subjects, our conclusions cannot be extended to individuals with underlying diseases. Conventional echocardiography and Doppler echocardiography are considered as less accurate non-invasive methods to assess pulmonary hemodynamics and cardiac function compared to invasive techniques (Fisher et al., 2009). Invasive methods, such as right heart catheterization, are less suitable due to ethical considerations in healthy individuals and challenging logistics in remote areas (Fagenholz et al., 2012; Feletti et al., 2018). Nevertheless, numerous studies have validated echocardiography by comparing it with invasive measurements of pulmonary hemodynamics at high-altitude (Allemann et al., 2000; Fagenholz et al., 2012).

Some studies included in the review reported similar number of subjects from the same authors, which might be the case that the same subject's data might have been used twice in two different publications. Although, we did not contact the authors regarding this issue, we have been very careful to screen the included studies if the authors have mentioned that the data presented in their studies had been used in previous publications.

CONCLUSION

This systematic review demonstrated that the reports on the effects of acute exposure to hypoxia on the RV are controversial and inconclusive. This may be due to significantly different study designs and non-optimal reporting of multiple RV parameters as recommended by international guidelines. Moreover, the potential impact of other factors such as gender, age, mode of ascent and physical activity on RV responses to hypoxia largely remained neglected. Larger-scale studies and longer follow-up are needed to explore RV adaptation to hypoxia and associated increased afterload and its clinical relevance. Future research should study RV physiology by assessing multiple conventional echocardiography parameters along with the recently developed techniques, such as speck-tracking and 3D echocardiography. Thus, this comprehensive overview will promote reproducible research with improved study design and methods for the future large-scale prospective studies assessing RV function in accordance with the international guidelines, which eventually may provide important insights into the RV response to acute hypoxia exposure.

AUTHOR CONTRIBUTIONS

ArM, MS, NK, and AkpS conceived and designed the study, drafted the manuscript, and provided overall supervision. ArM, MS, NK, MD, AbM, and AkyS performed data acquisition, analysis, or interpretation. ArM, MS, NK, MD, AbM, AkyS, and AkpS critically revised important intellectual content in the manuscript and approved the final version of the manuscript. All authors contributed to the article and approved the submitted version.

REFERENCES

Allemann, Y., Sartori, C., Lepori, M., Pierre, S., Mélot, C., Naeije, R., et al. (2000). Echocardiographic and invasive measurements of pulmonary artery pressure correlate closely at high altitude. *Am. J. Physiol. Heart Circul. Physiol.* 279, H2013–H2016 doi: 10.1152/ajpheart.2000.279.4.H2013

Anand, I., Chandrashekhar, Y., Bali, H., Wahi, P., Jindal, S., Malhotra, R., et al. (1990). Adult subacute mountain sickness—a syndrome of congestive heart failure in man at very high altitude. *Lancet* 335, 561–565 doi: 10.1016/0140-6736(90)90348-9

B?rtsch, P., and Gibbs, J. S. R. (2007). Effect of altitude on the heart and the lungs. *Circulation* 116, 2191–2202 doi: 10.1161/CIRCULATIONAHA.106.650796

Badagliacca, R., Papa, S., Valli, G., Pezzuto, B., Poscia, R., Reali, M., et al. (2017). Right ventricular dyssynchrony and exercise capacity in idiopathic pulmonary arterial hypertension. *Eur. Respir. J.* 49:1601419. doi: 10.1183/13993003.01419-2016

Badagliacca, R., Poscia, R., Pezzuto, B., Papa, S., Gambardella, C., Francone, M., et al. (2015). Right ventricular dyssynchrony in idiopathic pulmonary arterial hypertension: determinants and impact on pump function. *J. Heart Lung Transplant.* 34, 381–389. doi: 10.1016/j.healun.2014.06.010

Baggish, A. L., Fulco, C. S., Muza, S., Rock, P. B., Beidleman, B., Cymerman, A., et al. (2010). The impact of moderate-altitude staging on pulmonary arterial hemodynamics after ascent to high altitude. *High Alt. Med. Biol.* 11, 139–145. doi: 10.1089/ham.2009.1073

Baggish, A. L., Wolfel, E. E., and Levine, B. D. (2014). "Cardiovascular System," in *High Altitude: Human Adaptation to Hypoxia*, eds. E. R. Swenson and P. Bärtsch (New York, NY: Springer New York), 103–139. doi: 10.1007/978-1-4614-8772-2_6

Berger, M. M., Macholz, F., Schmidt, P., Fried, S., Perz, T., Dankl, D., et al. (2018). Inhaled budesonide does not affect hypoxic pulmonary vasoconstriction at 4559 meters of altitude. *High Alt. Med. Biol.* 19, 52–59. doi: 10.1089/ham.2017.0113

Boehme, J., Le Moan, N., Kameny, R. J., Loucks, A., Johengen, M. J., Lesneski, A. L., et al. (2018). Preservation of myocardial contractility during acute hypoxia with OMX-CV, a novel oxygen delivery biotherapeutic. *PLoS Biol.* 16:e2005924. doi: 10.1371/journal.pbio.2005924

Boos, C. J., Hodkinson, P. D., Mellor, A., Green, N. P., Bradley, D., Greaves, K., et al. (2013). The effects of prolonged acute hypobaric hypoxia on novel measures of biventricular performance. *Echocardiography* 30, 534–541. doi: 10.1111/echo.12088

Boos, C. J., Mellor, A., Begley, J., Stacey, M., Smith, C., Hawkins, A., et al. (2014). The effects of exercise at high altitude on high-sensitivity cardiac troponin release and associated biventricular cardiac function. *Clin. Res. Cardiol.* 103, 291–299 doi: 10.1007/s00392-013-0654-2

Boos, C. J., Mellor, A., O'hara, J. P., Tsakirides, C., and Woods, D. R. (2016). The effects of sex on cardiopulmonary responses to acute normobaric hypoxia. *High Alt. Med. Biol.* 17, 108–115. doi: 10.1089/ham.2015.0114

De Boeck, B. W., Toma, A., Kiencke, S., Dehnert, C., Zugel, S., Siebenmann, C., et al. (2018). Altered left ventricular geometry and torsional mechanics in high altitude-induced pulmonary hypertension: a three-dimensional echocardiographic study. *J. Am. Soc. Echocardiogr.* 31, 314–322. doi: 10.1016/j.echo.2017.12.001

de Vries, S. T., Kleijn, S. A., Van 'T Hof, A. W., Snaak, H., Van Enst, G. C., Kamp, O., et al. (2010). Impact of high altitude on echocardiographically determined cardiac morphology and function in patients with coronary artery disease and healthy controls. *Eur. J. Echocardiogr.* 11, 446–450. doi: 10.1093/ejechocard/jep237

Dedobbeleer, C., Hadefi, A., Pichon, A., Villafuerte, F., Naeije, R., and Unger, P. (2015). Left ventricular adaptation to high altitude: speckle tracking echocardiography in lowlanders, healthy highlanders and highlanders with chronic mountain sickness. *Int. J. Cardiovasc. Imaging* 31, 743–752. doi: 10.1007/s10554-015-0614-1

Ewalts, M., Dawkins, T., Boulet, L. M., Thijssen, D., and Stembridge, M. (2021). The influence of increased venous return on right ventricular dyssynchrony during acute and sustained hypoxaemia. *Exp. Physiol.* 106, 925–937. doi: 10.1113/EP088657

Fagenholz, P. J., Murray, A. F., Noble, V. E., Baggish, A. L., and Harris, N. S. (2012). Ultrasound for high altitude research. *Ultrasound Med. Biol.* 38, 1–12. doi: 10.1016/j.ultrasmedbio.2011.10.004

Faoro, V., Boldingh, S., Moreels, M., Martinez, S., Lamotte, M., Unger, P., et al. (2009). Bosentan decreases pulmonary vascular resistance and improves exercise capacity in acute hypoxia. *Chest* 135, 1215–1222. doi: 10.1378/chest.08-2222

Feletti, F., Mucci, V., and Aliverti, A. (2018). Chest ultrasonography in modern day extreme settings: from military setting and natural disasters to space flights and extreme sports. *Can. Respir. J.* 2018:8739704. doi: 10.1155/2018/8739704

Fisher, M. R., Forfia, P. R., Chamera, E., Housten-Harris, T., Champion, H. C., Girgis, R. E., et al. (2009). Accuracy of Doppler echocardiography in the hemodynamic assessment of pulmonary hypertension. *Am. J. Respir. Crit. Care Med.* 179, 615–621. doi: 10.1164/rccm.200811-1691OC

Fulco, C. S., Rock, P. B., and Cymerman, A. (1998). Maximal and submaximal exercise performance at altitude. *Aviat. Space Environ. Med.* 69, 793–801.

Galie, N., Humbert, M., Vachiery, J. L., Gibbs, S., Lang, I., Torbicki, A., et al. (2016). 2015 ESC/ERS Guidelines for the diagnosis and treatment of pulmonary hypertension: the joint task force for the diagnosis and treatment of pulmonary hypertension of the European Society of Cardiology (ESC) and the European Respiratory Society (ERS): endorsed by: Association for European Paediatric and Congenital Cardiology (AEPC), International Society for Heart and Lung Transplantation (ISHLT). *Eur. Heart J.* 37, 67–119. doi: 10.1093/eurheartj/ehv317

Gaur, P., Sartmyrzaeva, M., Maripov, A., Muratali Uulu, K., Saini, S., Ray, K., et al. (2021). Cardiac acclimatization at high altitude in two different ethnicity groups. *High Alt. Med. Biol.* 22, 58–69. doi: 10.1089/ham.2020.0035

Ghofrani, H. A., Reichenberger, F., Kohstall, M. G., Mrosek, E. H., Seeger, T., Olschewski, H., et al. (2004). Sildenafil increased exercise capacity during hypoxia at low altitudes and at Mount Everest base camp: a randomized, double-blind, placebo-controlled crossover trial. *Ann. Intern. Med.* 141, 169–177 doi: 10.7326/0003-4819-141-3-200408030-00005

Gibbs, J. S. (2007). Biventricular function at high altitude: implications for regulation of stroke volume in chronic hypoxia. *Adv. Exp. Med. Biol.* 618, 13–24 doi: 10.1007/978-0-387-75434-5_2

Goebel, B., Handrick, V., Lauten, A., Fritzenwanger, M., Schutze, J., Otto, S., et al. (2013). Impact of acute normobaric hypoxia on regional and global myocardial function: a speckle tracking echocardiography study. *Int. J. Cardiovasc. Imaging* 29, 561–570. doi: 10.1007/s10554-012-0117-2

Greiner, S., Jud, A., Aurich, M., Hess, A., Hilbel, T., Hardt, S., et al. (2014). Reliability of noninvasive assessment of systolic pulmonary artery pressure by Doppler echocardiography compared to right heart catheterization: analysis in a large patient population. *J. Am. Heart Assoc.* 3:e001103. doi: 10.1161/JAHA.114.001103

Groves, B. M., Reeves, J. T., Sutton, J. R., Wagner, P. D., Cymerman, A., Malconian, M. K., et al. (1987). Operation Everest II: elevated high-altitude pulmonary resistance unresponsive to oxygen. *J. Appl. Physiol.* 63, 521–530 doi: 10.1152/jappl.1987.63.2.521

Hanaoka, M., Kogashi, K., Droma, Y., Urushihata, K., and Kubo, K. (2011). Myocardial performance index in subjects susceptible to high-altitude pulmonary edema. *Intern. Med.* 50, 2967–2973 doi: 10.2169/internalmedicine.50.5942

He, C., Liu, C., Yu, S., Yang, J., Ding, X., Bian, S., et al. (2021). Atrial performance in healthy subjects following high altitude exposure at 4100 m: 2D speckle-tracking strain analysis. *Int. J. Cardiovasc. Imaging* 37, 1891–1902. doi: 10.1007/s10554-021-02173-8

Hilty, M. P., Merz, T. M., Hefti, U., Ince, C., Maggiorini, M., and Pichler Hefti, J. (2019). Recruitment of non-perfused sublingual capillaries increases microcirculatory oxygen extraction capacity throughout ascent to 7126 m. *J. Physiol.* 597, 2623–2638. doi: 10.1113/JP277590

Hilty, M. P., Müller, A., Flück, D., Siebenmann, C., Rasmussen, P., Keiser, S., et al. (2016). Effect of increased blood flow on pulmonary circulation before and during high altitude acclimatization. *High Alt. Med. Biol.* 17, 305–314 doi: 10.1089/ham.2016.0004

Holloway, C. J., Montgomery, H. E., Murray, A. J., Cochlin, L. E., Codreanu, I., Hopwood, N., et al. (2011). Cardiac response to hypobaric hypoxia: persistent changes in cardiac mass, function, and energy metabolism after a trek to Mt. *Everest Base Camp. FASEB J.* 25, 792–796. doi: 10.1096/fj.10-172999

Huez, S., Faoro, V., Guenard, H., Martinot, J. B., and Naeije, R. (2009). Echocardiographic and tissue Doppler imaging of cardiac adaptation to high altitude in native highlanders versus acclimatized lowlanders. *Am. J. Cardiol.* 103, 1605–1609. doi: 10.1016/j.amjcard.2009.02.006

Huez, S., Faoro, V., Vachiery, J. L., Unger, P., Martinot, J. B., and Naeije, R. (2007). Images in cardiovascular medicine. High-altitude-induced right-heart failure. *Circulation* 115, e308–e309. doi: 10.1161/CIRCULATIONAHA.106.650994

Huez, S., Retailleau, K., Unger, P., Pavelescu, A., Vachiery, J. L., Derumeaux, G., et al. (2005). Right and left ventricular adaptation to hypoxia: a tissue Doppler imaging study. *Am. J. Physiol. Heart Circ. Physiol.* 289, H1391–H1398. doi: 10.1152/ajpheart.00332.2005

Judge, E. P., Fabre, A., Adamali, H. I., and Egan, J. J. (2012). Acute exacerbations and pulmonary hypertension in advanced idiopathic pulmonary fibrosis. *Eur. Respir. J.* 40, 93–100. doi: 10.1183/09031936.00115511

Kalogeropoulos, A. P., Georgiopoulou, V. V., Howell, S., Pernetz, M. A., Fisher, M. R., Lerakis, S., et al. (2008). Evaluation of right intraventricular dyssynchrony by two-dimensional strain echocardiography in patients with pulmonary arterial hypertension. *J. Am. Soc. Echocardiogr.* 21, 1028–1034. doi: 10.1016/j.echo.2008.05.005

Kholdani, C., Fares, W. H., and Mohsenin, V. (2015). Pulmonary hypertension in obstructive sleep apnea: is it clinically significant? A critical analysis of the association and pathophysiology. *Pulm. Circ.* 5, 220–227. doi: 10.1086/679995

Kjaergaard, J., Snyder, E. M., Hassager, C., Olson, T. P., Oh, J. K., Johnson, B. D., et al. (2007). Right ventricular function with hypoxic exercise: effects of sildenafil. *Eur. J. Appl. Physiol.* 102, 87–95. doi: 10.1007/s00421-007-0560-2

Kossaify, A. (2015). Echocardiographic assessment of the right ventricle, from the conventional approach to speckle tracking and three-dimensional imaging, and insights into the "Right Way" to explore the forgotten chamber. *Clin. Med. Insights Cardiol.* 9, 65–75. doi: 10.4137/CMC.S27462

Lichtblau, M., Bader, P. R., Carta, A. F., Furian, M., Muralt, L., Saxer, S., et al. (2021). Extravascular lung water and cardiac function assessed by echocardiography in healthy lowlanders during repeated very high-altitude exposure. *Int. J. Cardiol.* 332, 166–174 doi: 10.1016/j.ijcard.2021.03.057

Luks, A. M., Levett, D., Martin, D. S., Goss, C. H., Mitchell, K., Fernandez, B. O., et al. (2017). Changes in acute pulmonary vascular responsiveness to hypoxia during a progressive ascent to high altitude (5300 m). *Exp. Physiol.* 102, 711–724. doi: 10.1113/EP086083

Maggiorini, M., Mélot, C., Pierre, S., Pfeiffer, F., Greve, I., Sartori, C., et al. (2001). High-altitude pulmonary edema is initially caused by an increase in capillary pressure. *Circulation* 103, 2078–2083. doi: 10.1161/01.CIR.103.16.2078

Maufrais, C., Rupp, T., Bouzat, P., Doucende, G., Verges, S., Nottin, S., et al. (2017). Heart mechanics at high altitude: 6 days on the top of Europe. *Eur. Heart J. Cardiovasc. Imaging* 18, 1369–1377. doi: 10.1093/ehjci/jew286

Maufrais, C., Rupp, T., Bouzat, P., Esteve, F., Nottin, S., Walther, G., et al. (2019). Medex 2015: the key role of cardiac mechanics to maintain biventricular function at high altitude. *Exp. Physiol.* 104, 667–676. doi: 10.1113/EP087350

Mounier, R., and Brugniaux, J. V. (2012). Counterpoint: hypobaric hypoxia does not induce different responses from normobaric hypoxia. *J. Appl. Physiol.* 112, 1784–1786 doi: 10.1152/japplphysiol.00067.2012a

Naeije, R. (2010). Physiological adaptation of the cardiovascular system to high altitude. *Prog. Cardiovasc. Dis.* 52, 456–466. doi: 10.1016/j.pcad.2010.03.004

Naeije, R., and Dedobbeleer, C. (2013). Pulmonary hypertension and the right ventricle in hypoxia. *Exp. Physiol.* 98, 1247–1256. doi: 10.1113/expphysiol.2012.069112

Naeije, R., Huez, S., Lamotte, M., Retailleau, K., Neupane, S., Abramowicz, D., et al. (2010). Pulmonary artery pressure limits exercise capacity at high altitude. *Eur. Respir. J.* 36, 1049–1055. doi: 10.1183/09031936.00024410

Netzer, N. C., Strohl, K. P., Hogel, J., Gatterer, H., and Schilz, R. (2017). Right ventricle dimensions and function in response to acute hypoxia in healthy human subjects. *Acta Physiol.* 219, 478–485. doi: 10.1111/apha.12740

Osculati, G., Revera, M., Branzi, G., Faini, A., Malfatto, G., Bilo, G., et al. (2016). Effects of hypobaric hypoxia exposure at high altitude on left ventricular twist in healthy subjects: data from HIGHCARE study on Mount Everest. *Eur. Heart J.* 17, 635–643 doi: 10.1093/ehjci/jev166

Page, M., Sauve, C., Serri, K., Page, P., Yin, Y., and Schampaert, E. (2013). Echocardiographic assessment of cardiac performance in response to high altitude and development of subclinical pulmonary edema in healthy climbers. *Can. J. Cardiol.* 29, 1277–1284. doi: 10.1016/j.cjca.2013.04.025

Pavelescu, A., and Naeije, R. (2012). Effects of epoprostenol and sildenafil on right ventricular function in hypoxic volunteers: a tissue Doppler imaging study. *Eur. J. Appl. Physiol.* 112, 1285–1294. doi: 10.1007/s00421-011-2085-y

Pena, E., Brito, J., El Alam, S., and Siques, P. (2020). Oxidative stress, kinase activity and inflammatory implications in right ventricular hypertrophy and heart failure under hypobaric hypoxia. *Int. J. Mol. Sci.* 21:6421. doi: 10.3390/ijms21176421

Pezzuto, B., Forton, K., Badagliacca, R., Motoji, Y., Faoro, V., and Naeije, R. (2018). Right ventricular dyssynchrony during hypoxic breathing but not during exercise in healthy subjects: a speckle tracking echocardiography study. *Exp. Physiol.* 103, 1338–1346. doi: 10.1113/EP087027

Pratali, L., Cavana, M., Sicari, R., and Picano, E. (2010). Frequent subclinical high-altitude pulmonary edema detected by chest sonography as ultrasound lung comets in recreational climbers. *Crit. Care Med.* 38, 1818–1823 doi: 10.1097/CCM.0b013e3181e8ae0e

Pugh, L. (1964). Blood volume and haemoglobin concentration at altitudes above 18,000 ft. (5500 m). *J. Physiol.* 170, 344–354 doi: 10.1113/jphysiol.1964.sp007335

Qiu, Y., Li, M., Li, S., Yang, T., Liu, Y., Zheng, S., et al. (2017). Physiological responses to acute hypoxia and indictors of acute mountain sickness in males. *Int. J. Clin. Exp. Pathol.* 10, 1466–1476.

Rademakers, F. E., Buchalter, M. B., Rogers, W. J., Zerhouni, E. A., Weisfeldt, M. L., Weiss, J. L., et al. (1992). Dissociation between left ventricular untwisting and filling. Accentuation by catecholamines. *Circulation* 85, 1572–1581 doi: 10.1161/01.CIR.85.4.1572

Reeves, J. T., Groves, B. M., Sutton, J. R., Wagner, P. D., Cymerman, A., Malconian, M. K., et al. (1987). Operation Everest II: preservation of cardiac function at extreme altitude. *J. Appl. Physiol.* 63, 531–539 doi: 10.1152/jappl.1987.63.2.531

Reichenberger, F., Kohstall, M. G., Seeger, T., Olschewski, H., Grimminger, F., Seeger, W., et al. (2007). Effect of sildenafil on hypoxia-induced changes in pulmonary circulation and right ventricular function. *Respir. Physiol. Neurobiol.* 159, 196–201. doi: 10.1016/j.resp.2007.07.005

Richalet, J.-P., and Pichon, A. (2014). "Right ventricle and high altitude," in *The Right Heart*, eds. S. P. Gaine, R. Naeije, and A. J. Peacock (London: Springer London), 117–129. doi: 10.1007/978-1-4471-2398-9_9

Richalet, J. P., Gratadour, P., Robach, P., Pham, I., Dechaux, M., Joncquiert-Latarjet, A., et al. (2005). Sildenafil inhibits altitude-induced hypoxemia and pulmonary hypertension. *Am. J. Respir. Crit. Care Med.* 171, 275–281. doi: 10.1164/rccm.200406-804OC

Ronkainen, V. P., Skoumal, R., and Tavi, P. (2011). Hypoxia and HIF-1 suppress SERCA2a expression in embryonic cardiac myocytes through two interdependent hypoxia response elements. *J. Mol. Cell Cardiol.* 50, 1008–1016. doi: 10.1016/j.yjmcc.2011.02.017

Rudski, L. G., Lai, W. W., Afilalo, J., Hua, L., Handschumacher, M. D., Chandrasekaran, K., et al. (2010). Guidelines for the echocardiographic assessment of the right heart in adults: a report from the American Society of Echocardiography endorsed by the European Association of Echocardiography, a registered branch of the European Society of Cardiology, and the Canadian Society of Echocardiography. *J. Am. Soc. Echocardiogr.* 23, 685–713. doi: 10.1016/j.echo.2010.05.010

Salvo, G. D., Pergola, V., Fadel, B., Bulbul, Z. A., and Caso, P. (2015). strain echocardiography and myocardial mechanics: from basics to clinical applications. *J. Cardiovasc. Echogr.* 25, 1–8. doi: 10.4103/2211-4122.158415

Sareban, M., Perz, T., Macholz, F., Reich, B., Schmidt, P., Fried, S., et al. (2019). Impairment of left atrial mechanics does not contribute to the reduction in stroke volume after active ascent to 4559 m. *Scand. J. Med. Sci. Sports* 29, 223–231 doi: 10.1111/sms.13325

Sareban, M., Perz, T., Macholz, F., Reich, B., Schmidt, P., Fried, S., et al. (2020). Preserved right ventricular function but increased right atrial contractile demand in altitude-induced pulmonary hypertension. *Int. J. Cardiovasc. Imaging* 36, 1069–1076. doi: 10.1007/s10554-020-01803-x

Savourey, G., Launay, J.-C., Besnard, Y., Guinet, A., and Travers, S. (2003). Normo- and hypobaric hypoxia: are there any physiological differences? *Eur. J. Appl. Physiol.* 89, 122–126 doi: 10.1007/s00421-002-0789-8

Seccombe, L. M., Chow, V., Zhao, W., Lau, E. M., Rogers, P. G., Ng, A. C., et al. (2017). Right heart function during simulated altitude in patients with pulmonary arterial hypertension. *Open Heart* 4:e000532. doi: 10.1136/openhrt-2016-000532

Silverman, H. S., Wei, S., Haigney, M. C., Ocampo, C. J., and Stern, M. D. (1997). Myocyte adaptation to chronic hypoxia and development of tolerance to subsequent acute severe hypoxia. *Circ. Res.* 80, 699–707. doi: 10.1161/01.RES.80.5.699

Singh, M., Rawal, S., and Tyagi, A. (1990). Body fluid status on induction, reinduction and prolonged stay at high altitude of human volunteers. *Int. J. Biometeorol.* 34, 93–97 doi: 10.1007/BF01093454

Soria, R., Egger, M., Scherrer, U., Bender, N., and Rimoldi, S. F. (2016). Pulmonary artery pressure and arterial oxygen saturation in people living at high or low altitude: systematic review and meta-analysis. *J. Appl. Physiol.* 121, 1151–1159. doi: 10.1152/japplphysiol.00394.2016

Soria, R., Egger, M., Scherrer, U., Bender, N., and Rimoldi, S. F. (2019). Pulmonary arterial pressure at rest and during exercise in chronic mountain sickness: a meta-analysis. *Eur. Respir. J.* 53:1802040. doi: 10.1183/13993003.02040-2018

Spahn, D. R. (2018). Artificial oxygen carriers: a new future? *Crit. Care* 22:46. doi: 10.1186/s13054-018-1949-5

Stembridge, M., Ainslie, P. N., Boulet, L. M., Anholm, J., Subedi, P., Tymko, M. M., et al. (2019). The independent effects of hypovolaemia and pulmonary vasoconstriction on ventricular function and exercise capacity during acclimatisation to 3800 m. *J. Physiol.* 597, 1059–1072. doi: 10.1113/JP275278

Stembridge, M., Ainslie, P. N., Hughes, M. G., Stohr, E. J., Cotter, J. D., Nio, A. Q., et al. (2014). Ventricular structure, function, and mechanics at high altitude: chronic remodeling in Sherpa vs. short-term lowlander adaptation. *J. Appl. Physiol.* 117, 334–343. doi: 10.1152/japplphysiol.00233.2014

Stembridge, M., Ainslie, P. N., Hughes, M. G., Stöhr, E. J., Cotter, J. D., Tymko, M. M., et al. (2015). Impaired myocardial function does not explain reduced left ventricular filling and stroke volume at rest or during exercise at high altitude. *J. Appl. Physiol.* 119, 1219–1227 doi: 10.1152/japplphysiol.00995.2014

Stembridge, M., Ainslie, P. N., and Shave, R. (2016). Mechanisms underlying reductions in stroke volume at rest and during exercise at high altitude. *Eur. J. Sport Sci.* 16, 577–584. doi: 10.1080/17461391.2015.1071876

Stewart, G. M., Wheatley-Guy, C. M., Morris, N. R., Coffman, K. E., Stepanek, J., Carlson, A. R., et al. (2020). Myocardial adaptability in young and older-aged sea-level habitants sojourning at Mt Kilimanjaro: are cardiac compensatory limits reached in older trekkers? *Eur. J. Appl. Physiol.* 120, 799–809. doi: 10.1007/s00421-020-04319-3

Swenson, E. R. (2013). Hypoxic pulmonary vasoconstriction. *High Alt. Med. Biol.* 14, 101–110. doi: 10.1089/ham.2013.1010

Sydykov, A., Mamazhakypov, A., Maripov, A., Kosanovic, D., Weissmann, N., Ghofrani, H. A., et al. (2021). Pulmonary hypertension in acute and chronic high altitude maladaptation disorders. *Int. J. Environ. Res. Public Health* 18:1692. doi: 10.3390/ijerph18041692

Taleb, M., Khuder, S., Tinkel, J., and Khouri, S. J. (2013). The diagnostic accuracy of Doppler echocardiography in assessment of pulmonary artery systolic pressure: a meta-analysis. *Echocardiography* 30, 258–265. doi: 10.1111/echo.12061

Tian, J. D., Liu, C., Yang, Y. Q., Yu, S. Y., Yang, J., Zhang, J. H., et al. (2020). Effects of baseline heart rate at sea level on cardiac responses to high-altitude exposure. *Int. J. Cardiovasc. Imaging* 36, 799–810. doi: 10.1007/s10554-020-01769-w

Tucker, C. E., James, W. E., Berry, M. A., Johnstone, C. J., and Grover, R. F. (1976). Depressed myocardial function in the goat at high altitude. *J. Appl. Physiol.* 41, 356–361 doi: 10.1152/jappl.1976.41.3.356

Wagner, P. D. (2000). Reduced maximal cardiac output at altitude–mechanisms and significance. *Respir. Physiol.* 120, 1–11. doi: 10.1016/S0034-5687(99)00101-2

Wang, Q., Hu, L., Hu, Y., Gong, G., Tan, H., Deng, L., et al. (2017). Carbon monoxide-saturated hemoglobin-based oxygen carriers attenuate high-altitude-induced cardiac injury by amelioration of the inflammation response and mitochondrial oxidative damage. *Cardiology* 136, 180–191. doi: 10.1159/000448652

Weitzenblum, E. (1994). The pulmonary circulation and the heart in chronic lung disease. *Monaldi. Arch. Chest. Dis.* 49, 231–234.

Yang, J., Zhang, L., Liu, C., Zhang, J., Yu, S., Yu, J., et al. (2019). Trimetazidine attenuates high-altitude fatigue and cardiorespiratory fitness impairment: a randomized double-blinded placebo-controlled clinical trial. *Biomed. Pharmacother.* 116:109003. doi: 10.1016/j.biopha.2019.109003

Yang, T., Li, X., Qin, J., Li, S., Yu, J., Zhang, J., et al. (2015). High altitude-induced borderline pulmonary hypertension impaired cardiorespiratory fitness in healthy young men. *Int. J. Cardiol.* 181, 382–388 doi: 10.1016/j.ijcard.2014.12.044

Yang, Y., Liu, C., Tian, J., Ding, X., Yu, S., Bian, S., et al. (2020a). Preliminary study of right ventricular dyssynchrony under high-altitude exposure: determinants and impacts. *Front. Physiol.* 11: 703. doi: 10.3389/fphys.2020.00703

Yang, Y., Liu, C., Yu, S., Qin, Z., Yang, J., Bian, S., et al. (2020b). Pulmonary function tests at low altitude predict pulmonary pressure response to short-term high altitude exposure. *Respir. Physiol. Neurobiol.* 282:103534. doi: 10.1016/j.resp.2020.103534

Yuan, F., Liu, C., Yu, S., Bian, S., Yang, J., Ding, X., et al. (2021). The association between notching of the right ventricular outflow tract flow velocity doppler envelope and impaired right ventricular function after acute high-altitude exposure. *Front. Physiol.* 12:39761. doi: 10.3389/fphys.2021.639761

Zhang, J., Wu, Y., Peng, X. Y., Li, Q. H., Xiang, X. M., Zhu, Y., et al. (2021). The protective effect of a novel cross-linked hemoglobin-based oxygen carrier on hypoxia injury of acute mountain sickness in rabbits and goats. *Front. Physiol.* 12:690190. doi: 10.3389/fphys.2021.690190

6

Crucial Role of Stromal Interaction Molecule-Activated TRPC-ORAI Channels in Vascular Remodeling and Pulmonary Hypertension Induced by Intermittent Hypoxia

Sebastián Castillo-Galán[1†], Bárbara Riquelme[1] and Rodrigo Iturriaga[1,2*†]

[1] Laboratorio de Neurobiología, Facultad de Ciencias Biológicas, Pontificia Universidad Católica de Chile, Santiago, Chile,
[2] Centro de Excelencia en Biomedicina de Magallanes (CEBIMA), Universidad de Magallanes, Punta Arenas, Chile

***Correspondence:**
Rodrigo Iturriaga
riturriaga@bio.puc.cl

† These authors have contributed equally to this work

Obstructive sleep apnea (OSA), a sleep breathing disorder featured by chronic intermittent hypoxia (CIH), is associate with pulmonary hypertension. Rats exposed to CIH develop lung vascular remodeling and pulmonary hypertension, which paralleled the upregulation of stromal interaction molecule (STIM)-activated TRPC-ORAI Ca^{2+} channels (STOC) in the lung, suggesting that STOC participate in the pulmonary vascular alterations. Accordingly, to evaluate the role played by STOC in pulmonary hypertension we studied whether the STOC blocker 2-aminoethoxydiphenyl borate (2-APB) may prevent the vascular remodeling and the pulmonary hypertension induced by CIH in a rat model of OSA. We assessed the effects of 2-APB on right ventricular systolic pressure (RVSP), pulmonary vascular remodeling, α-actin and proliferation marker Ki-67 levels in pulmonary arterial smooth muscle cells (PASMC), mRNA levels of STOC subunits, and systemic and pulmonary oxidative stress (TBARS) in male Sprague-Dawley (200 g) rats exposed to CIH (5% O_2, 12 times/h for 8h) for 28 days. At 14 days of CIH, osmotic pumps containing 2-APB (10 mg/kg/day) or its vehicle were implanted and rats were kept for 2 more weeks in CIH. Exposure to CIH for 28 days raised RVSP > 35 mm Hg, increased the medial layer thickness and the levels of α-actin and Ki-67 in PASMC, and increased the gene expression of TRPC1, TRPC4, TRPC6 and ORAI1 subunits. Treatment with 2-APB prevented the raise in RVSP and the increment of the medial layer thickness, as well as the increased levels of α-actin and Ki-67 in PASMC, and the increased gene expression of STOC subunits. In addition, 2-APB did not reduced the lung and systemic oxidative stress, suggesting that the effects of 2-APB on vascular remodeling and pulmonary hypertension are independent on the reduction of the oxidative stress. Thus, our results supported that STIM-activated TRPC-ORAI Ca^{2+} channels contributes to the lung vascular remodeling and pulmonary hypertension induced by CIH.

Keywords: 2-APB, STIM-activated TRPC-ORAI channels, chronic intermittent hypoxia, pulmonary hypertension, pulmonary vascular remodeling, hypoxia, obstructive sleep apnea

INTRODUCTION

Obstructive sleep apnea (OSA) characterized by cyclic episodes of intermittent hypoxia is a health problem that affect a large worldwide adult population (Somers et al., 2008; Dempsey et al., 2010; Floras, 2018). Obstructive sleep apnea is associated with somnolence, sleep fragmentation and cognitive dysfunction, but it is also considered as an independent risk factor for systemic diurnal hypertension (Somers et al., 2008; Dempsey et al., 2010; Iturriaga et al., 2021). Furthermore, OSA is associated with mild pulmonary hypertension with an incidence ranging from 20-50% (Sajkov and McEvoy, 2009; Floras, 2018). Chronic intermittent hypoxia (CIH) is the main factor for develop systemic hypertension in OSA patients (Somers et al., 2008; Dempsey et al., 2010) and animal exposed to CIH (Del Rio et al., 2010, 2014; Iturriaga et al., 2014, 2021; Iturriaga, 2018; Harki et al., 2021). In addition, CIH produces vascular pulmonary remodeling and increases right ventricular systolic pressure (RVSP) in rodents (Nisbet et al., 2009; Jin et al., 2014, 2016; Iturriaga and Castillo-Galán, 2019; Castillo-Galán et al., 2020). Recently, we found that CIH progressively increased the right ventricular systolic pressure (RVSP) over 35 mm Hg in the rat, enhanced the vasoconstrictor response of small pulmonary arteries to KCl and endothelin-1 (ET-1), increased the medial layer thickness, and increased the right-ventricular wall thickness and the right-ventricular end systolic volume related to the control rats (Castillo-Galán et al., 2020). However, even though the link between OSA and pulmonary hypertension is well recognized, the underlying pathogenic mechanisms are not completely known. The pathological pulmonary vascular alterations induced by CIH has been attributed to Ca^{2+}−dependent enhanced contractility and proliferation of pulmonary arterial smooth muscle cells (PASMC) induced by the activation of hypoxic inducible factors (HIFs) and oxidative stress (Nisbet et al., 2009: Jin et al., 2014, 2016; Iturriaga and Castillo-Galán, 2019). Thus, it is likely that the activation of HIFs and reactive oxygen species (ROS)-dependent signaling pathways may increase intracellular PASMC calcium levels contributing to the development of the CIH-induced enhanced vasoconstriction, cell proliferation and pulmonary hypertension (Waypa et al., 2002; Sylvester et al., 2012).

Among channels and transporters involved in Ca^{2+} intracellular homeostasis, it has been proposed that store operated calcium entry contributes to enhance the PASMC contractility in sustained hypoxia (Kuhr et al., 2012; Wang et al., 2012, 2017; Reyes et al., 2018). The binding of endothelin-1 (ET-1) or serotonin (5-HT) to their receptors coupled to G-protein evokes the release of the second messenger IP_3, which in turn activates intracellular calcium channels (IP3R) depleting the Ca^{2+} stores of the sarcoplasmic reticulum (Zhang et al., 2003; Wang et al., 2012). STOC are activated by a depletion of Ca^{2+} stores in the sarcoplasmic reticulum, which allow the entry of calcium from the extracellular space. A growing body of evidence supports the contribution of STOC in the contraction of pulmonary arteries in response to acute and sustained hypoxia (Weigand et al., 2005; Lu et al., 2008, 2009; Ng et al., 2008; Guibert et al., 2011). Furthermore, STOC-mediated calcium entry participates in pathological pulmonary vascular remodeling process, such as hypercontractility, proliferation and differentiation of PASMC (Golovina et al., 2001; Hou et al., 2013; Reyes et al., 2018). From a structural point of view, STOC are composed by homo or heterotetramer pore-forming subunits from the TRPC family (TRPC 1 to 7), or to the ORAI family (ORAI 1 to 3) (Reyes et al., 2018). On the other hand, an auxiliary subunit of the family of stromal interaction molecules [stromal interaction molecule (STIM) 1 and 2] acts as a calcium sensor activating pore-forming subunits in response to calcium depletion from sarcoplasmic reticulum deposits (Fuchs et al., 2010; Johnstone et al., 2010; Wray and Burdyga, 2010; Yang et al., 2010). Indeed, a growing body of evidence suggests that STIM-activated TRPC-ORAI Ca^{2+} channels (STOC) play a key role in PASMC remodeling and hypercontractility, which led to pulmonary hypertension in animals exposed to sustained hypoxia (Weigand et al., 2005; Ng et al., 2008; Castillo-Galán et al., 2016, 2022)

Recently, we found that CIH produced the upregulation of mRNA and protein levels of TRPC1, TRPC4, TRPC6, ORAI1, and STIM1 subunits in the rat lung tissue, which paralleled the vascular remodeling and pulmonary hypertension (Castillo-Galán et al., 2020), suggesting that STOC participate in the vascular alterations induced by CIH. Accordingly, to assess the contribution of STOC on the CIH-induced pulmonary vascular alterations, we study the effects of the STOC non-selective inhibitor 2-aminoethyldiphenylborinate (2-APB) (Bootman et al., 2002; Smith et al., 2015; Castillo-Galán et al., 2016, 2022; Jain et al., 2021) on the development of pulmonary hypertension and vascular remodeling induced by CIH in a well stablished preclinical model of OSA (Del Rio et al., 2010, 2012, 2014; Iturriaga et al., 2014, Iturriaga and Castillo-Galán, 2019). We also determined the effects of 2-APB on systemic and lung oxidative stress induced by CIH, because 2-APB ameliorates the oxidative stress in a heart ischemia-reperfusion model in mice (Morihara et al., 2017) and rat (Shen et al., 2021).

MATERIALS AND METHODS

Animal Model and Intermittent Chronic Hypoxia Protocols

The experimental protocols were approved by the Scientific Ethical Committee for the Animal and Environment Care from the Pontificia Universidad Católica de Chile, Santiago, Chile (ID:180803006), and were performed according to the National Institutes of Health Guide (NIH, United States) for the care and use of animals. The experiments were performed in 19 male Sprague-Dawley rats (∼ 200 g) from the Center from Innovation in Biomedical Experimental Models (CIBEM) of the Pontificia Universidad Católica de Chile. Rats were fed with a standard diet and access to food and water *ad libitum* and the room temperature was maintained between 23 and 25°C. Rats were exposed to CIH (5% O_2 for 20 s, followed by 290 s of normoxia, 12 time for 8 h/day, from 9:00 AM. to 5:00 PM. for 28 days. The O_2 levels in the chambers were regulated with a computerized system, which open and close solenoid valves that control the entry of N_2 and its removal by a fan (Del Rio et al., 2010, 2012, Castillo-Galán et al., 2020).

2-Aminoethyl Diphenylborinate Administration

Rats were randomized divided into 3 groups (n = 6–7). At 14 days of CIH, rats were anesthetized with isoflurane 2% in 100% O_2, and mini osmotic-pumps (2ML4, Alzet Scientific Products, MD, United States) were implanted subcutaneously in the back. Pumps were loaded with 2-APB (Sigma-Aldrich, United States) to produce a continuous release of 10 mg/kg/day or its vehicle (Dimethyl sulfoxide: ETOH: Saline 1: 5: 4). After surgery, both groups were exposed to CIH for 14 more days, and the results were compared with the control group of rats exposed to normoxia.

Right Ventricular Systolic Pressure Measurement

At the end of 28 days of CIH, rats were anesthetized with urethane/α-chloralose (40/800 mg/kg, i.p.), tracheostomized and artificially ventilated with a RoVent Jr ventilator (Kent Scientific, Torrington, CT, United States). A thoracotomy was performed to expose the heart, and the right ventricular systolic pressure (RVSP) was recorded with a heparinized catheter inserted into the right ventricle connected to a Statham P23 transducer (Hato Rey, Puerto Rico, United States). The heart rate was derived from the pressure signal recorded with a PowerLab 16 channels acquisition system (ADInstruments, Castle Hill, Australia) (Castillo-Galán et al., 2020).

mRNA Extraction and RT-qPCR

Frozen left lung samples (~100 mg) were homogenized in TRIzol (Thermo Fisher Scientific, Waltham, MA, United States). The RNA was resuspended in nuclease-free water (20 μl) to later determination of its concentration and purity by spectrophotometry, being the 260/280 ratio of all samples in the range of 1.9–2.0. The RNA was stored at −80°C until later use. Synthesis to cDNA was performed using the cDNA Synthesis Kit (ABM, Richmond, Canada). The gene expression of TRPC1, TRPC4, TRPC6, ORAI1, ORAI2 and 18S was determined by real-time PCR (qPCR) in a StepOne Plus equipment (Applied Biosystems, Foster City, CA, United States), using a KicqStart kit (Sigma-Aldrich, United States) with the primers sequence used by Castillo-Galán et al. (2020). Relative gene expression was calculated with the $2^{-\Delta\Delta Ct}$ method using 18S gene.

Malondialdehyde Concentration

The malondialdehyde (MDA) concentration was measured using a specific enzyme immunoassay thiobarbituric acid reactive substances (TBARS) kit (Cayman Chemical, Ann Arbor, MI, United States) Briefly, 25 mg of fresh lung tissue were homogenized in RIPA Buffer Concentrate (Cayman Chemical, Ann Arbor, MI United States) and centrifuged at 1600 x g for 10 min at 4°C. The supernatant were collected for analysis. Blood samples were collected from the left ventricle using a syringe with heparin. Blood samples were centrifuged at 1000 x g for 10 min at 4°C and the fresh plasma (supernatant) were use for analysis.

Vascular Remodeling and Immunohistochemistry

Samples of ~1 cm of the external portion of the medium lobe from the left lung containing distal pulmonary arterioles were collected. The lung tissue was fixed by immersion in Paraformaldehyde 4%, included in paraffin blocks, and cut in 3–5 μm slides. For the morphological analysis, the slides were deparaffinized, dehydrated and stained with Van Gieson. Using a trinocular microscope (Olympus BX41, Japan) with a digital camera (Jenoptik Progres C3), 10–15 images of 150–300 μm internal diameter pulmonary arteries were acquired per lung from each animal. The area of the muscle layer and the artery lumen were measured using the Image Pro6.3 Software (Sigma-imaging, United Kingdom). The percentage of muscle layer was determined using the following formula: (muscle area - lumen area)/muscle area * 100, according to Castillo-Galán et al. (2020).

Immunohistochemical detection of α-actin and Ki-67 (α-actin-r and KI-67-ir) was performed with the smooth muscle α-actin antibody (Clone RM253, Sigma-Aldrich, Misuri, United States, dilution: 1:400) and the Ki-67 antibody (Clone MIB-1, Dako, Glostrup, Denmark, dilution 1:100). For all procedures, the antigen retrieval was performed at 100°C with citrate buffer at pH 6.0. Primary antibody incubations were performed overnight at 4°C in a wet chamber. The labeling was developed using a HRP-diaminobenzidine kit (Envision, Dako, CA, United States). Lung tissue imagen were digitally acquired at 40×. The α-actin-ir in the muscle layer of small pulmonary arteries was measured as pixel count per area. The percentage of KI-67-ir positive nuclei in the medial layer of PMASC was calculated as the percentage of positive KI-67 nuclei (Castillo-Galán et al., 2016).

Vascular Luminal Surface and Vascular Density

In histological sections of lung stained with Van Gieson, 6 images were captured with a magnification of 10×. Subsequently, the vascular luminal surface (luminal area/total area) and the vascular density (number of arteries/total area) were determined in arteries of 150–300 μm of internal diameter.

Statistical Analysis

Data were expressed as mean ± standard standard desviation (SD). One-way or two way ANOVA followed by a Newman-Keuls post-test was used for the analysis. Results were analyzed and plotted in GraphPad Prism 8 software (GraphPad Software Inc., San Diego, CA, United States). For all comparisons, differences were considered statistically significant when $P < 0.05$.

RESULTS

Animal Weight Gain

All groups showed a similar gain of weight during the experiments ($P < 0.001$, two-way ANOVA, between initial and final weight in each group). However, we did not find differences in the initial and final weight between the groups ($P = 0.063$, two way-ANOVA) (**Table 1**).

2-Aminoethyl Diphenylborinate Prevented the Increased Right Ventricular Systolic Pressure in Rats Exposed to Intermittent Chronic Hypoxia

Following 28 days to CIH, the mean RVSP of the vehicle-treated CIH rats (Vehicle + 28d-CIH) was significantly higher related to the control rats (36.5 ± 3.2 mmHg vs. 19.4 ± 5.5 mmHg, $P = 0.0001$ for Vehicle + 28d-CIH vs. Control rats). Remarkably, 2-APB applied by osmotic pumps from day 14 of CIH (2-APB + 28d-CIH), prevented the increase of RVSP (24.7 ± 5.0 mmHg vs. 36.5 ± 3.2 mmHg, $P = 0.004$ for 2-APB + 28d-CIH vs. Vehicle + 28d-CIH, respectively, see **Figure 1A**). The heart rate was similar among all groups (**Figure 1B**).

2-Aminoethyl Diphenylborinate Prevented the Pulmonary Vascular Remodeling and the Proliferative Phenotype of PASCM Induced by Intermittent Chronic Hypoxia

Exposure to CIH for 28 days increased the thickness of the medial layer of pulmonary arteries (150–300 μm internal diameter) in the vehicle CIH-treated animals related to the control rats (67.4 ± 7.3% vs. 45.2 ± 2.5%, for Vehicle + 28d-CIH and control rats, respectively, $P < 0.0001$). In addition, 2-APB treatment prevented the increase of the medial layer thickness to 47.8 ± 3.5% related to its Vehicle ($P < 0.0001$) (**Figure 2A**). 2-APB treatment also prevented the increase of α-actin-ir in the medial layer of pulmonary arteries induced by CIH (7.38 ± 1.5 pixels/μm^2, 14.33 ± 1.6 pixels/μm^2 and 8.83 ± 0.6 pixels/μm^2, for Control group, Vehicle + 28d-CIH and 2-APB + 28d-CIH, respectively. $P < 0.0001$) (**Figure 2B**). Similarly, the percentage of Ki-67 positive cells in the pulmonary medial layer of vehicle-treated rats exposed to CIH was higher in CIH-treated rats than the control rats (6.3 ± 2.7% vs. 1.5 ± 0.8% for Vehicle + 28d-CIH vs. Control group, *respectively*. $P = 0.0003$). 2-APB treatment prevented the increased of PASMC proliferation marker Ki-67 (6.3 ± 2.7% vs. 3.9 ± 1.1% Vehicle + 28d-CIH vs. 2APB-28d-CIH, respectively. $P = 0.0051$) (**Figure 2C**).

TABLE 1 | Initial and final weights of the rats during the experiments.

Group	Initial weight (g)	Final weight (g)
Control	207.7 ± 14.5	290.0 ± 18.8 ##
Vehicle + 28 d CIH	199.5 ± 10.5	302.8 ± 24.9 ##
2-APB + 28 d CIH	209.5 ± 7.0	303.7 ± 24.6 ##

Mean ± SD. Two-way-ANOVA followed by Newman-Keuls tests. ##P > 0.001 vs. initial weight. No differences were found in the initial or final weight between the groups, two way-ANOVA, P = 0.063.

2-Aminoethyl Diphenylborinate Prevented the Reduction of the Luminal Vascular Surface Induced by Exposure to Chronic Intermittent Hypoxia

Exposure to CIH for 28 days increased the number of small pulmonary arteries of 150–300 μm of internal diameter compared to the control rats (12.7 ± 2.3 arteries/mm^2 vs. 7.2 ± 1.9 arteries/mm^2, for Vehicle + 28-CIH vs. control rats, respectively. $P = 0.0005$). Treatment with 2-APB normalized the number of arteries (7.9 ± 2.5 arteries/mm^2 in 2APB + 28-CIH, $P = 0{,}001$) (**Figure 3A**). In addition, CIH decreased the vascular luminal surface in the Vehicle-treated animals exposed to CIH as compared to the control group. Nevertheless, 2-APB prevented this decrease despite that rats were exposed to CIH, reaching similar values compared to control group (1497.0 ± 190.9 $\mu m^2/mm^2$, 797 ± 117.3 $\mu m^2/mm^2$ and 1632 ± 222.8 $\mu m^2/mm^2$, for control, Vehicle + 28d-CIH and 2-APB + 28d-CIH, respectively. $P < 0.0001$) (**Figure 3B**).

2-Aminoethyl Diphenylborinate Did Not Prevent the Systemic and Pulmonary Oxidative Stress Induced by Chronic Intermittent Hypoxia

Exposure to 28 days to CIH increase both systemic and pulmonary MDA concentration in Vehicle-treated rats related to control animals, but 2-APB treatment did not prevent the increase in both the systemic and pulmonary MDA concentration (**Figure 4**).

2-Aminoethyl Diphenylborinate Reduced the Relative Pulmonary Gene Expression of TRPC 1, 4, and 6 but Increased ORAI 1

CIH for 28 days increased the relative pulmonary gene expression of TRPC1, TRPC4, TRPC6, and ORAI 1, but not ORAI 2 as compared to control animals (**Figure 5**). 2-APB-treated rats did not shown an increase in the relative pulmonary gene expression of TRPC 1, TRPC 4 and TRPC6 induced by CIH, being these values similar to control animals (**Figures 5A–C**). On the contrary, the treatment with 2-APB induced an increase in the relative pulmonary gene expression of ORAI1, which was greater than the one found in the control animals and Vehicle-28d CIH-treated rats (**Figure 5D**). The expression of ORAI2 remained unchanged among the groups (**Figure 5E**).

DISCUSSION

We studied the effects of 2-APB, a drug with inhibitory actions on STOC (Bootman et al., 2002, Castillo-Galán et al., 2016, 2022),

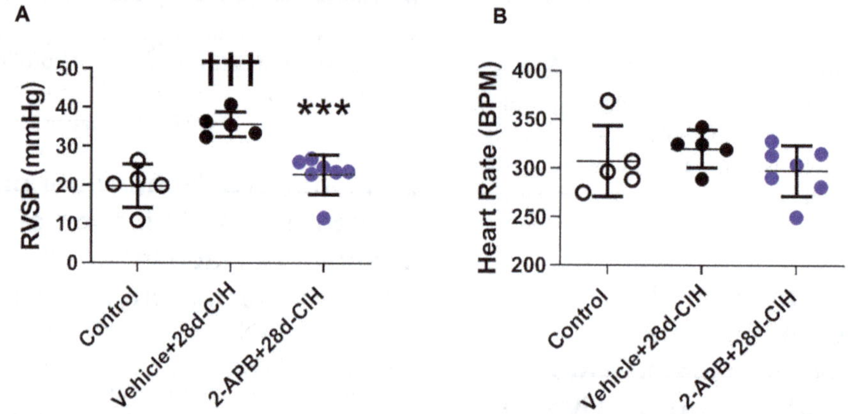

FIGURE 1 | Effect of 2-APB on right ventricular systolic pressure and heart rate in rats exposed to chronic intermittent hypoxia. 2-APB was infused from 14 days of CIH exposure with osmotic pumps at a rate of 10 mg/kg/day. **(A)** Right ventricular systolic pressure (RVSP) (ANOVA $P = 0.0002$). **(B)** Heart rate (HR) (ANOVA $P = 0.41$) in control (empty circles, $n = 5$), Vehicle + 28d-CIH (black circles, $n = 5$), and 2-APB + 28d-CIH rats (blue circles, $n = 7$). Mean ± SD. $^{\dagger\dagger\dagger}P < 0.001$ vs. all groups, $^{***}P < 0.001$ vs. Vehicle + 28d-CIH. One way ANOVA-followed by Newman Keuls tests.

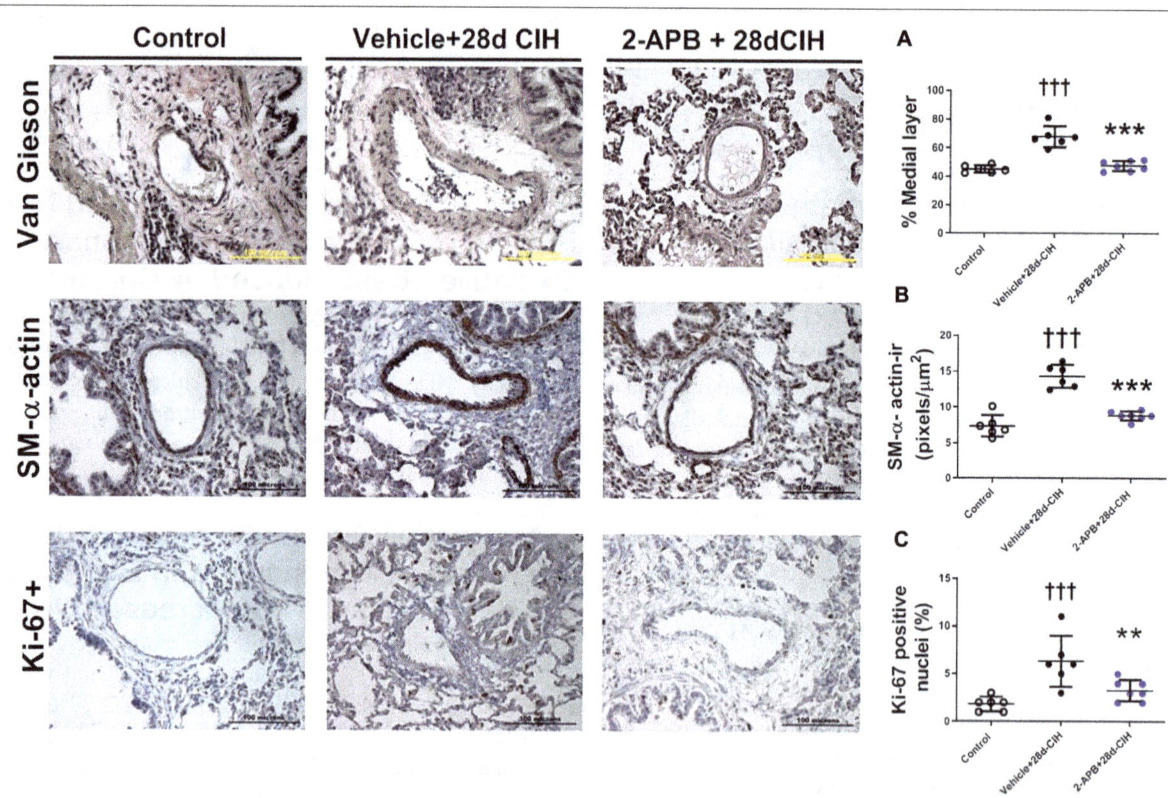

FIGURE 2 | Effect of 2-APB on pulmonary vascular remodeling induced by chronic intermittent hypoxia. **(A)** Medial layer (ANOVA $P < 0.0001$). **(B)** α-actin immunoreactivity in the medial layer (ANOVA $P < 0.0001$). **(C)** Ki-67 positive cells in PASMC (ANOVA $P = 0.0009$) of control (empty circles, $n = 6$), Vehicle + 28d-CIH (black circles, $n = 6$), and 2-APB + 28d-CIH rats (blue circles, $n = 7$). The % of medial layer was measured as (muscle area - lumen area)/(muscle area * 100). Scale bar = 100 μm. $^{\dagger\dagger\dagger}P < 0.001$ vs. all groups, $^{**}P < 0.01$ vs. Vehicle + 28d-CIH $^{***}P < 0.001$ vs. Vehicle + 28d-CIH, One way ANOVA-followed by Newman Keuls test.

in a rat model of CIH-induced pulmonary hypertension (Del Rio et al., 2010, 2012, 2014; Iturriaga et al., 2014; Castillo-Galán et al., 2020). Consistently with previous studies, rats exposed to CIH for 28 days, develop vascular remodeling characterized by an increased thickness of the medial layer in pulmonary arteries and an elevated right ventricular systolic pressure (Nisbet et al., 2009; Jin et al., 2014, 2016; Iturriaga and Castillo-Galán, 2019; Castillo-Galán et al., 2020). The main findings of this study are that 2-APB treatment prevented the raise of RVSP, the pulmonary vascular remodeling characterized by an increased medial layer

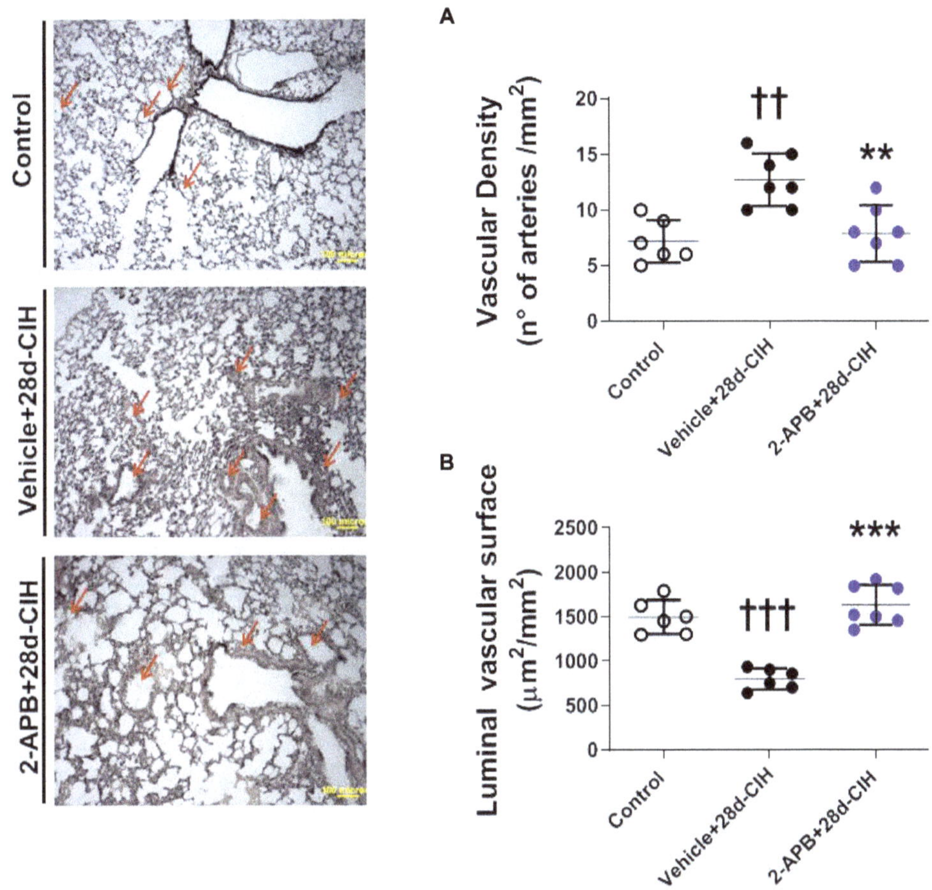

FIGURE 3 | Effect of 2-APB on vascular density and luminal surface in lungs of rats subjected to chronic intermittent hypoxia. Left panel, Reconstruction of 6 lung parenchyma slices stained with Van Gieson. **(A)** Vascular density (ANOVA, $P = 0.0007$). **(B)** Luminal vascular surface (ANOVA, $P < 0.0001$) in controls (empty circles, $n = 6$), Vehicle + 28d-CIH (black circles, $n = 6$), and 2-APB + 28d-CIH rats (blue circles, $n = 7$). Scale bar = 100 µm. Mean ± SD. $^{††}P < 0.01$ vs. all groups, $^{†††}P < 0.001$ vs. all groups, $^{**}P < 0.01$ vs. Vehicle + 28d-CIH, $^{***}P < 0.001$ vs. Vehicle + 28d-CIH. One way ANOVA-followed by Newman Keuls tests.

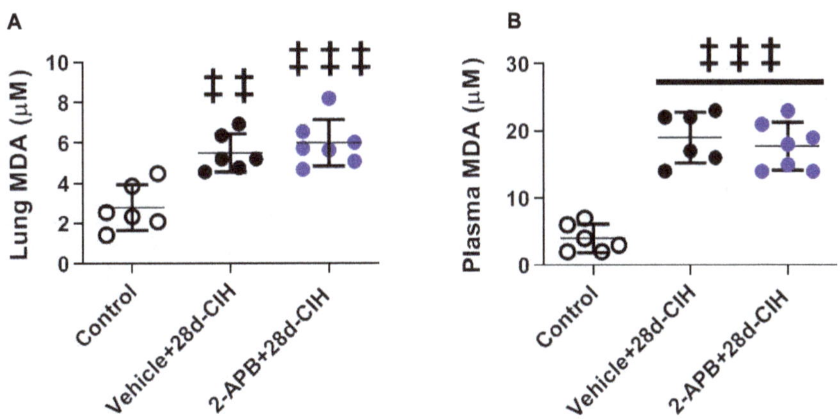

FIGURE 4 | Effect of 2-APB on pulmonary and systemic MDA concentration (TBARS) following chronic intermittent hypoxia. **(A)** MDA lung concentration (ANOVA, $P = 0.0002$). **(B)** Systemic plasma concentration (ANOVA, $P < 0.0001$) in control (empty circles, $n = 6$), exposed to Vehicle + 28d-CIH (black circles, $n = 6$), and 2-APB + 28d-CIH rats (blue circles, $n = 7$). Mean ± SD. $^{‡‡}P < 0.01$ vs. Control, $^{‡‡‡}P < 0.001$ vs. Control. One way ANOVA-Newman followed by Keuls tests.

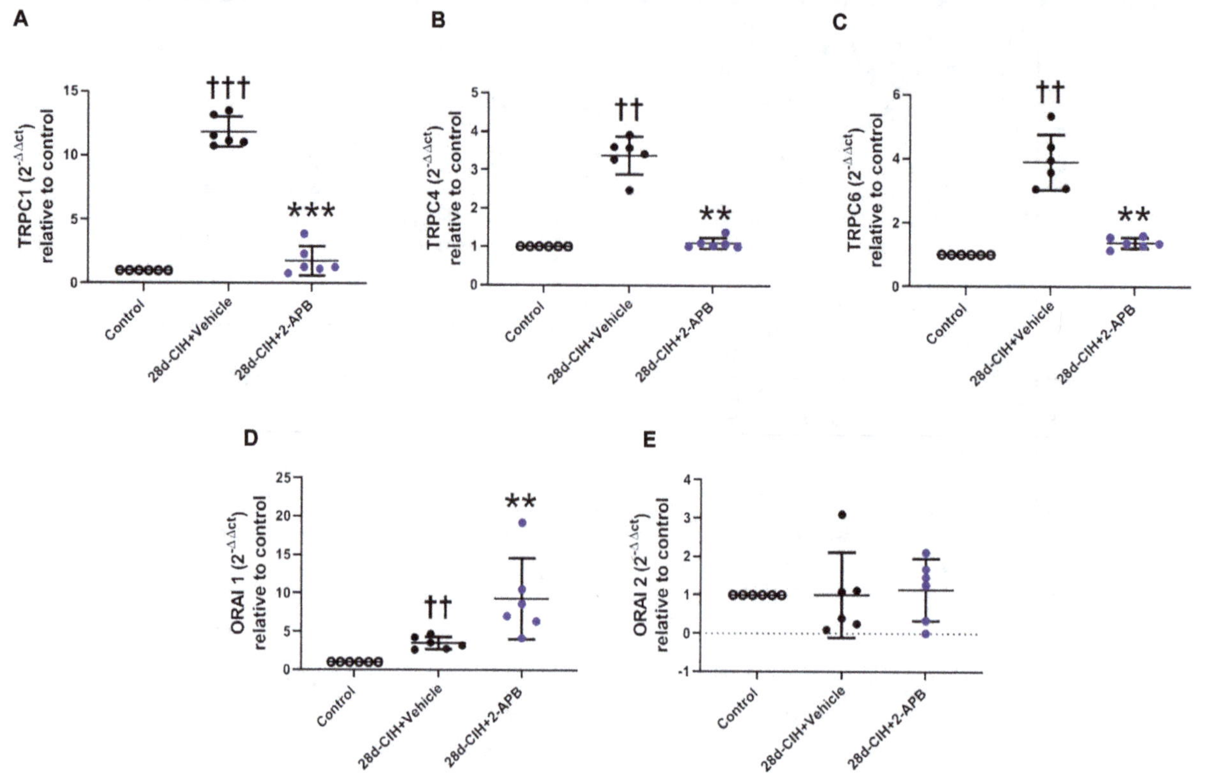

FIGURE 5 | Effect of 2-APB on the relative gene expression of STOC following chronic intermittent hypoxia. **(A)** relative lung gene expression of TRPC1 (ANOVA, $P = 0.0001$). **(B)** TRPC4 (ANOVA, $P = 0.0017$). **(C)** TRPC6 (ANOVA, $P = 0.0003$). **(D)** ORAI1 (ANOVA, $P = 0.0005$), and **(E)** ORAI2 (ANOVA, $P = 0.9612$) in control (empty circles, $n = 6$), Vehicle + 28d-CIH (black circles, $n = 6$), and 2-APB + 28d-CIH rats (blue circles, $n = 6$). Values expressed as $2^{-\Delta\Delta CT}$ related to the control. Mean ± SD. $^{††}P < 0.01$ vs. all groups, $^{†††}P < 0.001$ vs. all groups $^{**}P < 0.01$ vs. Vehicle + 28d-CIH, $^{***}P < 0.001$ vs. Vehicle + 28d-CIH, One way ANOVA-followed by Newman Keuls tests.

thickness, the increased α-actin-it and Ki-67 immunoreactive levels, and the lumen vascular surface reduction. In addition, we found that 2-APB did not reduce the lung and plasma oxidative stress, suggesting that the effects of 2-APB on vascular remodeling and pulmonary hypertension are independent of the oxidative stress action. Thus, present results strongly suggest that STOC contribute to the pulmonary hypertension and vascular remodeling in a pre-clinical model of OSA.

Present results showing that 2-APB infusion prevented the increase of RVSP induced by CIH, agree and extended previous studies, which found that 2-APB treatment attenuated the pulmonary vascular remodeling, the increased RVSP and the Fulton index in mice exposed for 4 weeks to sustained hypoxia, as compared to hypoxic animals treated with Vehicle (Smith et al., 2015). Similarly, the daily infusion of 2-APB reduced the vascular remodeling and pulmonary hypertension induced by pregestational hypoxia in newborn lambs in high altitude (Castillo-Galán et al., 2016). Interestingly, our results showed that 2-APB prevented the over-expression of TRPC subunits 1, 4 and 6 induced by CIH in the lung tissue. On the other hand, CIH activates the ET-1 – IP3R pathway in PASMC, releasing Ca^{2+} from the reticulum, which in turn activate STOC (Wang et al., 2012; Castillo-Galán et al., 2020) and raise the intracellular Ca^{2+} concentration (Reyes et al., 2018). In addition, Ca^{2+} activates or stabilized transcription factors that upregulated STOC subunits such as HIFs, NFAT, AP-1, NF-KB and the Platelet Derived Growth Factor (Shibasaki et al., 1996; Timmerman et al., 1996; Dolmetsch et al., 1997; Chen et al., 1998; Salnikow et al., 2002; Mottet et al., 2003; Ogawa et al., 2012; Jiang et al., 2014; Domínguez-Rodríguez et al., 2015; Wang et al., 2015, 2017). Taken together, the evidence suggests that 2-APB would induce a decrease in intracellular calcium (Parrau et al., 2013), which may inhibit the upregulation of TRPC1, TRPC4 and TRPC6. However, more studies are required to determine if all of these factors that regulated STOC changed in the lung tissue following CIH.

In this study, 2-APB was administered with osmotic pumps at a delivery rate of 10 mg/kg per day, which is similar to the daily dose range used by Smith et al. (2015), Castillo-Galán et al. (2016, 2022) and Jain et al. (2021) to block STOC *in vivo*. Indeed, Smith et al. (2015) treated chronic hypoxic mice with 2-APB (1 mg/kg/day i.p.) to reduce pulmonary hypertension and right ventricular enlargement. Castillo-Galán et al. (2016, 2022), administered 2-APB (10 mg/kg/day i.v.) to neonatal lambs with a partial or full gestation in high altitude to ameliorate the pulmonary hypertension and vascular remodeling, and Jain et al. (2021) administrated 2-APB (1 mg/kg per day i.p.) to attenuate pulmonary hypertension in hypoxic mice. We did not measure the plasma concentrations of 2-APB after its administration, but Parrau et al. (2013) estimated that a single dose of 2-APB (8 mg/kg i.v.) would reach a concentration in the extracellular space in the range of 10–100 μM, assuming a distribution volume of 40% of the body weight. The same order of 2-APB concentration blocks STOC in isolated pulmonary arteries from hypoxic lambs (Parrau et al., 2013) and in HEK293 cells transfected with Orai/Stim or TRPC subunits (Lievremont et al., 2005; Peinelt et al., 2008).

Since 2-APB is a non-selective STOC blocker, we cannot preclude effects of 2-APB at the IP3R level. This make it uncertain to determine to what extent the effects of 2-APB on pulmonary vascular remodeling and hypertension are due to its effects on any of these targets. The participation of IP3R on the response of pulmonary arteries to hypoxia is controversial and depend on the species and type of vessel studied. While in rat distal pulmonary artery PASMC, both Ca^{2+} release from intracellular stores and Ca^{2+} entry from the extracellular space induced by hypoxia are abolished by IP3R blockade with xestonpongin-C (Wang et al., 2012), in canine pulmonary artery PASMC, Ca^{2+} entry mediated by STOC in response to hypoxia is unaffected by IP3R blockade (Ng et al., 2008). On the other hand, in rat main pulmonary arteries, both cytosolic Ca^{2+} increase and contraction in response to hypoxia are biphasic, with a rapid transient fast response followed by a slowly developing and sustained response. In these arteries, the contraction in response to hypoxia develop without changes in IP3 content (Jin et al., 1993), Indeed, it has been proposed that STOC account for the sustained Ca^{2+} increase in response to hypoxia (Sylvester et al., 2012). Moreover, in isolated pulmonary arteries of newborn lambs, the relaxation elicited by SKF-96365, a specific STOC blocker without effect on IP3R is similar to the relaxation induced by 2-APB, and both of them increased in pulmonary arteries from hypoxic lambs (Parrau et al., 2013). Taken together these observations suggest that 2-APB may act on IP3R and STOC, but the final effect is an indirect or a direct reduction of Ca^{2+} entry mediated by STOC in pulmonary PASMC from animals exposed to hypoxia. Considering that 2-APB is not a selective STOC blocker, new drugs with a selective effects on ORAI1/STIM1 interaction are needed to evaluate the role of the STOC in OSA patients with pulmonary hypertension (Reyes et al., 2018; Waldron et al., 2019).

Chronic intermittent hypoxia induces oxidative stress at the pulmonary and systemic level, which may affect calcium homeostasis and contribute to the lung vascular remodeling (Del Rio et al., 2010, 2012; Jin et al., 2014, 2016; Iturriaga and Castillo-Galán, 2019; Castillo-Galán et al., 2020). Antioxidants such as procyanidin and melatonin reduced the elevated RVSP and the vascular remodeling induced by CIH (Jin et al., 2014, 2016). The activation of TRPC1 and TRPC6 by the transcription factor BMP4 in rat PASMC depended on the increased ROS levels mediated by NOX4 (Jiang et al., 2014). In addition, it has been proposed that the increase in ROS levels induced by hypoxia, activates the ryanodine receptors (RyR), which in turn induces the release of the reticular Ca^{2+}, activating STIM1, and allowing the interaction with ORAI in the plasma membrane and subsequent activation of the STOC (Suresh and Shimoda, 2016). These results suggest that the effects of antioxidants may be related with the inactivation of STOC and subsequently decrease in intracellular calcium. Although an antioxidant action of 2-APB has been shown in ischemia/reperfusion damage in mice and rat cardiomyocytes (Morihara et al., 2017; Shen et al., 2021), our results showed that 2-APB did not prevent the systemic and lung oxidative stress, suggesting that the effects of 2-APB on PASMC in the lung are not related by a reduction in oxidative stress. Thus, it is likely that the effects of 2-APB were related to its inhibitory action on the increased intracellular Ca^{2+} concentrations induced by STOC (Bootman et al., 2002). Thus, the treatment of hypoxic pulmonary hypertensive rats with 2-APB, has a strong effect preventing the increase of RVSP and the pulmonary vascular remodeling without any significant action on the oxidative stress markers.

CONCLUSION

Present results indicated that 2-APB treatment to rats exposed to CIH prevented the increased RVPS and the pulmonary vascular remodeling, without effects on both systemic and pulmonary oxidative stress markers, suggest that STOC are and attractive therapeutic target to prevent pulmonary hypertension in OSA. In summary, present results showed that 2-APB strongly ameliorated the pulmonary vascular alterations induced by CIH, indicates that the STOC inhibition may potentially be used to treat the pulmonary hypertension induced by OSA.

ETHICS STATEMENT

The animal study was reviewed and approved by Scientific Ethical Committee for the Animal and Environment Care Pontificia Universidad Católica de Chile, Santiago, Chile (ID:180803006).

AUTHOR CONTRIBUTIONS

SC-G and BR performed the experiments. SC-G and RI contributed to the conception and design of research, analyzed the data, interpreted the results, and drafted the manuscript. All authors revised the manuscript and approved final version of the manuscript.

REFERENCES

Bootman, M. D., Collins, T. J., Mackenzie, L., Roderick, H. L., Berridge, M. J., and Peppiatt, C. M. (2002). 2-aminoethoxydiphenyl borate (2-APB) is a reliable blocker of store-operated Ca^{2+} entry but an inconsistent inhibitor of InsP3-induced Ca^{2+} release. *FASEB J.* 10, 1145–1150. doi: 10.1096/fj.02-0037rev

Castillo-Galán, S., Arenas, G. A., Reyes, R. V., Krause, B. J., and Iturriaga, R. (2020). Stim- activated TRPC-ORAI channels in pulmonary hypertension induced by chronic intermittent hypoxia. *Pulm. Circ.* 10, 13–22. doi: 10.1177/2045894020941484

Castillo-Galán, S., Parrau, D., Hernández, I., Quezada, S., Díaz, M., Ebensperger, G., et al. (2022). The action of 2-aminoethyldiphenyl borinate on the pulmonary arterial hypertension and remodeling of high-altitude hypoxemic lambs. *Front. Physiol.* 12:765281. doi: 10.3389/fphys.2021.765281

Castillo-Galán, S., Quezada, S., Moraga, F. A., Ebensperger, G., Herrera, E. A., Beñaldo, F., et al. (2016). 2-aminoethyldiphenylborinate modifies the pulmonary circulation in pulmonary hypertensive newborn lambs with partial gestation at high altitude. *Am. J. Physiol. Lung. Cell Mol. Physiol.* 311, L788–L799. doi: 10.1152/ajplung.00230.2016

Chen, C. Y., Del Gatto-Konczak, F., Wu, Z., and Karin, M. (1998). Stabilization of interleukin-2 mRNA by the c-Jun NH2-terminal kinase pathway. *Science* 280, 1945–1949.

Del Rio, R., Moya, E. A., and Iturriaga, R. (2010). Carotid body and cardiorespiratory alterations in intermittent hypoxia: the oxidative link. *Eur. Respir. J.* 36, 143–150. doi: 10.1183/09031936.00158109

Del Rio, R., Moya, E. A., and Iturriaga, R. (2014). Carotid body potentiation during chronic intermittent hypoxia: implication for hypertension. *Front. Physiol.* 5:434. doi: 10.3389/fphys.2014.00434

Del Rio, R., Moya, E. A., Parga, M. J., Madrid, C., and Iturriaga, R. (2012). Carotid body inflammation and cardiorespiratory alterations in intermittent hypoxia. *Eur. Respir. J.* 39, 1492–1500. doi: 10.1183/09031936.00141511

Dempsey, J. A., Veasey, S. C., Morgan, B. R., and O'Donnell, C. P. (2010). Pathophysiology of sleep apnea. *Physiol. Rev.* 90, 47–112. doi: 10.1152/physrev.00043.2008

Dolmetsch, R. E., Lewis, R. S., Goodnow, C. C., and Healy, J. I. (1997). Differential activation of transcription factors induced by Ca^{2+} response amplitude and duration. *Nature* 386, 855–858.

Domínguez-Rodríguez, A., Ruiz-Hurtado, G., Sabourin, J., Gómez, A. M., Alvarez, J. L., and Benitah, J. P. (2015). Proarrhythmic effect of sustained EPAC activation on TRPC3/4 in rat ventricular cardiomyocytes. *J. Mol. Cell. Cardiol.* 87, 74–78.

Floras, J. S. (2018). Sleep apnea and cardiovascular disease. *Circ Res.* 122, 1741–1764. doi: 10.1161/CIRCRESAHA.118.310783

Fuchs, B., Dietrich, A., Gudermann, T., Kalwa, H., Grimminger, F., and Weissmann, N. (2010). The role of classical transient receptor potential channels in the regulation of hypoxic pulmonary vasoconstriction. *Adv Exp Med Biol.* 661, 187–200. doi: 10.1007/978-1-60761-500-2_12

Golovina, V. A., Platoshyn, O., Bailey, C. L., Wang, J., Limsuwan, A., Sweeney, M., et al. (2001). Upregulated TRP and enhanced capacitative Ca(2+) entry in human pulmonary artery myocytes during proliferation. *Am. J. Physiol. Heart Circ. Physiol.* 280, H746–H755. doi: 10.1152/ajpheart.2001.280.2.H746

Guibert, C., Ducret, T., and Savineau, J. P. (2011). Expression and physiological roles of TRP channels in smooth muscle cells. *Adv. Exp. Med. Biol.* 704, 687–706. doi: 10.1007/978-94-007-0265-3_36

Harki, O., Boete, Q., Pépin, J. L., Arnaud, C., Belaidi, E., Faury, G., et al. (2021). Intermittent hypoxia-related alterations in vascular structure and function: a systematic review and meta-analysis of rodent data. *Eur. Respir. J.* 19:2100866. doi: 10.1183/13993003.00866-2021

Hou, X., Chen, J., Luo, Y., Liu, F., Xu, G., and Gao, Y. (2013). Silencing of STIM1 attenuates hypoxia-induced PASMCs proliferation via inhibition of the SOC/Ca2+/NFAT pathway. *Respir. Res.* 14:2. doi: 10.1186/1465-9921-14-2

Iturriaga, R. (2018). Translating carotid body function into clinical medicine. *J. Physiol.* 596, 3067–3077. doi: 10.1113/JP275335

Iturriaga, R., Alcayaga, J., Chapleau, M. W., and Somers, V. K. (2021). Carotid body chemoreceptors: physiology, pathology, and implications for health and disease. *Physiol Rev.* 101, 1177–1235. doi: 10.1152/physrev.00039.2019

Iturriaga, R., and Castillo-Galán, S. (2019). Potential contribution of carotid body-induced sympathetic and renin-angiotensin system overflow to pulmonary hypertension in intermittent hypoxia. *Curr. Hypertens. Rep.* 21:89. doi: 10.1007/s11906-019-0995-y

Iturriaga, R., Andrade, D. C., and Del Rio, R. (2014). Enhanced carotid body chemosensory activity and the cardiovascular alterations induced by intermittent hypoxia. *Front. Physiol.* 5:468. doi: 10.3389/fphys.2014.00468

Jain, P., Lai, N., Xiong, M., Chen, J., Babicheva, A., Zhao, T., et al. (2021). TRPC6, a therapeutic target for pulmonary hypertension. *Am. J. Physiol. Lung Cell Mol. Physiol.* 321, L1161–L1182. doi: 10.1152/ajplung.00159.2021

Jiang, Q., Fu, X., Tian, L., Chen, Y., Yang, K., Chen, X., et al. (2014). NOX4 mediates BMP4-induced upregulation of TRPC1 and 6 protein expressions in distal pulmonary arterial smooth muscle cells. *PLoS One* 9:e107135. doi: 10.1371/journal.pone.0107135

Jin, H., Liu, M., Zhang, X., Pan, J., Han, J., Wang, Y., et al. (2016). Grape seed procyanidin extract attenuates hypoxic pulmonary hypertension by inhibiting oxidative stress and pulmonary arterial smooth muscle cells proliferation. *J. Nutr. Biochem.* 36, 81–88. doi: 10.1016/j.jnutbio.2016.07.006

Jin, H., Wang, Y., Zhou, L., Liu, L., Zhang, P., Deng, W., et al. (2014). Melatonin attenuates hypoxic pulmonary hypertension by inhibiting the inflammation and the proliferation of pulmonary arterial smooth muscle cells. *J. Pineal. Res.* 57, 442–450. doi: 10.1111/jpi.12184

Jin, N., Packer, C. S., English, D., and Rhoades, R. A. (1993). Inositol trisphosphate is involved in norepinephrine-but not in hypoxia-induced pulmonary arterial contraction. *Am. J. Physiol.* 264, L160–L164. doi: 10.1152/ajplung.1993.264.2.L160

Johnstone, L. S., Graham, S. J., and Dziadek, M. A. (2010). STIM proteins: integrators of signalling pathways in development, differentiation and disease. *J. Cell. Mol. Med.* 14, 1890–1903. doi: 10.1111/j.1582-4934.2010.01097.x

Kuhr, F. K., Smith, K. A., Song, M. Y., Levitan, I., and Yuan, J. X. (2012). New mechanisms of pulmonary arterial hypertension: role of Ca^{2+} signaling. *Am. J. Physiol. Heart Circ. Physiol.* 302, H1546–H1562. doi: 10.1152/ajpheart.00944.2011

Lievremont, J. P., Bird, G. S., and Putney, J. W. (2005). Mechanism of inhibition of TRPC cation channels by 2- aminoethoxydiphenylborane. *Mol. Pharmacol.* 68, 758–762. doi: 10.1124/mol.105.012856

Lu, W., Wang, J., Peng, G., Shimoda, L. A., and Sylvester, J. T. (2009). Knockdown of stromal interaction molecule 1 attenuates store-operated Ca^{2+} entry and Ca^{2+} responses to acute hypoxia in pulmonary arterial smooth muscle. *Am. J. Physiol. Lung Cell Mol. Physiol.* 297, L17–L25. doi: 10.1152/ajplung.00063.2009

Lu, W., Wang, J., Shimoda, L. A., and Sylvester, J. T. (2008). Differences in STIM1 and TRPC expression in proximal and distal pulmonary arterial smooth muscle are associated with differences in Ca^{2+} responses to hypoxia. *Am. J. Physiol. Lung Cell Mol. Physiol.* 295, L104–L113. doi: 10.1152/ajplung.00058.200

Morihara, H., Obana, M., Tanaka, S., Kawakatsu, I., Tsuchiyama, D., Mori, S., et al. (2017). 2-aminoethoxydiphenyl borate provides an anti-oxidative effect and mediates cardioprotection during ischemia reperfusion in mice. *PLoS One* 12:e0189948. doi: 10.1371/journal.pone.0189948

Mottet, D., Michel, G., Renard, P., Ninane, N., Raes, M., and Michiels, C. (2003). Role of ERK and calcium in the hypoxia-induced activation of HIF-1. *J. Cell. Physiol.* 194, 30–44. doi: 10.1002/jcp.10176

Ng, L. C., Kyle, B. D., Lennox, A. R., Shen, X. M., Hatton, W. J., and Hume, J. R. (2008). Cell culture alters Ca^{2+} entry pathways activated by store-depletion or hypoxia in canine pulmonary arterial smooth muscle cells. *Br. J. Pharmacol.* 152, 101–111. doi: 10.1152/ajpcell.00258.2007

Nisbet, R. E., Graves, A. S., Kleinhenz, D. J., Rupnow, H. L., Reed, A. L., Fan, T. H., et al. (2009). The role of NADPH oxidase in chronic intermittent hypoxia-induced pulmonary hypertension in mice. *Am. J. Respir. Cell Mol. Biol.* 40, 601–609. doi: 10.1165/2008-0145OC

Ogawa, A., Firth, A. L., Smith, K. A., Maliakal, M. V., and Yuan, J. X. (2012). PDGF enhances store-operated Ca^{2+} entry by upregulating STIM1/Orai1 via activation of Akt/mTOR in human pulmonary arterial smooth muscle cells. *Am. J. Physiol. Cell Physiol.* 302, C405–C411. doi: 10.1152/ajpcell.00337.2011

Parrau, D., Ebensperger, G., Herrera, E. A., Moraga, F., Riquelme, R. A., Ulloa, C. E., et al. (2013). Store-operated channels in the pulmonary circulation of high- and low-altitude neonatal lambs. *Am. J. Physiol. Lung Cell Mol. Physiol.* 304, L540–L548. doi: 10.1152/ajplung.00024.2012

Peinelt, C., Lis, A., Beck, A., Fleig, A., and Penner, R. (2008). 2-Aminoethoxydiphenyl borate directly facilitates and indirectly inhibits STIM1-dependent gating of CRAC channels. *J. Physiol.* 586, 3061–3073. doi: 10.1113/jphysiol.2008.151365

Reyes, R. V., Castillo-Galán, S., Hernandez, I., Herrera, E. A., Ebensperger, G., and Llanos, A. J. (2018). Revisiting the Role of TRP, Orai, and ASIC channels in the pulmonary arterial response to hypoxia. *Front. Physiol.* 9:486. doi: 10.3389/fphys.2018.00486

Sajkov, D., and McEvoy, R. D. (2009). Obstructive sleep apnea and pulmonary hypertension. *Prog. Cardiovasc. Dis.* 51, 363–370. doi: 10.1016/j.pcad.2008.06.001

Salnikow, K., Kluz, T., Costa, M., Piquemal, D., Demidenko, Z. N., Xie, K., et al. (2002). The regulation of hypoxic genes by calcium involves c-Jun/AP-1, which cooperates with hypoxia-inducible factor 1 in response to hypoxia. *Mol. Cell. Biol.* 22, 1734–1741. doi: 10.1128/MCB.22.6.1734-1741

Shen, Y. C., Shen, Y. J., Lee, W. S., Chen, M. Y., Tu, W. C., and Yang, K. T. (2021). Two benzene rings with a boron atom comprise the core structure of 2-APB responsible for the anti-oxidative and protective effect on the ischemia/reperfusion-induced rat heart Injury. *Antioxidants* 10:1667. doi: 10. 3390/antiox10111667

Shibasaki, F., Price, E. R., Milan, D., and McKeon, F. (1996). Role of kinases and the phosphatase calcineurin in the nuclear shuttling of transcription factor NF-AT4. *Nature* 382, 370–373. doi: 10.1038/382370a0

Smith, K. A., Voiriot, G., Tang, H., Fraidenburg, D. R., Song, S., Yamamura, H., et al. (2015). Notch activation of Ca(2+) signaling in the development of hypoxic pulmonary vasoconstriction and pulmonary hypertension. *Am. J. Respir. Cell Mol. Biol.* 53, 355–367. doi: 10.1165/rcmb.2014-0235OC

Somers, V. K., White, D. P., Amin, R., Abraham, W. T., Costa, F., Culebras, A., et al. (2008). Sleep apnea and cardiovascular disease: an American heart association/American college of cardiology foundation scientific statement from the american heart association council for high blood pressure research professional education committee, council on clinical cardiology, stroke council, and council on cardiovascular nursing. In collaboration with the national heart, lung, and blood institute national center on sleep disorders research (National Institutes of Health). *Circulation* 118, 1080–1111. doi: 10. 1161/CIRCULATIONAHA.107.189375

Suresh, K., and Shimoda, L. A. (2016). Lung circulation. *Compr. Physiol.* 6, 897–943. doi: 10.1002/cphy.c140049

Sylvester, J. T., Shimoda, L. A., Aaronson, P. I., and Ward, J. P. (2012). Hypoxic pulmonary vasoconstriction. *Physiol. Rev.* 92, 367–520. doi: 10.1152/physrev. 00041.2010

Timmerman, L. A., Clipstone, N. A., Ho, S. N., Northrop, J. P., and Crabtree, G. R. (1996). Rapid shuttling of NF-AT in discrimination of Ca^{2+} signals and immunosuppression. *Nature* 383, 837–840. doi: 10.1038/383837a0

Waldron, R. T., Chen, Y., Pham, H., Go, A., Su, H. Y., Hu, C., et al. (2019). The Orai Ca^{2+} channel inhibitor CM4620 targets both parenchymal and immune cells to reduce inflammation in experimental acute pancreatitis. *J. Physiol.* 597, 3085–3105. doi: 10.1113/JP277856

Wang, J., Fu, X., Yang, K., Jiang, Q., Chen, Y., Jia, J., et al. (2015). Hypoxia inducible factor-1-dependent up-regulation of BMP4 mediates hypoxia-induced increase of TRPC expression in PASMCs. *Cardiovasc. Res.* 107, 108–118. doi: 10.1093/ cvr/cvv122

Wang, J., Shimoda, L. A., and Sylvester, J. T. (2012). Ca^{2+} responses of pulmonary arterial myocytes to acute hypoxia require release from ryanodine and inositol trisphosphate receptors in sarcoplasmic reticulum. *Am. J. Physiol. Lung Cell. Mol. Physiol.* 303, 161–168. doi: 10.1152/ajplung.00348.2011

Wang, J., Xu, C., Zheng, Q., Yang, K., Lai, N., Wang, T., et al. (2017). Orai1, 2, 3 and STIM1 promote store-operated calcium entry in pulmonary arterial smooth muscle cells. *Cell. Death. Discov.* 3:17074. doi: 10.1038/cddiscovery.2017.74

Waypa, G. B., Marks, J. D., Mack, M. M., Boriboun, C., Mungai, P. T., and Schumacker, P. T. (2002). Mitochondrial reactive oxygen species trigger calcium increases during hypoxia in pulmonary arterial myocytes. *Circ Res.* 91, 719–726. doi: 10.1161/01.res.0000036751.04896.f1

Weigand, L., Foxson, J., Wang, J., Shimoda, L. A., and Sylvester, J. T. (2005). Inhibition of hypoxic pulmonary vasoconstriction by antagonists of store-operated Ca^{2+} and nonselective cation channels. *Am. J. Physiol. Lung Cell Mol. Physiol.* 289, L5–L13. doi: 10.1152/ajplung.00044.2005

Wray, S., and Burdyga, T. (2010). Sarcoplasmic reticulum function in smooth muscle. *Physiol. Rev.* 90, 113–178. doi: 10.1152/physrev.00018.2008

Yang, X. R., Lin, M. J., and Sham, J. S. (2010). Physiological functions of transient receptor potential channels in pulmonary arterial smooth muscle cells. *Adv. Exp. Med. Biol.* 661, 109–122. doi: 10.1007/978-1-60761-500-2_7

Zhang, W. M., Yip, K. P., Lin, M. J., Shimoda, L. A., Li, W. H., and Sham, J. S. (2003). ET-1 activates Ca^{2+} sparks in PASMC: local Ca^{2+} signaling between inositol trisphosphate and ryanodine receptors. *Am. J. Physiol. Lung Cell Mol. Physiol.* 3, L680–L690. doi: 10.1152/ajplung.00067.2003

7

The mTORC1/eIF4E/HIF-1α Pathway Mediates Glycolysis to Support Brain Hypoxia Resistance in the Gansu Zokor, *Eospalax cansus*

Jinyan Lin, Lele Fan, Yuming Han, Juanjuan Guo, Zhiqiang Hao, Lingna Cao, Jiamin Kang, Xiaoqin Wang, Jianping He and Jingang Li**

National Engineering Laboratory for Resource Development of Endangered Crude Drugs in Northwest China, Key Laboratory of the Ministry of Education for Medicinal Resources and Natural Pharmaceutical Chemistry, College of Life Science, Shaanxi Normal University, Xi'an, China

***Correspondence:**
Jianping He
hejianping@snnu.edu.cn
Jingang Li
jingang@snnu.edu.cn

The Gansu zokor (*Eospalax cansus*) is a subterranean rodent species that is unique to China. These creatures inhabit underground burrows with a hypoxia environment. Metabolic energy patterns in subterranean rodents have become a recent focus of research; however, little is known about brain energy metabolism under conditions of hypoxia in this species. The mammalian (mechanistic) target of rapamycin complex 1 (mTORC1) coordinates eukaryotic cell growth and metabolism, and its downstream targets regulate hypoxia inducible factor-1α (HIF-1α) under conditions of hypoxia to induce glycolysis. In this study, we compared the metabolic characteristics of hypoxia-tolerant subterranean Gansu zokors under hypoxic conditions with those of hypoxia-intolerant Sprague-Dawley rats with a similar-sized surface area. We exposed Gansu zokors and rats to hypoxia I (44 h at 10.5% O_2) or hypoxia II (6 h at 6.5% O_2) and then measured the transcriptional levels of mTORC1 downstream targets, the transcriptional and translational levels of glycolysis-related genes, glucose and fructose levels in plasma and brain, and the activity of key glycolysis-associated enzymes. Under hypoxia, we found that *hif-1α* transcription was upregulated *via* the mTORC1/eIF4E pathway to drive glycolysis. Furthermore, Gansu zokor brain exhibited enhanced fructose-driven glycolysis under hypoxia through increased expression of the GLUT5 fructose transporter and ketohexokinase (KHK), in addition to increased KHK enzymatic activity, and utilization of fructose; these changes did not occur in rat. However, glucose-driven glycolysis was enhanced in both Gansu zokor and rat under hypoxia II of 6.5% O_2 for 6 h. Overall, our results indicate that on the basis of glucose as the main metabolic substrate, fructose is used to accelerate the supply of energy in Gansu zokor, which mirrors the metabolic responses to hypoxia in this species.

Keywords: brain, hypoxia, mTORC1, fructose-driven glycolysis, Gansu zokor (*Eospalax cansus*)

INTRODUCTION

Although mammals are largely intolerant of hypoxia and their brains exhibit exquisite sensitivity to hypoxia, a few species, such as subterranean rodents, inhabit hypoxic niches and are able to survive hypoxia (Su et al., 2013; Nayak et al., 2016; Grimes et al., 2017; Altwasser et al., 2019; Li et al., 2019; Pamenter et al., 2019; Dong et al., 2020). These subterranean rodents have evolved various strategies to cope with the harsh environmental pressures of the hypoxic environment. All six African mole-rat species have sufficient antioxidant capacity to respond to dynamic hypoxia (Logan et al., 2020), *Lasiopodomys mandarinus*, *Spalax ehrenbergi* (the blind mole rat) and *Heterocephalus glaber* (the naked mole rat) all show hypoxia adaptation as an enhanced capacity for DNA repair and damage prevention (Shams et al., 2013; Lewis et al., 2016; Dong et al., 2020). *Eospalax fontanierii* exhibits reduced blood circulation resistance under hypoxia, which has a protective effect of myocardial function (Xu et al., 2019). These adaptations indicate that subterranean rodents have evolved hypoxic defense mechanisms, which confer protection against a low-oxygen environment.

Hypoxia is an environmental challenge for fossorial species that inhabit underground burrows. One of the greatest challenges in this environment is the high energy cost of burrowing in order to find limited food resources underground and maintain the burrow structure (Vleck, 1979, 1981; Šumbera et al., 2007; Barčiová et al., 2009). Maintaining the balance between energy production and consumption is the key to hypoxia tolerance, which protects against cell death (Staples and Buck, 2009; Speers-Roesch et al., 2010). The mammalian (or mechanistic) target of rapamycin (mTOR), which is a serine/threonine protein kinase in the PI3K-related kinase (PIKK) family, plays a vital role in energy metabolism and cell growth. It exists in two complexes: mTORC1 and mTORC2 (Saxton and Sabatini, 2017; Yan et al., 2017). mTORC1 controls the balance of metabolism in response to hypoxic conditions. The mTORC1/eIF4E pathway regulates hypoxia inducible factor 1α (HIF-1α), which plays an important role in glycolysis (Cheng et al., 2016; Chi et al., 2017; Saxton and Sabatini, 2017). HIF-1α stimulates the expression of transporters, glycolytic enzymes and glycolytic-inducing factors to regulate glycolysis (Zhang and Sadek, 2014). Glucose and fructose enter cells *via* the GLUT1 and GLUT5 transporters, respectively. GLUT5 is a highly selective transporter for fructose (Inukai et al., 1995). In the glucose-driven glycolysis pathway, phosphofructokinase (PFK) catalyzes the rate-limiting step from fructose-6-phosphate to fructose-1,6-bisphosphate (Real-Hohn et al., 2010). In the fructose-driven glycolysis pathway, ketohexokinase (KHK) catalyzes the direct phosphorylation of fructose to form fructose 1-phosphate, thus bypassing the PFK regulatory block and allowing continued glycolytic flux independent of cellular energy status (Park et al., 2017).

There have been some studies on the mechanisms underlying adaptive responses to hypoxia in subterranean rodents in recent years (Park et al., 2017; Schmidt et al., 2017; Faulkes et al., 2019; Pamenter et al., 2019; Farhat et al., 2020), but these have been mainly limited to naked mole rats and blind mole rats and further studies on other subterranean rodent species are needed. The family Spalacidae includes a group of naturally subterranean rodents known as zokors. Zokors (*Eospalax*) spend 85–90% of their time in self-constructed underground burrows, rarely venturing out on the ground surface; on the one hand, the burrows offer shelter from extreme climatic conditions and predators, while on the other hand, zokors must withstand the stress of a hypoxic and hypercapnic environment in almost total darkness burrows (Zhou and Dou, 1990; Zhang et al., 2003; Lacey et al., 2010; Xu et al., 2019). Furthermore, these animals require large amounts of energy digging to locate unpredictably and unevenly scattered food resources (Begall et al., 2007). Zokors have a marked influence on the soil texture and water-holding capacity by excavating vast burrow systems, which play an important role in the ecosystem structure and development (Zhang et al., 2003). The Gansu zokor (*Eospalax cansus*) is unique to China and endemic to the Loess plateau, inhabiting prairie, forest, meadow and farmland habitats (Su et al., 2014; Xu et al., 2019). The foraging activity of Gansu zokor is conducted mainly at a depth of 8–13 cm under the ground, and they rest in nest at the bottom of the burrow, which are usually 1–2 m deep. Their burrow systems are approximately 10 cm in diameter, with extending to approximately 100 m (Chen and Huang, 2012; Pleštilová et al., 2018). During the recent decades, studies have been conducted on the population age of Gansu zokor (Li and Wang, 1992) and seismic communication (Li et al., 2001), as well as harms and their prevention (Yang and Wang, 1992; Wang, 2010). Recently, hypoxia adaptation in Gansu zokor has received increasing attention to provide a theoretical basis for hypoxic injury treatment (Tang et al., 2013; Shan et al., 2016; Zhang et al., 2016; Meng et al., 2017). In the laboratory, Gansu zokor tolerates 3% O_2 for more than 1 h and 4% O_2 for more than 10 h. As a hypoxia-intolerant species, rats survive for only 16 min at 3% O_2 and 4 h at 4% O_2 (Yan et al., 2012). Moreover, studies have shown that Gansu zokor have higher red blood cell (RBC) counts, hemoglobin concentration (HGB), hematocrit (HCT), and vessel density (Xie et al., 2012; Shan et al., 2016) as well as higher cardiac activities of superoxide dismutase (SOD), catalase (CAT), and glutathione reductase (GR) compared with rats under hypoxic conditions (Tang et al., 2013). These findings indicate that Gansu zokor maintains hypoxia tolerance through increased oxygen-carrying capacity and antioxidant enzyme activity. The hypoxia tolerance capacity of Gansu zokor may be the result of adaptations to the putatively mild hypoxic environment in their sealed burrows. Furthermore, these rodents probably experience several hours of severe hypoxia in their deep nests during periods of extreme weather, such as rainy season.

Due to its almost completely aerobic metabolism, the brain is the most hypoxia-sensitive organ and requires a higher oxygen consumption and energy demand than other tissues (Buck and Pamenter, 2018; Sun et al., 2018; Logan et al., 2020). Studies showed that the naked mole rat brain has evolved the ability to alter glycolytic substrates using fructose in near-anaerobic metabolism, which supports the viability of this species under conditions of oxygen deprivation (Park et al., 2017). Furthermore, energy metabolism is suppressed and the lipid composition of membranes is altered in the naked mole rat brain in response to moderate hypoxia (Farhat et al., 2020).

These findings indicate that metabolic "rewiring" may be a mechanism by which hypoxic brain damage is minimized. However, little is known about the underlying mechanism of brain energy metabolism in subterranean rodents *in vivo* under the hypoxic conditions that might occur in subterranean burrows. Gansu zokor represents an ideal natural model of subterranean rodents that can be used to study the mechanism of hypoxia tolerance. Here we hypothesize that under the hypoxic condition of subterranean burrow, Gansu zokor could also mediate the rewired glycolysis to support its brain hypoxia resistance. Thus, we focused on brain glycolysis mediated *via* the mTORC1/eIF4E/HIF-1α pathway under hypoxia (**Figure 1**) and investigated the mechanisms by which Gansu zokor cope with these conditions. We addressed these issues by performing an *in vivo* comparison of the subterranean hypoxia-tolerant Gansu zokor and the surface hypoxia-intolerant Sprague-Dawley rat under normoxic (21% O_2) and hypoxic (10.5% O_2 or 6.5% O_2) conditions. The hypoxic conditions used reflect the relatively mild hypoxia to which Gansu zokor might be exposed while rebuilding collapsed burrows (10.5% O_2), and the relative acute hypoxia that might occur at the bottom of the subterranean burrow during the rainy season (6.5% O_2) (Shams et al., 2005; Band et al., 2010; Moskovitz et al., 2012). Whole brain RNA and protein were extracted to detect the transcriptional levels of mTORC1/eIF4E/HIF-1α pathway genes, and the transcriptional and translational levels of glycolysis-related genes. We then tested the activity of key enzymes involved in glucose-driven and fructose-driven glycolysis, with the aim of revealing the molecular mechanisms involved in energy supply in subterranean rodents under hypoxic conditions.

MATERIALS AND METHODS

Animals and Hypoxia Treatment

Gansu zokors (**Figure 2A**, bottom) were captured from the wild during the month of June in Weinan, Shaanxi Province, China (35°4′N, 109°16′E). Animals were housed in individual cages (47.5 cm × 35.0 cm × 20.0 cm) at room temperature under a 12:12 h light-dark cycle and acclimated to laboratory conditions for 3 weeks prior to exposure to hypoxia. Sprague-Dawley rats (rats; **Figure 2A**, top) were obtained from the Xi'an Jiaotong University and group-housed (three rats per cage) under the same environmental conditions. All animals were fed *ad libitum* (Gansu zokors, carrots; rats, standard rat feed and water).

To mimic hypoxia, nine healthy adult male Gansu zokors (230 ± 25 g) and nine healthy adult female Gansu zokors (210 ± 25 g) were randomly divided into three groups (n = 6 animals per species per group; three male and three female): (1) normoxia group (21% O_2); (2) hypoxia I group (44 h at 10.5% O_2) and (3) hypoxia II group (6 h at 6.5% O_2). A hypoxic cabin was used to simulate hypoxia, and an O_2 analyzer (Junfang, Beijing, China) was used to measure and maintain the O_2 level at 6.5% O_2/10.5% O_2. The O_2 level was maintained by delivering N_2 and two plates containing soda-lime were placed in the chamber to absorb the CO_2 released by the animals. Eighteen healthy adult rats (nine male and nine female; 200 ± 15 g) were treated in the same groups under the same experimental conditions. All experimental animals were sacrificed by injection with pentobarbital sodium at a dose of 45 mg/kg of body weigh. Cardiac blood samples were drawn from the right ventricle, and heparin-plasma was collected after centrifugation (3,000 rpm, 10 min, 4°C). Brain samples were removed and immediately frozen in liquid nitrogen. Plasma and brain samples were stored at −80°C until analyzed.

RNA Extraction and Quantitative Real-Time PCR Verification

Total RNA was extracted from brain tissues using TRIzol reagent (TaKaRa, Beijing, China) according to the manufacturer's instructions. The RNA samples were then reverse transcribed to cDNA using a Prime Script II 1st Strand cDNA Synthesis kit (TaKaRa, Beijing, China). Primers were designed using Primer-BLAST, and the sequences are shown in **Table 1**. Six technical replicates were prepared for the analysis of each gene by quantitative real-time PCR verification (qRT-PCR) using a Step One Real-Time System (ABI). The samples were analyzed in a 25 μl reaction volume, which consisted of 12.5 μl SYBR® Premix Ex TaqII (Tli RNaseH Plus) (2×), 1 μl each primer (10 μM), 8.5 μl nuclease-free water, and 2 μl template cDNA (diluted 30 times). The qRT-PCR conditions were as follows: 95°C for 30 s, followed by 39 cycles of 95°C for 15 s and 60°C for 30 s. Relative gene expression levels were normalized to that of an internal reference gene (β-*actin*) and calculated according to the $2^{-\Delta\Delta Ct}$ method.

Western Blot Analysis

Brain samples were homogenized and transferred to a separate tube containing RIPA buffer for 35 min on ice. After centrifugation (13,000 rpm, 30 min, 4°C), protein concentrations were measured in the resulting supernatants using a BCA kit (Coolaber, Beijing, China). Protein lysates (20 μg per well) were separated by sodium dodecyl sulfate-polyacrylamide gel (10%) electrophoresis (SDS-PAGE) and transferred to polyvinylidene fluoride (PVDF) membranes. After blocking in 5% skimmed milk for 2 h at room temperature on a shaking platform, the membranes were incubated overnight at 4°C with primary antibodies for the detection of GLUT1 (1:8,000; Abcam, Cambridge, MA, United States), PFK (1:1,000; Abcam, Cambridge, MA, United States), GLUT5 (1:500; Affinity Biosciences, Cincinnati, OH, United States), KHK (1:2,500; Abcam, Cambridge, MA, United States) and β-actin (1:8,000; ABclonal, Wuhan, China). The membranes were then washed and incubated with the secondary detection antibody (1:3,000; horseradish peroxidase-conjugated anti-rabbit IgG; ABclonal, Wuhan, China). Immunoreactive protein bands were visualized using an ECL Western blot substrate (Pierce, Rockford, IL, United States) and images were captured on an Alpha Innotech ChemiImager (Alpha Innotech, San Leandro, CA, United States). Quantification of the proteins was carried out using Image J Software.

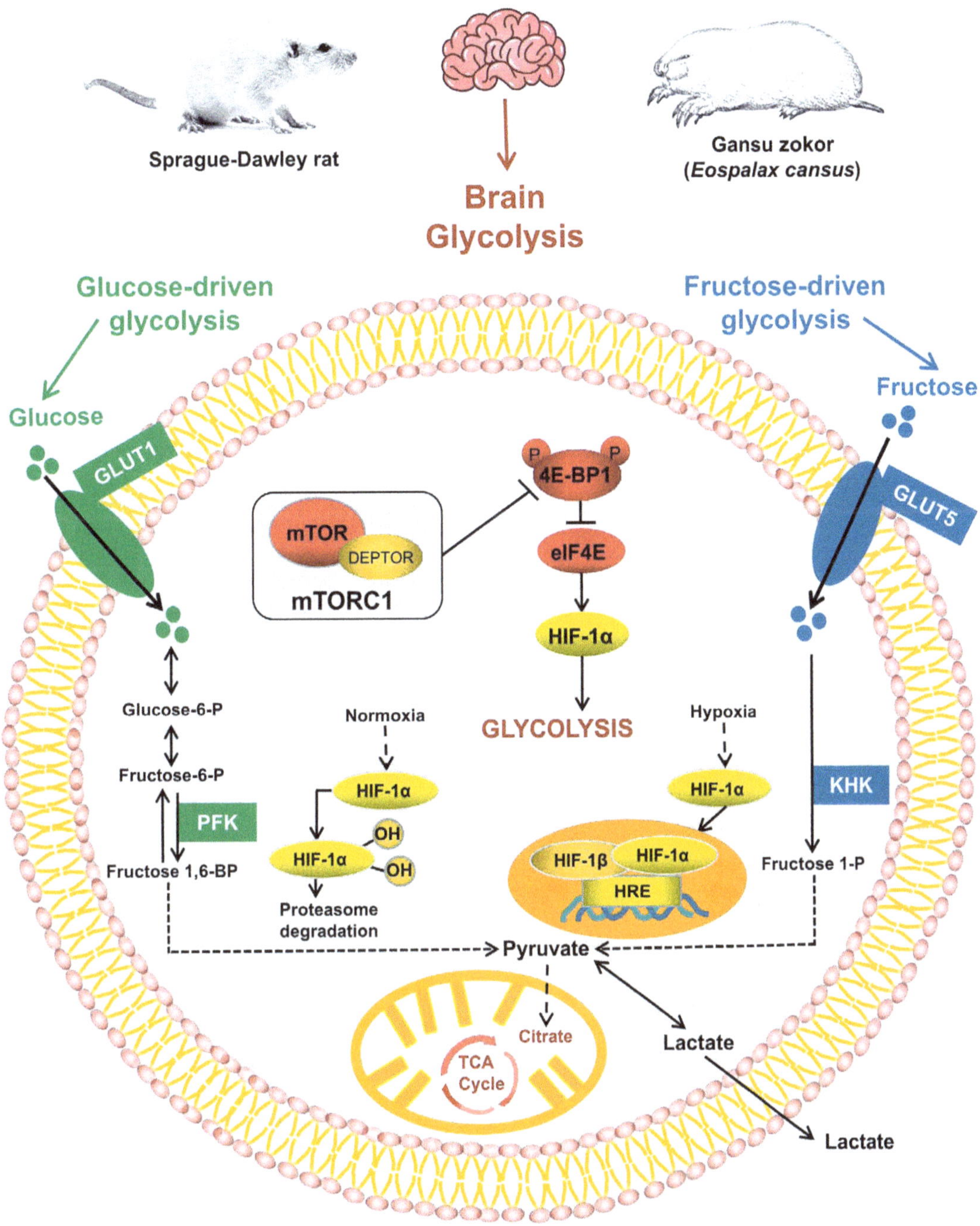

FIGURE 1 | The mTORC1 signaling and glycolysis pathways. mTORC1 controls the activity of several transcription factors (shown in red) that drive HIF-1α expression. Glucose enters the brain *via* GLUT1 and is converted *via* phosphofructokinase (PFK; shown in green); fructose enters cells *via* GLUT5 and is phosphorylated by ketohexokinase (KHK; shown in blue).

Immunohistochemical Staining

Brain sections were incubated in 3% H_2O_2 for 20 min to quench endogenous peroxidase activity. Then sections were incubated with 5% goat serum to block non-specific staining. The sections were incubated overnight at 4°C with primary antibodies for the detection of GLUT1 (1:500; Abcam, Cambridge, MA, United States), PFK (1:50; Abcam, Cambridge, MA, United States), GLUT5 (1:100; Affinity Biosciences, Cincinnati, OH, United States), and KHK (1:500; Abcam, Cambridge, MA, United States). The sections were then washed and incubated with horseradish peroxidase (Maixin, Fuzhou, China) for 50 min at room temperature. Signals were visualized using the diaminobenzidine (DAB) chromogenic kit. The negative control was treated with PBS in place of primary antibodies.

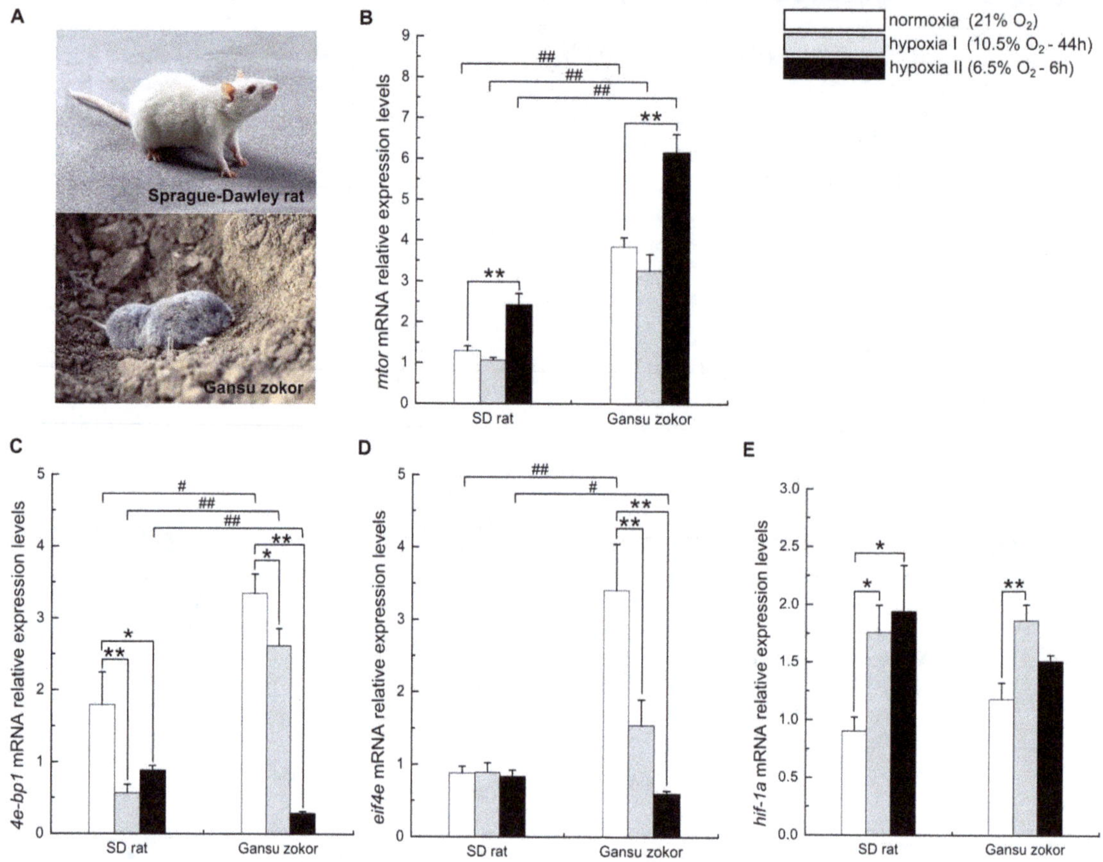

FIGURE 2 | Transcription level analysis of the mTORC1/eIF4E/HIF-1α pathway in Sprague-Dawley rat [**(A)**, top; this image from the network: https://baike.baidu.com/item/%E5%A4%A7%E7%99%BD%E9%BC%A0/6868090?fr=aladdin] and Gansu zokor [**(A)**, bottom; this image from the network: https://news.qq.com/a/20150330/064242.htm?pc#p=2]. *mtor* **(B)**, *4e-bp1* **(C)**, *eif4e* **(D)**, and *hif-1α* **(E)** mRNA expression. All data are presented as mean ± SEM (n = 6 animals per species). Statistical symbols: #P < 0.05 and ##P < 0.01 between two species under the same oxygen treatments; *P < 0.05 and **P < 0.01 between different oxygen treatments in the same species.

Then sections were counterstained with hematoxylin and were viewed by optical microscopy. The Image Pro Plus 6.0 software was applied to determine the integral optical density (IOD) values of proteins.

Enzymatic Activity Assay

Brain samples were placed at room temperature for 1 h after storage at 4°C for 12 h. PBS (10 times the volume of brain tissue) was then added for homogenization. The supernatant samples were collected after centrifugation (5,000 rpm, 15 min, room temperature) and the activity of PFK and KHK enzymes was measured immediately using enzyme-linked immunoassay (ELISA) kits (PFK kit, Kete, Yancheng, China and KHK kit, Meimian, Yancheng, China), according to the manufacturers' instructions, with six biological replicates per treatment.

Glucose and Fructose Determination

Approximately 0.1 g brain tissue was placed into 1 ml dd H_2O, homogenized and centrifuged to collect the supernatant (8,000 × g, 10 min, room temperature). The glucose and fructose contents in supernatant samples and plasma were assessed using a glucose content kit (Feiya, Yancheng, China) and a fructose content kit (Feiya, Yancheng, China) according to the manufacturers' instructions.

Statistical Analysis

Data were presented as mean values ± standard error of mean (SEM). Differences between two species at the same oxygen concentration were evaluated using independent sample t-tests, and differences within the same species at different oxygen concentrations were evaluated using *post hoc* tests. P-values < 0.05 were considered to indicate statistical significance.

RESULTS

Quantitative Analysis of the Expression of Genes Related to the mTORC1/eIF4E/HIF-1α Pathway

We first analyzed the expression levels of the *mtor*, *4e-bp1*, *eif4e* and *hif-1α* genes in Gansu zokor under conditions of hypoxia compared with those under normoxia by qRT-PCR using the primers shown in **Table 1**. We observed that the expression of *mtor* mRNA was significantly increased in the hypoxia II group ($P < 0.01$) (**Figure 2B**), while the expression levels of *4e-bp1* and *eif4e*, which are downstream genes in the mTORC1 pathway, decreased gradually with as the oxygen concentration was reduced (**Figures 2C,D**). Expression of *hif-1α* mRNA was significantly increased in the hypoxia I group ($P < 0.01$), with a slight increase in the hypoxia II group (**Figure 2E**).

We then made a major observation by comparing the expression of these genes expression in Gansu zokor and the hypoxia-intolerant rat; the expression levels of *mtor* mRNA in Gansu zokor were significantly higher than those in rat under conditions of normoxia as well as the two hypoxia conditions ($P < 0.01$) (**Figure 2B**). Compared with rats, the expression levels of *4e-bp1* and *eif4e* mRNA in Gansu zokors were significantly higher in the normoxia group and significantly lower in the hypoxia II group (**Figures 2C,D**). Furthermore, there were no significant differences in *hif-1α* mRNA expression between the two species in all groups (**Figure 2E**).

TABLE 1 | Primers for qRT-PCR analysis.

Gene	Primer	Primer sequence (5′–3′)	Tm (°C)
Mtor Eospalax cansus	Forward	CCTCTCTCACCATCACACCA	64
	Reverse	GGCTCTTCACAAAGGACACC	
Mtor Sprague-Dawley rat	Forward	GAAGTGAAGCGAGCCTTGGA	62
	Reverse	AATCAGACAGGCACGAAGGG	
4e-bp1 Eospalax cansus	Forward	TGAGCCTCCCATGAAAACCA	62
	Reverse	TGCTATGGCTCTCCTCCCAA	
4e-bp1 Sprague-Dawley rat	Forward	ATTCCTGATGGAGTGTCGGAA	60
	Reverse	CCACCTGCCCGCTTATCTT	
Eif4e Eospalax cansus	Forward	GGGAGCAGTTCATGGTTGG	60
	Reverse	TGGTGTTGGGAGGTAGGTTA	
Eif4e Sprague-Dawley rat	Forward	GGGAGCAGTTCATGGTTGG	60
	Reverse	TGGTGTTGGGAGGTAGGTTA	
hif-1α Eospalax cansus	Forward	CTCATTTTGCCGCAGTGCCT	62
	Reverse	CGCACCATTCCTCGCCATAA	
Hif-1α Sprague-Dawley rat	Forward	CCAGATTCAAGATCAGCCAGCA	62
	Reverse	GCTGTCCACATCAAAGCAGTACTCA	
glut1 Eospalax cansus	Forward	ATTGTGCTGCTGACCTTACC	58
	Reverse	GTTCCTAAATGGATGGAGCCTA	
glut1 Sprague-Dawley rat	Forward	ATTGTGCTGCTGACCTTACC	58
	Reverse	GTTCCTAAATGGATGGAGCCTA	
Pfk Eospalax cansus	Forward	CGACCGTATCTTGAGCAGCAA	62
	Reverse	CGTCAAACCTCTTGTCATCCA	
Pfk Sprague-Dawley rat	Forward	CGACCGTATCTTGAGCAGCAA	62
	Reverse	CGTCAAACCTCTTGTCATCCA	
glut5 Eospalax cansus	Forward	AATCCGGAAGGAGGATGAGG	61
	Reverse	TGCGCTGAGGTAGATCTGGT	
glut5 Sprague-Dawley rat	Forward	AATCCGGAAGGAGGATGAGG	61
	Reverse	TGCGCTGAGGTAGATCTGGT	
Khk Eospalax cansus	Forward	AAGCAGATCCTGTGCGTGG	62
	Reverse	CCAGCGAGCCCATGAAGG	
Khk Sprague-Dawley rat	Forward	AAGCAGATCCTGTGCGTGG	62
	Reverse	CCAGCGAGCCCATGAAGG	
β-actin	Forward	CTAAGGCCAACCGTGAAAAGAT	60 ± 5
	Reverse	GACCAGAGGCATACAGGGACA	

Quantitative Analysis of Glycolysis-Related Gene Expression

We first analyzed the expression levels of *glut1* and *pfk* (glucose-driven glycolysis pathway) and *glut5* and *khk* (fructose-driven glycolysis pathway) in Gansu zokor under conditions of hypoxia compared with those under normoxia by qRT-PCR using the primers shown in **Table 1**. In the glucose-driven glycolysis pathway, hypoxia II significantly decreased *glut1* mRNA expression (**Figure 3A**), whereas GLUT1 protein expression was significantly increased (**Figure 4A**). Hypoxia did not significantly change the *pfk* expression at either the mRNA or protein levels (**Figures 3B, 4B**). In the fructose-driven glycolysis pathway, both hypoxia I and hypoxia II induced increases in the expression of *glut5* and *khk* mRNA in Gansu zokor (**Figures 3C,D**), with the protein levels corresponding with the mRNA levels (**Figures 4C,D**).

The mRNA levels of these glycolysis-related genes were then compared between Gansu zokor and rat and the results revealed differences between the two species. In the glucose-driven glycolysis pathway, *glut1* mRNA expression in Gansu zokor was significantly higher than that in rat both under normoxia and the two hypoxia conditions ($P < 0.01$) (**Figure 3A**). However, at the protein expression level, this differential expression was found only in the hypoxia II group (**Figure 4A**). The *pfk* mRNA expression in Gansu zokor was significantly higher than that in rat both under normoxia and hypoxia I conditions ($P < 0.01$) (**Figure 3B**), but this differential in PFK protein expression was found only under normoxic condition (**Figure 4B**). In the fructose-driven glycolysis pathway, although the *glut5* and *khk* mRNA expression levels were significantly higher in Gansu zokor than those in rat only in some groups (**Figures 3C,D**), the GLUT5 and KHK protein expression levels in Gansu zokor were significantly higher than those in rat in all groups ($P < 0.01$) (**Figures 4C,D**), showing a high degree of consistency. Surprisingly, KHK protein was almost totally absent in rat brain tissue; however, like the PFK protein in the glucose-driven glycolysis pathway, this protein was expressed normally in Gansu zokor, at levels hundreds of times higher than that in rat (**Figure 4D**), this was an important and interesting finding in our study.

We further verified the glycolysis-related protein expression by immunohistochemistry staining (**Figure 5E**). We analyzed the protein immunoreactivity of GLUT1, PFK, GLUT5, and KHK in Gansu zokor under conditions of hypoxia compared with those under normoxia. In the glucose-driven glycolysis pathway, only the hypoxia II significantly increased GLUT1 protein immunoreactivity ($P < 0.01$) (**Figure 5A**), and hypoxia did not significantly change the PFK protein immunoreactivity (**Figure 5B**). In the fructose-driven glycolysis pathway, both hypoxia I and hypoxia II significantly increased GLUT5 and KHK protein immunoreactivity (**Figures 5C,D**). Furthermore, we also found that the GLUT5 and KHK protein immunoreactivity in Gansu zokor was significantly higher than those in rat in all

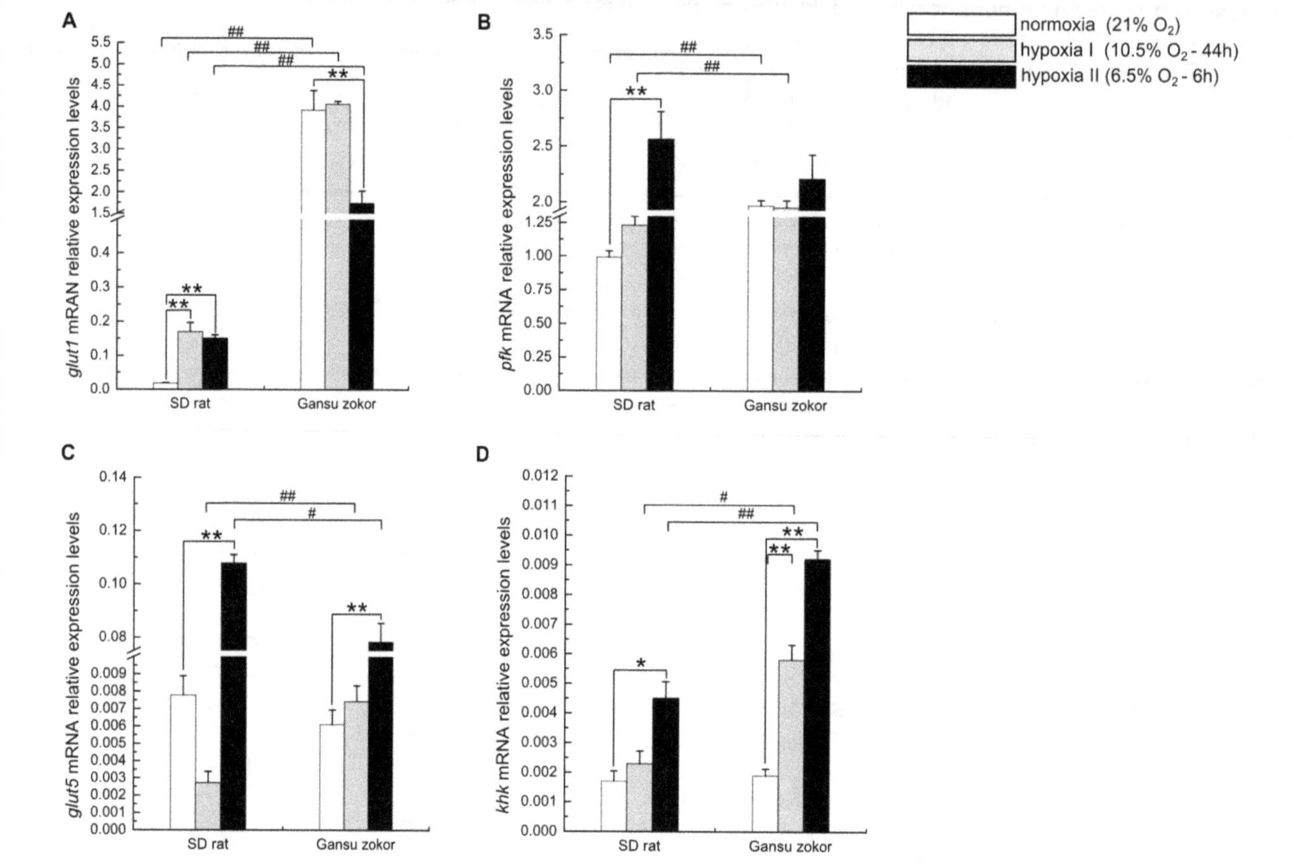

FIGURE 3 | Transcription level analysis of glycolysis-related transporters and enzymes in Sprague-Dawley rat and Gansu zokor. *glut1* glucose transporter **(A)**, *pfk* **(B)**, *glut5* glucose transporter **(C)**, and *khk* **(D)** mRNA expression. All data are presented as mean ± SEM (n = 6 animals per species). Statistical symbols: #$P < 0.05$ and ##$P < 0.01$ between two species under the same oxygen treatment; *$P < 0.05$ and **$P < 0.01$ between different oxygen treatments in the same species.

groups ($P < 0.01$) (**Figures 5C,D**). These results were consistent with those detected by the Western blot method.

Quantitative Analysis of Glycolysis-Related Enzymatic Activity

We first observed that hypoxia exposure did not significantly change the enzymatic activity of PFK in Gansu zokor brain (**Figure 6A**), whereas KHK enzymatic activity was significantly increased (**Figure 6B**). Then compared with rat, PFK enzymatic activity in Gansu zokor was significantly lower than that in rat in hypoxia I group, whereas the activity was significantly higher in hypoxia II group (**Figure 6A**). In contrast, KHK enzymatic activity in Gansu zokor was significantly higher in all groups than that in rat (**Figure 6B**). Thus, we observed differences in the activity of glycolysis-related of Gansu zokor compared with hypoxia-intolerant rats under both normoxic and hypoxic conditions.

Hypoxia Affects Glucose and Fructose Levels

To evaluate whether hypoxia affects glucose or fructose levels, we detected the levels of these sugars in plasma and brain. Surprisingly, the plasma glucose levels in Gansu zokor were significantly lower than those in rat both at normoxia and under the two hypoxia conditions ($P < 0.01$) (**Figure 7A**). In contrast, the plasma fructose levels in Gansu zokor were significantly higher than those in rat under normoxia ($P < 0.05$) and hypoxia II conditions ($P < 0.01$) (**Figure 7B**). Furthermore, unlike rats, Gansu zokors exhibited raised plasma levels of both glucose and fructose under hypoxia II condition (**Figures 7A,B**).

Interestingly, although the plasma glucose levels in Gansu zokor were significantly lower than those in rat, there were no significant differences in brain glucose levels between the two species under normoxia and hypoxia I conditions (**Figure 7C**). Furthermore, rats showed unchanged brain fructose levels after hypoxic exposure (**Figure 7D**), although Gansu zokors showed significant decreases in two hypoxia groups when compared with normoxia (**Figure 7D**).

DISCUSSION

In humans, hypoxia leads to loss of consciousness within minutes. Furthermore, hypoxic-ischemic brain injury has devastating impacts, especially in patients who are comatose

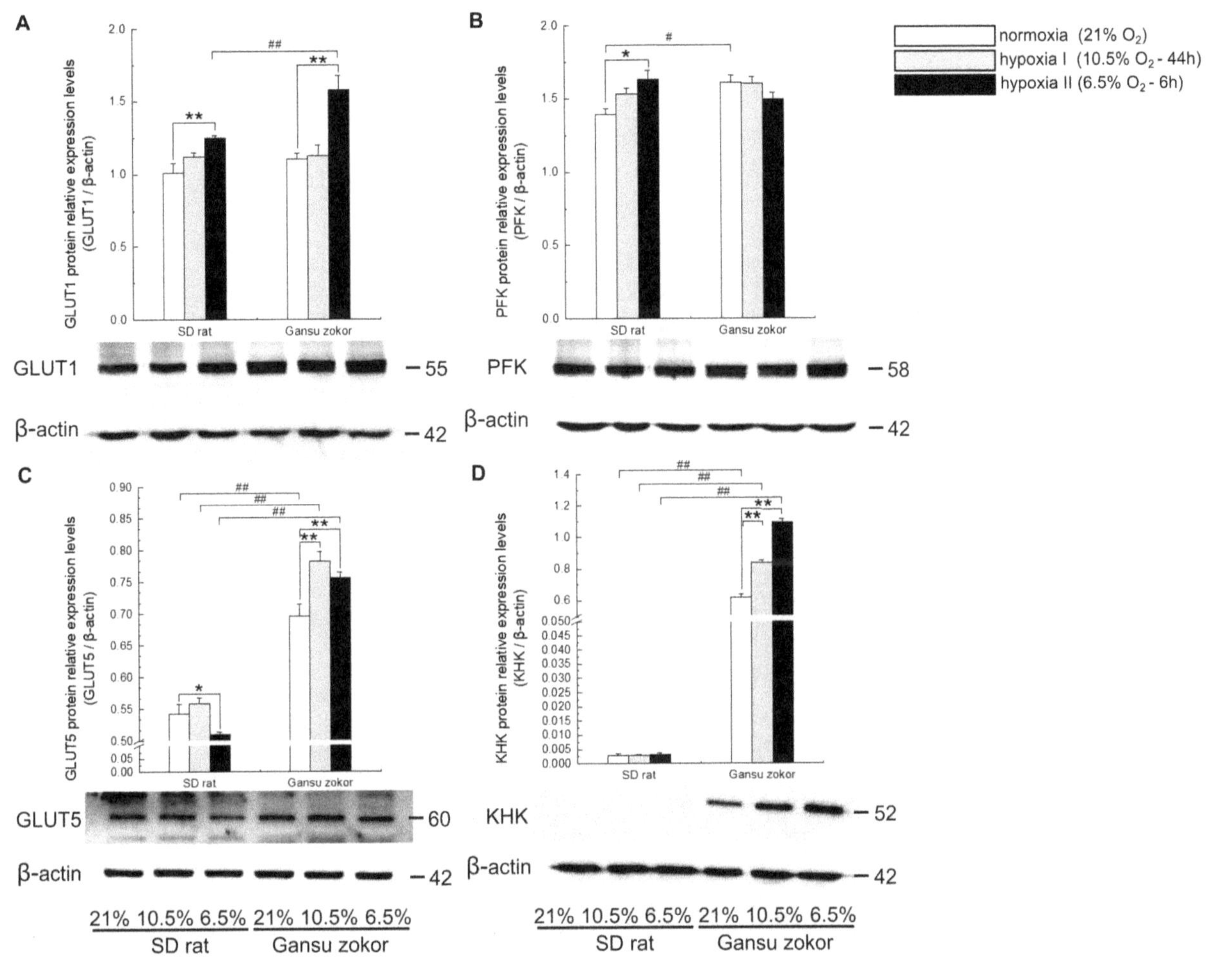

FIGURE 4 | Translation level analysis of glycolysis-related transporters and enzymes in Sprague-Dawley rat and Gansu zokor. GLUT1 glucose transporter **(A)**, PFK **(B)**, GLUT5 glucose transporter **(C)**, and KHK **(D)** protein expression. Representative images of at least three separate blots below each bar graph showing expression of the proteins. All data are presented as mean ± SEM. Statistical symbols: $\#P < 0.05$ and $\#\#P < 0.01$ between two species under the same oxygen treatment; $^{*}P < 0.05$ and $^{**}P < 0.01$ between different oxygen treatments in the same species.

after resuscitation from cardiac arrest (Weil et al., 2008; Avivi et al., 2010; Sandroni et al., 2018). However, some subterranean rodent species can tolerate the ambient hypoxia in their underground burrows for prolonged periods (Band et al., 2010; Pamenter et al., 2019). The native subterranean rodent species used in current hypoxia studies have some limitations, and are mainly limited in naked mole rats and blind mole rats. The molecular mechanisms underlying the brain adaptations of subterranean rodents to hypoxic condition, especially in the Gansu zokor, remain to be elucidated. In this study, we investigated the mechanisms underlying brain glycolysis in Gansu zokor under hypoxic conditions by revealing the regulatory effects of the mTORC1/eIF4E/HIF-1α pathway on glycolysis. Our study yielded the following important findings: (i) As a downstream transcription factor in the mTORC1/eIF4E pathway, *hif-1α* gene expression in the brain of both Gansu zokor and rat under hypoxic conditions was increased when compared with normoxia. (ii) Expression of the GLUT5 transmembrane protein, which is a highly selective fructose transporter (Park et al., 2017), was significantly higher in Gansu zokor than that in rat in all the groups. (iii) Under the two different degrees of hypoxia, expression of *khk* in Gansu zokor brain was significantly higher than in rat at both the mRNA and its protein levels. In particular, KHK protein expression was extremely significantly higher in Gansu zokor than that in rat in all the groups. Furthermore, in Gansu zokor, but not in rat, KHK protein expression was upregulated in parallel with the decrease in oxygen concentration. Finally, in terms of enzymatic activity, KHK activity was significantly higher in Gansu zokor than that in rat in all the groups. (*iv*) On the whole, in Gansu zokor, hypoxia exposure significantly increased blood fructose levels, while brain fructose levels were significantly decreased; however, no significant changes in blood or brain fructose levels were observed in rats exposed to hypoxia stress. Based on these findings, we postulated that Gansu zokor have a glycometabolism pattern in response to hypoxia that differs from that of hypoxia-intolerant animals.

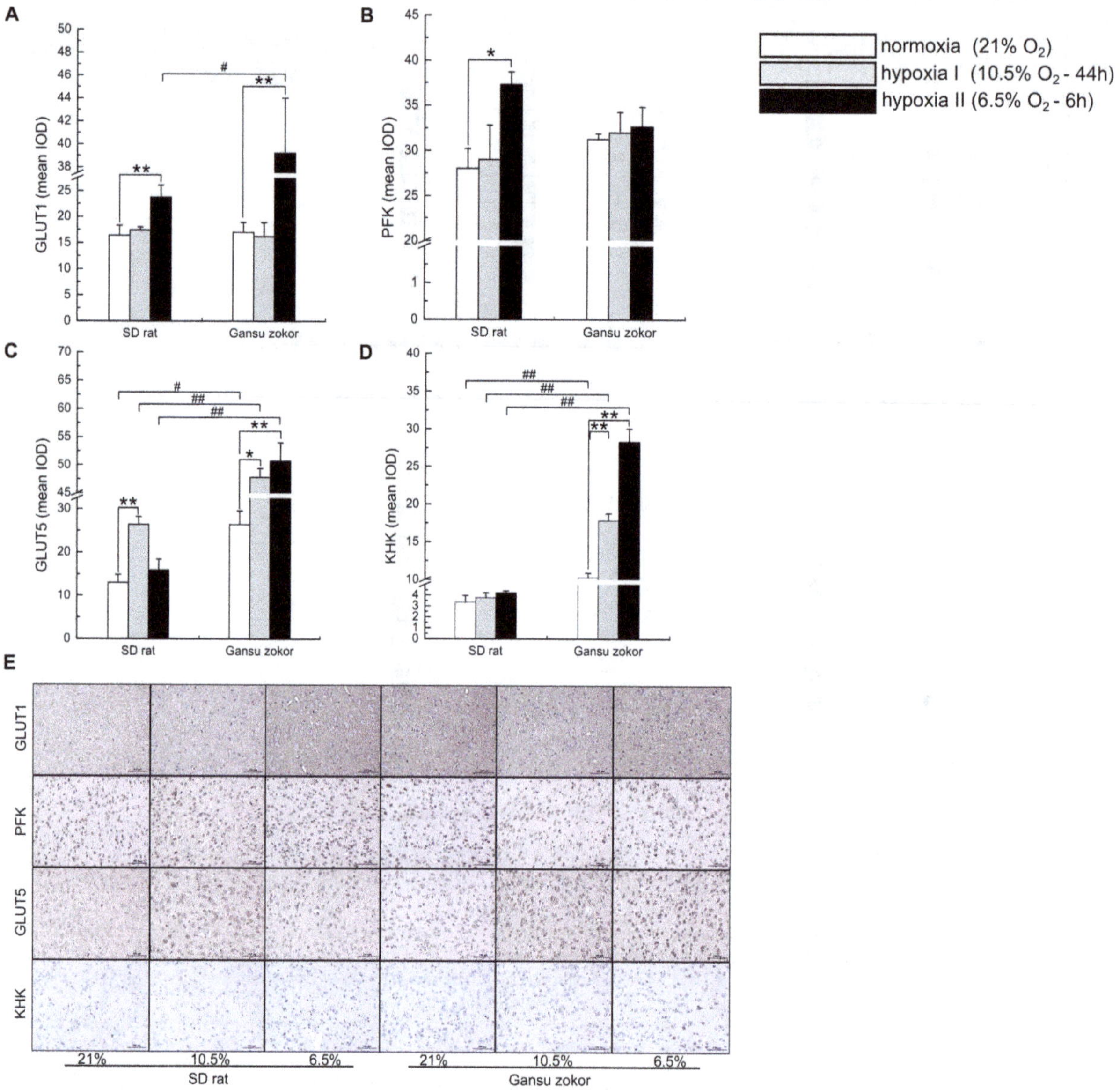

FIGURE 5 | Immunohistochemical analysis of glycolysis-related transporters and enzymes in Sprague-Dawley rat and Gansu zokor. GLUT1 glucose transporter **(A)**, PFK **(B)**, GLUT5 glucose transporter **(C)**, and KHK **(D)** protein immunoreactivity. Representative images **(E)** of immunostaining, scale bar represents: 100 μm, magnification: 200×. All data are presented as mean ± SEM. Statistical symbols: #$P < 0.05$ and ##$P < 0.01$ between two species under the same oxygen treatment; *$P < 0.05$ and **$P < 0.01$ between different oxygen treatments in the same species.

The mTOR controls cellular growth and energy (Hall, 2008; Saxton and Sabatini, 2017). In this study, we found significantly higher levels of *mtor* mRNA in Gansu zokor compared with those in rat under all treatment conditions, indicating that Gansu zokors have a high capacity for energy metabolism or/and growth compared with the surface dwelling rat. HIF-1α is known to regulate the expression of downstream genes with roles in the process of glycolysis (Shams et al., 2004; Zhang and Sadek, 2014). Our data support the conclusions of previous studies, showing that mTORC1 signaling promotes *hif-1α* transcription (Dodd et al., 2015; Chi et al., 2017). To gain a better understanding of this process in subterranean rodents *in vivo* under conditions of hypoxia, we designed this study to explore mTORC1-mediated metabolism under hypoxia.

Fructose-Driven Glycolysis Capability Is Reinforced in Hypoxic Gansu Zokor Brain

Fructolysis occurs primarily in the liver, small intestine, and kidney (Mirtschink et al., 2018); in part because GLUT5, a highly selective fructose transporter, and KHK, which catalyzed the first step in fructose metabolism, are primarily expressed in these organs (Funari et al., 2005; Diggle et al., 2009;

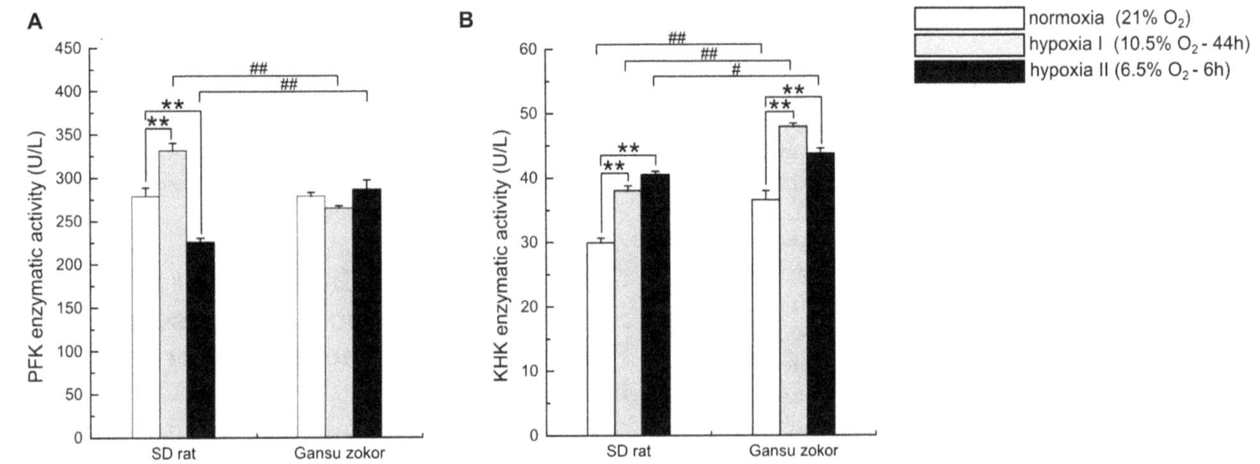

FIGURE 6 | Enzymatic activity analysis of glycolysis in Sprague-Dawley rat and Gansu zokor. The activity of PFK (glucose enzyme) **(A)** and KHK (fructose enzyme) **(B)**. All data are presented as mean ± SEM (n = 6 animals per species). Statistical symbols: #P < 0.05 and ##P < 0.01 between two species under the same oxygen treatment; **P < 0.01 between different oxygen treatments in the same species.

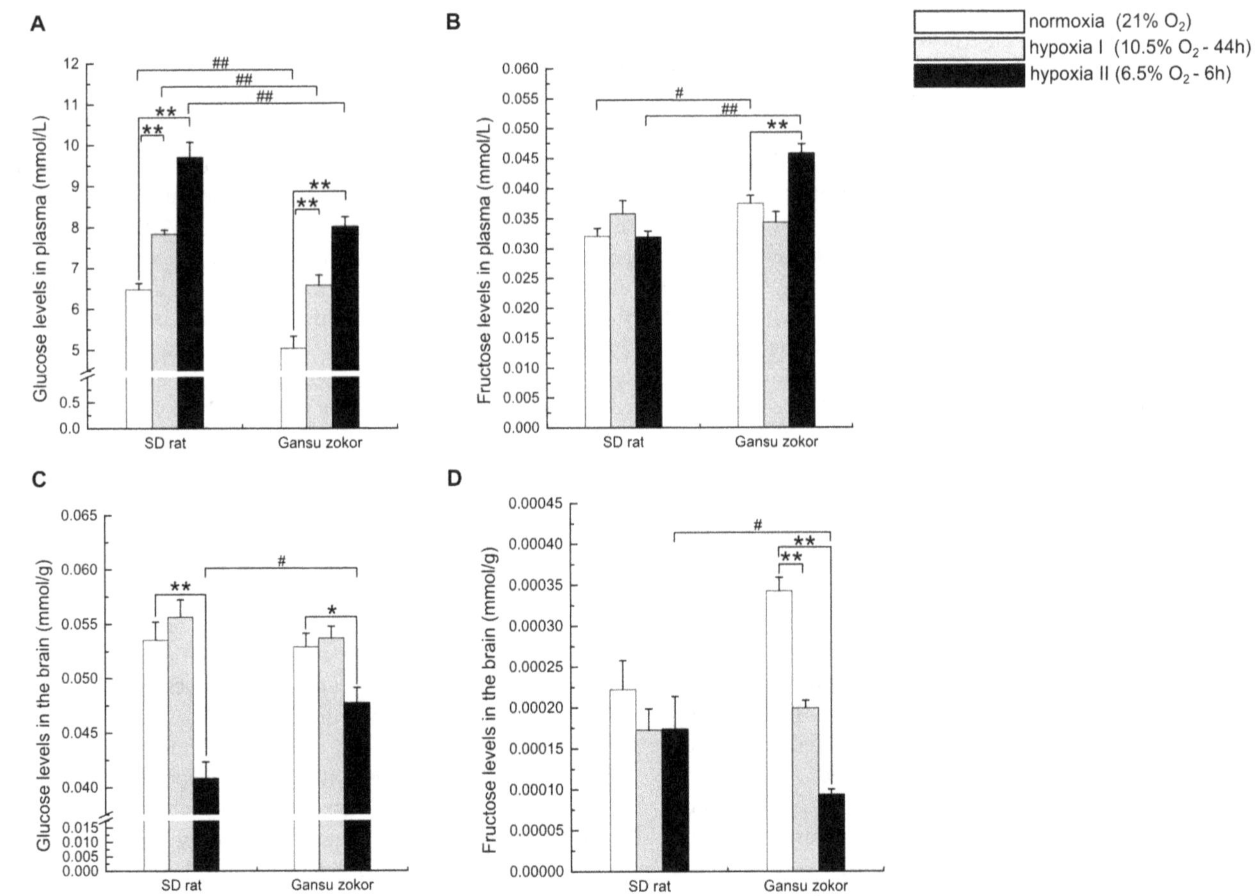

FIGURE 7 | Glucose and fructose levels in the plasma and brain in Sprague-Dawley rat and Gansu zokor. Plasma glucose **(A)**, plasma fructose **(B)**, brain glucose **(C)**, and brain fructose **(D)** levels. All data are presented as mean ± SEM (n = 6 animals per species). Statistical symbols: #P < 0.05 and ##P < 0.01 between two species under the same oxygen treatment; *P < 0.05 and **P < 0.01 between different oxygen treatments in the same species.

Gonzalez and Betts, 2018). However, in an important study, Park et al. showed that naked mole rats have the ability to use fructose to fuel the brain under near anaerobic conditions (Park et al., 2017). This led us to suspect that this fructose metabolism pattern exists in other subterranean rodents living in burrows under conditions of hypoxia, even if this environment is not as extreme as near-anaerobic conditions. Therefore, we exposed Gansu zokors to hypoxic conditions that might occur in underground habitats (Shams et al., 2005). Similar to naked mole rats (Park et al., 2017), we found that Gansu zokor brain showed increased fructose-driven glycolysis in response to hypoxia stress.

GLUT5 expression in Gansu zokor brains is higher than that in the surface-dwelling rat, which is consistent with the previous report in naked mole rat brain (Park et al., 2017). It is also worth noting that under hypoxia II condition, Gansu zokor has lower *glut5* mRNA but higher protein expression than that in rat, which suggests that substrates for fructose-driven glycolysis are rapidly transported in Gansu zokor by improving the translation efficiency of *glut5* mRNA. This mechanism clearly facilitates the rapid activation of the fructose metabolism pathway in Gansu zokor under hypoxia. Furthermore, hypoxia increased GLUT5 protein levels in Gansu zokor brain, which is similar to the stimulation observed in rat rostral ventrolateral medulla (RVLM) in response to a high fructose diet (Wu et al., 2014). This seems to suggest that hypoxia in Gansu zokor produces similar results to that caused by high fructose intake in rat. We then found that plasma fructose is increased to statistically significant levels in the Gansu zokor during hypoxia II condition. Although the source of this fructose is not clear, it is probably produced by endogenous synthesis (Patel et al., 2015). On the other hand, KHK initiates fructose-driven glycolysis to bypass the PFK regulatory block in glucose-driven glycolysis (Diggle et al., 2009; Park et al., 2017). In this study, we showed that KHK protein is expressed at negligible levels in the rat brain, but can be expressed in the Gansu zokor brain. Furthermore, KHK activity in Gansu zokor was significantly higher than that in rat, and was upregulated under hypoxia; consistent results occurred in the expression of the enzyme at both the mRNA and protein levels. These results indicated that Gansu zokor has the capacity to initiate fructose metabolism, especially under conditions of hypoxia; which meant that the fructose-fueled glycolysis pattern occurred in Gansu zokor. Thus, experimental results confirmed our initial hypothesis that Gansu zokor could mediate the rewired glycolysis. This rewired fructose metabolism pathway bypasses metabolic block at PFK, it involves equipping brain with fructose transporter and fructose enzyme for fructose metabolism. Besides, we observed marked differences in the fructose-driven glycolysis pathway between Gansu zokor and rat, suggesting that Gansu zokor has different metabolic patterns from those of the surface-dwelling rat. Fructose enters the glycolysis pathway at a much higher rate than glucose (Park et al., 2017; Liu et al., 2020). The rapid metabolism of fructose is critical for maintaining normal brain metabolism activity in Gansu zokor under hypoxia. This metabolic pattern can circumvent the lethal effects of hypoxia, thus providing a mechanism for survival in the subterranean burrow. Our findings suggested that Gansu zokor brain could adapt to subterranean hypoxia through rewiring the metabolism of glycolysis, which may be attributed to the long-term evolution of Gansu zokor inhabiting hypoxic environments. The adaptive evolution of subterranean rodents is both degenerative and compensatory, thus providing a model of the nature of adaptation through modifications at the molecular and organism levels (Nevo, 1999; Begall et al., 2007). The unique insights in to the glycolysis characteristics in Gansu zokor obtained in our study will be useful for further studies on evolution in subterranean rodents.

Glycolysis Fuel in Gansu Zokor Brain Strengthen Reliance on Glucose and Fructose Simultaneously Under Hypoxia II Condition

As described previously, Gansu zokors may rely upon fructose-driven glycolysis under hypoxia, as a mechanism that allows continued glycolytic flux (Park et al., 2017). This mechanism may also represent an adaptation strategy in subterranean rodents that allows rapid energy supply in hypoxic environments. Our results also seemed to suggest that Gansu zokor increased the fructose-driven glycolysis in hypoxia. Interestingly, we also observed that Gansu zokors exhibit a simultaneous enhancement of glucose-driven glycolysis and fructose-driven glycolysis in hypoxia II group, while hypoxia I did not significantly change glucose-driven glycolysis. This regulation of glycolysis imply differences in the energy responses of Gansu zokor brain under different hypoxia conditions.

Glucose is the obligatory energy source in the brain, and is transported into the brain *via* GLUT1 (Bélanger et al., 2011; Koch and Weber, 2019; Pragallapati and Manyam, 2019), where it is converted by PFK, PFK is the first irreversible reaction in glucose-driven glycolysis, playing an important role in the control of the glycolysis pathway (Nakajima, 1995; Moreno-Sánchez et al., 2007; Real-Hohn et al., 2010). We found that GLUT1 protein levels were increased in Gansu zokor brain under hypoxia II condition, which is consistent with similar hypoxia responses reported in some tumor cells (Chen et al., 2010; Cretenet et al., 2016). GLUT1 overexpression increases glucose metabolism (Freemerman et al., 2014), indicating that Gansu zokor brain has the capacity for increased glucose-driven glycolysis to cope with hypoxia II. Moreover, the plasma glucose levels of Gansu zokor rose approximately 50% in hypoxia II compared with the levels in normoxia, which consistent with results observed in the naked mole rat, healthy adults, and Oriental river prawn (Newhouse et al., 2017; Sun et al., 2018; Pamenter et al., 2019); however, brain glucose levels in Gansu zokor were significantly decreased under hypoxia II condition. Thus, even with the increase in plasma glucose levels under hypoxia II condition, concentrations of the glucose substrate in the brain decline, suggesting that hypoxia II promotes cerebral glycolysis (Vannucci and Vannucci, 2000; Mergenthaler et al., 2013).

Similar to Gansu zokors, rats showed the same enhancement in glucose-driven glycolysis in response to hypoxia II; however, it is interesting to note that this enhancement in rats was due to the overexpression of both GLUT1 and PFK. We observed that only in rats, *pfk* expression at both the mRNA and its protein levels was significantly increased after exposure to hypoxia II condition; thus, even though its levels in rats was significantly lower than those in Gansu zokor under normoxia, there were no significant differences in *pfk* expression between two species under hypoxia II condition. These results suggest that the enhancement of glucose-driven glycolysis in Gansu zokor brain under hypoxia II condition may be less marked than that in rats. However, rats did not show the same capacity for fructolysis in the brain. This indicates that Gansu zokor has evolved a strategy for coping with hypoxia that is different from that of rats, in that Gansu zokor utilize fructose metabolism to provide energy rapidly. To sum up, Gansu zokor brain may increase both glucose-driven and fructose-driven simultaneously when exposed to hypoxia II, suggesting greater requirement for energy supply in the brain under conditions of hypoxia II of 6.5% O_2 for 6 h. Finally, it is important to note that the elevation of plasma glucose induced in Gansu zokor exposed to hypoxia is considerably greater than the increase in plasma fructose, which is consistent with the pattern reported in the naked mole rat (Park et al., 2017). Furthermore, whether in normoxia or hypoxia, the levels of glucose in Gansu zokor are much higher than the fructose levels, indicating that, on the basis of glucose as the main metabolic substrate, fructose is used to accelerate the supply of energy in Gansu zokor.

Study Limitations

This study has some limitations. First, we did not collect the oxygen concentration data for Gansu zokor in their wild underground burrows at different depths, seasons, and weather; our selection of the hypoxia treatment conditions (hypoxia I: 44 h at 10.5% O_2; hypoxia II: 6 h at 6.5% O_2) was based mainly on laboratory tests of hypoxia tolerance in Gansu zokor and previous studies of *Spalax* (Shams et al., 2005; Band et al., 2010; Moskovitz et al., 2012; Yan et al., 2012). Second, the duration time of hypoxic II treatment can ensure the survival of rats for tissue sampling, and the hypoxic I treatment is a relatively long-mild form of hypoxia; these two hypoxic treatment conditions, including oxygen concentration and duration time, reflect the different hypoxic environments that may occur in the burrows inhabited by Gansu zokor in the wild; but even these rigorous simulations can not totally represent the burrow environment. Besides, more hypoxic experimental groups will be required to perfect the design of experiment. Finally, we have investigated glycolysis differences in Gansu zokor and Sprague-Dawley rat; our aim was to reveal the hypoxic tolerance mechanism in subterranean rodent through exploring the different hypoxic response in hypoxia-tolerant subterranean Gansu zokor and hypoxia-intolerant surface rat. However, in the current study, although Sprague-Dawley rats are non-burrowing rodents, they are not the best controls because of not living in the wild environment; therefore, our discussion of the comparison between two species remains limited.

CONCLUSION

Gansu zokor has evolved the capacity to utilize fructose to fuel the brain on the basis of glucose metabolism. This metabolic rewiring of glycolysis seems to be an adaptive that underlies the hypoxia tolerance of this species. Gansu zokor exhibited significantly higher levels of GLUT5 and KHK proteins, as well as increased KHK enzymatic activity compared with the levels in the hypoxia-intolerant surface-dwelling rat. GLUT5 and KHK represent molecular signatures of fructose metabolism that are also upregulated by hypoxia stress. Thus, these results reveal the mechanism underlying hypoxia tolerance in Gansu zokor. Further studies of energy metabolism in "natural" hypoxia tolerance in an animal model will provide an important supplement to hypoxia adaptation studies and highlight potential strategies to mitigate hypoxic brain damage, which can provide theoretical basis and novel strategies for hypoxic brain injury treatment of human beings.

ETHICS STATEMENT

The animal study was reviewed and approved by Animal Management Committee and Ethical Review Committee of Experimental Animal Welfare, Shaanxi Normal University.

AUTHOR CONTRIBUTIONS

JGL and JH designed the study. JYL wrote the manuscript with help of JGL. LF, LC, JK, and XW contributed to experimental work. JYL, YH, JG, and ZH performed the data analysis. All authors contributed to the revision of the manuscript and approved the final version of the manuscript.

ACKNOWLEDGMENTS

The authors would like to thank all the reviewers who participated in the review and MJEditor (www.mjeditor.com) for its linguistic assistance during the preparation of this manuscript.

REFERENCES

Altwasser, R., Paz, A., Korol, A., Manov, I., Avivi, A., and Shams, I. (2019). The transcriptome landscape of the carcinogenic treatment response in the blind mole rat: insights into cancer resistance mechanisms. *BMC Genomics* 20:17. doi: 10.1186/s12864-018-5417-z

Avivi, A., Gerlach, F., Joel, A., Reuss, S., Burmester, T., and Hankeln, N. T. (2010). Neuroglobin, cytoglobin, and myoglobin contribute to hypoxia adaptation of the subterranean mole rat Spalax. *Proc. Natl. Acad. Sci. U.S.A.* 107, 21570–21575. doi: 10.1073/pnas.1015379107

Band, M., Joel, A., and Avivi, A. (2010). The muscle ankyrin repeat proteins are hypoxia-sensitive: in vivo mRNA expression in the hypoxia-tolerant blind subterranean mole rat, *Spalax ehrenbergi*. *J. Mol. Evol.* 70, 1–12. doi: 10.1007/s00239-009-9306-6

Barčiová, L., Šumbera, R., and Burda, H. (2009). Variation in the digging apparatus of the subterranean silvery mole-rat, *Heliophobius argenteocinereus* (Rodentia, Bathyergidae): the role of ecology and geography. *Biol. J. Linn. Soc.* 97, 822–831. doi: 10.1111/j.1095-8312.2009.01228.x

Begall, S., Burda, H., and Schleich, C. E. (2007). *Subterranean Rodents: News From Underground*. Berlin: Springer, 3–9.

Bélanger, M., Allaman, I., and Magistretti, P. J. (2011). Brain energy metabolism: focus on astrocyte-neuron metabolic cooperation. *Cell Metab.* 14, 724–738. doi: 10.1016/j.cmet.2011.08.016

Buck, L. T., and Pamenter, M. E. (2018). The hypoxia-tolerant vertebrate brain: arresting synaptic activity. *Comp. Biochem. Physiol. B Biochem. Mol. Biol.* 224, 61–70. doi: 10.1016/j.cbpb.2017.11.015

Chen, C. L., Chu, J. S., Su, W. C., Huang, S. C., and Lee, W. Y. (2010). Hypoxia and metabolic phenotypes during breast carcinogenesis: expression of HIF-1α, GLUT1, and CAIX. *Virchows Arch.* 457, 53–61. doi: 10.1007/s00428-010-0938-0

Chen, Y., and Huang, G. (2012). Biological study of gansu zokor in Yuanzhou District in Guyuan City. *Modern Agric. Sci. Technol.* 17, 149–151. doi: 10.3969/j.issn.1007-5739.2012.17.091 (in Chinese),

Cheng, K. J., Bao, Y. Y., and Zhou, S. H. (2016). The role of hypoxia inducible factor in nasal inflammations. *Eur. Rev. Med. Pharmacol. Sci.* 20, 5067–5076.

Chi, P. I., Huang, W. R., Chiu, H. C., Li, J. Y., Nielsen, B. L., and Liu, H. J. (2017). Avian reovirus σA-modulated suppression of lactate dehydrogenase and upregulation of glutaminolysis and the mTOC1/eIF4E/HIF-1α pathway to enhance glycolysis and the TCA cycle for virus replication. *Cell. Microbiol.* 20:e12946. doi: 10.1111/cmi.12946

Cretenet, G., Clerc, I., Matias, M., Loisel, S., Craveiro, M., Oburoglu, L., et al. (2016). Cell surface Glut1 levels distinguish human CD4 and CD8 T lymphocyte subsets with distinct effector functions. *Sci. Rep.* 6:24129. doi: 10.1038/srep24129

Diggle, C. P., Shires, M., Leitch, D., Brooke, D., Carr, I. M., Markham, A. F., et al. (2009). Ketohexokinase: expression and localization of the principal fructose-metabolizing enzyme. *J. Histochem. Cytochem.* 57, 763–774. doi: 10.1369/jhc.2009.953190

Dodd, K. M., Yang, J., Shen, M. H., Sampson, J. R., and Tee, A. R. (2015). mTORC1 drives HIF-1α and VEGF-A signalling via multiple mechanisms involving 4E-BP1, S6K1 and STAT3. *Oncogene* 34, 2239–2250. doi: 10.1038/onc.2014.164

Dong, Q., Wang, Z., Jiang, M., Sun, H., Wang, X., Li, Y., et al. (2020). Transcriptome analysis of the response provided by *Lasiopodomys mandarinus* to severe hypoxia includes enhancing DNA repair and damage prevention. *Front. Zool.* 17:9. doi: 10.1186/s12983-020-00356-y

Farhat, E., Devereaux, M. E. M., Pamenter, M. E., and Weber, J. M. (2020). Naked mole-rats suppress energy metabolism and modulate membrane cholesterol in chronic hypoxia. *Am. J. Physiol. Regul. Integr. Comp. Physiol.* 319, R148–R155. doi: 10.1152/ajpregu.00057.2020

Faulkes, C. G., Eykyn, T. R., and Aksentijevic, D. (2019). Cardiac metabolomic profile of the naked mole-rat-glycogen to the rescue. *Biol. Lett.* 15:20190710. doi: 10.1098/rsbl.2019.0710

Freemerman, A. J., Johnson, A. R., Sacks, G. N., Milner, J. J., Kirk, E. L., Troester, M. A., et al. (2014). Metabolic reprogramming of macrophages: glucose transporter 1 (GLUT1)-mediated glucose metabolism drives a proinflammatory phenotype. *J. Biol. Chem.* 289, 7884–7896. doi: 10.1074/jbc.M113.522037

Funari, V. A., Herrera, V. L. M., Freeman, D., and Tolan, D. R. (2005). Genes required for fructose metabolism are expressed in Purkinje cells in the cerebellum. *Brain Res. Mol. Brain Res.* 142, 115–122. doi: 10.1016/j.molbrainres.2005.09.019

Gonzalez, J. T., and Betts, J. A. (2018). Dietary fructose metabolism by splanchnic organs: size matters. *Cell Metab.* 27, 483–485. doi: 10.1016/j.cmet.2018.02.013

Grimes, K. M., Barefield, D. Y., Kumar, M., Mcnamara, J. W., Weintraub, S. T., De Tombe, P. P., et al. (2017). The naked mole-rat exhibits an unusual cardiac myofilament protein profile providing new insights into heart function of this naturally subterranean rodent. *Pflugers Arch.* 469, 1603–1613. doi: 10.1007/s00424-017-2046-3

Hall, M. N. (2008). mTOR-what does it do? *Transplant. Proc.* 40, S5–S8. doi: 10.1016/j.transproceed.2008.10.009

Inukai, K., Katagiri, H., Takata, K., Asano, T., Anai, M., Ishihara, H., et al. (1995). Characterization of rat GLUT5 and functional analysis of chimeric proteins of GLUT1 glucose transporter and GLUT5 fructose transporter. *Endocrinology* 136, 4850–4857. doi: 10.1210/endo.136.11.7588216

Koch, H., and Weber, Y. G. (2019). The glucose transporter type 1 (Glut1) syndromes. *Epilepsy Behav.* 91, 90–93. doi: 10.1016/j.yebeh.2018.06.010

Lacey, E., Patton, J., and Cameron, G. (2010). Life underground: the biology of subterranean rodents. *Ethology* 107, 559–560. doi: 10.1046/j.1439-0310.2001.00684.x

Lewis, K. N., Soifer, I., Melamud, E., Roy, M., Mcisaac, R. S., Hibbs, M., et al. (2016). Unraveling the message: insights into comparative genomics of the naked mole-rat. *Mamm. Genome* 27, 259–278. doi: 10.1007/s00335-016-9648-5

Li, J., Wang, T., and He, J. (2001). Seismic communication in subterranean Gansu zokor (*Myospalax cansus*). *Acta Theriol. Sin.* 21, 152–154. doi: 10.16829/j.slxb.2001.02.011 (in Chinese),

Li, S., Xu, B., An, Z., Wang, Z., and Wei, D. (2019). Evolutionary analysis of TSP-1 gene in Plateau zokor (Myospalax Baileyi) and its expression pattern under hypoxia. *Cell Mol. Biol. (Noisy-le-Grand)* 65, 48–57. doi: 10.14715/cmb/2019.65.3.7

Li, X., and Wang, T. (1992). Studies on the population age of Gansu zokor. *Acta Theriol. Sin.* 12, 193–199. doi: 10.16829/j.slxb.1992.03.007 (in Chinese),

Liu, L., Li, T., Liao, Y., Wang, Y., Gao, Y., Hu, H., et al. (2020). Triose kinase controls the lipogenic potential of fructose and dietary tolerance. *Cell Metab.* 32, 605–618. doi: 10.1016/j.cmet.2020.07.018

Logan, S. M., Szereszewski, K. E., Bennett, N. C., Hart, D. W., Jaarsveld, B. V., Pamenter, M. E., et al. (2020). The brains of six African mole-rat species show divergent responses to hypoxia. *J. Exp. Biol.* 223:jeb215905. doi: 10.1242/jeb.215905

Meng, T., Wang, Q., Ge, B., Pan, Q., Li, J., and He, J. (2017). The harderian gland of the Gansu Zokor (*Myospalax cansus*): a structural and antioxidant study. *Chin. J. Zool.* 52, 283–293. doi: 10.13859/j.cjz.201702012 (in Chinese),

Mergenthaler, P., Lindauer, U., Dienel, G. A., and Meisel, A. (2013). Sugar for the brain: the role of glucose in physiological and pathological brain function. *Trends Neurosci.* 36, 587–597. doi: 10.1016/j.tins.2013.07.001

Mirtschink, P., Jang, C., Arany, Z., and Krek, W. (2018). Fructose metabolism, cardiometabolic risk, and the epidemic of coronary artery disease. *Eur. Heart. J.* 39, 2497–2505. doi: 10.1093/eurheartj/ehx518

Moreno-Sánchez, R., Rodríguez-Enríquez, S., Marín-Hernández, A., and Saavedra, E. (2007). Energy metabolism in tumor cells. *FEBS J.* 274, 1393–1418. doi: 10.1111/j.1742-4658.2007.05686.x

Moskovitz, J., Malik, A., Hernandez, A., Band, M., and Avivi, A. (2012). Methionine sulfoxide reductases and methionine sulfoxide in the subterranean mole rat (Spalax): characterization of expression under various oxygen conditions. *Comp. Biochem. Physiol. A Mol. Integr. Physiol.* 161, 406–414. doi: 10.1016/j.cbpa.2011.12.014

Nakajima, H. (1995). [Phosphofructokinase (PFK)]. *Nihon Rinsho* 53, 1241–1246.

Nayak, G., Prentice, H. M., and Milton, S. L. (2016). Lessons from nature: signalling cascades associated with vertebrate brain anoxic survival. *Exp. Physiol.* 101, 1185–1190. doi: 10.1113/ep085673

Nevo, E. (1999). *Mosaic Evolution of Subterranean Mammals: Regression, Progression and Global Convergence*. New York, NY: Oxford University Press.

Newhouse, L. P., Joyner, M. J., Curry, T. B., Laurenti, M. C., Man, C. D., Cobelli, C., et al. (2017). Three hours of intermittent hypoxia increases circulating glucose levels in healthy adults. *Physiol. Rep.* 5:e13106. doi: 10.14814/phy2.13106

Pamenter, M. E., Dzal, Y. A., Thompson, W. A., and Milsom, W. K. (2019). Do naked mole rats accumulate a metabolic acidosis or an oxygen debt in severe hypoxia? *J. Exp. Biol.* 222:jeb.191197. doi: 10.1242/jeb.191197

Park, T. J., Reznick, J., Peterson, B. L., Blass, G., Omerbašić, D., Bennett, N. C., et al. (2017). Fructose-driven glycolysis supports anoxia resistance in the naked mole-rat. *Science* 356, 307–311. doi: 10.1126/science.aab3896

Patel, C., Sugimoto, K., Douard, V., Shah, A., Inui, H., Yamanouchi, T., et al. (2015). Effect of dietary fructose on portal and systemic serum fructose levels in rats and in KHK-/- and GLUT5-/- mice. *Am. J. Physiol. Gastrointest Liver Physiol.* 309, G779–G790. doi: 10.1152/ajpgi.00188.2015

Pleštilová, L., Hrouzková, E., Burda, H., Hua, L., and Šumbera, R. (2018). Additional row of outer hair cells - the unique pattern of the Corti organ in a subterranean rodent, the Gansu zokor (*Eospalax cansus*). *Mamm. Biol.* 94, 11–17. doi: 10.1016/j.mambio.2018.11.003

Pragallapati, S., and Manyam, R. (2019). Glucose transporter 1 in health and disease. *J. Oral. Maxillofac. Pathol.* 23, 443–449. doi: 10.4103/jomfp.JOMFP_22_18

Real-Hohn, A., Zancan, P., Da Silva, D., Martins, E. R., Salgado, L. T., Mermelstein, C. S., et al. (2010). Filamentous actin and its associated binding proteins are the stimulatory site for 6-phosphofructo-1-kinase association within the membrane of human erythrocytes. *Biochimie* 92, 538–544. doi: 10.1016/j.biochi.2010.01.023

Sandroni, C., D'Arrigo, S., and Nolan, J. P. (2018). Prognostication after cardiac arrest. *Crit. Care* 22, 150. doi: 10.1186/s13054-018-2060-7

Saxton, R. A., and Sabatini, D. M. (2017). mTOR signaling in growth, metabolism, and disease. *Cell* 168, 960–976. doi: 10.1016/j.cell.2017.02.004

Schmidt, H., Malik, A., Bicker, A., Poetzsch, G., Avivi, A., Shams, I., et al. (2017). Hypoxia tolerance, longevity and cancer-resistance in the mole rat Spalax - a liver transcriptomics approach. *Sci. Rep.* 7:14348. doi: 10.1038/s41598-017-13905-z

Shams, I., Avivi, A., and Nevo, E. (2004). Hypoxic stress tolerance of the blind subterranean mole rat: expression of erythropoietin and hypoxia-inducible factor 1 alpha. *Proc. Natl. Acad. Sci. U.S.A.* 101, 9698–9703. doi: 10.1073/pnas.0403540101

Shams, I., Avivi, A., and Nevo, E. (2005). Oxygen and carbon dioxide fluctuations in burrows of subterranean blind mole rats indicate tolerance to hypoxic-hypercapnic stresses. *Comp. Biochem. Physiol. A Mol. Integr. Physiol.* 142, 376–382. doi: 10.1016/j.cbpa.2005.09.003

Shams, I., Malik, A., Manov, I., Joel, A., Band, M., and Avivi, A. (2013). Transcription pattern of p53-targeted DNA repair genes in the hypoxia-tolerant subterranean mole rat Spalax. *J. Mol. Biol.* 425, 1111–1118. doi: 10.1016/j.jmb.2013.01.007

Shan, M., Wang, W., Ge, B., Li, J., and He, J. (2016). Muscle fiber types and metabolic characteristics of Gansu zoker (*Myospalax cansus*) in adaptation to hypoxia. *J. Northwest J. Northwest A&F University (Nat. Sci. Ed.)* 44, 18–24. doi: 10.13207/j.cnki.jnwafu.2016.10.004 (in Chinese),

Speers-Roesch, B., Sandblom, E., Lau, G. Y., Farrell, A. P., and Richards, J. G. (2010). Effects of environmental hypoxia on cardiac energy metabolism and performance in tilapia. *Am. J. Physiol. Regul. Integr. Comp. Physiol.* 298, R104–R119. doi: 10.1152/ajpregu.00418.2009

Staples, J. F., and Buck, L. T. (2009). Matching cellular metabolic supply and demand in energy-stressed animals. *Comp. Biochem. Physiol. A Mol. Integr. Physiol.* 153, 95–105. doi: 10.1016/j.cbpa.2009.02.010

Su, J., Hua, L., Wang, J., Gleeson, D. M., Wei, Y., Howitt, R., et al. (2014). Abundance and characteristics of microsatellite markers in Gansu zokor (*Eospalax cansus*), a fossorial rodent endemic to the Loess plateau. *China. J. Genet.* 93, e25–e28. doi: 10.1007/s12041-014-0352-5

Su, J., Wang, J., Hua, L., Gleeson, D., and Ji, W. (2013). Complete mitochondrial genome of the Gansu zokor, *Eospalax cansus* (Rodentia, Spalacidae). *Mitochondrial DNA* 24, 651–653. doi: 10.3109/19401736.2013.772166

Šumbera, R., Chitaukali, W. N., and Burda, H. (2007). *Biology of the Silvery Mole-rat (Heliophobius argenteocinereus). Why Study a Neglected Subterranean Rodent Species?* Berlin: Springer, 221–236.

Sun, S., Guo, Z., Fu, H., Zhu, J., and Ge, X. (2018). Integrated metabolomic and transcriptomic analysis of brain energy metabolism in the male Oriental river prawn (*Macrobrachium nipponense*) in response to hypoxia and reoxygenation. *Environ. Pollut.* 243, 1154–1165. doi: 10.1016/j.envpol.2018.09.072

Tang, Y., Wang, J., Li, J., Xie, H., Li, T., and He, J. (2013). Comparision of antioxidase and ATPase activity in heart between *Myospalax cansus* and *Rattus norvegicus* under acute hypoxia. *Acta Theriol. Sin.* 33, 178–185. doi: 10.16829/j.slxb.2013.02.011 (in Chinese),

Vannucci, R. C., and Vannucci, S. J. (2000). Glucose metabolism in the developing brain. *Semin. Perinatol.* 24, 107–115. doi: 10.1053/sp.2000.6361

Vleck, D. (1979). The energy cost of burrowing by the pocket gopher *Thomomys bottae*. *Physiol. Zool.* 52, 122–136. doi: 10.2307/30152558

Vleck, D. (1981). Burrow structure and foraging costs in the fossorial rodent, *Thomomys bottae*. *Oecologia* 49, 391–396. doi: 10.1007/BF00347605

Wang, Z. (2010). Present situation of harm and prevention measure for Gansu zokor (*Myospalax cansus*). *Anhui Agri. Sci. Bull.* 16, 189–190. doi: 10.16377/j.cnki.issn1007-7731.2010.07.021 (in Chinese),

Weil, Z. M., Norman, G. J., DeVries, A. C., and Nelson, R. J. (2008). The injured nervous system: a Darwinian perspective. *Prog. Neurobiol.* 86, 48–59. doi: 10.1016/j.pneurobio.2008.06.001

Wu, K. L., Hung, C. Y., Chan, J. Y., and Wu, C. W. (2014). An increase in adenosine-5′-triphosphate (ATP) content in rostral ventrolateral medulla is engaged in the high fructose diet-induced hypertension. *J. Biomed. Sci.* 21:8. doi: 10.1186/1423-0127-21-8

Xie, F., Li, T., and He, J. (2012). Effect of Hypoxia on ACTH and Blood Parameters in Gansu Zokor. *Chin. J. Zool.* 47, 119–123. doi: 10.13859/j.cjz.2012.05.015 (in Chinese),

Xu, L., Hao, Z., Lin, J., Zhao, Q., Zhang, B., Li, G., et al. (2019). Transcriptome sequencing of *Eospalax fontanierii* to determine hypoxia regulation of cardiac fibrinogen. *Mol. Biol. Rep.* 46, 5671–5683. doi: 10.1007/s11033-019-04690-1

Yan, T., Fan, W., and He, J. (2012). The effect of hypoxia tolerance on cardiac muscle structure of Gansu zokor (*Myospalax cansus*). *J. Shaanxi Normal University (Natural Sci. Ed.)* 40, 62–66. doi: 10.15983/j.cnki.jsnu.2012.02.020 (in Chinese),

Yan, T., Zhang, J., Tang, D., Zhang, X., Jiang, X., Zhao, L., et al. (2017). Hypoxia regulates mTORC1-mediated keratinocyte motility and migration via the AMPK pathway. *PLoS One* 12:e0169155. doi: 10.1371/journal.pone.0169155

Yang, H., and Wang, T. (1992). Studies on the degree of injury by zoker and economic threshold of its control. *Acta Phytophylacica Sinica* 19, 283–287. doi: 10.13802/j.cnki.zwbhxb.1992.03.020 (in Chinese),

Zhang, C. C., and Sadek, H. A. (2014). Hypoxia and metabolic properties of hematopoietic stem cells. *Antioxid. Redox Signal.* 20, 1891–1901. doi: 10.1089/ars.2012.5019

Zhang, J., Wang, Q., Qian, L., Yang, J., and He, J. (2016). Variety of cardiac functions of *Eospalax cansus* after hypoxia acclimatization. *Sichuan J. Zool.* 35, 421–425. doi: 10.11984/j.issn.1000-7083.20150335 (in Chinese),

Zhang, Y., Zhang, Z., and Liu, J. (2003). Burrowing rodents as ecosystem engineers: the ecology and management of plateau zokors *Myospalax fontanierii* in alpine meadow ecosystems on the Tibetan plateau. *Mamm. Rev.* 33, 284–294. doi: 10.1046/j.1365-2907.2003.00020.x

Zhou, W., and Dou, F. (1990). Studies on activity and home range of plateau zokor. *Acta Theriol. Sin.* 10, 31–39. doi: 10.16829/j.slxb.1990.01.006 (in Chinese),

8

Physiological Effects of Intermittent Passive Exposure to Hypobaric Hypoxia and Cold in Rats

Garoa Santocildes[1], Ginés Viscor[1], Teresa Pagès[1], Sara Ramos-Romero[1,2], Josep Lluís Torres[2] and Joan Ramon Torrella[1]*

[1] Secció de Fisiologia, Departament de Biologia Cel·lular, Fisiologia i Immunologia, Facultat de Biologia, Universitat de Barcelona, Barcelona, Spain, [2] Departament de Química Biològica, Institut de Química Avançada de Catalunya (IQAC-CSIC), Barcelona, Spain

***Correspondence:**
Ginés Viscor
gviscor@ub.edu

The benefits of intermittent hypobaric hypoxia (IHH) exposure for health and its potential use as a training tool are well-documented. However, since hypobaric hypoxia and cold are environmental factors always strongly associated in the biosphere, additive or synergistic adaptations could have evolved in animals' genomes. For that reason, the aim of the present study was to investigate body composition and hematological and muscle morphofunctional responses to simultaneous intermittent exposure to hypoxia and cold. Adult male rats were randomly divided into four groups: (1) control, maintained in normoxia at 25°C (CTRL); (2) IHH exposed 4 h/day at 4,500 m (HYPO); (3) intermittent cold exposed 4 h/day at 4°C (COLD); and (4) simultaneously cold and hypoxia exposed (COHY). At the end of 9 and 21 days of exposure, blood was withdrawn and gastrocnemius (GAS) and tibialis anterior muscles, perigonadal and brown adipose tissue, diaphragm, and heart were excised. GAS transversal sections were stained for myofibrillar ATPase and succinate dehydrogenase for fiber typing and for endothelial ATPase to assess capillarization. Hypoxia-inducible factor 1α (HIF-1α), vascular endothelial growth factor (VEGF), and glucose transporter 1 (GLUT1) from GAS samples were semi-quantified by Western blotting. COLD and HYPO underwent physiological adjustments such as higher brown adipose tissue weight and increase in blood-related oxygen transport parameters, while avoiding some negative effects of chronic exposure to cold and hypoxia, such as body weight and muscle mass loss. COHY presented an additive erythropoietic response and was prevented from right ventricle hypertrophy. Intermittent cold exposure induced muscle angiogenesis, and IHH seems to indicate better muscle oxygenation through fiber area reduction.

Keywords: cold, erythropoiesis, skeletal muscle, rats, intermittent hypoxia, hypobaria, capillarization

INTRODUCTION

More than 140 million people worldwide live at high altitude (above 2,500 m) and 40 million people are also exposed to altitude environment due to recreational or other reasons (Moore et al., 1998; West et al., 2012). Altitude is characterized by low barometric pressure and, hence, reduced atmospheric oxygen partial pressure (PO_2), which in turn results in a decrease in arterial oxygen content leading to tissue hypoxia (Lundby et al., 2009). Mammalian cells are able to sense oxygen changes and to respond to maintain adequate oxygen levels and homeostasis and, thus, ensure cell function and survival (Semenza, 1998). Organisms can react with a wide range of responses to low PO_2 (Breen et al., 2008; Lundby et al., 2009), but the magnitude of this response to hypoxia is directly related to the dose because the severity of the hypoxemia, the duration of the hypoxic exposure, and its frequency are responsible for the subsequent beneficial or pathological reaction (hormesis) (Navarrete-Opazo and Mitchell, 2014).

Intermittent hypoxia is characterized by long periods of normoxia alternated with periods in hypoxia, resulting in a potentially cumulative effect that begins with the first exposure (Neubauer, 2001; Viscor et al., 2018). During the last few decades, it has been well documented that intermittent hypobaric hypoxia (IHH) could elicit beneficial responses in the organism without detectable adverse consequences. Among other things, it has been shown that IHH enhances erythropoiesis and aerobic capacity, improves muscle capillarization and metabolism, controls hypertension, accelerates tissue repair, ameliorates bronchial asthma, regulates metabolic syndrome, and improves altitude acclimatization (see for review Viscor et al., 2018).

Despite numerous studies focused on the effect of hypobaric hypoxia, very few works have considered the fact that high altitude in natural environments always involves a simultaneous exposure to hypobaric hypoxia and cold stimuli. Exposure to cold is characterized by increased metabolic rate and blood flow in order to respond to the higher oxygen needs by tissues during thermogenesis. However, during hypoxia, cellular oxygen availability is reduced due to a low PO_2, triggering physiological responses oriented to maintain oxygen supply at the tissue level. Interestingly, during concurrent cold and hypoxia, increased oxygen demands and compromised oxygen availability occur simultaneously (Banchero et al., 1985; Jackson et al., 1987).

Mammals have the ability to respond and adapt to different environmental stressors to guarantee their survival (Breen et al., 2008; Maekawa et al., 2013). During acclimatization to hypoxia, increased ventilation and enhanced oxygen transport and delivery are aimed at improving oxygen extraction and use in cells (Neubauer, 2001). Hypoxia-inducible factor 1α (HIF-1α) is the main mediator of cellular hypoxia, regulating more than 100 genes involved in key processes such as erythropoiesis and iron metabolism, angiogenesis, glucose metabolism, cell proliferation and survival, and apoptosis (Ke and Costa, 2006). When homeotherms are exposed to a cold environment, different behavioral responses, morphological adjustments, and physiological adaptations take place in order to reduce heat loss and increase endogenous heat production and, therefore, maintain a stable core temperature (Deveci et al., 2001b; Deveci and Egginton, 2002; Deveci and Egginton, 2003; Maekawa et al., 2013). The hypothalamic–pituitary–adrenal and hypothalamic–pituitary–thyroid axes play a significant role by means of the upregulation of sympathetic effect over the metabolism of carbohydrates and lipids and increasing the expression of beta-adrenergic receptors in hepatic, adipose, and cardiac cells (Zhang Z. et al., 2018). Shivering thermogenesis, which takes place exclusively in the skeletal muscle, is the primary source of heat in the early phase of cold exposure (Suzuki et al., 1997; Egginton et al., 2001; Deveci and Egginton, 2002; Egginton, 2002; Sepa-Kishi et al., 2017; Mahalingam et al., 2020), while during subsequent cold acclimatization, there is a progressive increase of non-shivering thermogenesis *via* brown adipose tissue (BAT) activation (Suzuki et al., 1997; Deveci and Egginton, 2002; Sepa-Kishi et al., 2017; Mahalingam et al., 2020). Moreover, skeletal muscle is also involved in non-shivering thermogenesis based on the activity of Ca^{2+}-ATPase in the sarcoplasmic reticulum (SR) (Sepa-Kishi et al., 2017). Thermogenesis in skeletal muscle is supported by increased oxidative metabolism (Egginton et al., 2001; Egginton, 2002) and mitochondrial plasticity (Mahalingam et al., 2020) and requires adaptive changes to improve the oxygen transport system and, thereby, support oxygen demands (Suzuki et al., 1997; Deveci and Egginton, 2002).

In the 1980s, the group led by Natalio Banchero pioneered several studies investigating the effect of concurrent hypobaric hypoxia and cold in muscle tissue, showing that when cold and hypoxia were applied simultaneously, a greater capillarity was found in the gastrocnemius (GAS) muscle than that observed after acclimation to these two factors separately (Banchero et al., 1985; Jackson et al., 1987). Later on, other researchers studied the possible cross-adaptation between cold and hypoxia on the autonomous nervous system (Lunt et al., 2010). Moreover, we have recently shown that simultaneous exposure to IHH and intermittent cold counteracts the pro-inflammatory effect and the body weight (BW) loss produced by isolated hypobaric hypoxia exposure (Ramos-Romero et al., 2020).

The aim of the present study was to investigate the physiological responses to IHH and intermittent cold when they were applied separately or simultaneously. We used rats as a widespread animal model having in mind that an in-depth study on hematological and muscular responses to these two environmental factors could help to better understand the altitude acclimatization process and find out the usefulness of both stimuli as a non-pharmacological therapeutic treatment for injury recovery or as a tool for training in sport performance.

MATERIALS AND METHODS

Animals

A total of 108 adult male Sprague–Dawley rats (Envigo, Casatenovo, Italy) with an initial weight of 211 ± 28 g (mean ± SD) were used in the study. Animals were housed at 25°C ± 2°C and maintained on a 12-h light–dark cycle, with *ad libitum* access to water and food (even during cold and hypoxia exposures). After 1 week of quarantine, rats were randomly divided into four groups: (1) control (CTRL), maintained in normoxia at 25°C; (2) intermittent cold exposed (COLD); (3) IHH exposed (HYPO); and (4) rats simultaneously submitted to intermittent cold and hypobaric hypoxia (COHY). Animals from these different groups were submitted to the assigned intervention procedure for 9 or 21 days.

All procedures were performed in accordance with European Union guidelines for the care and management of laboratory animals and were under license from the Catalan authorities (reference no. 1899), as approved by the University of Barcelona's Ethical Committee for Animal Experimentation.

Intervention Protocols

A hypobaric chamber was used to expose rats to IHH. The hypobaric chamber had 136-L capacity, allowing for two rat cages to be placed inside it. The chamber walls were made of polymethyl methacrylate plastic, allowing for the animals' behavior to be observed during the protocol. A relative vacuum (low pressure) in the chamber was produced by a rotational vacuum pump (TRIVAC D5E; Leybold-Oerlikon, Köln, Germany) by regulating the airflow rate at the inlet with a micrometric valve. Inner pressure was controlled by two differential pressure sensors (ID 2000; Leybold-Oerlikon, Köln, Germany) connected to a vacuum controller (Combivac IT23; Leybold-Oerlikon, Köln, Germany) driving a diaphragm (DIA) pressure regulator (MR16; Leybold-Oerlikon, Köln, Germany). The target pressure of 577 hPa (equivalent to 4,500 m of altitude) was achieved steadily over ~15 min. Once this desired level was reached, the internal barometric pressure of the chamber was regulated and maintained by the control system for 4 h. A continuous entry of air through the inlet valve avoided the accumulation of humidity and CO_2 into the hypobaric chamber. At the end of the session, pressurization to normal barometric pressure was gradually restored over ~15 min. The intermittent cold exposure (ICE) was performed by introducing the rats into their own cages in a cold room at 4°C. Finally, simultaneous cold and hypobaric hypoxia exposure was carried out by placing the hypobaric chamber in the cold room. All intervention consisted of 4 h/day sessions.

Blood and Tissue Sampling

Animals from the different groups were sampled the day after the last intervention at two different points in time (9 or 21 days). After being anesthetized, a blood sample was drawn from the abdominal cava vein and analyzed by a hematological analyzer (Coulter Spincell 3; Spinreact, Girona, Spain). Then, both GAS, both tibialis anterior (TA), perigonadal (epididymal) adipose tissue (PAT), interscapular BAT, DIA, and heart were excised from each rat, rinsed in saline solution, and weighed. Skeletal muscles were frozen in precooled isopentane (Sigma-Aldrich) and stored at −80°C until further analysis. At the end, the animals were euthanized by anesthetic overdose.

Histochemical Procedures

Frozen GAS muscles were embedded in a mounting medium (Tissue-Tek; Sakura Finitek Europe, Zoeterwoude, The Netherlands) and cut in serial transverse sections (14–16 μm) using a cryostat (Leica CM3050S, Wetzlar, Germany) at −22°C. Sections were mounted on gelatinized slides (0.02%), incubated for 5 min in a fixing *buffer* (Viscor et al., 1992) in order to prevent shrinkage or wrinkling and finally stained for: (1) myofibrillar adenosine triphosphatase (mATPase), following preincubation in alkaline solution (pH 10.7), to differentiate between slow- and fast-twitch fibers (Brooke and Kaiser, 1970); (2) succinate dehydrogenase (SDH), to identify aerobic and anaerobic fibers (Nachlas et al., 1957); (3) endothelial adenosine triphosphatase (eATPase), to reveal muscle capillaries (Fouces et al., 1993). A representative combined image can be seen in **Figure 1**. A complete set of representative images for all the histochemical assays from the four experimental groups at the two sampling time points is included as **Supplementary Material** (**Supplementary Figure 1**).

Morphofunctional Measurements

Morphofunctional measurements were performed on microphotographs of stained sections, obtained with a light microscope (BX61; Olympus, Tokyo, Japan) connected to a digital camera (DP70; Olympus, Tokyo, Japan) at × 20 magnification. Since GAS muscle has a heterogeneous muscle fiber type distribution and morphometry, three different zones from each muscle (red, intermediate, and white), as previously described by Armstrong and Phelps (1984), were photographed and further analyzed (Armstrong and Phelps, 1984). All the parameters listed below were measured or calculated from transverse cross-section tissues with an area of 5.5×10^5 μm^2 using ImageJ software (v. 1.51n; National Institutes of Health, United States).

All muscle fibers were typified according to their metabolic and contractile character (**Figures 1B,C**) and classified as slow-twitch oxidative (SO), fast-twitch oxidative glycolytic (FOG), fast-twitch glycolytic (FG), or fast-twitch intermediate glycolytic (FIG). SO fibers were unstained for mATPase (pH 10.7) and presented high SDH activity; FOG fibers displayed a dark mATPase and SDH stain; FG fibers presented moderate mATPase stain and remained unstained for SDH assay; and FIG fibers presented moderate to high mATPase and intermediate SDH stain (higher than FG fibers but lower than FOG fibers). Images from eATPase (**Figure 1A**) were used to measure or calculate the following parameters: fiber cross-sectional area (FCSA), Feret diameter, number of capillaries per 1,000 μm^2 of FCSA ($CCA = NCF \cdot 10^3/FCSA$), number of capillaries per fiber (NCF), fiber density (FD), capillary density (CD), and capillary-to-fiber ratio (C/F = CD/FD). The mean total number of fibers per rat included for the analysis was 477 ± 112 (±SD). The same researcher performed fiber typing and identification of the capillaries to guarantee that the same criteria were used in all the analyzed images.

Protein Extraction and Western Blotting

HIF-1α protein expression and two of its target proteins, vascular endothelial growth factor (VEGF) and glucose transporter 1 (GLUT1), were semi-quantified using Western blot technique. Whole GAS muscles were homogenized in urea lysis buffer [6 M urea, 1% sodium dodecyl sulfate (SDS)], supplemented with protease and phosphatase inhibitors (Complete Protease Inhibitor Cocktail and PhosphoSTOP, Sigma-Aldrich), using the Precellys® Evolution tissue homogenizer (Bertin Technologies, Montignt-le-Bretonneux, France). The lysates were centrifuged at 25,000 g for 15 min at 4°C to remove cell debris, and total protein content of the collected supernatants was quantified by the bicinchoninic acid assay (Thermo Fisher Scientific). Muscle protein extracts were solubilized in an electrophoresis loading buffer (62.5 mM Tris·HCl, pH 6.8; 2.3% SDS; 10% glycerol; 5% mercaptoethanol; and bromophenol blue), and equal amounts of

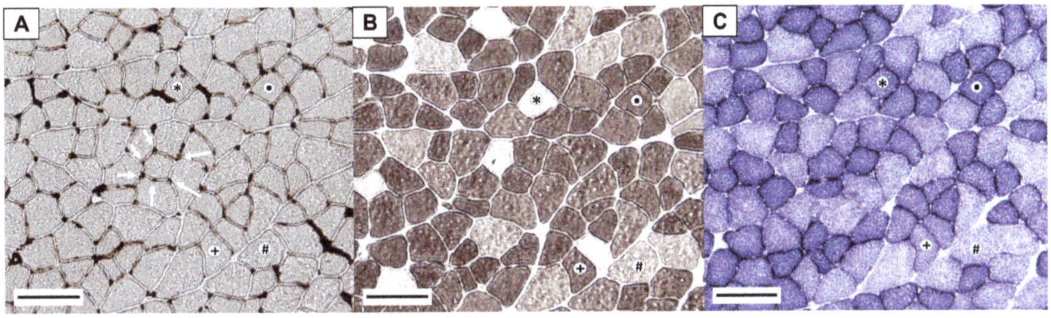

FIGURE 1 | Representative microphotographs of gastrocnemius cross-section histochemical assays. **(A)** Endothelial ATPase stain (arrows indicate muscle capillaries); **(B)** myosin ATPase stain; **(C)** succinate dehydrogenase stain. (*) Slow oxidative fiber (SO); (·) fast oxidative glycolytic fiber (FOG); (+) fast intermediate glycolytic fiber (FIG); # fast glycolytic fiber (FG). Bar represents 100 μm.

protein (between 10 and 55 μg) were loaded onto each lane of the gel, and electrophoresis was run on 10% SDS–polyacrylamide gel electrophoresis (PAGE) gels. Ten study samples and one control sample in triplicate (to verify the possible variability between samples across each membrane) were loaded onto each gel. The following internal quality control criteria were used to consider a valid blot: the variation between the control samples had to be less than 20%, and the same control sample was loaded in all the gels to compensate for the variability between gels and to be able to compare them, as described by Martin-Rincon et al. (2019).

After electrophoresis, proteins were transferred to an Immun-Blot polyvinylidene fluoride (PVDF) membrane for protein blotting (Bio-Rad Laboratories). To verify that equal amounts of muscle protein were charged in each well and the efficiency of transference, the membranes were stained with Ponceau S stain (Sigma-Aldrich). For immunoblotting, membranes were blocked with 4% bovine serum albumin (BSA) in TBS-T (Tris-buffered saline containing 0.1% Tween 20) for 1 h at room temperature. To detect our target proteins, membranes were incubated overnight at 4°C with primary antibodies against HIF-1α (MA1-516; Thermo Fisher Scientific), VEGF (MA1-16629; Thermo Fisher Scientific), and GLUT1 (#12939; Cell Signaling Technology) diluted 1:1,000 in 4% BSA-TBS-T. Following this, the membranes were incubated with the corresponding secondary horseradish peroxidase (HRP)-conjugated antibody (#31460 and #31430; Thermo Fisher Scientific) diluted 1:5,000 in 5% Blotto in TBS-T for 1 h at room temperature. The specific bands were visualized with the Clarity TM Western ECL Substrate Kit (Bio-Rad Laboratories), and the chemiluminescence signal was measured using the Odyssey Fc Imaging System (LI-COR Inc. Biotechnology, Lincoln, Nebraska, United States) and quantified with the Image Studio Software (v. 5.2.5, LI-COR Inc. Biotechnology). Muscle signaling data were reported (in arbitrary units) as the sample band intensity relative to Ponceau S stain, and the final data were normalized to the mean value (band densities) of the three control samples loaded on all the gels.

Statistical Analysis

Data were analyzed using a one-way ANOVA test followed by the Holm–Sidak *post hoc* test or Student's *t* when appropriate. Statistical comparisons were only tested by comparing groups within the same time point. Statistical significance was set at $p < 0.05$. The results are reported as mean ± standard error (SE) in histograms, tables, and throughout the text, unless otherwise indicated. Most figures are represented through box-and-whisker plots. The box represents the first and third quartiles separated by the median. Whisker end points represent minimum and maximum values, and the mean is represented with a black dot. All statistical tests were performed using the statistical package SigmaPlot 11 (Systat Software, Inc., San Jose, CA, United States, 2008–2009).

RESULTS

Animal Body Weight, Time Course, and Body Composition

Rats' BW was monitored throughout the study, and the weight change percentage was calculated every 2 days (**Figure 2**). The weight of all the animals increased gradually over time, but with some differences between experimental groups at some time points. On day 2 of intervention, animals exposed to IHH (HYPO and COHY) suffered a significant ($p < 0.001$ and $p < 0.001$, respectively) BW loss compared to CTRL, whose BW increased slightly respective to its initial values. Moreover, HYPO presented a significantly reduced BW gain in relation to COLD ($p < 0.001$). Between days 2 and 4 of the study, COHY exhibited significant lower growth than the other groups ($p < 0.001$), while no differences were found across the rest of the experimental groups. On day 8, COHY presented, compared to the previous day, a significantly lower BW increase than CTRL and COLD ($p = 0.005$ and $p = 0.009$, respectively). Nevertheless, from days 10 to 12, only COLD exhibited changes, specifically, larger BW increase than CTRL and COHY ($p = 0.006$ and $p = 0.001$, respectively). No more statistical differences were found among the different experimental groups in the remaining measures. Data showing the percentage changes in BW from the start to the end of the study are shown in **Table 1**. After 9 days, a statistically significant lower BW gain in animals exposed to hypoxia (alone or combined with cold) when compared to CTRL was evident. COHY also

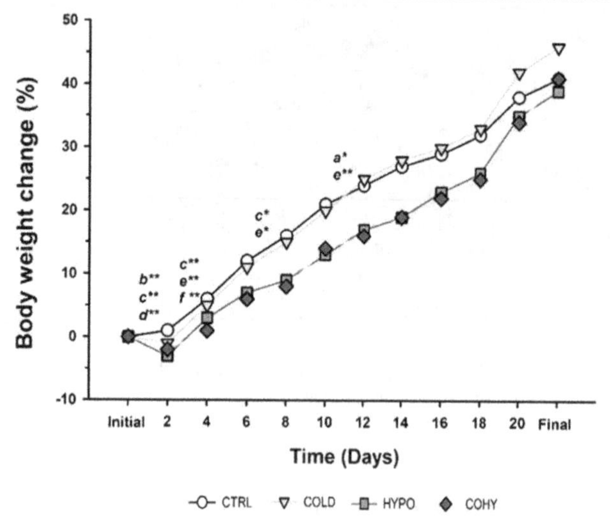

FIGURE 2 | Body weight change during the study. Statistically significant differences are indicated as follows: *$p < 0.05$, **$p < 0.001$ between the following pairs: a, CTRL vs. COLD; b, CTRL vs. HYPO; c, CTRL vs. COHY; d, COLD vs. HYPO; e, COLD vs. COHY; f, HYPO vs. COHY. CTRL, control; COLD, intermittent cold; HYPO, intermittent hypoxia; COHY, intermittent cold + hypoxia.

presented reduced BW gain compared to COLD ($p < 0.026$). However, after 21 days, COLD presented a significantly higher weight gain than the rest of the groups.

Rats exposed to hypoxia for 9 days exhibited higher limb lean mass (GAS+TA weight) than COLD and CTRL, although these differences were only statistically significant when hypoxia was applied alone (HYPO) ($p < 0.001$ vs. COLD; $p = 0.006$ vs. CTRL). After 21 days, all animals submitted to any intervention sessions (cold and/or hypoxia) showed a significantly higher GAS+TA weight than CTRL ($p < 0.001$). There were also significant differences in lean mass weight between HYPO and COHY (3.35 ± 0.11 g vs. 3.01 ± 0.06 g, $p = 0.001$). Regarding adipose tissue, IHH alone induced a statistically significant decrease in BAT/BW ratio, which was already appreciated after 9 days and was maintained throughout the whole time that the intervention lasted. Furthermore, after 9 days of ICE sessions, COLD presented a significantly higher BAT/BW ratio than CTRL, HYPO, and COHY ($p < 0.001$, $p < 0.001$, and $p = 0.005$, respectively). Nevertheless, after 21 days, COLD group only presented significant differences in BAT weight when compared to CTRL and HYPO ($p = 0.003$ and $p < 0.001$, respectively). Regarding PAT, no statistical differences were found among the different groups on day 9 of the study, but a significant reduction in PAT/BW ratio was found in HYPO compared with the other three groups after 21 days of IHH sessions.

No changes were found in DIA or in heart weight between different experimental groups at any time point (**Table 1**). Nevertheless, a significant increase in the right ventricular index (calculated as the ratio of right ventricle to whole heart weight) was found in HYPO at day 9 of the experimental period (vs. CTRL, $p = 0.003$; vs. COLD, $p = 0.012$; vs. COHY, $p = 0.004$).

Hematological Parameters

Oxygen-related transport hematological parameters are shown in **Figure 3**. After 9 days of IHH exposure, alone (HYPO) or combined with cold (COHY), animals had a significantly higher hemoglobin concentration ([Hb]) and hematocrit (Htc) compared to CTRL. COHY also exhibited a significantly higher [Hb] and Htc than COLD after 9 days ([Hb]: $p = 0.024$, Htc: $p = 0.007$) and significantly higher Htc ($p = 0.001$) after 21 days. COLD compared to CTRL increased [Hb] significantly ($p = 0.021$) within the first 9 days of exposure and had non-significantly higher [Hb] after 21 days. Regarding red blood cell (RBC) count, COHY presented significantly higher values than CTRL both after 9 and 21 days of exposure and higher than COLD after 21 days ($p = 0.007$). An almost significantly greater RBC count ($p = 0.058$) was found in HYPO when compared to CTRL on both days 9 and 21.

Table 2 shows hematimetric indices and white blood cell (WBC) and platelet counts. Statistically significant differences were only found after 9 days in COHY when compared to CTRL and COLD in mean corpuscular volume (MCV) and after 21 days in mean corpuscular hemoglobin concentration (MCHC),

TABLE 1 | Rats' body composition parameters.

	9 days				21 days			
	CTRL $n = 14$	COLD $n = 15$	HYPO $n = 11$	COHY $n = 16$	CTRL $n = 14$	COLD $n = 13$	HYPO $n = 11$	COHY $n = 14$
BW (Δ%)	24.8 ± 1.2	22.6 ± 1.7	18.7 ± 1.5*	16.5 ± 1.6**#	41.7 ± 3.2	48.9 ± 1.9*	37.7 ± 2.6##	36.1 ± 1.9##
Muscle (GAS+TA)/ 100 g BW	1.68 ± 0.01	1.64 ± 0.03	1.80 ± 0.09**##	1.74 ± 0.03	2.62 ± 0.04	3.08 ± 0.0**	3.35 ± 0.11**##	3.01 ± 0.06**$$
PAT/BW (mg/g)	8.98 ± 0.41	8.13 ± 0.37	7.81 ± 0.46	8.47 ± 0.62	10.00 ± 0.39	10.07 ± 0.37	8.38 ± 0.38*#	10.3 ± 0.43$
BAT/BW (mg/g)	1.31 ± 0.08	1.73 ± 0.10**	0.76 ± 0.04**##	1.43 ± 0.04#$$	1.12 ± 0.06	1.38 ± 0.05*	0.89 ± 0.03*##	1.33 ± 0.27*$$
Diaphragm/ BW (mg/g)	1.93 ± 0.05	1.90 ± 0.05	1.80 ± 0.04	1.74 ± 0.13	1.81 ± 0.08	1.82 ± 0.05	1.83 ± 0.09	2.03 ± 0.10
Heart/BW (mg/g)	3.35 ± 0.04	3.34 ± 0.06	3.48 ± 0.10	3.43 ± 0.07	3.37 ± 0.08	3.41 ± 0.10	3.40 ± 0.07	3.59 ± 0.07
Right ventricle/ total heart (%)	24.4 ± 0.8	25.0 ± 0.7	28.3 ± 1.4*#	24.5 ± 0.5$	25.6 ± 1.2	26.3 ± 1.2	28.8 ± 0.8	26.4 ± 0.9

Data are presented as mean ± standard error. BW, body weight; GAS, gastrocnemius muscle; TA, tibialis anterior muscle; PAT, perigonadal adipose tissue; BAT, brown adipose tissue. CTRL, control; COLD, intermittent cold; HYPO, intermittent hypoxia; COHY, intermittent cold + hypoxia. Statistically significant differences are indicated as follows: *$p < 0.05$ *vs. CTRL,* **$p < 0.001$ *vs. CTRL,* #$p < 0.05$ *vs. COLD,* ##$p < 0.001$ *vs. COLD,* \$$p < 0.05$ *vs. HYPO,* \$\$$p < 0.001$ *vs. HYPO.*

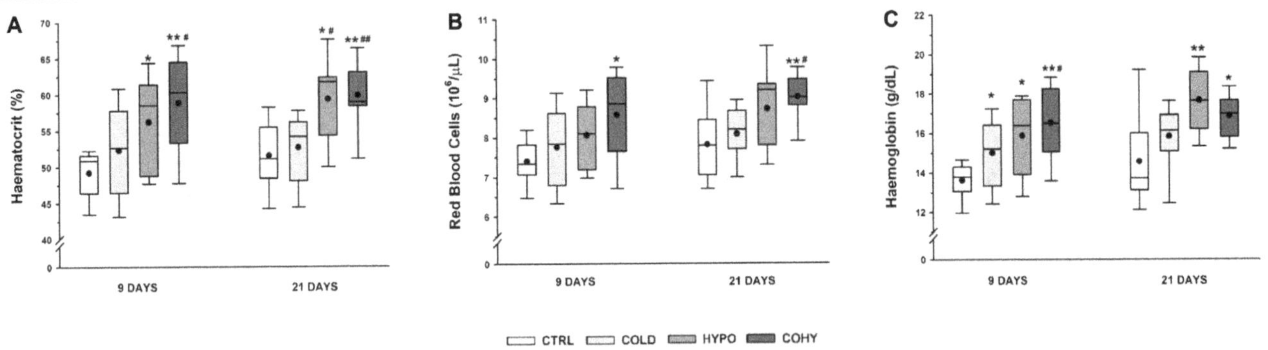

FIGURE 3 | Hematological parameters after 9 and 21 days. **(A)** Hematocrit; **(B)** red blood cell counts; **(C)** hemoglobin concentration. CTRL, control; COLD, intermittent cold; HYPO, intermittent hypoxia; COHY, intermittent cold + hypoxia. Statistically significant differences are indicated as follows: $^{*}p < 0.05$ vs. CTRL, $^{**}p < 0.001$ vs. CTRL, $^{\#}p < 0.05$ vs. COLD, $^{\#\#}p < 0.001$ vs. COLD. Sample size: n = 8–13 per group at each temporal time point.

TABLE 2 | Rats' blood haematimetric parameters.

	9 days				21 days			
	CTRL $n = 11$	**COLD** $n = 13$	**HYPO** $n = 8$	**COHY** $n = 12$	**CTRL** $n = 9$	**COLD** $n = 12$	**HYPO** $n = 9$	**COHY** $n = 11$
MCV (fL)	66.7 ± 0.7	67.6 ± 0.6	68.6 ± 0.4	$70.4 \pm 1.1^{*\#}$	65.2 ± 0.9	65.2 ± 0.8	66.6 ± 0.3	66.5 ± 0.6
MHC (pg)	18.4 ± 0.3	18.8 ± 0.6	19.4 ± 0.2	19.6 ± 0.2	18.5 ± 0.5	19.1 ± 0.3	19.22 ± 0.3	18.68 ± 0.2
MCHC (g/dL)	27.7 ± 0.3	28.6 ± 0.3	28.3 ± 0.3	28.1 ± 0.3	27.5 ± 0.1	$29.9 \pm 0.5^{*}$	$29.0 \pm 0.5^{*}$	$28.4 \pm 0.3^{\#}$
WBC (10^9/L)	7.0 ± 0.5	$12.5 \pm 0.5^{*}$	$10.9 \pm 1.4^{*}$	$11.3 \pm 1.3^{*}$	6.4 ± 1.7	6.9 ± 0.6	$10.4 \pm 1.7^{*\#}$	$6.8 \pm 0.6^{\$}$
Platelets (10^9/L)	522 ± 22	603 ± 71	$392 \pm 34^{*\#}$	$406 \pm 31^{\#}$	497 ± 37	587 ± 44	488 ± 34	451 ± 32

Data are presented as mean ± standard error. MCV, mean corpuscular volume; MHC, mean corpuscular hemoglobin; MCHC, mean corpuscular hemoglobin concentration; WBC, white blood cells. CTRL, control; COLD, intermittent cold; HYPO, intermittent hypoxia; COHY, intermittent cold + hypoxia. Statistically significant differences are indicated as follows: $^{*}p < 0.05$ *vs. CTRL,* $^{\#}p < 0.05$ *vs. COLD,* $^{\$}p < 0.05$ *vs. HYPO.*

all groups having higher values than CTRL. All intervened groups showed higher WBC than CTRL after 9 days, while after 21 days, only HYPO presented significantly higher values than the other groups. Regarding platelets, CTRL and COLD had statistically significant higher counts than HYPO and COHY after 9 days, which was not observed after 21 days.

Fiber Cross-Sectional Area and Feret Diameter

Figures 4A–D show the FCSA measurements of the different fiber types presented separately. All rats subjected to any treatment for 9 days presented a slight FCSA reduction relative to CTRL group in SO fiber type, which is statistically significant (p = 0.049) in COHY. After 21 days, SO fibers in COLD-treated animals presented a similar mean FCSA to CTRL (3,314 ± 258 μm^2 vs. 3,400 ± 225 μm^2), while both hypoxic groups had a non-significant FCSA reduction (**Figure 4A**). After 9 days, FOG and FIG fibers (**Figures 4B,C**) had very similar values in all groups. However, after 21 days, a consistent trend in FOG and FIG fiber size reduction was evident in groups exposed to intermittent hypoxia (HYPO and COHY). These reductions were not statistically significant and ranged from 16 to 18% in FOG fibers and from 10 to 24% in FIG fibers. Finally, no changes were found in FG fibers FCSA among the different groups at any time point.

Feret diameter parameter shows the longest distance between any two points along the section boundary, also known as maximum caliper. As shown in **Figures 4E–H**, COLD, HYPO, and COHY showed smaller maximum Feret diameter than CTRL in SO fiber type after day 9 (p = 0.095, p = 0.043, and p = 0.007, respectively). After 21 days, only HYPO and COHY presented smaller mean maximum Feret diameter than CTRL, but without reaching significant differences (80.1 ± 6.6 and 80.1 ± 4.5 vs. 88.3 ± 4.0) (**Figure 4E**). No changes on Feret diameter were found in FOG and FIG fibers at 9 days of intervention protocols (**Figures 4F,G**). However, at 21 days, a trend toward smaller mean maximum Feret diameter was found in FOG fibers of all treated groups, and smaller mean was observed in FIG fibers of COHY. No changes were found in FG fibers in any group at any temporal point.

Individual Fiber Capillarization

After 9 days, the intervened groups showed in all fiber types a trend to reduce the NCF compared to CTRL (**Figures 5A–D**). This reduction was statistically significant in FG fibers of the animals exposed to IHH (HYPO and COHY) with a higher significant reduction in COHY (p = 0.003) than in HYPO

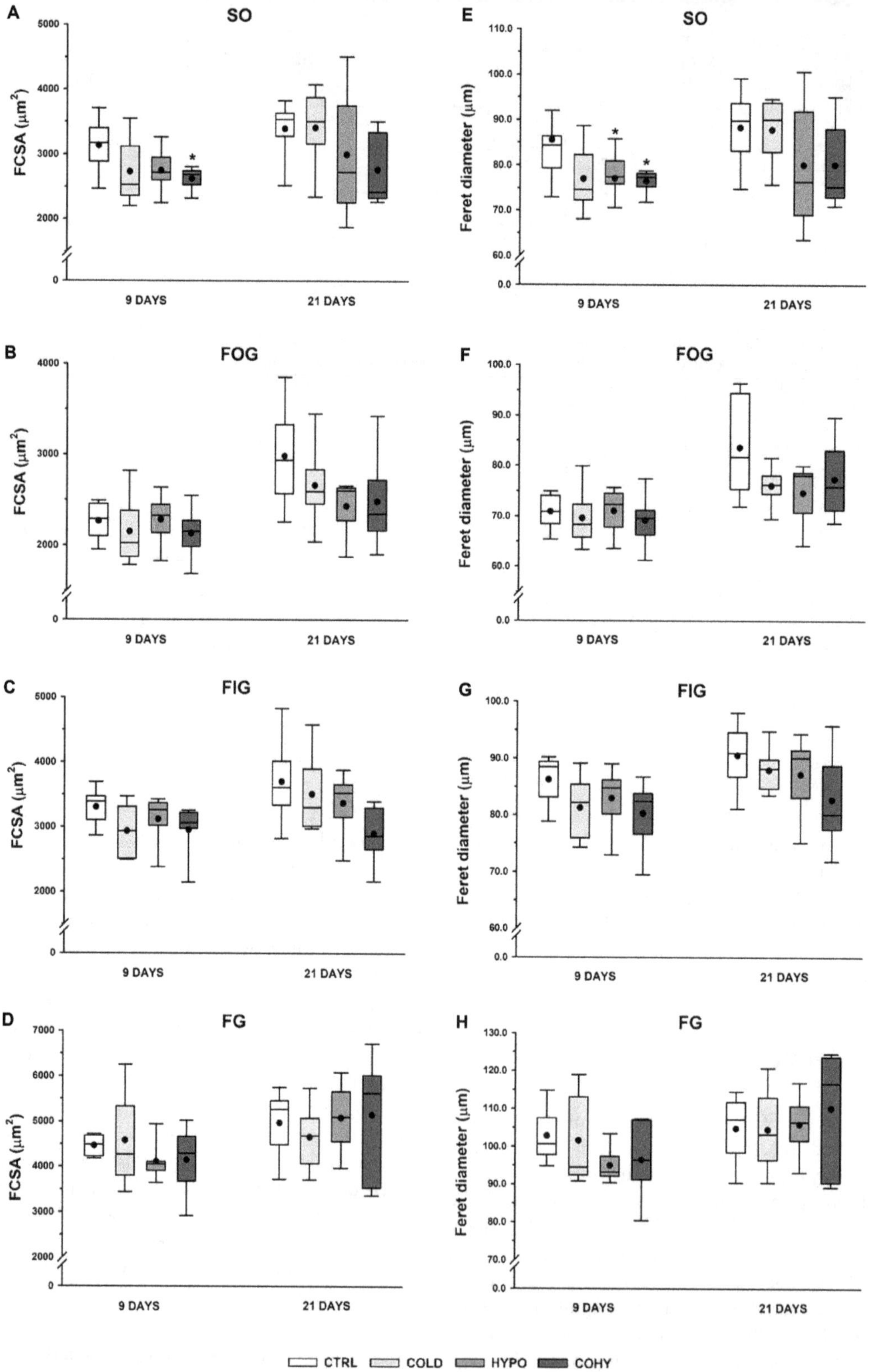

FIGURE 4 | Gastrocnemius muscle fiber morphometry after 9 and 21 days in the different fiber types. **(A–D)** Fiber cross-sectional area (FCSA), **(E–H)** Feret diameter. SO, slow oxidative; FOG, fast oxidative glycolytic; FIG, fast intermediate glycolytic; FG, fast glycolytic. CTRL, control; COLD, intermittent cold; HYPO, intermittent hypoxia; COHY, intermittent cold + hypoxia. Statistically significant differences are indicated as follows: $^{*}p < 0.05$ vs. CTRL. Sample size: $n = 6$ per group at each temporal time point.

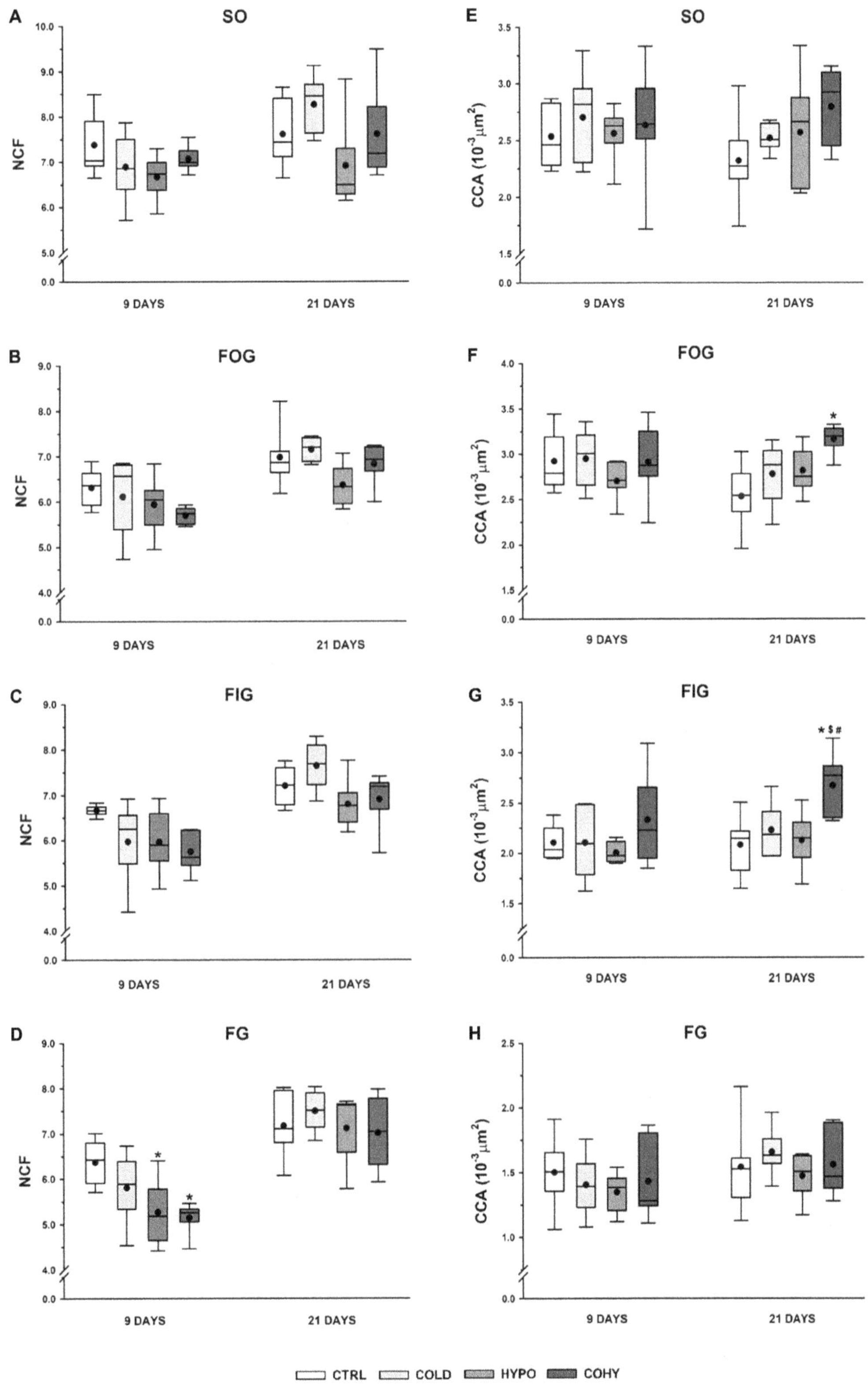

FIGURE 5 | Gastrocnemius individual fiber capillarization after 9 and 21 days in the different fiber types. **(A–D)** Number of capillaries per fiber (NCF), **(E–H)** fiber capillarization index (CCA). SO, slow oxidative; FOG, fast oxidative glycolytic; FIG, fast intermediate glycolytic; FG, fast glycolytic. CTRL, control; COLD, intermittent cold; HYPO, intermittent hypoxia; COHY, intermittent cold + hypoxia. Statistically significant differences are indicated as follows: $^{*}p < 0.05$ vs. CTRL, $^{\#}p < 0.05$ vs. COLD, $^{\$}p < 0.05$ vs. HYPO. Sample size: $n = 6$ per group at each temporal time point.

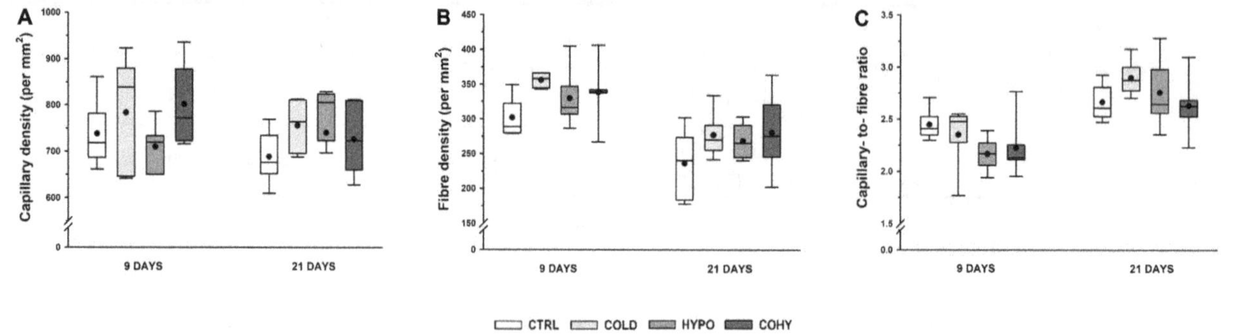

FIGURE 6 | Gastrocnemius global capillarization and morphometric parameters after 9 and 21 days. **(A)** Capillary density, **(B)** fiber density, **(C)** capillary-to-fiber ratio. Sample size: $n = 6$ per group at each temporal time point.

($p = 0.022$). However, after 21 days, COLD had non-significant increases in the NCF (ranging from 2 to 8%) in all fiber types compared to CTRL. Conversely, HYPO presented a non-significantly lower NCF than CTRL in SO, FOG, and FIG fibers, while COHY did show similar values than CTRL in all fiber types.

The NCF parameter is highly influenced by fiber size. To correct this influence, CCA index was calculated. CCA could be seen as an estimate of the average area to which each adjacent capillary supplies oxygen. After 9 days of any treatment, no changes were found in any fiber type nor between groups for this index (**Figures 5E–H**), but after the longer exposure period of 21 days, COLD, HYPO, and COHY showed a tendency to increase CCA in SO, FOG, and FIG fiber types. This increase was statistically significant in COHY for FOG and FIG fiber types.

Fiber Density, Capillary Density, and Capillary-to-Fiber Ratio

No statistical differences were found in CD between the different groups at any time point, although the COLD group showed a slight increase (6 and 9%) at 9 and 21 days (**Figure 6A**). Non-significant increases in FD were observed in all intervened groups at both temporal points (**Figure 6B**). To analyze the relationship between the capillary and fiber densities, the C/F ratio was calculated. At 9 days, the results showed similar values to CTRL for COLD and non-significant reductions (10–13%) for both hypoxic groups (**Figure 6C**). After 21 days, COLD had 9% higher values than CTRL, while HYPO and COHY remained unaltered.

Fiber Type Distribution

Fiber type proportions in different groups are shown in **Figure 7**. After 9 days, the proportion of SO fibers remained unaltered in all conditions studied (averaging 22%), while a significant 10% reduction relative to CTRL was found on day 21 in HYPO. A higher significant percentage of FOG fibers was found in COLD compared to CTRL and COHY and in HYPO compared to COHY after 9 days. Similar percentages of FOG were shown (between 30 and 35%) for all groups after 21 days. FIG and FG fiber proportions remained unchanged in the different groups at both temporal points.

Hypoxia-Inducible Factor 1α Pathway Protein Expression

After 9 days, the expression of the three proteins analyzed had its higher values in COLD (**Figure 8**). For HIF-1α and GLUT1, the differences were statistically significant compared to COHY and non-significantly higher compared to CTRL (25 and 27%, respectively) (**Figures 8A,B**), while for VEGF, these were additionally significant with respect to CTRL (**Figure 8C**). VEGF also had a significantly higher expression in HYPO compared to COHY and a trend to higher values than CTRL (26%). The results obtained for HIF-1α and GLUT1 after 9 days contrasted with the absence of significant differences between groups obtained after 21 days. The significant reduction in VEGF expression in COHY was also evident after 21 days.

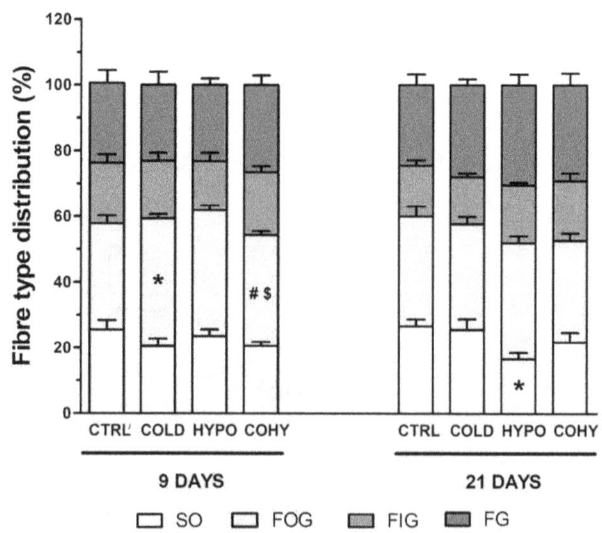

FIGURE 7 | Gastrocnemius fiber type distribution after 9 and 21 days. SO, slow oxidative; FOG, fast oxidative glycolytic; FIG, fast intermediate glycolytic; and FG, fast glycolytic. CTRL, control; COLD, intermittent cold; HYPO, intermittent hypoxia; COHY, intermittent cold + hypoxia. Data are presented as mean ± standard error. $^{*}p < 0.05$ vs. CTRL, $^{\#}p < 0.05$ vs. COLD, $^{\$}p < 0.05$ vs. HYPO. Sample size: $n = 6$ per group at each temporal time point.

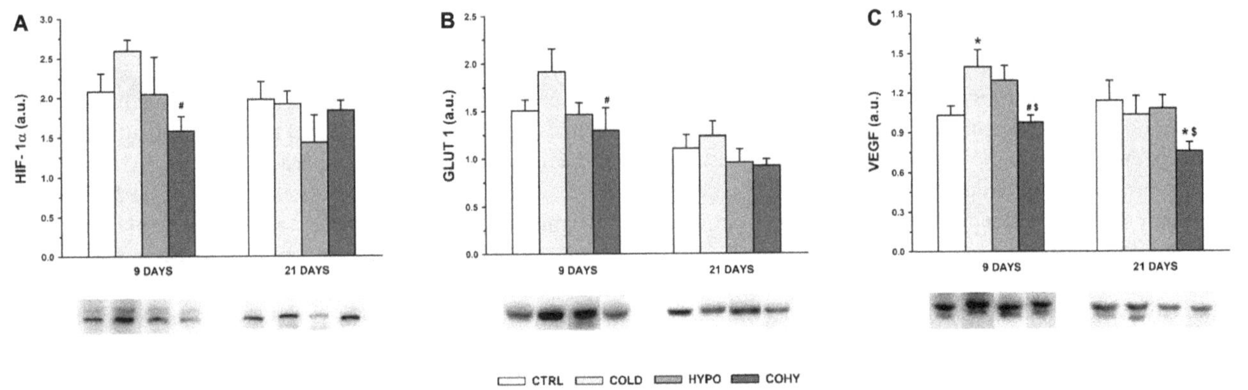

FIGURE 8 | Hypoxia-inducible factor 1α (HIF-1α) signaling pathway protein expression in gastrocnemius muscle after 9 and 21 days. **(A)** HIF-1α; **(B)** glucose transporter 1 (GLUT 1); **(C)** vascular endothelial growth factor (VEGF). CTRL, control; COLD, intermittent cold; HYPO, intermittent hypoxia; COHY, intermittent cold + hypoxia. Data are presented as mean ± standard error and expressed in arbitrary units (a.u.). Statistically significant differences are indicated as follows: $^{*}p < 0.05$ vs. CTRL, $^{\#}p < 0.05$ vs. COLD, $^{\$}p < 0.05$ vs. HYPO. Sample size: $n = 6$ per group at each temporal time point.

DISCUSSION

Body Weight and Body Composition Time Course

We have found a significant increment of BW and higher BAT/BW ratio in animals submitted to ICE (COLD) and lower PAT/BW and BAT/BW ratios in animals exposed to IHH alone (HYPO). This adipose tissue reduction could account for the increased skeletal muscle/BW ratio (**Table 1**). Two more interesting conclusions are derived from our results: (i) simultaneous exposure to intermittent cold and hypoxia (COHY) reverted the decrease of adipose tissue/BW ratios to control values; and (ii) these changes were already evident from 9 days of exposure to the treatment. Although previous studies in non-hibernator rodents have reported that chronic cold exposure either does not produce any changes (Deveci et al., 2001b; Egginton et al., 2001; Deveci and Egginton, 2002, 2003; Sepa-Kishi et al., 2017) or does produce a significant BW reduction (Suzuki et al., 1997; Mizunoya et al., 2014; Tsibul'nikov et al., 2016), our results agree with those reported by others who found that ICE caused an increase in rodents' BW (Yoo et al., 2014; Tsibul'nikov et al., 2016), which was accompanied by inguinal adipose tissue and BAT weight increase, as well as by the activation of proteins involved in thermogenesis and energy balance, such as uncoupling protein 1 (UCP-1) and proliferator-activated receptor-γ coactivator 1α (PGC-1) (Egginton et al., 2001; Ravussin et al., 2014; Yoo et al., 2014; Tsibul'nikov et al., 2016). These results suggest that intermittent exposure to cold induces adaptive responses preconditioning thermogenic mechanisms for subsequent cold exposures (Yoo et al., 2014; Tsibul'nikov et al., 2016) and did not compromise tissue metabolism and function, maintaining the increase of animal growth and muscle mass (Ravussin et al., 2014; Yoo et al., 2014; Tsibul'nikov et al., 2016).

"Altitude anorexia" has been well documented in high-altitude sojourns. It is characterized by BW loss (muscle mass waste and fat mass reduction), increased metabolic rate, loss of water, and food intake reduction due to a reduced appetite and an increased energy expenditure at altitude (Mathieu-Costello, 2001; Debevec et al., 2014; Dünnwald et al., 2019). The changes of body composition occurring at altitude depend on the severity and the duration of the exposure, as well as the intensity of the physical activity performed. This has been observed in animals housed in both a well-controlled environment (cold, humidity, food availability, activity) and high-altitude expeditions (Kayser et al., 1993; Hoppeler and Vogt, 2001; Mathieu-Costello, 2001; Cabrera-Aguilera et al., 2018; Dünnwald et al., 2019; Flores et al., 2020). Thus, different response patterns have been found depending on the exposure protocols, ranging from the reduction of animals' weight and retarded animals' growth (Mathieu-Costello, 2001; Siqués et al., 2006; Cabrera-Aguilera et al., 2018; Flores et al., 2020) to the absence of changes and increase of muscle mass (Deveci et al., 2002; Rizo-Roca et al., 2017, 2018). In concordance with the results of the present study, previous studies carried out in our laboratory based on similar IHH protocols have shown no significant changes in BW (Panisello et al., 2007, 2008; Rizo-Roca et al., 2017, 2018) and in soleus and TA muscle weight (Rizo-Roca et al., 2017) and GAS muscle weight after 3–4 weeks of intermittent hypoxic exposure (Cabrera-Aguilera et al., 2018). Moreover, our results suggest that the lower BW gain observed during the first week of hypoxic stimulus (HYPO) could be directly related to a reduction of fat mass (Mathieu-Costello, 2001). Finally, no reductions in food intake during IHH have been registered in a previous study (Ramos-Romero et al., 2020). Taking all these results together, it seems that 4 h/day of IHH exposure below 5,000 m of altitude and during 9–33 days did not disturb the animals' growth, preserving muscle mass.

One of the main objectives of this work was to assess the different physiological responses to intermittent cold and hypoxia when they act simultaneously or separately. Regarding registered anatomical measurements, we can observe that COHY presented a reduction in growth-related BW gain during the first days of intervention sessions. Moreover, this reduction was slightly greater than that observed when hypoxia was applied alone (**Table 1**). However, these differences disappeared in the following days in agreement with previous findings (Banchero et al., 1985), suggesting acclimation of the animals to the stressful environment. Additionally, the high muscle mass suggests that no catabolic process related to physiological stress has occurred. COHY, as well as COLD, presented adaptations to cold exposure by increasing BAT mass.

Another widely known consequence of hypoxia is pulmonary arterial hypertension (PAH) (Ma et al., 2015; Mirrakhimov and Strohl, 2016; Brito et al., 2020), which finally resulted in right ventricle hypertrophy (Ma et al., 2015; Rizo-Roca et al., 2017). This hypoxia-related PAH is produced by pulmonary vasoconstriction and subsequently increased pulmonary vascular resistance and is accompanied by pulmonary vascular remodeling (Pak et al., 2007; Ma et al., 2015; Mirrakhimov and Strohl, 2016; Brito et al., 2020). Our results show a significant increase in right ventricle relative mass (**Table 1**) after 9 days of intermittent hypoxic exposure, which is in accordance with recent publications (Rizo-Roca et al., 2017). After 21 days, the higher values found in the right ventricle/BW ratio in HYPO were not significant compared to CTRL, which could indicate acclimatization to hypoxic environment as was already suggested by Panisello et al. (2007). Interestingly, the absence of right ventricular hypertrophy when cold and hypoxia stressful stimuli acted simultaneously (COHY, **Table 1**) suggests a protection against hypoxia-related PAH (Banchero et al., 1985). The mechanism for this phenomenon can be the generalized peripheral constriction induced by cold (Granberg, 1991) that causes a higher vascular resistance in peripheral vessels, thus balancing both vascular resistance and cardiac work in the pulmonary and systemic circuits.

Hematological Parameters

Our results indicate that intermittent exposure to cold (COLD) induces a moderate increase in blood oxygen transport-related parameters such as Hct, RBC, and [Hb] (**Figure 3**) and in the hematimetric indices (**Table 2**), this increase being statistically significant in [Hb] after 9 days and in MCHC after 21 days. The high interquartile variation shown by the box plots depicted in **Figure 2**, especially after 9 days, could explain why the increase in some parameters failed to show statistical significance. These results match the current knowledge on prolonged exposures to cold, where non-shivering thermogenesis and higher metabolic heat production lead to enhanced oxygen consumption and, hence, the need to increase oxygen-carrying capacity (Deveci et al., 2001b; Maekawa et al., 2013). The results also agree with the studies performed in chronic exposure to cold, where increases of [Hb], RBC, and Htc in non-hibernator rodents were reported (Deveci et al., 2001b; Maekawa et al., 2013).

Regarding intermittent exposure to hypoxia (HYPO), a more consistent, statistically significant and greater response was evident. The hematological responses already took place after the shorter exposure period (9 days) and lasted while the hypoxic stimulus was present at least until day 21 (**Figure 2**). These results agree with previous studies where similar intermittent exposure protocols were applied (Casas et al., 2000; Esteva et al., 2009; Núñez-Espinosa et al., 2014, 2015). It has been widely known that exposure to high altitude *per se* produces an increase of oxygen transport capacity both in humans and animals except for those adapted to life at high altitude (Vinegar and Hillyard, 1972; León-Velarde et al., 1993; Heinicke et al., 2003; Zhang H. et al., 2018; Laguë et al., 2020). Moreover, intermittently exposed subjects can achieve [Hb], RBC, and Htc values close to those observed in high-altitude residents or in chronically exposed subjects (Heinicke et al., 2003). In fact, it has been previously reported that single exposure to altitude during 90 min is enough to produce a significant increase of EPO in humans (Rodríguez et al., 2000) and that nine alternate sessions of 90 min at 4,000–5,000 m are enough to induce significant hematological adaptive responses to hypoxia (Casas et al., 2000).

Interestingly, we have found that the greatest erythropoietic response appeared when intermittent cold and hypoxia were simultaneously applied (COHY), with significant differences not only to CTRL but also to COLD and greater non-significant values than HYPO, indicating a synergistic effect of cold and hypoxia on erythropoiesis. These results were in contrast to those obtained by Lechner et al. (1981) who reported reduced erythropoietic response after exposure to cold and hypoxia compared to hypoxia alone.

Fiber Morphometry and Muscle Oxidative Capacity

Intermittent Cold Exposure

In the current study, we have seen that ICE produced a tendency toward smaller FCSA, as it happens with chronic exposure (Suzuki et al., 1997). This trend to lower FCSA has been observed even after a short period of ICE (9 days) and was accompanied by light reduction of fiber Feret diameter, which indicates that muscle fibers became smaller and more rounded to reduce oxygen diffusion distance and their capillary domain area, facilitating homogeneous oxygen delivery to whole fiber (Suzuki et al., 1997; Egginton et al., 2001). Regarding individual fiber capillarization, our results show that despite the observed trend to lower NCF compared to CTRL after 9 days of ICE, there were no changes in CCA, suggesting that muscle fiber oxygenation was maintained due to fiber size reduction in the first days of ICE (Suzuki et al., 1997; Egginton et al., 2001; Deveci and Egginton, 2003). However, after 21 days of cold exposure, we found a slightly higher NCF, which in turn was translated into higher CCA, which would lead to an improvement in oxygen delivery per fiber area (Suzuki et al., 1997; Deveci and Egginton, 2002). In the same way, regarding whole-muscle capillarization, a higher C/F ratio was observed at day 21 in COLD, indicating that an angiogenic process occurs after ICE. To ensure adequate oxygen supply, an increase in vascularity is needed (Jackson et al., 1987), but capillary bed is not only important to supply oxygen and fuel to the fibers, it is also relevant to remove metabolic end products and to maintain local thermal balance (Deveci and Egginton, 2002). These observed increases in NCF and in C/F ratio after

21 days of ICE could be directly related to the increase of VEGF protein expression observed in day 9 samples. These results match the hypothesis that angiogenesis is a progressive event in rats (Deveci and Egginton, 2003). Thus, the observed increase in VEGF expression on the first days of ICE underwent histological evidence after 21 days. Additionally, we observed an overexpression of GLUT1 protein in COLD after 9 days of ICE, in accordance with previous findings that suggested that cold adaptation facilitates glucose uptake by skeletal muscle and upregulates oxidative pathway by an insulin-independent manner (Bukowieckh, 1989; Vallerand et al., 1990; Sepa-Kishi et al., 2017). Taken together, all these results indicate that ICE could upregulate HIF-1α signaling pathway based on the higher HIF-1α protein expression and the consequent overexpression of its targets VEGF and GLUT1.

Intermittent Hypoxia Exposure

In the present study, we have seen that IHH applied alone (HYPO) produced a trend to smaller FCSA in SO and FG fibers after 9 days, this reduction being accompanied by smaller Feret diameter. After 21 days, the oxidative fibers (SO, FOG, and FIG) largely respond to the hypoxic stimulus, presenting a clear trend to decrease their FCSA and Feret diameter. On the other hand, fibers from HYPO showed the lowest NCF. Considering that NCF and fiber size are closely related, this finding is not surprising because HYPO had smaller fibers overall. It is interesting to note that after 21 days, SO and FOG fibers presented a clear trend to higher CCA probably mostly due to the reduced FCSA found in these fibers. These changes in SO and FOG fiber morphometry indicate that the hypoxic stimulus reduced capillary domain area and diffusion distance in fibers with a predominant oxidative metabolism. It has been shown that hypoxia *per se* is not able to produce angiogenesis in the skeletal muscle, exercise or activity being necessary to activate the angiogenic process (Jackson et al., 1987; Deveci et al., 2001a; Deveci and Egginton, 2002; Rizo-Roca et al., 2018). Deveci et al. (2001a) conducted some experiments in which chronic normobaric hypoxia was applied during different time periods. They found that after 3 weeks of hypoxia, only the active muscles such as DIA (respiratory muscle) and soleus (postural muscle) showed an increased capillarity, while the locomotor muscles such as extensor digitorum longus (EDL) and TA did not show any increase in C/F ratio. Moreover, they did not report changes in FCSA in any of the muscles studied (Deveci et al., 2001a). Nevertheless, after a longer period of hypoxia (6 weeks), fiber capillarity increased in all studied muscles (DIA, SOL, EDL, and TA), and no changes or increases in FCSA were reported (Deveci et al., 2002), confirming the importance of hypoxic dose (exposure time) and the activity in the muscle responses. Thus, our results confirm that IHH at rest did not produce angiogenesis, which may be due to the lack of adequate metabolic or mechanical stimuli necessary to show capillary growth (Deveci et al., 2001a, 2002; Rizo-Roca et al., 2018). Analyzing HIF-1α signaling pathway modulation in HYPO, VEGF protein presented a tendency toward higher expression than CTRL. Despite the higher VEGF expression, we did not find an increase in C/F ratio nor in NCF after IHH at any time point, suggesting that new capillaries there were not generated. Capillary bed arrangement is the result of a combination of continuous and simultaneous angiogenesis, remodeling, and pruning processes in response to hemodynamic and metabolic stimuli (Pries and Secomb, 2014). Therefore, it is important to underline that one role of VEGF is to protect and preserve the capillary bed, even when there is muscle mass loss (Breen et al., 2008). VEGF could be modulated by the HIF-1α signaling pathway (when PO_2 is low), but also it could be regulated by inflammatory cytokines, high oxidative stress, and energy balance-related AMP-activated protein kinase (AMPK) (Breen et al., 2008). From our results, we are not able to differentiate or identify which stimulus has induced higher VEGF expression after IHH, since HIF-1α pathway upregulation was not clear (**Figure 8**). Interestingly, the local and systemic adaptations carried out during hypoxic adaptation could attenuate the degree of hypoxia in some tissue cells (Lundby et al., 2009), and maybe our stimulus was not intense enough at muscle to induce angiogenesis. Moreover, HIF-1α is only slightly altered during hypoxic stimulus due to a preexisting high level of this protein in skeletal muscle (Lundby et al., 2009).

Simultaneous Intermittent Cold and Hypoxia Exposure

Similarly to what was observed in HYPO, simultaneous exposure to intermittent cold and hypoxia (COHY) showed a reduction of FCSA and Feret diameter in SO fibers within the first days of exposure (9 days). These reductions also affected FOG and FIG fibers, indicating that fibers having the more oxidative profile had a greater response to IHH and ICE, confirming the differential behavior of each fiber type when facing the stressful environmental stimuli (Banchero et al., 1985; Deveci et al., 2002; Panisello et al., 2007; Rizo-Roca et al., 2017, 2018). It is noteworthy that FCSA reductions were larger in COHY than in HYPO and COLD. NCF was reduced in all fibers within the first 9 days, but the absence of changes in CCA indicates that fiber irrigation was maintained. However, after 21 days, COHY presented similar NCF as CTRL, but CCA was significantly increased, reducing the capillary domain in oxidative fibers (SO, FOG, FIG) through fiber area reductions. In contrast to what Banchero et al. (1985) observed after chronic exposure to concurrent cold and hypoxia, intermittent COHY acclimation did not produce increases in CD nor in C/F ratio in any of the time points studied. Moreover, the VEGF angiogenic factor appeared significantly reduced compared to HYPO and COLD, and HIF-1α signaling pathway remained inactivated after COHY exposure (**Figure 8**). As well as during IHH exposure alone, other systemic and local adaptations, such as increased RBC and [Hb], could attenuate skeletal muscle hypoxia and, hence, would have reduced subsequent muscle adaptive responses.

Fiber Type Distribution

We found an increase of FOG fiber type proportion in HYPO and COLD after 9 days. In the case of HYPO, this increase was at the expense of reducing FIG proportion, which would be explained by the metabolic flexibility of these fibers to shift to a more oxidative or a more glycolytic character. Surprisingly, increased proportion of FOG percentage in COLD was accompanied by reduced SO fiber type proportion. After 21 days, however, only HYPO presented changes in fiber type composition, showing reduced SO fiber type percentage. This increase of FOG fiber type proportion in HYPO has been previously well documented and could be the cause of the observed reduction in SO percentage due to an inhibition of the well-known type shift from FOG to SO fiber type that takes place during growth in normoxic rats (Ishihara et al., 2000). Moreover, a higher FG fiber type proportion in HYPO and COHY is also observed (22 and 17%, respectively), which would be a more efficient path to produce energy when oxygen availability is compromised (Jackson et al., 1987).

CONCLUSION

In conclusion, ICE produced adaptive changes in the physiology of the animals to afford thermogenesis, increasing BAT mass, muscle capillarity, and glucose transport capacity. IHH elicited a reduction in FCSA to enhance blood oxygen transport and preserve muscle fiber oxygenation. Concurrent intermittent cold and hypoxia induced increased BAT, RBC count, and [Hb] and reduced right ventricle hypertrophy but, in contrast to our initial hypothesis, did not produce angiogenesis in skeletal muscle, although reduced capillary supply domain area to facilitate oxygen delivery to the muscle fibers.

ETHICS STATEMENT

The animal study was reviewed and approved by the University of Barcelona's Ethical Committee for Animal Experimentation.

AUTHOR CONTRIBUTIONS

GV, TP and JRT conceived the study. GS and JRT obtained the data. GS, GV, TP, SRR, JLT, and JRT participated in data treatment and discussed the results. GS prepared the manuscript draft. JRT and GV edited the manuscript. All authors approved the submitted version of the document.

ACKNOWLEDGMENTS

We are grateful to the contribution of Santiago Ruvira, Ignacio Cabrera, Silvia Lara, Marc Comas, Leticia I. Millán, Laura F. Espitia, Deisy C. Ortiz, Cristian A. Guzmán, and Ana M. Ortega. We would also like to thank Jonny English for his assistance in proofreading the English text.

REFERENCES

Armstrong, R., and Phelps, R. (1984). Muscle fiber type composition of the rat hindlimb. *Am. J. Anat.* 171, 259–272. doi: 10.1002/aja.1001710303

Banchero, N., Kayar, S., and Lechner, A. (1985). Increased capillarity in skeletal muscle of growing guinea pigs acclimated to cold and hypoxia. *Respir. Physiol.* 62, 245–255. doi: 10.1016/0034-5687(85)90118-5

Breen, E., Tang, K., Olfert, M., Knapp, A., and Wagner, P. (2008). Skeletal muscle capillarity during hypoxia: VEGF and its activation. *High Alt. Med. Biol.* 9, 158–166. doi: 10.1089/ham.2008.1010

Brito, J., Siques, P., and Pena, E. (2020). Long-term chronic intermittent hypoxia: a particular form of chronic high-altitude pulmonary hypertension. *Pulm. Circ.* 10, 5–12. doi: 10.1177/2045894020934625

Brooke, M. H., and Kaiser, K. K. (1970). Muscle fiber types: how many and what kind? *Arch. Neurol.* 23, 369–379. doi: 10.1001/archneur.1970.00480280083010

Bukowieckh, J. L. (1989). Energy balance and diabetes, The effects of cold exposure, exercise training, and diet composition on glucose tolerance and glucose metabolism in rat peripheral tissues. *Can. J. Physiol. Pharmacol.* 67, 382–393.

Cabrera-Aguilera, I., Rizo-Roca, D., Marques, E. A., Santocildes, G., Pagès, T., Viscor, G., et al. (2018). Additive effects of intermittent hypobaric hypoxia and endurance training on bodyweight, food intake, and oxygen Consumption in Rats. *High Alt. Med. Biol.* 19, 278–285. doi: 10.1089/ham.2018.0013

Casas, H., Casas, M., Ricart, A., Rama, R., Ibáñez, J., Palacios, L., et al. (2000). Effectiveness of three short intermittent hypobaric hypoxia protocols hematological responses. *J. Exerc. Physiol.* 3, 38–45.

Debevec, T., Bali, T. C., Simpson, E. J., Macdonald, I. A., Eiken, O., and Mekjavic, I. B. (2014). Separate and combined effects of 21-day bed rest and hypoxic confinement on body composition. *Eur. J. Appl. Physiol.* 114, 2411–2425. doi: 10.1007/s00421-014-2963-1

Deveci, C., and Egginton, S. (2003). Cold exposure differentially stimulates angiogenesis in glycolytic and oxidative muscles of rats and hamsters. *Exp. Physiol.* 88, 741–746. doi: 10.1113/eph8802630

Deveci, D., and Egginton, S. (2002). Differing mechanisms of cold- induced changes in capillary supply in m. tibialis anterior of rats and hamsters. *J. Exp. Biol.* 205, 829–840.

Deveci, D., Marshall, J. M., and Egginton, S. (2001a). Relationship between capillary angiogenesis, fiber type, and fiber size in chronic systemic hypoxia. *Am. J. Physiol.* 281, H241–H252. doi: 10.1152/ajpheart.2001.281.1.H241

Deveci, D., Stone, P. C. W., and Egginton, S. (2001b). Differential effect of cold acclimation on blood composition in rats and hamsters. *J. Comp. Physiol. B* 171, 135–143. doi: 10.1007/s003600000156

Deveci, D., Marshall, J. M., and Egginton, S. (2002). Chronic hypoxia induces prolonged angiogenesis in skeletal muscles of rat. *Exp. Physiol.* 87, 287–291. doi: 10.1113/eph8702377

Dünnwald, T., Gatterer, H., Faulhaber, M., Arvandi, M., and Schobersberger, W. (2019). Body composition and body weight changes at different altitude levels: a systematic review and meta-analysis. *Front. Physiol.* 10:430. doi: 10.3389/fphys.2019.00430

Egginton, S. (2002). Temperature and angiogenesis: the possible role of mechanical factors in capillary growth. *Comp. Biochem. Physiol. A Mol. Integr. Physiol.* 132, 773–787. doi: 10.1016/s1095-6433(02)00047-8

Egginton, S., Fairney, J., and Bratcher, J. (2001). Differential effects of cold exposure on muscle fibre composition and capillary supply in hibernator and non-hibernator rodents. *Exp. Physiol.* 86, 629–639. doi: 10.1113/eph8602260

Esteva, S., Panisello, P., Torrella, J. R., Pagés, T., and Viscor, G. (2009). Blood rheology adjustments in rats after a program of intermittent exposure to hypobaric hypoxia. *High Alt. Med. Biol.* 10, 275–281. doi: 10.1089/ham.2008.1086

Flores, K., Siques, P., Brito, J., Ordenes, S., Arriaza, K., Pena, E., et al. (2020). Lower body weight in rats under hypobaric hypoxia exposure would lead to reduced right ventricular hypertrophy and increased AMPK activation. *Front. Physiol.* 11:342. doi: 10.3389/fphys.2020.00342

Fouces, V., Torrella, J. R., Palomeque, J., and Viscor, G. (1993). A histochemical ATPase method for the demonstration of the muscle capillary network. *J. Histochem. Cytochem.* 41, 283–289. doi: 10.1177/41.2.7678272

Granberg, P. O. (1991). Human physiology under cold exposure. *Arctic Med. Res.* 50, 23–27.

Heinicke, K., Prommer, N., Cajigal, J., Viola, T., Behn, C., and Schmidt, W. (2003). Long-term exposure to intermittent hypoxia results in increased hemoglobin mass, reduced plasma volume, and elevated erythropoietin plasma levels in man. *Eur. J. Appl. Physiol.* 88, 535–543. doi: 10.1007/s00421-002-0732-z

Hoppeler, H., and Vogt, M. (2001). Muscle tissue adaptations to hypoxia. *J. Exp. Biol.* 204, 3133–3139.

Ishihara, A., Itoh, K., and Hirofuji, C. (2000). Effect of hypobaric hypoxia on rat soleus muscle fibers and their innervating motoneurons: a review. *Jpn. J. Physiol.* 50, 561–568. doi: 10.2170/jjphysiol.50.561

Jackson, C. G. R., Sillau, A., and Banchero, N. (1987). Fiber composition and capillarity in growing guinea pigs acclimated to cold and cold plus hypoxia. *Proc. Soc. Exp. Biol. Med.* 185, 101–106. doi: 10.3181/00379727-185-42524

Kayser, B., Narici, M., Milesi, S., Grassi, B., and Cerretelli, P. (1993). Body composition and maximum alactic anaerobic performance during a one month stay at high Altitude. *Int. J. Sports Med.* 14, 244–247. doi: 10.1055/s-2007-1021171

Ke, Q., and Costa, M. (2006). Hypoxia-Inducible Factor-1 (HIF-1). *Mol. Pharmacol.* 70, 1469–1480. doi: 10.1124/mol.106.027029

Laguë, S. L., Ivy, C. M., York, J. M., Chua, B. A., Alza, L., Cheek, R., et al. (2020). Cardiovascular responses to progressive hypoxia in ducks native to high altitude in the Andes. *J. Exp. Biol.* 223:jeb211250. doi: 10.1242/jeb.211250

Lechner, A., Salvato, V., and Banchero, N. (1981). The hematological response to hypoxia in growing guinea pigs is blunted during concomitant cold stress. *Comp. Biochem. Physiol. A Physiol.* 70, 321–327.

León-Velarde, F., Sanchez, J., Bigard, A. X., Brunet, A., Lesty, C., and Monge-C, C. (1993). High altitude tissue adaptation in Andean coots: capillarity, fibre area, fibre type and enzymatic activities of skeletal muscle. *J. Comp. Physiol. B* 163, 52–58. doi: 10.1007/BF00309665

Lundby, C., Calbet, J. A. L., and Robach, P. (2009). The response of human skeletal muscle tissue to hypoxia. *Cell. Mol. Life Sci.* 66, 3615–3623. doi: 10.1007/s00018-009-0146-8

Lunt, H. C., Barwood, M. J., Corbett, J., and Tipton, M. J. (2010). "Cross-adaptation": habituation to short repeated cold-water immersions affects the response to acute hypoxia in humans. *J. Physiol.* 588, 3605–3613. doi: 10.1113/jphysiol.2010.193458

Ma, T.-T., Wang, Y., Zhou, X.-L., Jiang, H., Guo, R., Jia, L.-N., et al. (2015). Research on rat models of hypobaric hypoxia-induced pulmonary hypertension. *Eur. Rev. Med. Pharmacol. Sci.* 19, 3723–3730.

Maekawa, S., Iemura, H., and Kato, T. (2013). Enhanced erythropoiesis in mice exposed to low environmental temperature. *J. Exp. Biol.* 216, 901–908. doi: 10.1242/jeb.076760

Mahalingam, S., Cheviron, Z. A., Storz, J. F., McClelland, G. B., and Scott, G. R. (2020). Chronic cold exposure induces mitochondrial plasticity in deer mice native to high altitudes. *J. Physiol.* 598, 5411–5426. doi: 10.1113/JP280298

Martin-Rincon, M., Pérez-López, A., Morales-Alamo, D., Perez-Suarez, I., de Pablos-Velasco, P., Perez-Valera, M., et al. (2019). Exercise mitigates the loss of muscle mass by attenuating the activation of autophagy during severe energy deficit. *Nutrients* 11:2824. doi: 10.3390/nu11112824

Mathieu-Costello, O. (2001). Muscle adaptation to altitude: tissue capillarity and capacity for aerobic metabolism. *High Alt. Med. Biol.* 2, 413–425. doi: 10.1089/15270290152608598

Mirrakhimov, A. E., and Strohl, K. P. (2016). High-altitude pulmonary hypertension: an update on disease pathogenesis and management. *Open Cardiovasc. Med. J.* 10, 19–27. doi: 10.2174/1874192401610010019

Mizunoya, W., Iwamoto, Y., Sato, Y., Tatsumi, R., and Ikeuchi, Y. (2014). Cold exposure increases slow-type myosin heavy chain 1 (MyHC1) composition of soleus muscle in rats. *Anim. Sci. J.* 85, 293–304. doi: 10.1111/asj.12143

Moore, L. G., Niermeyer, S., and Zamudio, S. (1998). Human adaptation to high altitude: regional and life-cycle perspectives. *Am. J. Phys. Anthropol.* 107, 25–64.

Nachlas, M. M., Tsou, K., De Souza, E., Cheng, C., and Seligman, A. M. (1957). Cytochemical demostration of succinic dehydrogenase by the use of new p-nitrophenyl substituted ditetrazole. *J. Histochem. Cytochem.* 5, 420–436. doi: 10.1177/5.4.420

Navarrete-Opazo, A., and Mitchell, G. S. (2014). Therapeutic potential of intermittent hypoxia: a matter of dose. *Am. J. Physiol.* 307, R1181–R1197. doi: 10.1152/ajpregu.00208.2014

Neubauer, J. A. (2001). Invited Review: physiological and pathophysiological responses to intermittent hypoxia. *J. Appl. Physiol.* 90, 1593–1599.

Núñez-Espinosa, C., Douziech, A., Ríos-Kristjánsson, J. G., Rizo, D., Torrella, J. R., Pagès, T., et al. (2014). Effect of intermittent hypoxia and exercise on blood rheology and oxygen transport in trained rats. *Respir. Physiol. Neurobiol.* 192, 112–117. doi: 10.1016/j.resp.2013.12.011

Núñez-Espinosa, C., Ferreira, I., Ríos-Kristjánsson, J. G., Rizo-Roca, D., Dolors, M., Godoy, G., et al. (2015). Effects of intermittent hypoxia and light aerobic exercise on circulating stem cells and side population, after strenuous eccentric exercise in trained rats. *Curr. Stem Cell Res. Ther.* 10, 132–139. doi: 10.2174/1574888x09666140930130048

Pak, O., Aldashev, A., Welsh, D., and Peacock, A. (2007). The effects of hypoxia on the cells of the pulmonary vasculature. *Eur. Respir. J.* 30, 364–372. doi: 10.1183/09031936.00128706

Panisello, P., Torrella, J. R., Esteva, S., Pagés, T., and Viscor, G. (2008). Capillary supply, fibre types and fibre morphometry in rat tibialis anterior and diaphragm muscles after intermittent exposure to hypobaric hypoxia. *Eur. J. Appl. Physiol.* 103, 203–213. doi: 10.1007/s00421-008-0691-0

Panisello, P., Torrella, J. R., Pagés, T., and Viscor, G. (2007). Capillary supply and fiber morphometry in rat myocardium after intermittent exposure to hypobaric hypoxia. *High Alt. Med. Biol.* 8, 322–330. doi: 10.1089/ham.2007.1030

Pries, A. R., and Secomb, T. W. (2014). Making microvascular networks work: angiogenesis, remodeling, And pruning. *Physiology* 29, 446–455. doi: 10.1152/physiol.00012.2014

Ramos-Romero, S., Santocildes, G., Piñol-Piñol, D., Rosés, C., Pagés, T., Hereu, M., et al. (2020). Implication of gut microbiota in the physiology of rats intermittently exposed to cold and hypobaric hypoxia. *PLoS One* 15:e0240686. doi: 10.1371/journal.pone.0240686

Ravussin, Y., Xiao, C., Gavrilova, O., and Reitman, M. L. (2014). Effect of intermittent cold exposure on brown fat activation, obesity, and energy homeostasis in mice. *PLoS One* 9:e85876. doi: 10.1371/journal.pone.0085876

Rizo-Roca, D., Bonet, J. B., Ínal, B., Ríos-Kristjánsson, J. G., Pagès, T., Viscor, G., et al. (2018). Contractile activity is necessary to trigger intermittent hypobaric hypoxia-induced fiber size and vascular adaptations in skeletal muscle. *Front. Physiol.* 9:481. doi: 10.3389/fphys.2018.00481

Rizo-Roca, D., Ríos-Kristjánsson, J. G., Núñez-Espinosa, C., Santos-Alves, E., Gonçalves, I. O., Magalhães, J., et al. (2017). Intermittent hypobaric hypoxia combined with aerobic exercise improves muscle morphofunctional recovery after eccentric exercise to exhaustion in trained rats. *J. Appl. Physiol.* 122, 580–592. doi: 10.1152/japplphysiol.00501.2016

Rodríguez, F. A., Ventura, J. L., Casas, M., Casas, H., Pagés, T., Rama, R., et al. (2000). Erythropoietin acute reaction and haematological adaptations to short, intermittent hypobaric hypoxia. *Eur. J. Appl. Physiol.* 82, 170–177. doi: 10.1007/s004210050669

Semenza, G. (1998). Hypoxia-inducible factor 1 and the molecular physiology of oxygen homeostasis. *J. Lab. Clin. Med.* 131, 207–214. doi: 10.1016/s0022-2143(98)90091-9

Sepa-Kishi, D. M., Sotoudeh-Nia, Y., Iqbal, A., Bikopoulos, G., and Ceddia, R. B. (2017). Cold acclimation causes fiber type-specific responses in glucose and fat metabolism in rat skeletal muscles. *Sci. Rep.* 7:15430. doi: 10.1038/s41598-017-15842-3

Siqués, P., Brito, J., León-Velarde, F., Barrios, L., Cruz, J. J., López, V., et al. (2006). Time course of cardiovascular and hematological responses in rats exposed to chronic intermittent hypobaric hypoxia (4600 m). *High Alt. Med. Biol.* 7, 72–80. doi: 10.1089/ham.2006.7.72

Suzuki, J., Gao, M., Ohinata, H., Kuroshima, A., and Koyama, T. (1997). Chronic cold exposure stimulates microvascular remodeling prefentially in oxidative muscles in rats. *Jpn. J. Physiol.* 47, 513–520. doi: 10.2170/jjphysiol.47.513

Tsibul'nikov, S. Y., Maslov, L. N., Naryzhnaya, N. V., Ivanov, V. V., and Lishmanov, Y. B. (2016). Specific features of adaptation of rats to chronic cold treatment. *Dokl. Biol. Sci.* 470, 214–216. 10.1134/S00124966160 50033

Vallerand, A. L., Pfirusse, F., and Bukowiecki, L. J. (1990). Stimulatory effects of cold exposure and cold acclimation on glucose uptake in rat peripheral tissues. *Am. J. Physiol.* 259, R1043–R1049. doi: 10.1152/ajpregu.1990.259.5.R1043

Vinegar, A., and Hillyard, S. D. (1972). The effects of altitude on oxygen-binding parameters of the blood of the iguanid lizards, Sceloporus jarrovi and Sceloporus occidentals. *Comp. Biochem. Physiol. A Comp. Physiol.* 43, 317–320. doi: 10.1016/0300-9629(72)90190-9

Viscor, G., Torrella, J. R., Corral, L., Ricart, A., Javierre, C., Pages, T., et al. (2018). Physiological and biological responses to short-term intermittent hypobaric hypoxia exposure: from sports and mountain medicine to new biomedical applications. *Front. Physiol.* 9:814. doi: 10.3389/fphys.2018.00814

Viscor, G., Torrella, J. R., Fouces, V., and Palomeque, J. (1992). Skeletal muscle capillarization and fiber types in urban and homing pigeons (*Columba livia*). *Comp. Biochem. Physiol. Comp. Physiol.* 101, 751–757. doi: 10.1016/0300-9629(92)90354-s

West, J., Schoene, R., Luks, A., and Milledge, J. (2012). *High Altitude Medicine And Physiology*, 5th Edn. London: CRC Press.

Yoo, H. S., Qiao, L., Bosco, C., Leong, L.-H., Lytle, N., Feng, G.-S., et al. (2014). Intermittent cold exposure enhances fat accumulation in mice. *PLoS One* 9:e96432. doi: 10.1371/journal.pone.0096432

Zhang, H., Dong, H., Mehmood, K., Li, K., Nabi, F., Chang, Z., et al. (2018). Physiological variations among blood parameters of domestic cats at high- and low-altitude regions of China. *Arch. Physiol. Biochem.* 124, 458–460. doi: 10.1080/13813455.2018.1423623

Zhang, Z., Boelen, A., Kalsbeek, A., and Fliers, E. (2018). TRH neurons and thyroid hormone coordinate the hypothalamic response to cold. *Eur. Thyroid J.* 7, 279–288. doi: 10.1159/000493976

9

The Action of 2-Aminoethyldiphenyl Borinate on the Pulmonary Arterial Hypertension and Remodeling of High-Altitude Hypoxemic Lambs

*Sebastián Castillo-Galán[1], Daniela Parrau[2], Ismael Hernández[2], Sebastián Quezada[3], Marcela Díaz[4], Germán Ebensperger[2,5], Emilio A. Herrera[2,5], Fernando A. Moraga[6], Rodrigo Iturriaga[1,7], Aníbal J. Llanos[2,5] and Roberto V. Reyes[2,5]**

[1] Laboratorio de Neurobiología, Facultad de Ciencias Biológicas, Pontificia Universidad Católica de Chile, Santiago, Chile, [2] Unidad de Fisiología y Fisiopatología Perinatal, Programa de Fisiopatología, Facultad de Medicina, Instituto de Ciencias Biomédicas, Universidad de Chile, Santiago, Chile, [3] School of Health and Biomedical Sciences, RMIT University, Bundoora, VIC, Australia, [4] Departamento de Promoción de la Salud de la Mujer y el Recién Nacido, Facultad de Medicina, Universidad de Chile, Santiago, Chile, [5] International Center for Andean Studies, Universidad de Chile, Santiago, Chile, [6] Laboratorio de Fisiología, Hipoxia y Función Vascular, Departamento de Ciencias Biomédicas, Facultad de Medicina, Universidad Católica del Norte, Coquimbo, Chile, [7] Centro de Excelencia en Biomedicina de Magallanes, Universidad de Magallanes, Punta Arenas, Chile

***Correspondence:**
Roberto V. Reyes
virreyc@gmail.com;
vicreyes@med.uchile.cl;
vreyes@uchile.cl

Calcium signaling is key for the contraction, differentiation, and proliferation of pulmonary arterial smooth muscle cells. Furthermore, calcium influx through store-operated channels (SOCs) is particularly important in the vasoconstrictor response to hypoxia. Previously, we found a decrease in pulmonary hypertension and remodeling in normoxic newborn lambs partially gestated under chronic hypoxia, when treated with 2-aminoethyldiphenyl borinate (2-APB), a non-specific SOC blocker. However, the effects of 2-APB are unknown in neonates completely gestated, born, and raised under environmental hypoxia. Accordingly, we studied the effects of 2-APB-treatment on the cardiopulmonary variables in lambs under chronic hypobaric hypoxia. Experiments were done in nine newborn lambs gestated, born, and raised in high altitude (3,600 m): five animals were treated with 2-APB [intravenous (i.v.) 10 mg kg^{-1}] for 10 days, while other four animals received vehicle. During the treatment, cardiopulmonary variables were measured daily, and these were also evaluated during an acute episode of superimposed hypoxia, 1 day after the end of the treatment. Furthermore, pulmonary vascular remodeling was assessed by histological analysis 2 days after the end of the treatment. Basal cardiac output and mean systemic arterial pressure (SAP) and resistance from 2-APB- and vehicle-treated lambs did not differ along with the treatment. Mean pulmonary arterial pressure (mPAP) decreased after the first day of 2-APB treatment and remained lower than the vehicle-treated group until the third day, and during the fifth, sixth, and ninth day of treatment. The net mPAP increase in response to acute hypoxia did not change, but the pressure area under the curve (AUC) during hypoxia was slightly lower in 2-APB-treated lambs than in vehicle-treated lambs. Moreover, the 2-APB treatment decreased the pulmonary arterial wall thickness and the α-actin immunoreactivity and increased the luminal area with no changes in the vascular density. Our findings show that 2-APB treatment partially reduced the contractile hypoxic response and reverted the pulmonary vascular remodeling, but this is not enough to normalize the pulmonary hemodynamics in chronically hypoxic newborn lambs.

Keywords: neonatal pulmonary hypertension, hypoxia, high altitude, 2-APB, store operated channels

INTRODUCTION

The failure in the fetal-to-neonatal transition ensuing in a functional pulmonary circulation after birth results in pulmonary hypertension of the newborn, a syndrome that affects up to 6.8 per 1,000 of the births in lowlands (Walsh-Sukys et al., 2000), but whose prevalence could reach ~10% of neonates under hypobaric hypoxia of the Andean Altiplano (Keyes et al., 2003; Peñaloza and Arias-Stella, 2007; Herrera et al., 2015). The pulmonary hypertension of the newborn is characterized by high postnatal mean pulmonary arterial pressure (mPAP), pulmonary vascular resistance (PVR), and contractility, resulting from an imbalance between vasoconstrictor and vasodilator mechanisms, and a pathological remodeling involving hyperplasic/hypertrophic growth of the wall of distal pulmonary arteries (Gao and Raj, 2011; Suresh and Shimoda, 2016; Mathew and Lakshminrusimha, 2017). The persistent high mPAP can lead to right ventricle hypertrophy, cardiac failure, and death. Moreover, survivors may have impaired neurological development and recurrent pulmonary hypertension later in life (Nair and Lakshminrusimha, 2014). Both fetal and postnatal pulmonary arteries quickly contract and develop a pathological remodeling in response to hypoxia (Gao and Raj, 2011; Dunham-Snary et al., 2017; Hussain et al., 2017). Therefore, the high-altitude chronic hypoxia during pregnancy and early after birth results in pulmonary hypertension of the newborn and associated cardiopulmonary risk later in life (Herrera et al., 2015; Gonzaléz-Candia et al., 2020). We have previously established two ovine models of neonatal pulmonary hypertension induced by high-altitude hypoxia. In the first model, conception, 100% of gestation, birth, and postnatal study were conducted at 3,600 meters above sea level (m.a.s.l) (Herrera et al., 2007). In the second model, conception and first 30% of gestation occurred at lowland; the last 70% of gestation and birth at 3,600 m.a.s.l. to return to the lowland at 2 days of postnatal age for the study (Herrera et al., 2010). Both models of perinatal hypoxia exposure showed increased mPAP, PVR, and hypoxic pulmonary vasoconstriction, right ventricular hypertrophy, and thickened pulmonary arterial walls compared with lowland healthy controls. Nevertheless, the first model is hypoxemic (Herrera et al., 2007), while the second is normoxemic after birth, simulating in the latter, the human neonatal pulmonary hypertension that persists despite oxygenation (Herrera et al., 2010). Store-operated Ca^{2+} entry (SOCE) is a Ca^{2+} influx across the plasma membrane, which is activated by a decrease in intraluminal Ca^{2+} of sarcoplasmic reticulum released through inositol triphosphate receptors (IP_3R) or ryanodine receptors. SOCE allows replenishment of Ca^{2+} stores, but it can itself generate long-term Ca^{2+} signals.

The major components of store-operated channels (SOCs) are Orai1 and stromal interacting molecule 1 (Stim1) that form the pore at the plasma membrane and the Ca^{2+} sensor of the sarcoplasmic reticulum, respectively. In resting cells, Stim1 is uniformly found in the sarcoplasmic reticulum. Fall of Ca^{2+} from sarcoplasmic reticulum results in oligomerization and redistribution of Stim1 near the plasma membrane to activate Orai1 and initiate an inwardly rectifying and Ca^{2+}-selective current known as Ca^{2+}-release-activated Ca^{2+} current (Icrac). In both pulmonary artery smooth muscle and endothelial cells, this Ca^{2+} entry through Orai1 allows recruitment, and activation of transient receptor potential canonical (TRPC), mainly TRPC1 to provide additional and less selective Ca^{2+} influx. The sum of both Orai- and TRPC-mediated currents generates a sustained Ca^{2+} influx termed store-operated Ca^{2+} current (Isoc) (Fernandez et al., 2012; Earley and Brayden, 2015; Ambudkar et al., 2017; Putney, 2018; Reyes et al., 2018a). There is great evidence about the involvement of this Ca^{2+} signaling complex in adults forms hypoxic pulmonary over-constriction and remodeling, the main components of pulmonary hypertension (Reyes et al., 2018a). Our group has also found evidence on the participation of these channels on neonatal pulmonary hypertension in ovine models. Thus, the treatment of normoxic pulmonary hypertensive newborn lambs with 2-aminoethyldiphenyl borinate (2-APB), a non-selective inhibitor of store-operated Ca^{2+} signaling, results in a partial reversal of pulmonary hypertension (Castillo-Galán et al., 2016). In contrast, we have observed that these channels are functionally upregulated in the pulmonary circulation of hypoxic high-altitude newborn lambs where they contribute to increased vasoconstrictor response to acute hypoxia (Parrau et al., 2013). Nevertheless, in addition to their hypoxemia, highland lambs also differ from lambs with partial gestation at high altitude in their greater pulmonary arterial medial layer thickening (Quezada et al., 2014). The window of perinatal hypoxia exposure also determines differences in key proteins involved in vascular contraction and remodeling: soluble guanylate cyclase (sGC) is downregulated in the high-altitude lambs but is unchanged in lambs with partial gestation at highlands, while big conductance Ca^{2+}-dependent potassium channel (BKCa channels) expression is constant in the former and upregulated in the later (Herrera et al., 2008a, 2010, 2019). These differences could have a great influence on the response to treatments against pulmonary hypertension. The ability to reverse pulmonary hypertension has not been studied in lambs with gestation, birth, and postnatal development in high altitude. In this study, we evaluated the effect of treatment with 2-APB in hemodynamic variables and pulmonary vascular remodeling of lambs developed and raised at 3,600 m.a.s.l.

MATERIALS AND METHODS

All experimental protocols were reviewed and approved by the Faculty of Medicine Bioethics Committee of the University of Chile (CBA 0476 and 1172 FMUCH). Animal care, maintenance, procedures, and experimentation were performed in accordance with the Guide for the Care and Use of Laboratory Animals published by the National Institutes of Health (NIH Publication No. 85-23, Revised 1996) and adhered to the ARRIVE guidelines.

Animals

Experiments were performed on 10 newborn sheep (*Ovis aries*) gestated, born, and raised at Putre Research Station, International Center for Andean Studies (INCAS), at 3,600 m.a.s.l.

Surgical Preparation and *in vivo* Experiments

At 3 days old, newborn lambs were chronically instrumented for *in vivo* studies as reported previously (Herrera et al., 2007, 2010; Parrau et al., 2013; Castillo-Galán et al., 2016). Briefly, animals were anesthetized with a combination of ketamine [10 mg/kg, intramuscularly (i.m.)] and xylazine (0.05 mg/kg i.m.) and also an additional local infiltration of 2% lidocaine. Polyvinyl catheters were placed into the femoral artery to record systemic variables and a Swan–Ganz catheter was placed into the pulmonary artery to record cardiopulmonary variables. Oxytetracycline [20 mg/kg, subcutaneously (s.c.)] and sodium metamizole (0.1 mg/kg i.m.) were given for 3 days after surgery (Herrera et al., 2007, 2010; Parrau et al., 2013; Castillo-Galán et al., 2016).

At 4 days old, the lambs were randomly divided into two groups and submitted to 10-day treatment with a single daily dose of infusion vehicle [dimethyl sulfoxide (DMSO): NaCl 1:10 intravenous (i.v.), $n = 4$] or 2-APB infusion (10 mg/kg/day bolus in vehicle i.v., $n = 5$) every morning. A similar dose of 2-APB administered to lambs with partial gestation under chronic hypoxia induced marked hemodynamic improvement (Castillo-Galán et al., 2016). Pulmonary arterial pressure (PAP), systemic arterial pressure (SAP), and heart rate (HR) were recorded *via* a data acquisition system (PowerLab/8SP System, ADInstruments, Bella Vista, NSW, Australia and Lab Chart version 7.0 Software, ADInstruments, Castle Hill, NSW, Australia) connected to a computer. Cardiac output (CO) was determined using the thermodilution method by injecting 3 ml of chilled (0°C) 0.9% NaCl into the pulmonary artery through the Swan–Ganz catheter connected to a CO computer (COM-2, Baxter, Healthcare Corporation's Edwards Critical-Care Division, United States). mPAP, mean SAP (mSAP), PVR, and systemic vascular resistance (SVR) were calculated as described previously (Herrera et al., 2007, 2010, 2019; Parrau et al., 2013; Castillo-Galán et al., 2016). Arterial blood samples were taken daily to determine arterial pH, PO_2, PCO_2, hemoglobin saturation percentage (SaO_2), total hemoglobin (THb), and oxygen content (O_2ct) (IL-synthesis 25, Instrumentation Laboratories, AACC's Washington DC, United States; measurements corrected to 39°C). Cardiopulmonary variables and arterial blood gasses were measured every day, 5 min before the infusion, so that the first day corresponds to the basal condition before starting the treatment, and on the following days, values were recorded 24 h after the infusion of the previous day.

Twenty-four hours after the last infusion, animals were subjected to a 3-h experimental protocol of a superimposed acute hypoxic challenge as previously described (Herrera et al., 2010, 2019; Parrau et al., 2013; Castillo-Galán et al., 2016), consisting in 1 h of basal recording (breathing room air), 1 h of superimposed isocapnic hypoxia, and 1 h of recovery during which they returned to breath room air. Superimposed isocapnic hypoxia was induced *via* a transparent, loosely tied polyethylene bag placed over the head of the animal into which a known mixture of air, N_2, and CO_2 was passed at a rate of 20 L/min to reach an arterial PO_2 of ~30 mmHg with a constant PCO_2. Cardiopulmonary variables and arterial blood gasses were also recorded during this protocol. The contractile response of the pulmonary circulation to acute hypoxia after the end of the treatment was calculated as the mPAP/ΔPO_2 ratio or the area under the curve (AUC) as described previously (Castillo-Galán et al., 2016; Reyes et al., 2018b).

Euthanasia and Tissue Sampling

Twenty-four hours after the superimposed hypoxic challenge test, the lambs underwent euthanasia with an overdose of sodium thiopental (100 mg/kg i.v.), and lung samples were immediately obtained for *in vitro* analyses.

Histological Staining and Immunohistochemistry

Lungs were perfused at 25 mmHg through the pulmonary artery with saline for blood removal, and then the left lung was perfused-fixed in 4% paraformaldehyde (PFA) in PBS 1×. Then, ~1 cm^3 piece of pulmonary tissue was taken from the distal portion of the central lobe, close to the pleura, and immersed-fixed with 4% PFA for 24 h at 4°C, followed by conservation in sodium azide 0.01% in 1× PBS at 4°C. The fixed tissue was embedded in paraffin, cut in 4–5 μm serial slices.

A van Gieson staining was used to assess vascular morphometry. Images were captured at 10× and 40× with an optical microscope (Olympus BX-41, Shinjuku-ku, Tokyo, Japan) coupled with a digital camera and computer. Notably, 20–25 representative resistance pulmonary arteries (150–250 μm of internal diameter) from each animal were selected for these analyses. Vascular density (number of arteries/area), percentage luminal area (luminal area/total area), and the wall, media, and adventitia thicknesses were calculated as described previously (Herrera et al., 2008b; Torres et al., 2015; Castillo-Galán et al., 2016; Castillo-Galan et al., 2020). The analysis of the microphotographs was performed with the Image Pro-Plus 6.2 software (Media Cybernetics, Inc., Rockville, MD, United States).

The immunohistochemical detection for SM-α-actin was performed with commercial antibodies (Sigma-Aldrich, Saint Louis, MO, United States, dilution: 1:400). The antigen retrieval was performed at 100°C with citrate buffer pH: 6, 1×

(Dako, CA, United States). Primary antibody incubation was performed for 4 h for SM-α-actin at 4°C and labeling was developed using an HRP-diaminobenzidine kit (Envision TM+, Dako, CA, United States). The immunoreactivity of the small arteries muscle layer was calculated as described previously (Herrera et al., 2014).

Statistical Analysis

Data are expressed as mean ± SEM. The cardiovascular variables from the baseline time point (B), from the 2-APB- and vehicle-treated lambs, were analyzed using an unpaired *t*-test and the time course using two-way ANOVA for repeated measures and the *post hoc* Newman–Keuls test. The latter test was used to analyze the cardiovascular variables from the two groups in the systemic and pulmonary responses to a superimposed hypoxic challenge. The histological and immunohistochemistry data, from the 2-APB- and vehicle-treated lambs, were analyzed using an unpaired *t*-test. For all comparisons, differences were considered statistically significant when $P < 0.05$.

RESULTS

Animal Weight

The weight of the lambs used in the study was 4.90 ± 0.54–5.82 ± 0.67 kg for animals assigned to the vehicle-treated group and 4.85 ± 0.14–6.73 ± 0.29 kg for those assigned to the 2-APB-treated group at the beginning and the end of the study, respectively.

Effect of 2-Aminoethyldiphenyl Borinate Administration on Basal Systemic and Pulmonary Variables

The mSAP, HR, CO, and SVR were similar in control lambs and 2-APB-treated lambs along with the treatment (**Figure 1**). Before starting the infusion, the basal mPAP was similar in both animals assigned to the vehicle-treated group (34.04 ± 2.34 mmHg) and the 2-APB group (31.33 ± 8.55 mm Hg) (**Figure 2A**). However, after the first day of treatment, mPAP significantly decreased and remained lower in the 2-APB group than in the vehicle-treated group until the fourth day, and during the eighth and ninth day of treatment (**Figure 2A**). On the last day of treatment, the values of mPAP were similar in both groups (26.40 ± 2.83 vs. 20.85 ± 2.11 mmHg, for vehicle- and 2-APB-treated lambs, respectively) (**Figure 2A**). The daily recording of PVR showed similar values for both groups along the experimental period (**Figure 2C**). Nevertheless, the AUC along with the treatment for both mPAP and PVR, reflecting the integrated value for these variables, was lower in the 2-APB-treated lambs than in the vehicle-treated lambs (**Figures 2B,D**).

Cardiovascular Response to a Superimposed Hypoxic Challenge After the Treatment

Basal values for arterial pH, PO_2, PCO_2, THb, SaO_2, and O_2ct at the end of treatment were similar in both experimental groups. During the superimposed hypoxic challenge, PO_2, SaO_2, and O_2ct decreased to a similar degree reaching similar values in both experimental groups. During recovery, all these variables returned to basal values in both groups (**Table 1**).

In both experimental groups, mSAP was similar and remained stable along with the protocol (**Figure 3A**). HR and CO were similar in the control and 2-APB-treated lambs under basal conditions, and they showed a similar increase in both groups during acute hypoxia, and during recovery, they returned to baseline values (**Figures 3B,C**). The basal SVR was also similar in control and 2-APB-treated lambs decreased to similar values under acute hypoxic challenge and normalized during recovery (**Figure 3D**).

Basal mPAP was similar in control and 2-APB-treated lambs, increased during the hypoxemic challenge in both experimental groups, and decreased during recovery but remained slightly higher than the basal values (**Figure 4A**). The $\Delta mPAP/\Delta PO_2$ ratio did not change with the treatment (1.26 ± 0.22 vs. 1.25 ± 0.17, for vehicle- and 2-APB-treated group, respectively), but the AUC for mPAP during the hypoxic challenge was lower in the 2-APB-treated lambs (**Figure 4A** insert). PVR followed a similar pattern in both vehicle and 2-APB-treated groups: basal values were similar in the control and 2-APB treated groups and increased during the acute hypoxemic challenge but did not return to baseline values during recovery (**Figure 4B**).

Pulmonary Vascular Morphometry

The pulmonary vascular density was similar in both groups (**Figures 5A,B**), but the luminal vascular surface of the lung was increased in the 2-APB-treated lambs compared with the vehicle-treated lambs (**Figures 5A,C**). Pulmonary arteries from

TABLE 1 | Arterial pH and blood gasses during a superimposed hypoxic challenge.

	Basal	Hypoxia	Recovery
pH			
Vehicle	7.483 ± 0.011	7.457 ± 0.014	7.457 ± 0.014
2-APB	7.520 ± 0.020	7.497 ± 0.009	7.497 ± 0.011
PO_2, mmHg			
Vehicle	40.7 ± 2.3	30.0 ± 0.4†	39.9 ± 2.9
2-APB	42.4 ± 2.1	30.1 ± 0.4†	44.5 ± 2.5
PCO_2, mmHg			
Vehicle	32.7 ± 1.2	33.0 ± 1.5	31.5 ± 1.5
2-APB	31.8 ± 1.7	31.8 ± 1.3	30.8 ± 1.6
S_{O2}, %			
Vehicle	73.4 ± 3.5	52.9 ± 3.3†	70.3 ± 4.5
2-APB	70.5 ± 3.2	47.6 ± 2.5†	72.9 ± 3.5
THb, g/dl			
Vehicle	11.6 ± 1.1	12.1 ± 1.1	11.5 ± 1.1
2-APB	11.9 ± 0.5	12.4 ± 0.5	11.9 ± 0.6
O_2ct, ml O_2/dl			
Vehicle	11.0 ± 0.8	8.6 ± 0.9†	10.7 ± 0.8
2-APB	10.9 ± 0.3	7.9 ± 0.4†	11.2 ± 0.4

Values are the mean ± SEM for arterial pH, PO_2, PCO_2, hemoglobin saturation (S_{O2}), total hemoglobin (THb), and oxygen content (O_2ct). 2-APB, 2-aminoethyldiphenyl borinate.

†$P < 0.05$, significant differences vs. all in the same group, two-way ANOVA for repeated measures with Newman–Keuls post hoc test.

animals treated with 2-APB did not change the adventitial area but showed a decrease in the media layer area (**Figure 6A**) and in the immunoreactivity to SM-α-actin (**Figure 6B**) compared with the vehicle-treated lambs.

DISCUSSION

In this study, we tested whether treatment with 2-APB for 10 days can ameliorate the pulmonary arterial hypertension in hypoxic newborn lambs, conceived, gestated, born, and studied during their first 15 days of postnatal life at the Andean Altiplano at 3,600 m.a.s.l. This is a well-established model, showing increased basal mPAP and PVR, with also a greater increase in mPAP and PVR in response to acute hypoxia compared with the lowland controls (Herrera et al., 2007, 2019; Lopez et al., 2016; Gonzaléz-Candia et al., 2020). Our results showed that 2-APB-treated lambs had a lower mPAP between the first and the third day of treatment and during the fifth, the sixth, and the ninth day of treatment compared with the vehicle-treated lambs ($P < 0.001$ for the global effect of the factor treatment in two-way ANOVA), but at the end of the treatment, mPAP did not differ between groups. Nevertheless, the AUC for mPAP, as an integrated assessment of this variable along with the treatment, was lower in the 2-APB-treated group. The postnatal evolution of basal HR, CO, mSAP, and SVR was unaffected by the treatment, in agreement with previous findings on acute administration of a single dose of 2-APB (Parrau et al., 2013). The net basal PVR was similar in the vehicle- and 2-APB-treated high-altitude lambs at the end of the treatment, but in the latter, the AUC during the treatment was lower in agreement with analogous observation in mPAP. The increase in mPAP in response to acute hypoxic stress evaluated 24 h after the end of the treatment was slightly attenuated by the treatment, but neither PVR nor CO responses to hypoxia were modified despite a significant decrease in pulmonary vascular remodeling. In a previous study, our group observed that a single dose of 8 mg/kg of 2-APB did not modify the basal mPAP or PVR in either low- or high-altitude lambs, but it attenuated the hypoxic pulmonary vasoconstriction in both when measurements are carried out immediately after the drug infusion. Moreover, the inhibitory action of 2-APB in these responses was greater in the high-altitude lambs than in the low-altitude lambs (Parrau et al., 2013). The marked attenuation of hypoxic pulmonary vasoconstriction with a single dose of 2-APB observed in our previous study compared with its mild action observed with repetitive doses over 10 days may result from differences in the time spent between the drug infusion and the acute hypoxic challenge test. This is suggestive of rapid clearance of 2-APB away from the pulmonary circulation in high-altitude hypoxemic lambs. In our previous studies performed on highland lambs, we suggested that a similar single dose of this compound would allow reaching a concentration in the 10–100 μM range in the extracellular space, assuming a distribution volume of 40% of the body weight. The same concentration order blocks SOC in the pulmonary arteries isolated from those animals (Parrau et al., 2013) and in HEK293 cell lines transfected with Orai/Stim

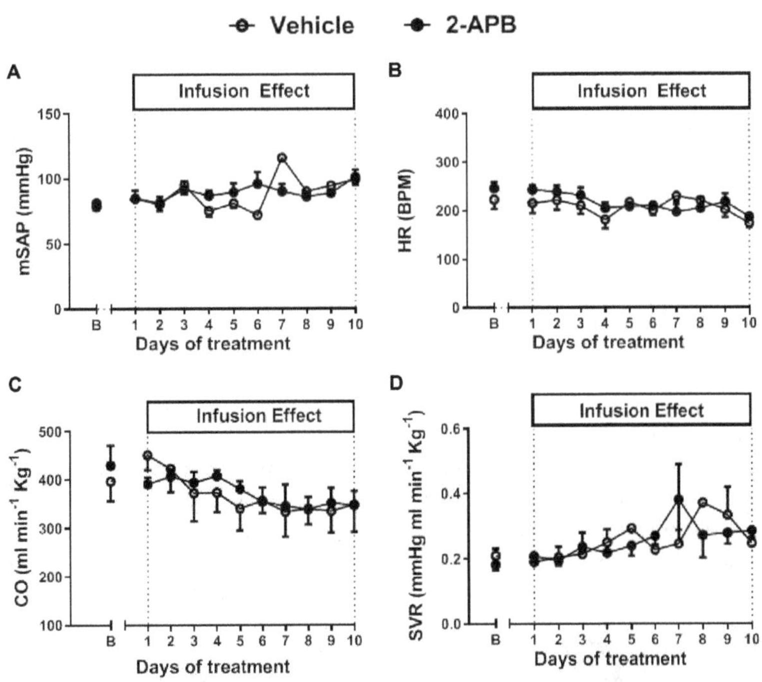

FIGURE 1 | Systemic cardiovascular variables during the experimental period. Basal values for mean systemic artery pressure (mSAP) **(A)**, heart rate (HR) **(B)**, cardiac output (CO) **(C)**, and systemic vascular resistance (SVR) **(D)** were recorded 5 min before the daily infusion of vehicle (white circles) or 2-APB (black circles). The B day corresponds to basal values before treatment and the following days to values recorded 24 h after the infusion of the previous day. Values are the mean ± SEM. Statistical analysis, unpaired *t*-test for basal values, two-way ANOVA for repeated measures with Newman–Keuls *post hoc* test, for daily treatment.

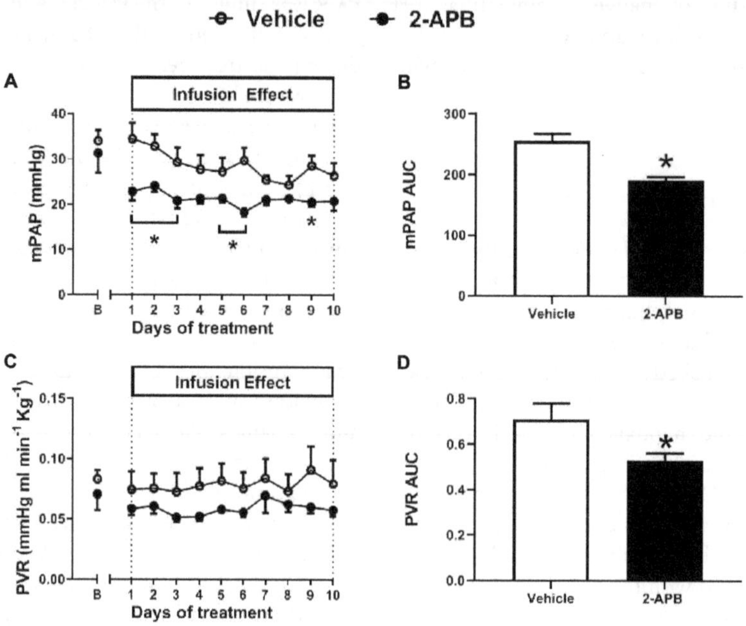

FIGURE 2 | Pulmonary variables during the experimental period. Basal values for mean pulmonary artery pressure (mPAP) **(A)**, the area under the curve for mPAP (mPAP AUC) **(B)**, pulmonary vascular resistance (PVR) **(C)**, and the AUC for PVR (PVR AUC) **(D)** were measured 5 min before the daily infusion of vehicle (white symbols) or 2-APB (black symbols). The B day corresponds to basal values before starting the treatment and the following days to values recorded 24 h after the infusion of the previous day. Values are the mean ± SEM. *$P \leq 0.05$, significant differences for vehicle vs. 2-APB, two-way ANOVA for repeated-measures with Newman–Keuls *post hoc* test for daily recording, unpaired *t*-test for basal values, and AUC.

or TRPC subunits (Lievremont et al., 2005; DeHaven et al., 2008; Peinelt et al., 2008). Nevertheless, a pharmacokinetic study is needed to elucidate the time needed to reach maximal plasma and tissue concentration and the clearance rate of 2-APB. In fact, when measured *ex vivo*, under conditions of blockade of voltage-dependent Ca^{2+} channels with nifedipine, the pulmonary arterial contraction elicited by voltage-independent Ca^{2+} entry from extracellular space was upregulated in high-altitude lambs, and the relaxation in response to either 2-APB or SKF-96365, another non-selective TRPC channels inhibitor was also greater. These responses are in agreement with the upregulation of Stim1 and TRPC4 transcripts in lungs from high-altitude lambs (Parrau et al., 2013). Taken together, these findings, in addition to extensive pharmacological characterization of 2-APB on Ca^{2+} signaling, suggest that cardiopulmonary actions of this drug in newborn lambs are the result of their action on SOC, even though we cannot preclude its targeting on intracellular Ca^{2+} sources, such as IP_3 receptors, as discussed below (reviewed in Putney, 2010; Parrau et al., 2013). 2-APB also inhibits TRPM7 channels and connexin proteins from GAP junctions. Nevertheless, it seems unlikely that cardiopulmonary actions observed here are related to these targets because neither TRPM7 nor 2-APB-sensitive connexins are upregulated in the pulmonary vasculature under chronic hypoxia, and the concentrations needed to inhibit the former are excessively high and related to acidification of intracellular milieu rather than direct action on the channel (Bai et al., 2006; Billaud et al., 2011; Chokshi et al., 2012). There is also evidence that 2-APB can act as a reactive oxygen species (ROS) scavenger, and in doing so, it protects cardiomyocytes, ovary, and testis tissue against ischemia/reperfusion damage (Taskin et al., 2014; Sari et al., 2015; Morihara et al., 2017). Inhibition of oxidative stress through melatonin administration increases NO bioavailability and NO-dependent vasodilation of pulmonary arteries in highland lambs (Torres et al., 2015). It is possible that 2-APB, under our experimental conditions, produces similar effects as melatonin, increasing NO bioavailability, but in that case, the NO-vasodilation would be limited by blunted sGC observed in highland lambs (Herrera et al., 2008a). Previously, we reported the effects of a similar treatment with 2-APB but in lambs with partial gestation and birth at high altitude, and postnatally raised at low altitude under normoxia (Castillo-Galán et al., 2016). These lambs have also increased PAP and resistance, enhanced pulmonary vasoconstrictor response to acute hypoxic pulmonary vasoconstriction and pulmonary arterial remodeling compared with the control lambs gestated, born, and studied at low altitude (Herrera et al., 2010). Nevertheless, these lambs are normoxemic, while the lambs used in this study are hypoxemic (Herrera et al., 2010, 2019). When the hemodynamic effects of the treatment with cumulative doses of 2-APB are compared in both models, we observed that basal mPAP decreases from ~31 mmHg at the beginning of this study to ~21 mmHg at the end, while the initial and final PVR were ~0.071 and ~0.058 mmHg ml kg^{-1} min^{-1}, respectively. In contrast, in lambs with partial gestation at high-altitude basal mPAP decreases from ~22 mmHg at the beginning of the treatment to ~15 mmHg at the end, while basal PVR lowers from ~ 0.06 to ~0.045 mmHg ml kg^{-1} min^{-1} (Castillo-Galán et al., 2016). In contrast, under acute hypoxic challenge after the end

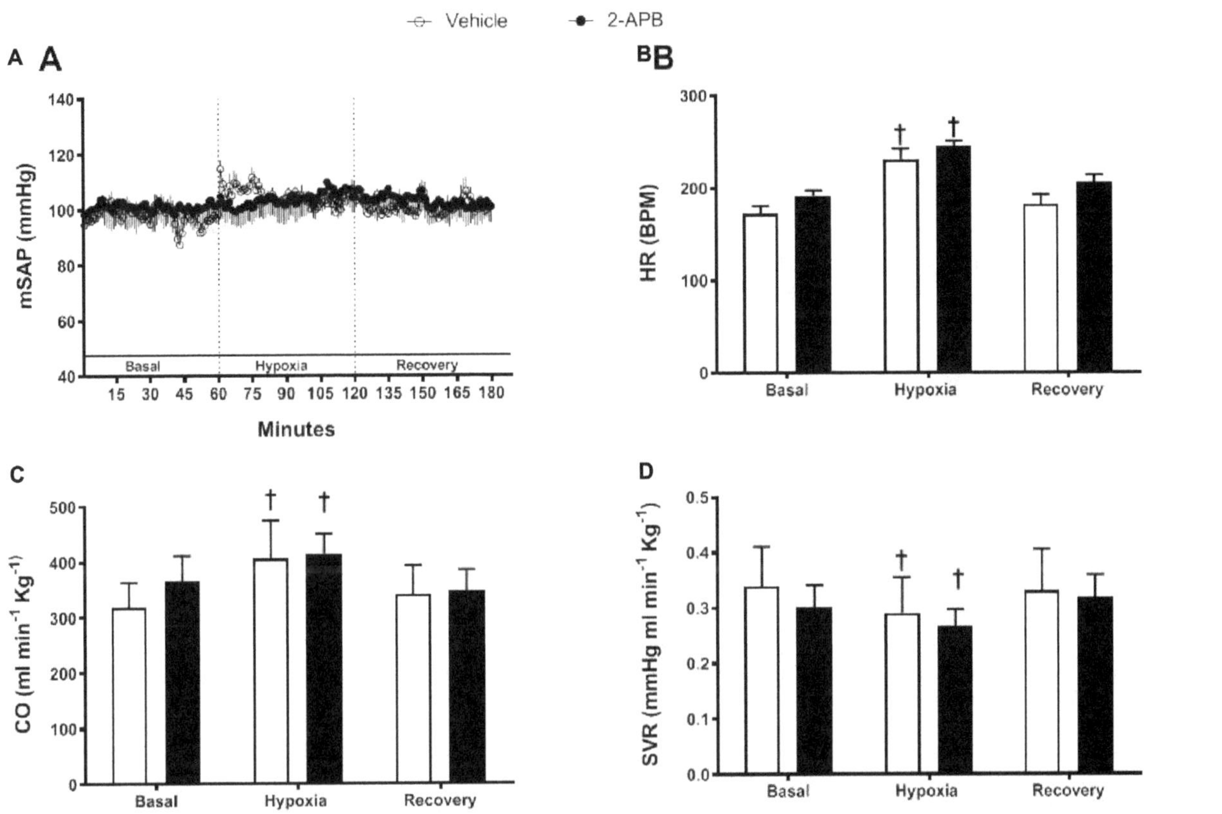

FIGURE 3 | Systemic cardiovascular responses to a superimposed hypoxic challenge. Vehicle-treated (white symbols) and 2-APB-treated (black symbols) lambs were submitted to a superimposed acute hypoxic challenge 1 day after the end of the treatment and mSAP **(A)**, HR **(B)**, CO **(C)**, and SVR **(D)** were evaluated and expressed as the mean ± SEM for each experimental period. $^{\dagger}P \leq 0.05$, significant differences vs. all in the same group, two-way ANOVA for repeated measures with Newman–Keuls *post hoc* test.

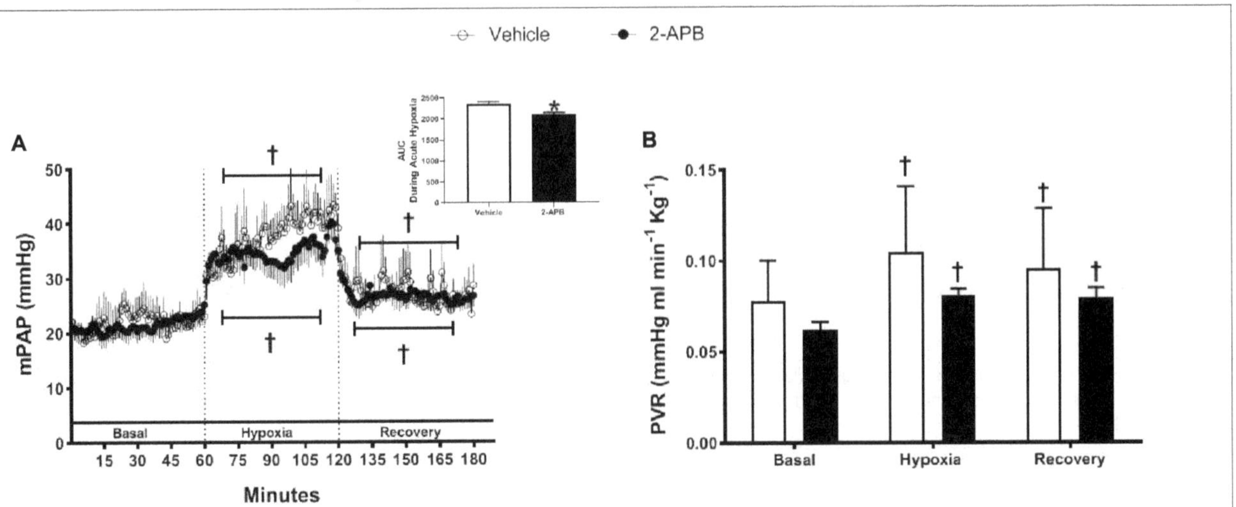

FIGURE 4 | Pulmonary responses to a superimposed hypoxic challenge. Vehicle-treated (white symbols) and 2-APB-treated (black symbols) animals were submitted to a superimposed acute hypoxic challenge 1 day after the end of the treatment and mPAP, PVR, and AUC during acute hypoxia were determined as indicated in section "Materials and Methods". **(A)** Continuous recording of mPAP, (**A**, insert) AUC during acute hypoxia, and **(B)** PVR expressed as the mean ± SEM for each experimental period. $^{*}P \leq 0.05$, significant differences for vehicle vs. 2-APB, unpaired *t*-test for AUC; $^{\dagger}P \leq 0.05$, significant differences vs. all in the same group, two-way ANOVA for repeated measures with Newman–Keuls *post hoc* test for acute hypoxia challenge test.

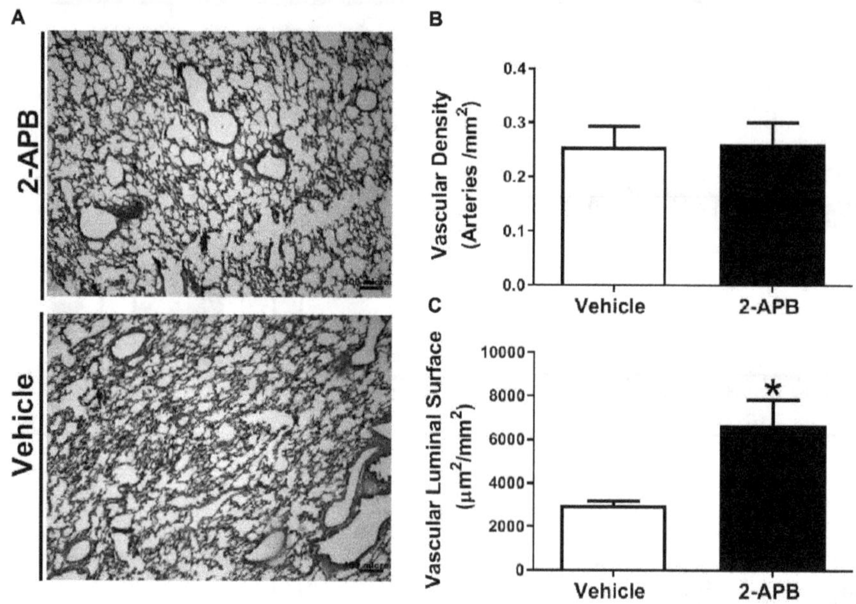

FIGURE 5 | Pulmonary vascular density and luminal surface. Representative micrographs of van Gieson-stained lung sections were performed in lung slices 48 h after the end of the treatment **(A)**, vascular density **(B)**, and luminal surface area **(C)**. Scale bar = 100 μm; magnification: 10×. Values are the mean ± SEM. *$P \leq 0.05$, significant differences for vehicle vs. 2-APB, unpaired *t*-test.

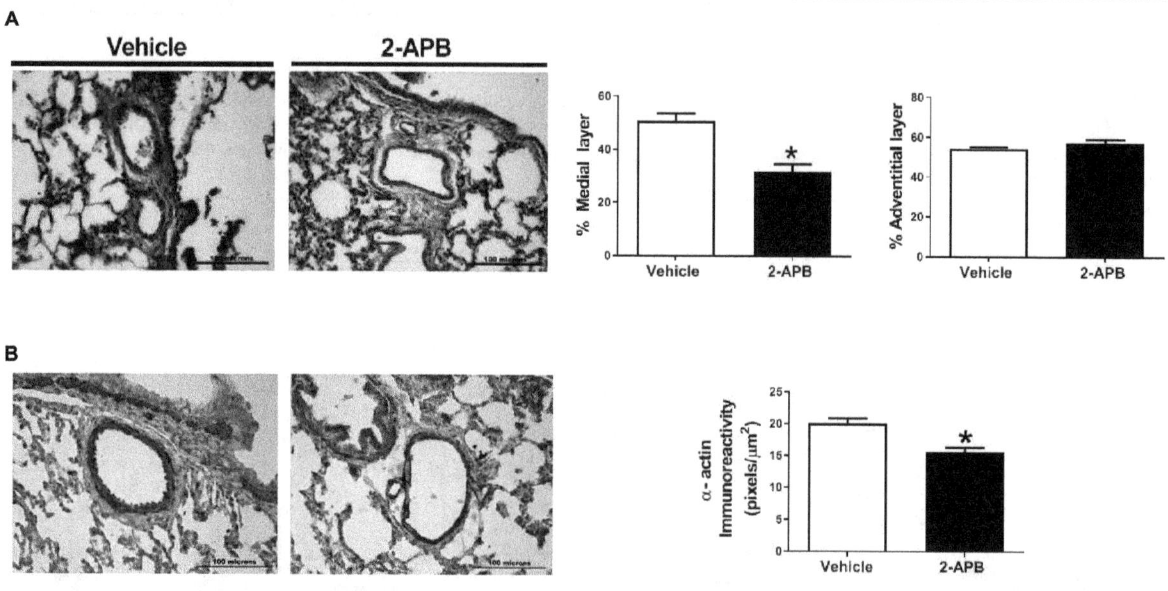

FIGURE 6 | Small pulmonary arteries remodeling. Medial and adventitial layer area **(A)** and SM-α-actin **(B)** immunostaining of pulmonary arteries, performed in lung slices 48 h after the end of the treatment. Scale bar = 100 μm; magnification: 40×. Values are the mean ± SEM. *$P \leq 0.05$, significant differences for vehicle vs. 2-APB, unpaired *t*-test.

of the treatment, mPAP and PVR reached ~38–40 mmHg and 0.105 mmHg ml kg^{-1} min^{-1} in high-altitude lambs from this study. A similar response is reported in previous studies (Parrau et al., 2013; Lopez et al., 2016; Herrera et al., 2019). After 2-APB treatment, hypoxic mPAP and PVR were ~35 mmHg and 0.081 mmHg ml kg^{-1} min^{-1}, respectively. In lambs with partial gestational hypoxia, the mPAP and PVR under acute hypoxia reached ~32 mmHg and ~0.085 mmHg ml kg^{-1} min^{-1}, respectively, while 2-APB treatment markedly lowered these values to ~22 mmHg and ~0.055 mmHg ml kg^{-1} min^{-1}, respectively (Herrera et al., 2010; Castillo-Galán et al., 2016). We speculate that the higher initial mPAP of lambs used in this study, as well as their hypoxemic state, compared with lambs with partial gestation at high altitude but treated under normoxia could partially explain these differences. Both pulmonary vasoconstriction and remodeling induced by the environmental hypoxia are related to the enhancement of store-operated Ca^{2+} signaling through rapid association and upregulation of their Stim, Orai, and TRPC protein components, respectively (Lin et al., 2004; Ng et al., 2012; Hou et al., 2013; Chen et al., 2017; Wang et al., 2017; He et al., 2018; Reyes et al., 2018a). Increased basal mPAP probably results from the combination of hypoxic pulmonary vasoconstriction together with the pulmonary arterial remodeling in the hypoxemic lambs, while it could mainly result from remodeling in our previous study with normoxemic lambs with less severe disease (Castillo-Galán et al., 2016). Therefore, the administration of the combination of postnatal reoxygenation and 2-APB results in a better reversal of pulmonary arterial hypertension. It is interesting to note that neither CO nor SAP and resistance was modified by 2-APB, under basal conditions or acute hypoxic challenge, reinforcing the idea that vasoactive mechanisms modified by 2-APB are functionally present in the pulmonary vessels than in other vascular beds as described for SOC (Snetkov et al., 2003). When the action of 2-APB on pulmonary vascular remodeling in both ovine models is compared, similarities and differences are found. In this study, we detected a decrease in pulmonary arterial medial layer area in 2-APB-treated lambs, associated with increased luminal vascular surface and decreased α-actin immunoreactivity, while the adventitial layer was not modified. In contrast, α-actin staining, medial, and adventitial layers are diminished in normoxemic pulmonary hypertensive lambs treated with 2-APB (Castillo-Galán et al., 2016). The attenuated regression of remodeling involving only the medial layer in hypoxic pulmonary hypertensive lambs against medial and adventitial layers in normoxic pulmonary hypertensive lambs could be also a partial explanation of the difference in pulmonary hypertension improvement after 2-APB treatment in both models, but this assumption needs further investigation. Regardless of the model, basal mPAP does not normalize to the ~10–12 mmHg and PVR does not reach the values of ~0.04 mmHg ml kg^{-1} min^{-1} or lower reported for healthy lowland lambs (Herrera et al., 2007, 2010, 2019). Moreover, in this study, we observed a rapid initial decrease in basal mPAP at the beginning of the treatment followed by stabilization on the following days. Various explanations are possible for this finding. First, other sources of Ca^{2+} influx, such as L-type or T-type Ca^{2+} channels, could be present and compensate as SOCE inhibition by 2-APB is taking place. Both L- and T-type channels are upregulated in pulmonary arteries from hypoxic adult mice and contribute to pulmonary hypertension (Rodman et al., 2005; Wan et al., 2013; Chevalier et al., 2014). Whether those channels contribute to neonatal pulmonary hypertension in hypoxic lambs remains to be established. Second, the lack of selectivity of this drug and its action on other targets, such as IP3 receptors, could play a role. IP3 receptors contribute to Ca^{2+} release, Ca^{2+} store depletion, and SOCE activation in pulmonary arterial smooth muscle. However, it has been recently reported that the type II IP3 receptor subtype can also play a counter-regulatory role by limiting excessive intracellular Ca^{2+} increase through inhibition of SOCE, vasoconstriction, and remodeling (Shibata et al., 2019). At micromolar concentration, 2-APB could simultaneously block Stim1/Orai1 interaction, and IP3 receptor II, and also activates Orai3 channels in a Stim-independent way (Reyes et al., 2018a; Rosenberg et al., 2019). Consequently, cumulative treatment with 2-APB may prevent both Stim1-dependent activation of Orai1 and subsequent SOCE, but it also could attenuate the counter-regulation dependent on type II IP3 receptors. In addition, this can stimulate Stim1-independent Ca^{2+} entry through Orai3, limiting, in this way, the regression of pulmonary hypertension. The use of emerging drugs blocking selectively Orai1, independently of its interaction with Stim1 or IP3 receptors, such as AnCoA4 or CM-4620, are needed to validate SOCE as a pharmacological target against hypoxic pulmonary hypertension can achieve normalization (Reyes et al., 2018a; Stauderman, 2018; Waldron et al., 2019).

CONCLUSION

The treatment of hypoxic pulmonary hypertensive lambs with 2-APB, a non-selective inhibitor of store-operated Ca^{2+} signaling, has a mild effect on pulmonary hypertension and PAP response to acute superimposed hypoxia, without any significant action on other systemic cardiovascular variables. Considering that 2-APB is not a specific blocker, new selective inhibitors for Orai1, the primary pore-forming subunit of store-operated Ca^{2+} channels, need to be assessed. The improvement promoted by 2-APB on hemodynamic variables in high-altitude hypoxemic newborn lambs is less marked than those previously documented by the same treatment on pulmonary hypertensive normoxemic lambs, despite significant regression of pulmonary vascular remodeling. Therefore, we suggest that oxygenation and 2-APB treatment could have additive actions in the reversal of pulmonary hypertension induced by perinatal hypoxia and validate this signaling pathway as a potential complementary treatment for hypoxic pulmonary arterial hypertension of the neonate.

ETHICS STATEMENT

The animal study was all experimental protocols were reviewed and approved by the Faculty of Medicine Bioethics Committee of the University of Chile (CBA 0476 and 1172 FMUCH Acceptance Protocols).

AUTHOR CONTRIBUTIONS

SC-G, DP, SQ, FM, MD, GE, EH, IH, and AL performed the experiments. SC-G, SQ, GE, EH, RI, and AL analyzed the data. SC-G, SQ, EH, AL, RI, and RR interpreted the results of experiments. SC-G, DP, RR, AL, and GE prepared the figures. SC-G and RR drafted the manuscript. RR contributed to conception and design of research. All authors edited and revised the manuscript and approved final version of the manuscript.

ACKNOWLEDGMENTS

The authors thank Carlos Brito, Juan Carlos Fuenzalida, and Gabino Llusco for excellent technical assistance.

REFERENCES

Ambudkar, I. S., de Souza, L. B., and Ong, H. L. (2017). TRPC1, Orai1, and STIM1 in SOCE: friends in tight spaces. *Cell Calcium* 63, 33–39. doi: 10.1016/j.ceca.2016.12.009

Bai, D., del Corsso, C., Srinivas, M., and Spray, D. C. (2006). Block of specific gap junction channel subtypes by 2-aminoethoxydiphenyl borate (2-APB). *J. Pharmacol. Exp. Ther.* 319, 1452–1458. doi: 10.1124/jpet.106.112045

Billaud, M., Dahan, D., Marthan, R., Savineau, J.-P., and Guibert, C. (2011). Role of the gap junctions in the contractile response to agonists in pulmonary artery from two rat models of pulmonary hypertension. *Respir. Res.* 12:30. doi: 10.1186/1465-9921-12-30

Castillo-Galan, S., Arenas, G. A., Reyes, R. V., Krause, B. J., and Iturriaga, R. (2020). Stim-activated TRPC-ORAI channels in pulmonary hypertension induced by chronic intermittent hypoxia. *Pulm. Circ.* 10, 13–22. doi: 10.1177/2045894020941484

Castillo-Galán, S., Quezada, S., Moraga, F., Ebensperger, G., Herrera, E. A., Beñaldo, F., et al. (2016). 2-Aminoethyldiphenylborinate modifies the pulmonary circulation in pulmonary hypertensive newborn lambs partially gestated at high altitude. *Am. J. Physiol. Lung Cell Mol. Physiol.* 311, L788–L799. doi: 10.1152/ajplung.00230.2016

Chen, T. X., Xu, X. Y., Zhao, Z., Zhao, F. Y., Gao, Y. M., Yan, X. H., et al. (2017). Hydrogen peroxide is a critical regulator of the hypoxia-induced alterations of store-operated Ca2+ entry into rat pulmonary arterial smooth muscle cells. *Am. J. Physiol. Lung Cell Mol. Physiol.* 312, L477–L487. doi: 10.1152/ajplung.00138.2016

Chevalier, M., Gilbert, G., Roux, E., Lory, P., Marthan, R., Savineau, J.-P., et al. (2014). T-type calcium channels are involved in hypoxic pulmonary hypertension. *Cardiovasc. Res.* 103, 597–606. doi: 10.1093/cvr/cvu166

Chokshi, R., Fruasaha, P., and Kozak, J. A. (2012). 2-aminoethyl diphenyl borinate (2-APB) inhibits TRPM7 channels through an intracellular acidification mechanism. *Channels (Austin)* 6, 362–369. doi: 10.4161/chan.21628

DeHaven, W. I., Smyth, J. T., Boyles, R. R., Bird, G. S., and Putney, J. W. Jr. (2008). Complex actions of 2-aminoethyldiphenyl borate on store-operated calcium entry. *J. Biol. Chem.* 283, 19265–19273. doi: 10.1074/jbc.M801535200

Dunham-Snary, K. J., Wu, D., Sykes, E. A., Thakrar, A., Parlow, L. R., Mewburn, J. D., et al. (2017). Hypoxic pulmonary vasoconstriction: from molecular mechanisms to medicine. *Chest* 151, 181–192. doi: 10.1016/j.chest.2016.09.001

Earley, S., and Brayden, J. E. (2015). Transient receptor potential channels in the vasculature. *Physiol. Rev.* 95, 645–690. doi: 10.1152/physrev.00026.2014

Fernandez, R. A., Sundivakkam, P., Smith, K. A., Zeifman, A. S., Drennan, A. R., and Yuan, J. X. J. (2012). Pathogenic role of store-operated and receptor-operated channels in pulmonary arterial hypertension. *J. Signal. Transduct.* 2012:951497. doi: 10.1155/2012/951497

Gao, Y., and Raj, J. U. (2011). Hypoxic pulmonary hypertension of the newborn. *Compr. Physiol.* 1, 61–79.

Gonzaléz-Candia, A., Candia, A. A., Ebensperger, G., Reyes, R. V., Llanos, A. J., and Herrera, E. A. (2020). The newborn sheep translational model for pulmonary arterial hypertension of the neonate at high altitude. *J .Dev. Orig. Health Dis.* 11, 452–463. doi: 10.1017/S2040174420000616

He, X., Song, S., Ayon, R. J., Balisterieri, A., Black, S. M., Makino, A., et al. (2018). Hypoxia selectively upregulates cation channels and increases cytosolic [Ca2+] in pulmonary, but not coronary, arterial smooth muscle cells. *Am. J. Physiol. Cell Physiol.* 314, C504–C517. doi: 10.1152/ajpcell.00272.2017

Herrera, E. A., Ebensperger, G., Hernández, I., Sanhueza, E. M., Llanos, A. J., and Reyes, R. V. (2019). The role of nitric oxide signaling in pulmonary circulation of high-and low-altitude newborn sheep under basal and acute hypoxic conditions. *Nitric Oxide* 89, 71–80. doi: 10.1016/j.niox.2019.05.003

Herrera, E. A., Reyes, R. V., Giussani, D. A., Riquelme, R. A., Sanhueza, E. M., Ebensperger, G., et al. (2008a). Carbon monoxide: a novel pulmonary artery vasodilator in neonatal llamas of the Andean altiplano. *Cardiovasc. Res.* 77, 197–201. doi: 10.1093/cvr/cvm013

Herrera, E. A., Farías, J. G., Ebensperger, G., Reyes, R. V., Llanos, A. J., and Castillo, R. L. (2015). Pharmacological approaches in either intermittent or permanent hypoxia: a tale of two exposures. *Pharmacol. Res.* 101, 94–101. doi: 10.1016/j.phrs.2015.07.011

Herrera, E. A., Macchiavello, R., Montt, C., Ebensperger, G., Díaz, M., Ramírez, S., et al. (2014). Melatonin improves cerebrovascular function and decreases oxidative stress in chronically hypoxic lambs. *J. Pineal. Res.* 57, 33–42. doi: 10.1111/jpi.12141

Herrera, E. A., Pulgar, V. M., Riquelme, R. A., Sanhueza, E. M., Reyes, R. V., Ebensperger, G., et al. (2007). High-altitude chronic hypoxia during gestation and after birth modifies cardiovascular responses in newborn sheep. *Am. J. Physiol. Regul. Integr. Comp. Physiol.* 292, R2234–R2240. doi: 10.1152/ajpregu.00909.2006

Herrera, E. A., Ebensperger, G., Krause, B. J., Riquelme, R. A., Reyes, R. V., Capetillo, M., et al. (2008b). Sildenafil reverses hypoxic pulmonary hypertension in highland and lowland newborn sheep. *Pediatr. Res.* 63, 169–175. doi: 10.1203/PDR.0b013e31815ef71c

Herrera, E. A., Riquelme, R. A., Ebensperger, G., Reyes, R. V., Ulloa, C. E., Cabello, G., et al. (2010). Long-term exposure to high-altitude chronic hypoxia during gestation induces neonatal pulmonary hypertension at sea level. *Am. J. Physiol. Regul. Integr. Comp. Physiol.* 299, R1676–R1684. doi: 10.1152/ajpregu.00123.2010

Hou, X., Chen, J., Luo, Y., Liu, F., Xu, G., and Gao, Y. (2013). Silencing of STIM1 attenuates hypoxia-induced PASMCs proliferation via inhibition of the SOC/Ca2+/NFAT pathway. *Respir. Res.* 14:2. doi: 10.1186/1465-9921-14-2

Hussain, A., Suleiman, M. S., George, S. J., Loubani, M., and Morice, A. (2017). Hypoxic pulmonary vasoconstriction in humans: tale or myth. *Open Cardiovasc. Med. J.* 11, 1–13. doi: 10.2174/1874192401711010001

Keyes, L. E., Armaza, F. J., Niermeyer, S., Vargas, E., Young, D. A., and Moore, L. G. (2003). Intrauterine growth restriction, preeclampsia, and intrauterine mortality at high altitude in Bolivia. *Pediatr. Res.* 54, 20–25. doi: 10.1203/01.PDR.0000069846.64389.DC

Lievremont, J.-P., Bird, G. S., and Putney, J. W. Jr. (2005). Mechanism of inhibition of TRPC cation channels by 2-aminoethoxydiphenylborane. *Mol. Pharmacol.* 68, 758–762. doi: 10.1124/mol.105.012856

Lin, M. J., Leung, G. P., Zhang, W. M., Yang, X. R., Yip, K. P., Tse, C. M., et al. (2004). Chronic hypoxia–induced upregulation of store-operated and receptor-operated Ca2+ channels in pulmonary arterial smooth muscle cells: a novel mechanism of hypoxic pulmonary hypertension. *Circ. Res.* 95, 496–505. doi: 10.1161/01.RES.0000138952.16382.ad

Lopez, N. C., Ebensperger, G., Herrera, E. A., Reyes, R. V., Calaf, G., Cabello, G., et al. (2016). Role of the RhoA/ROCK pathway in high-altitude associated neonatal pulmonary hypertension in lambs. *Am. J. Physiol. Regul. Integr. Comp. Physiol.* 310, R1053–R1063. doi: 10.1152/ajpregu.00177.2015

Mathew, B., and Lakshminrusimha, S. (2017). Persistent pulmonary hypertension in the newborn. *Children* 4:63. doi: 10.3390/children4080063

Morihara, H., Obana, M., Tanaka, S., Kawakatsu, I., Tsuchiyama, D., Mori, S., et al. (2017). 2-aminoethoxydiphenyl borate provides an anti-oxidative effect and mediates cardioprotection during ischemia reperfusion in mice. *PLoS One* 12:e0189948. doi: 10.1371/journal.pone.0189948

Nair, J., and Lakshminrusimha, S. (2014). Update on PPHN: mechanisms and treatment. *Semin. Perinatol.* 38, 78–91. doi: 10.1053/j.semperi.2013.11.004

Ng, L. C., O'Neill, K. G., French, D., Airey, J. A., Singer, C. A., Tian, H., et al. (2012). TRPC1 and Orai1 interact with STIM1 and mediate capacitative Ca2+ entry caused by acute hypoxia in mouse pulmonary arterial smooth muscle cells. *Am. J. Physiol. Cell Physiol.* 303, C1156–C1172. doi: 10.1152/ajpcell.00065.2012

Parrau, D., Ebensperger, G., Herrera, E. A., Moraga, F., Riquelme, R. A., Ulloa, C. E., et al. (2013). Store-operated channels in the pulmonary circulation of high-and low-altitude neonatal lambs. *Am. J. Physiol. Lung Cell Mol. Physiol.* 304, L540–L548. doi: 10.1152/ajplung.00024.2012

Peinelt, C., Lis, A., Beck, A., Fleig, A., and Penner, R. (2008). 2-Aminoethoxydiphenyl borate directly facilitates and indirectly inhibits STIM1-dependent gating of CRAC channels. *J. Physiol.* 586, 3061–3073. doi: 10.1113/jphysiol.2008.151365

Peñaloza, D., and Arias-Stella, J. (2007). The heart and pulmonary circulation at high altitudes. *Circulation* 115, 1132–1146. doi: 10.1161/CIRCULATIONAHA.106.624544

Putney, J. W. (2010). Pharmacology of store-operated calcium channels. *Mol. Interv.* 10, 209–218. doi: 10.1124/mi.10.4.4

Putney, J. W. (2018). Forms and functions of store-operated calcium entry mediators, STIM and Orai. *Adv. Biol. Regul.* 68, 88–96. doi: 10.16/j.jbior.2017.11006

Quezada, S., González-Candia, A., Araya, C., Castillo, S., Ebensperger, G., Herrera, E., et al. (2014). "PDGF expression and pulmonary artery remodeling in newborn lambs differentially exposed to perinatal hypoxia," in *Proccedings of the 41th annual FNPS*, (St. Vicent).

Reyes, R. V., Castillo-Galán, S., Hernandez, I., Herrera, E. A., Ebensperger, G., and Llanos, A. J. (2018a). Revisiting the role of TRP, orai, and ASIC channels in the pulmonary arterial response to hypoxia. *Front Physiol.* 9:486. doi: 10.3389/fphys.2018.00486

Reyes, R. V., Díaz, M., Ebensperger, G., Herrera, E. A., Quezada, S. A., Hernandez, I., et al. (2018b). The role of nitric oxide in the cardiopulmonary response to hypoxia in highland and lowland newborn llamas. *J. Physiol.* 596, 5907–5923. doi: 10.1113/JP274340

Rodman, D. M., Reese, K., Harral, J., Fouty, B., Wu, S., West, J., et al. (2005). Low-voltage-activated (T-type) calcium channels control proliferation of human pulmonary artery myocytes. *Circ. Res.* 96, 864–872. doi: 10.1161/01.RES.0000163066.07472.ff

Rosenberg, P., Katz, D., and Bryson, V. (2019). SOCE and STIM1 signaling in the heart: timing and location matter. *Cell Calcium* 77, 20–28. doi: 10.1016/j.ceca.2018.11.008

Sari, E., Aksit, H., Erken, H. A., Yay, A., Aksit, D., Amasyali, A. S., et al. (2015). Protective effect of 2-APB on testicular ischemia-reperfusion injury in rats. *J. Urol.* 193, 1036–1041. doi: 10.1016/j.juro.2014.09.120

Shibata, A., Uchida, K., Kodo, K., Miyauchi, T., Mikoshiba, K., Takahashi, T., et al. (2019). Type 2 inositol 1, 4, 5-trisphosphate receptor inhibits the progression of pulmonary arterial hypertension via calcium signaling and apoptosis. *Heart Vessels* 34, 724–734. doi: 10.1007/s00380-018-1304-4

Snetkov, V. A., Aaronson, P. I., Ward, J. P., Knock, G. A., and Robertson, T. P. (2003). Capacitive calcium entry as a pulmonary specific vasoconstrictor mechanism in small muscular arteries in the rat. *Br. J. Pharmacol.* 140, 97–106. doi: 10.1038/sj.bjp.0705408

Stauderman, K. A. (2018). CRAC channels as targets for drug discovery and development. *Cell Calcium* 74, 147–159. doi: 10.1016/j.ceca.2018.07.005

Suresh, K., and Shimoda, L. A. (2016). Lung circulation. *Compr. Physiol.* 6, 897–943. doi: 10.1002/cphy.c140049

Taskin, M. I., Hismiogullari, A. A., Yay, A., Adali, E., Gungor, A. C., Korkmaz, G. O., et al. (2014). Effect of 2-aminoethoxydiphenyl borate on ischemia-reperfusion injury in a rat ovary model. *Eur. J. Obstet. Gynecol. Reprod. Biol.* 178, 74–79. doi: 10.1016/j.ejogrb.2014.03.049

Torres, F., González-Candia, A., Montt, C., Ebensperger, G., Chubretovic, M., Serón-Ferré, M., et al. (2015). Melatonin reduces oxidative stress and improves vascular function in pulmonary hypertensive newborn sheep. *J. Pineal. Res.* 58, 362–373. doi: 10.1111/jpi.12222

Waldron, R. T., Chen, Y., Pham, H., Go, A., Su, H. Y., Hu, C., et al. (2019). The Orai Ca2+ channel inhibitor CM4620 targets both parenchymal and immune cells to reduce inflammation in experimental acute pancreatitis. *J. Physiol.* 597, 3085–3105. doi: 10.1113/JP277856

Walsh-Sukys, M. C., Tyson, J. E., Wright, L. L., Bauer, C. R., Korones, S. B., Stevenson, D. K., et al. (2000). Persistent pulmonary hypertension of the newborn in the era before nitric oxide: practice variation and outcomes. *Pediatrics* 105, 14–20. doi: 10.1542/peds.105.1.14

Wang, J., Xu, C., Zheng, Q., Yang, K., Lai, N., Wang, T., et al. (2017). Orai1, 2, 3 and STIM1 promote store-operated calcium entry in pulmonary arterial smooth muscle cells. *Cell Death Discov.* 3, 1–11. doi: 10.1038/cddiscovery.2017.74

Wan, J., Yamamura, A., Zimnicka, A. M., Voiriot, G., Smith, K. A., Tang, H., et al. (2013). Chronic hypoxia selectively enhances L- and T-type voltage-dependent Ca^{2+} channel activity in pulmonary artery by upregulating $Ca_V1.2$ and $Ca_V3.2$. *Am. J. Physiol. Lung Cell. Mol. Physiol.* 305, L154–L164. doi: 10.1152/ajplung.00313.2012

10

The Effect of Chronic Intermittent Hypobaric Hypoxia on Sleep Quality and Melatonin Serum Levels in Chilean Miners

*Rodrigo Calderon-Jofre[1], Daniel Moraga[2] and Fernando A. Moraga[1]**

[1] Laboratorio de Fisiología, Hipoxia y Función Vascular, Departamento de Ciencias Biomédicas, Facultad de Medicina, Universidad Católica del Norte, Coquimbo, Chile, [2] Departamento de Medicina, Facultad de Ciencias de la Salud, Universidad de Tarapacá, Arica, Chile

***Correspondence:**
Fernando A. Moraga
fmoraga@ucn.cl

High-altitude mining is an important economic resource for Chile. These workers are exposed to chronic intermittent hypobaric hypoxia (CIHH), which reduces their sleep quality and increases the risk of accidents and long-term illnesses. Melatonin, a hormone produced by the pineal gland, is a sleep inducer that regulates the circadian cycle and may be altered in populations subjected to CIHH. This work aimed to assess the relationship between altitude, sleep quality, and plasma melatonin concentrations in miners with CIHH exposure. 288 volunteers were recruited from five altitudes (0, 1,600, 2,500, 3,500, and 4,500 m). All volunteers worked for 7 days at altitude, followed by 7 days of rest at sea level. We performed anthropometric assessments, nocturnal oximetry, sleep quality and sleepiness surveys, and serum melatonin levels upon awakening. Although oxygen saturation progressively decreased and heart rate increased at higher altitudes, subjective perception of sleep quality was not significantly different, and sleepiness increased in all groups compared to population at sea level. Similarly, melatonin levels increased at all assessed altitudes compared to the population at sea level. These data confirm that sleep disturbances associated with CIHH increase morning melatonin levels. Therefore, this hormone and could potentially serve as a biomarker of sleep quality.

Keywords: melatonin, chronic intermittent hypobaric hypoxia, sleep quality, oxygen saturation, heart rate

INTRODUCTION

Approximately 140 million people worldwide live or work at altitudes over 2,500 m, exposing them to *hypoxia*, a condition where oxygen availability is reduced due to decreased atmospheric pressure (Moore et al., 2001). According to exposure time, hypoxia can be *acute* (exposure for hours or days), *chronic* (permanent exposure to low oxygen), or intermittent (alternated periods of exposure to normoxia and hypoxia, Viscor et al., 2018). The effects of hypoxia due to altitude on the human body depend on the altitude reached, the rate of ascent, the exposure time, and the personal response to altitude (Davis and Hackett, 2017).

Mining activity is one of the most important economic incomes in Chile. Most of the mining complexes are located at altitudes between 3,000 and 5,200 m. Most workers (estimated at 120,000 people in big mining companies) have to commute rapidly (within a few hours) from lowland cities to high altitude facilities (Consejo de Competencias Mineras, 2017). Miners with this type of working shift are exposed to a model of hypoxia called *chronic intermittent hypobaric hypoxia* (CIHH), also known as *The Chilean Model* (Richalet et al., 2002). This exposure pattern is gaining attention due to the potential adverse effects of long-term exposure on cardiovascular, respiratory, and metabolic health (Brito et al., 2007; Vearrier and Greenberg, 2011; Vinnikov et al., 2011; Pedreros-Lobos et al., 2021).

Several studies show sleep disturbances in people exposed to hypoxia. Climbers exposed to acute hypoxia show sleep disturbances due to low oxygen availability from an altitude of 2,400 m, like sleep apnea episodes, or *periodic breathing* (cyclic oscillations in ventilation amplitude including apnea episodes, also known as *Cheyne-Stokes breathing*, Waggener et al., 1984). These alterations are increased at very high altitudes (West et al., 1986) and are practically absent in natives (Lahiri et al., 1983). Using simulated normobaric hypoxia, acute exposure to 4,500 m resulted in a relationship between poor sleep quality and altered mood and cognitive function (De Aquino Lemos et al., 2012).

Richalet et al. (2002) showed perceived low sleep quality in a CIHH population during the first two nights of shift work, and this perception was kept with no acclimation during the time of study (almost 2 years). Previous data from our group showed that an acclimatized population exposed to 4,200 m presented reduced arterial oxygen saturation, periodic breathing, increased awakenings, and perceived poor sleep. These alterations were improved with oxygen supplementation during the night (Moraga et al., 2014). Poor sleep quality due to nocturnal hypoxia is an important threat to lifespan, because it is an important factor related to the increased frequency of occupational accidents and its relation with an increase in risk of road traffic accident at high altitude location (Behn and De Gregorio, 2020).

Regulation of sleep is dependent on secretion of melatonin, an hormone produced from tryptophan by the pineal gland at night (Arendt et al., 1982). Production of melatonin is synchronized by the photopigment melanopsin, contained in intrinsically photosensitive retinal ganglion cells, where light exposure in the range 460–480 nm initiates the signal transduction toward several regions in the brain, including the suprachiasmatic nuclei (Do, 2019). Activation of this structure is essential to synchronize pineal secretion of melatonin and initiate the nocturnal phase of the circadian cycle (Arendt, 1998). Effects of melatonin include regulation of metabolism and reduction of energy expenditure (Coomans et al., 2013; Peschke et al., 2013; Cipolla-Neto et al., 2014), thermoregulation (Gubin et al., 2009), and redox regulation, acting as a natural antioxidant (Tan et al., 1993, 2013) and inducing expression of antioxidant enzymes (KęKędziora-Kornatowska et al., 2007).

Previous studies show that hypoxia alters the circadian cycle. Acute exposure to hypoxia (2 h at 8,000 m) elevated melatonin levels in rats and resulted in remodeling of the pineal gland, which lasted between 14 and 21 days after exposure (Kaur et al., 2002). In humans, an expedition to the Himalayas shown an increase in the excretion of 6-hydroxymelatonin, a breakdown product of melatonin, indicating elevated hormone production during high altitude exposure (Frisch et al., 2004). Furthermore, patients with obstructive sleep apnea syndrome (OSAS), a clinical condition characterized by chronic and intermittent hypoxia during sleep, an elevated plasma melatonin concentration was observed, and the use of CPAP enhanced arterial oxygenation and reduced plasma melatonin concentration (Hernández et al., 2007). In this sense, acute hypoxia or high altitude exposure could affect melatonin rhythm by a delay the phase of melatonin rhythm (Coste et al., 2009) and exposure to CIHH affects circadian pattern in people exposed to 7 days of work at 4,000 m (Vargas et al., 2001). However, studies on melatonin production in miners exposed to CIHH are scarce. Therefore, the aim of this study was to evaluate melatonin levels in workers exposed to different altitudes in a model of CIHH exposure.

SUBJECTS, MATERIALS, AND METHODS

A cross-sectional study and descriptive scope were carried out in a acclimatized workers exposed to CIHH model with a time of exposure between 6 month at 4 years. We recruited 288 male workers who worked at different altitudes (0, 1,600, 2,500, 3,500, and 4,500 m) through their respective company headquarters. All volunteers had to be working for at least 6 months at the respective altitude and included mining operations and administrative employees in diurnal work shift (starting between 7 and 8 a.m.). Shift work in this population is characterized by 7 days of work at the indicated altitude followed by 7 days of rest at lower altitude (<1,000 m). All volunteers were healthy, without diagnosis of cardiorespiratory and metabolic illness. At the time of recruitment, the volunteers read the informed consent and were informed of possible risks and discomfort, according to guidelines of the Ethics Committee of University's Faculty of Medicine (CECFAMED# 01/09) and the Medical Director of the respective company. Once agreed, all evaluations were performed during the third day of respective shift work at high altitude as previously described (Moraga et al., 2014; Moraga et al., 2018; Pedreros-Lobos et al., 2021).

Anthropometric Measurement

Weight (kg) and height (m) were measured using a scale (SECA model 767), and body mass index (BMI) was calculated using formula BMI = weight/height^2 (kg/m^2). Waist circumference (WC, cm) was measured using inextensible metric tape (SECA model 201). Four skinfolds (biceps, triceps, subscapular, and suprailiac) were determined by skinfold caliper (Lang skinfold, Cambridge, Maryland), and body fat mass (BF, percentage) was calculated using a previous described formula (Durnin and Womersley, 1973). Additionally, to estimate physical activity in the workplace, an IPAQs survey (International Physical Activity Questionary short, Ainsworth et al., 2000) was used and lifestyle was classified as sedentary, light, moderate, and active. All measurements were carried out by the same evaluator as performed previously (Pedreros-Lobos et al., 2021).

Nocturnal Oximetry

Evaluation of nocturnal oximetry was performed using a pulse oximeter (WristOx 3100,^{TM} Nonin, Plymouth, MN, United States). To evaluate desaturation events during the night, we considered the following variables: arterial oxygen saturation (SaO_2, percentage), heart rate (bpm), number of events (NE), total time of events (TTE, min), average time per event (ATE, s), and oxygen desaturation index of 4% (ODI, events/h), defined by a reduction of oxygen saturation over 4% by at least 10 s.

Sleep Quality and Sleepiness Surveys

To determine sleep quality and sleepiness, translated self-reported surveys were performed. To evaluate sleep quality, we used the Spiegel Sleep Questionnaire (Spiegel, 1984; Moraga et al., 2014), considering sleep quality as *Normal* (score below 13 points), *Regular* (between 13 and 18 points), *Poor* (between 19 and 25 points), and *Very Poor* (over 26 points). To evaluate sleepiness, we used the Epworth Sleepiness Scale (Johns, 1991), considering sleepiness as *Normal* (below 6 points), *Mild* (score between 6 and 13 points), *Moderate* (between 14 and 19 points), and *Severe* (between 20 and 24 points).

Blood Sample and Melatonin Quantification

Blood samples were taken from the brachial vein before the work shift (between 7 and 8 am) and collected in tubes without anticoagulant. Afterward, blood samples were centrifugated (3,000 rpm by 20 min) and serum was frozen at −80°C until analysis. Melatonin levels were measured by enzyme-linked immunoassay using a commercial kit (RE54021; IBL-Hamburg GmbH, Hamburg, Germany), after treatment of samples following instructions from the manufacturer. All samples were measured in duplicate and level of melatonin was expressed in pg/mL.

Statistical Analysis

All data were analyzed using Prism 8.4 software (GraphPad Software, San Diego, United States), tables are presented as mean ± standard deviation (SD) and plots are expressed as box-and-whisker graphs. Differences between the population at each altitude were determined using Kruskal-Wallis for non-parametric variables, followed by *post hoc* Dunn's test. Linear regression analysis was performed to establish an association between nocturnal oximetry parameters, heart rate, sleep quality and sleepiness (as independent variables), and melatonin concentration, and correlation between parameters were performed using Pearson's correlation coefficient. Significant differences were set at $p < 0.05$.

RESULTS

From 288 volunteers recruited at all altitudes, 209 were analyzed and 79 were excluded. Exclusion criteria considered people who retracted or were absent at the time of assessment, or whose nocturnal oximetry data was inconsistent due to mechanical artifacts and lipemic or hemolyzed blood samples. According with inclusion criteria, there were no records of people with chronic diseases (hypertension, diabetes, or respiratory diseases). The summary of the physical characteristics of the study population is shown in **Supplementary Table 1**. Briefly, mean age of all participants is 38.9 ± 9.7 years, and most of them present overweight according to BMI (27.5 ± 3.3). No significant differences in age and anthropometrical data were found between groups at altitudes studied. In agree with the IPAQs survey, 75% of volunteers were declared sedentary, 17% did light or moderate training, and only 8% were considered active.

A progressive decrease in nocturnal oxygen saturation was observed, starting with 95.6 ± 1.2% in the population at 0 m, and reaching 88.5 ± 1.8% at 4,500 m (**Figure 1A**). Even though heart rate progressively rises with altitude, it was only significantly different at 4,500 m (78.9 ± 2.95 bpm, compared to 61.6 ± 7.8 bpm at 0 m, **Figure 1B**).

Nocturnal oximetry parameters trended to increase with altitude (**Table 1** and **Supplementary Figure 1**). Desaturation events significantly rose from 2,500 m (63.4 ± 48.0), reaching a mean of 359.3 ± 262.1 events at 4,500 m (compared to 44.7 ± 66.7 at 0 m, **Supplementary Figure 1A**). The total time (TTE) significantly increased from 3,500 m (72.5 ± 49.6 min) and 4,500 m (113.2 ± 76.3 min) compared to 0 m (33.6 ± 45.8 min, **Supplementary Figure 1B**). The average time per event (ATE) was progressively reduced from 47.5 ± 20.3 s at 0 m, reaching 24.9 ± 6.2 at 3,500 m and 20.3 ± 4.1 at 4,500 m (**Supplementary Figure 1C**). ODI, an estimate of desaturation events greater than 4% per hour, significantly increased at 2,500 m (9.2 ± 7.0 events/h), 3,500 m (25.1 ± 19.6 events/h), and 4,500 m (46.1 ± 33.6 events/h) compared to 0 m (6.8 ± 9.7, **Supplementary Figure 1D**).

Subjective sleep quality and sleepiness were analyzed using self-reported surveys at several altitudes. Although there is no significant difference in sleep quality between groups, the mean scores indicate that overall perception is "regular" (**Figure 2A**). However, when scores are pooled and expressed as percentages, there is a reduction in people with normal or regular sleep quality, and an increase in people with poor sleep quality at 4,500 m (**Figure 2B**). In addition, high altitude increased sleepiness scores, showing a significant difference at 3,500 (7.5 ± 4.1) and 4,500 m (7.8 ± 5.0) compared to 0 m (3.4 ± 3.1, **Figure 2C**), and although most people described sleepiness as mild, at 3,500 and 4,500 m there is an increase in the percentage of people with moderate somnolence (**Figure 2D**).

Melatonin concentration in miners at several altitudes was significantly increased at all altitudes compared to 0 m (8.8 ± 11.3 pg/mL). However, the mean melatonin values were similar and not significantly different between altitudes (**Figure 3A** and **Supplementary Table 2**). Compared with the parameters of nocturnal oximetry, heart rate or self-reported questionaries, we found an inverse correlation between melatonin concentration and nocturnal oxygen saturation (**Figure 3B**). Still, when data were separated by altitude, a significant correlation was found only at 4,500 m (**Supplementary Table 2**). In addition, no correlation between

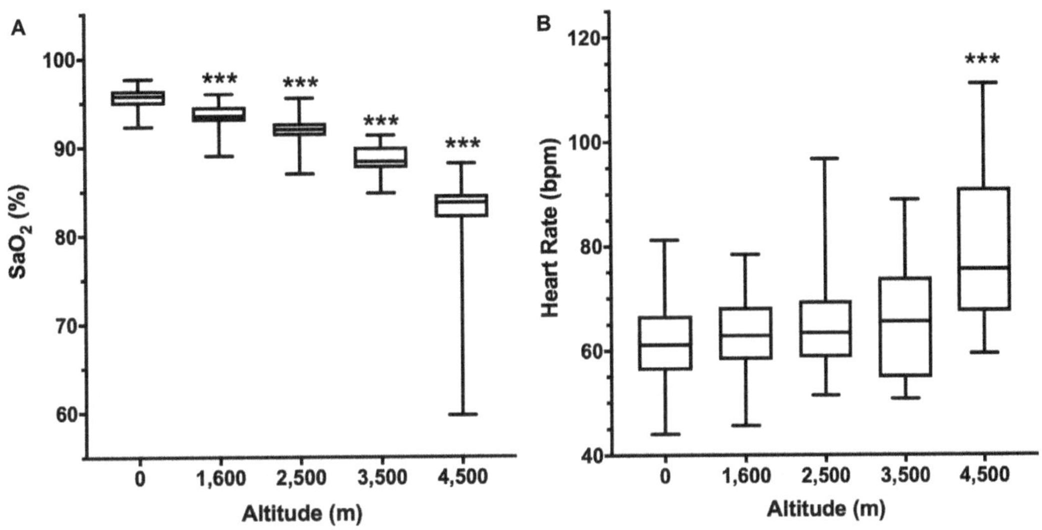

FIGURE 1 | Arterial oxygen saturation (SaO_2, **A**) and Heart rate **(B)** according to altitude. Data are presented as a box-and-whisker plot. Significant differences: $^{***}p < 0.001$ compared to the population at 0 m.

TABLE 1 | Nocturnal oximetry parameters according to altitude.

Altitude (m)	N	SaO_2 (%)	Heart rate (bpm)	NE	TTE (min)	ATE (s)	ODI (event/h)
0	60	95.6 ± 1.2	61.6 ± 7.8	44.7 ± 66.7	33.6 ± 45.8	47.5 ± 20.3	6.8 ± 9.7
1600	60	93.6 ± 1.3***	62.8 ± 7.1	61.1 ± 68.8	34.9 ± 34.2	37.7 ± 8.2	8.6 ± 9.6
2500	49	91.9 ± 1.7***	64.7 ± 9.0	63.4 ± 48.0*	32.6 ± 23.2	33.5 ± 11.4***	9.2 ± 7.0*
3500	19	88.5 ± 1.8***	66.6 ± 11.7	196.3 ± 157.3***	72.5 ± 49.6***	24.9 ± 6.2***	25.1 ± 19.6***
4500	21	82.3 ± 5.4***	78.9 ± 14.2***	359.3 ± 262.1***	113.2 ± 76.3***	20.3 ± 4.1***	46.1 ± 33.6***

Values are expressed such as mean ± SD. SaO_2, arterial oxygen saturation; NE, number of events; TTE, total time of events; ATE, Average time per event; ODI, Oxygen desaturation index of 4%. Significant differences: $^{*}p < 0.05$, $^{***}p < 0.001$ compared to the population at 0 m.

melatonin levels and anthropometric parameters (BMI, BF, WC) was found at any altitude studied (**Supplementary Table 3**).

DISCUSSION

This study provides new insights regarding melatonin levels in workers exposed to CIHH in Chile. The data shown here suggest that altitude could elevate melatonin levels, affecting sleep quality and increasing a risk of road traffic accidentality.

The melatonin levels observed at the time of sampling at 0 m are consistent with previous studies focused on its secretion profile, and correspond to approximately 25% of the maximum secretion level and could be used as a reference parameter (Arendt et al., 1982; Wehr, 1991; Benloucif et al., 2005). Elevation on melatonin levels at high altitude are in agree with previous reports observed in humans (Tapia et al., 2018) and rats (Kaur et al., 2002). In addition, an inverse relation was observed when arterial oxygen saturation was measured during sleep, showing that subjects that have a lower arterial oxygen saturation correlate with higher values of melatonin, especially at 4,500 m (**Figure 3** and **Supplementary Table 2**). A similar pattern was described in a previous study were exposure to normobaric hypoxia of 13.5% oxygen (equivalent to 4,500 m) showed that increased melatonin levels are inversely correlated with arterial oxygen saturation, and exercise partially reduces this increase, improving sleep (De Aquino Lemos et al., 2018).

Evidence for the effect of altitude on sleep was well documented but focused mainly on dwellers with acute exposure to extreme altitudes, where high altitude induces sleep apneas, periodic breathing, and sleep fragmentation (reviewed in Ainslie et al., 2013). Initial studies show that people exposed to CIHH in Chile presented values of sleep quality qualified as "regular" (13–18 points) during a 7-day shift at 4,500 m, with no changes in this pattern for at least for 18 months (Richalet et al., 2002). Similar values were described in our study, supporting that sleep quality is not acclimatized. In order to enhance sleep quality at high altitude we performed a study where room enrichment with oxygen at 24% was useful to reduce apneas and improve sleep quality (with a significant reduction in mean score equivalent to "normal," below 13 points) in a population working at 4,200 m (Moraga et al., 2014). In the present study, subjective perception of sleep was not significantly different between altitudes and did not directly correlate with arterial oxygen saturation. However, most people described regular sleep quality and mild somnolence. Possible explanations could be associated with the mining culture, where workers will not admit

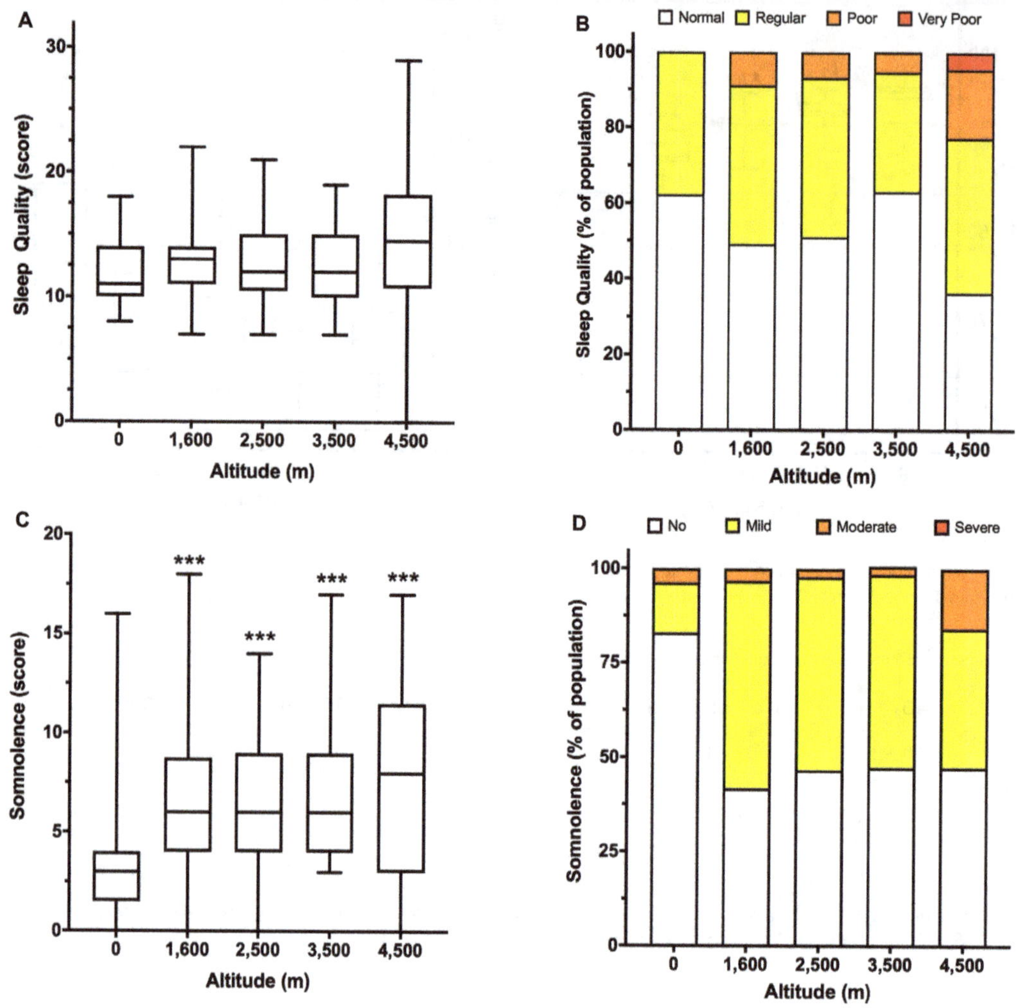

FIGURE 2 | Subjective evaluation of sleep quality and somnolence according to altitude. Sleep quality is expressed as a score **(A)** and percentage of people in the indicated category **(B)**. Somnolence is expressed as a score **(C)** and a percentage of people in the indicated category **(D)**. Data in panels **(A,C)** are presented as a box-and-whisker plot. Significant differences: $^{***}p < 0.001$ compared to the population at 0 m.

fatigue or sleep problems because of fears of being suspended or fired from work and a lack of objective methods to determine sleep quality. Therefore, an alternative to assess sleep quality or detect problems during sleep in the mining population is required. It is known that circadian dysregulation caused by hypoxia (Mortola, 2017) and desynchronization by shift work (Mirick et al., 2013) may represent a factor involved in the increase of risk of road traffic accidentality in high altitude activities, such as mining, border, or astronomical labor (Behn et al., 2014; Behn and De Gregorio, 2020).

Even though high altitude disturbs sleep, studies linking melatonin levels in people living or working in this condition are scarce and mostly focused on acute exposure. A simulation of 8,000 m exposure in rats showed increased melatonin production during the first 7 days, followed by a decrease to baseline levels between 14 and 21 days after exposure (Kaur et al., 2002). Another study focused on chronic and intermittent hypobaric hypoxia showed that rats exposed to 4,500 m for 32 days (in cycles of 96 h) increased melatonin levels, and this elevation was associated with antioxidant protection in the heart, lungs, and kidneys (Farías et al., 2012). However, the main source of information on melatonin production and hypoxia comes from studies related to obstructive sleep apnea syndrome (OSAS), a model of intermittent hypoxia related to upper airway obstruction. Previous studies in animals suggest that heart damage stimulated by OSAS can be prevented by treatment with melatonin (Xie et al., 2015). Additionally, the use of exogenous melatonin in rats exposed intermittently to 5% oxygen stimulates the expression of antioxidant enzymes and reduces the presence of oxidative damage markers (Hung et al., 2008). Also, the use of exogenous melatonin in rats chronically exposed to 10% hypoxia could attenuate elevated right ventricular systolic pressure, reduce pulmonary hypertension, and inhibit the expression of pro-inflammatory substances (Hung et al., 2017). Preliminary studies show decreased expression of pro-inflammatory cytokines interleukin

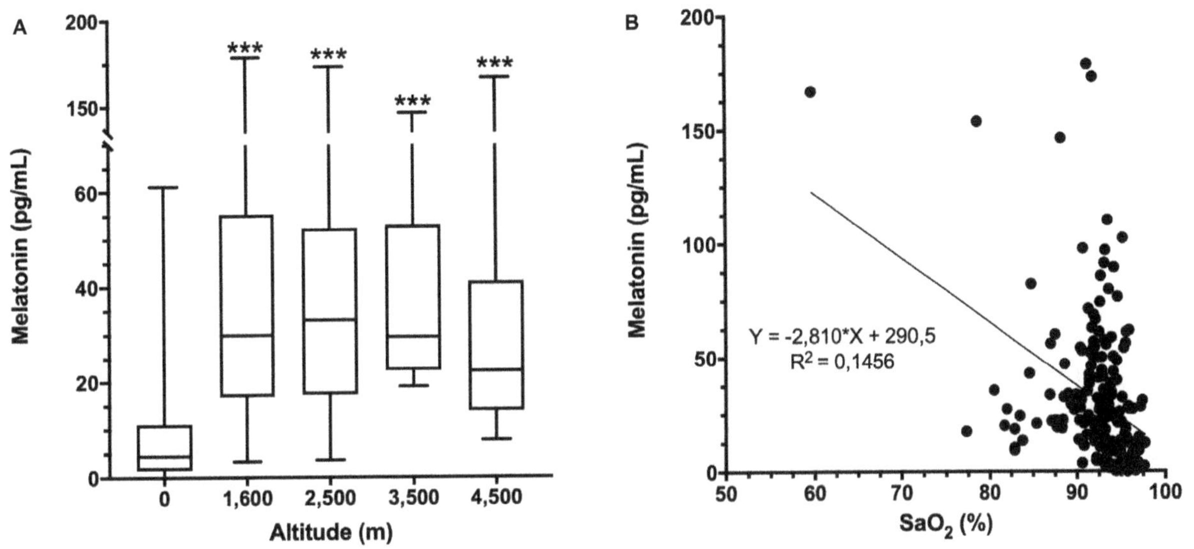

FIGURE 3 | Melatonin concentration and altitude. **(A)** Melatonin concentration in plasma at each altitude. Data are presented as a box-and-whisker plot. Significant differences: $^{***}p < 0.001$ compared to the population at 0 m. **(B)** Correlation of melatonin concentration with oxygen saturation (SaO_2) at all altitudes. Equation and the linear regression R^2 are shown.

2 (IL-2) and IL-6 measured in lymphocytes of rats exposed to CIHH of 4600 m, which could be associated with increased anti-inflammatory interleukin-10 levels (Bernal et al., 2009). In regard to sleep biomarkers and its regulation, supporting evidence shows that increased levels of IL-1 and tumor necrosis factor alfa (TNF-α) can modulate a complex biochemical cascade that regulates sleep in humans and animals, and IL10 exerts an inhibitory effect of over sleep control (to more details, see Clinton et al., 2011). Related with this, unpublished data from our group suggest increased anti-inflammatory interleukin-10 production in people with exposure to CIHH at 4,500 m. This cytokine could be part of a protective response to high altitude-mediated inflammation and oxidative damage, but more studies are needed to confirm the role of melatonin. One hypothesis could be related to alterations in sympathetic pathways promoted by hypoxia since melatonin synthesis is stimulated by norepinephrine in the absence of light (Arendt, 1998). Stressful stimuli, such as hypoxia itself or in combination with exercise, can stimulate interleukin-6 expression, mediated by the α-adrenergic pathway (Mazzeo et al., 2001). Furthermore, melatonin production can be peripherally enhanced in dendritic cells and macrophages by activating β-adrenoreceptors, turning them to an anti-inflammatory state (Pires-Lapa et al., 2018), supporting the idea of an interaction between hypoxia, the immune system, and melatonin production.

Another important factor associated with melatonin production is light exposure, which inhibits production and delays sleep induction (Lewy et al., 1980). Exposure to light at a wavelength between 446 and 477 nm (near blue light in the spectrum, as seen in electronic devices such as tablets or smartphones) suppresses melatonin production during the dark phase of the circadian cycle (Brainard et al., 2001). This phenomenon was evaluated as a potential regulator of the cycle, helping acclimatization during acute exposure to hypoxia (Silva-Urra et al., 2015). In this work, exposure to blue light during simulated hypoxia equivalent to 4,000 m increased systolic blood pressure and improved cognitive performance and alertness, associated with inhibited melatonin production. Another factor to consider is the time of light exposure, mainly associated with seasonal variation. Exposure to light is necessary to synchronize the cycle, affecting the duration of wakefulness, shortening the duration of sleep time in summer and extending it in winter. This seasonal pattern shifts melatonin production without modifying the amount of plasma melatonin (Wehr, 1991). Since all volunteers performed daytime work during the study and were exposed to similar artificial light in the common areas inside the complexes, most participants probably exhibited a similar photoperiod. Therefore, it would not be a relevant factor affecting hormone production, but personal habits in their bedrooms, including the use of television or mobile devices before sleeping, could affect melatonin production (Oh et al., 2015; Yasukouchi et al., 2019).

The limitations of the present study are associated with the melatonin production profile in miners during shift work. To precisely establish whether alterations in melatonin are associated with changes in the nocturnal phase, 24 h studies are necessary. However, taking blood samples during the shift is difficult, and we could not evaluate the nocturnal secretion profile or perform multiple blood sampling due to technical limitations and restrictions imposed by companies and labor unions. Although saliva samples are considered a good replacement for blood as a source of melatonin, daytime production could be too low to detect a significant amount unless alterations in secretion increase availability.

In conclusion, evaluation of melatonin levels in wakefulness could be used as a marker to analyze sleep quality at high altitude and a possible evidence of protection against oxidative damage in workers exposed to CIHH. Future studies should consider the long-term effect of CIHH exposure on melatonin levels and assess the potential prophylactic role of melatonin supplementation as an element that improves sleep quality and function as a cardiac and pulmonary protector associated to high altitude exposure.

ETHICS STATEMENT

The studies involving human participants were reviewed and approved by Ethics Committee of the Facultad de Medicina, Universidad Católica del Norte, Chile. The participants provided their written informed consent to participate in this study.

AUTHOR CONTRIBUTIONS

RC-J and FM conceived and designed the study, and performed the statistical analysis. DM and RC-J contributed to sample and data collections. FM was the guarantor. All authors drafted the report, interpreted the results, critically revised the manuscript, and approved the final manuscript.

ACKNOWLEDGMENTS

We thank Hervis Galleguillos for his permanent support in the laboratory work during the development of this project. We also thank the volunteers who participated in the study and the technical and logistical support provided by the participating companies' medical boards and trade unions.

REFERENCES

Ainslie, P. N., Lucas, S. J. E., and Burgess, K. R. (2013). Breathing and sleep at high altitude. *Respir. Physiol. Neurobiol.* 188, 233–256.

Ainsworth, B. E., Haskell, W. L., Whitt, M. C., Irwin, M. L., Swartz, A. M., Strath, S. J., et al. (2000). Compendium of physical activities: an update of activity codes and MET intensities. *Med. Sci. Sports Exerc.* 32, S498–S504. doi: 10.1097/00005768-200009001-00009

Arendt, J. (1998). Melatonin and the pineal gland: influence on mammalian seasonal and circadian physiology. *Rev. Reprod.* 3, 13–22.

Arendt, J., Hampton, S., English, J., Kwasowski, P., and Marks, V. (1982). 24-Hour profiles of melatonin. Cortisol, insulin, c-peptide and GIP following a meal and subsequent fasting. *Clin. Endocrinol.* 16, 89–95. doi: 10.1111/j.1365-2265.1982.tb03151.x

Behn, C., and De Gregorio, N. (2020). Melatonin relations with energy metabolism as possibly involved in fatal mountain road traffic accidents. *Int. J. Mol. Sci.* 21:2184. doi: 10.3390/IJMS21062184

Behn, C., Dinamarca, G. A., De Gregorio, N. F., Lips, V., Vivaldi, E. A., Soza, D., et al. (2014). Age-related arrhythmogenesis on ascent and descent: "autonomic conflicts" on hypoxia/reoxygenation at high altitude? *High Alt. Med. Biol.* 15, 356–363. doi: 10.1089/HAM.2013.1092

Benloucif, S., Guico, M. J., Reid, K. J., Wolfe, L. F., L'Hermite-Balériaux, M., and Zee, P. C. (2005). Stability of melatonin and temperature as circadian phase markers and their relation to sleep times in humans. *J. Biol. Rhythms* 20, 178–188. doi: 10.1177/0748730404273983

Bernal, G., Correa, C., Castillo, C., and Moraga, F. A. (2009). "Efecto de la hipoxia sobre la expresión de las citoquinas IL-2, IL-10e IL-2b en linfocitos de ratón," in *Proceedings of the V Workshop Internacional de Fisiología y Medicina de Altura: Medicina de Montaña y Neuropsicología Ambiental*, (La Serena: Facultad de Medicina, Universidad Catolica del Norte).

Brainard, G. C., Hanifin, J. R., Greeson, J. M., Byrne, B., Glickman, G., Gerner, E., et al. (2001). Action spectrum for melatonin regulation in humans: evidence for a novel circadian photoreceptor. *J. Neurosci.* 21, 6405–6412. doi: 10.1523/jneurosci.21-16-06405.2001

Brito, J., Siqués, P., León-Velarde, F., De La Cruz, J. J., López, V., and Herruzo, R. (2007). Chronic intermittent hypoxia at high altitude exposure for over 12 years: assessment of hematological, cardiovascular, and renal effects. *High Alt. Med. Biol.* 8, 236–244.

Cipolla-Neto, J., Amaral, F. G., Afeche, S. C., Tan, D. X., and Reiter, R. J. (2014). Melatonin, energy metabolism, and obesity: a review. *J. Pineal Res.* 56, 371–381. doi: 10.1111/JPI.12137

Clinton, J. M., Davis, C. J., Zielinski, M. R., Jewett, K. A., and Krueger, J. M. (2011). Biochemical regulation of sleep and sleep biomarkers. *J. Clin. Sleep Med.* 7, S38–S42. doi: 10.5664/JCSM.1360

Consejo de Competencias Mineras (2017). *Fuerza Laboral Gran Meneriìa 2017-2026. Diagnostico y Recomendaciones*, Vol. 148. http://www.ccm.cl/wp-content/uploads/2017/11/ReporteCCM_13-11_FINAL.pdf (accessed Novermber 4, 2021).

Coomans, C. P., Van Den Berg, S. A. A., Lucassen, E. A., Houben, T., Pronk, A. C. M., Van Der Spek, R. D., et al. (2013). The suprachiasmatic nucleus controls circadian energy metabolism and hepatic insulin sensitivity. *Diabetes* 62, 1102–1108. doi: 10.2337/DB12-0507/-/DC1

Coste, O., Van Beers, P., and Touitou, Y. (2009). Hypoxia-induced changes in recovery sleep, core body temperature, urinary 6-sulphatoxymelatonin and free cortisol after a simulated long-duration flight. *J. Sleep Res.* 18, 454–465. doi: 10.1111/J.1365-2869.2009.00744.X

Davis, C., and Hackett, P. (2017). Advances in the prevention and treatment of high altitude illness. *Emerg. Med. Clin. North Am.* 35, 241–260. doi: 10.1016/J.EMC.2017.01.002

De Aquino Lemos, V., Antunes, H. K. M., Dos Santos, R. V. T., Lira, F. S., Tufik, S., and De Mello, M. T. (2012). High altitude exposure impairs sleep patterns, mood, and cognitive functions. *Psychophysiology* 49, 1298–1306.

De Aquino Lemos, V., dos Santos, R. V. T., Antunes, H. K. M., Behn, C., Viscor, G., Lira, F. S., et al. (2018). Melatonin and sleep responses to normobaric hypoxia and aerobic physical exercise: a randomized controlled trial. *Physiol. Behav.* 196, 95–103. doi: 10.1016/j.physbeh.2018.08.016

Do, M. T. H. (2019). Melanopsin and the intrinsically photosensitive retinal ganglion cells: biophysics to behavior. *Neuron* 104, 205–226.

Durnin, B. Y. J. V. G. A., and Womersley, J. (1973). Body fat assessed from total body density and Its estimation from skinfold thickness: measurements on 481 men and women aged from 16 to 72 years. *Br. J. Nutr.* 32, 77–97. doi: 10.1079/BJN19740060

Farías, J. G., Zepeda, A. B., and Calaf, G. M. (2012). Melatonin protects the heart, lungs and kidneys from oxidative stress under intermittent hypobaric hypoxia in rats. *Biol. Res.* 45, 81–85. doi: 10.4067/S0716-976020120001 00011

Frisch, H., Waldhauser, F., Waldhör, T., Müllner-Eidenböck, A., Neupane, P., and Schweitzer, K. (2004). Increase in 6-hydroxymelatonin excretion in humans during ascent to high altitudes. *J. Clin. Endocrinol. Metab.* 89, 4388–4390. doi: 10.1210/jc.2003-032214

Gubin, D. G., Gubin, G. D., Waterhouse, J., and Weinert, D. (2009). The circadian body temperature rhythm in the elderly: effect of single daily melatonin dosing. *Chronobiol. Int.* 23, 639–658. doi: 10.1080/074205206006 50612

Hernández, C., Abreu, J., Abreu, P., Castro, A., and Jiménez, A. (2007). Nocturnal melatonin plasma levels in patients with OSAS: the effect of CPAP. *Eur. Respir. J.* 30, 496–500. doi: 10.1183/09031936.00 051906

Hung, M. W., Tipoe, G. L., Poon, A. M. S., Reiter, R. J., and Fung, M. L. (2008). Protective effect of melatonin against hippocampal injury of rats with intermittent hypoxia. *J. Pineal Res.* 44, 214–221.

Hung, M. W., Yeung, H. M., Lau, C. F., Poon, A. M. S., Tipoe, G. L., and Fung, M. L. (2017). Melatonin attenuates pulmonary hypertension in chronically hypoxic rats. *Int. J. Mol. Sci.* 18:1125. doi: 10.3390/ijms18061125

Johns, M. W. (1991). A new method for measuring daytime sleepiness: the Epworth sleepiness scale. *Sleep* 14, 540–545. doi: 10.1093/sleep/14.6.540

Kaur, C., Srinivasan, K. N., Singh, J., Peng, C. M., and Ling, E. A. (2002). Plasma melatonin, pinealocyte morphology, and surface receptors/antigen expression on macrophages/microglia in the pineal gland following a high-altitude exposure. *J. Neurosci. Res.* 67, 533–543. doi: 10.1002/jnr.10136

Kędziora-Kornatowska, K., Szewczyk-Golec, K., Czuczejko, J., Lumen, K. V. M. D., Pawluk, H., Motyl, J., et al. (2007). Effect of melatonin on the oxidative stress in erythrocytes of healthy young and elderly subjects. *J. Pineal Res.* 42, 153–158. doi: 10.1111/j.1600-079X.2006.00394.x

Lahiri, S., Maret, K., and Sherpa, M. G. (1983). Dependence of high altitude sleep apnea on ventilatory sensitivty to hypoxia. *Respir. Physiol.* 52, 281–301. doi: 10.1016/0034-5687(83)90086-5

Lewy, A., Wehr, T., Goodwin, F., Newsome, D., and Markey, S. (1980). Light suppresses melatonin secretion in humans. *Science* 210, 1267–1269.

Mazzeo, R. S., Donovan, D., Fleshner, M., Butterfield, G. E., Zamudio, S., Wolfel, E. E., et al. (2001). Downloaded from journals.physiology.org/journal/jappl (190.163.176.171) on. *J. Appl. Physiol.* 91, 2143–2149.

Mirick, D. K., Bhatti, P., Chen, C., Nordt, F., Stanczyk, F. Z., and Davis, S. (2013). Night shift work and levels of 6-sulfatoxymelatonin and cortisol in men. *Cancer Epidemiol. Prev. Biomarkers* 22, 1079–1087.

Moore, L. G., Human, L. G., and Med, A. (2001). Abstract adaptation. *High Alt. Med. Biol.* 2, 257–279.

Moraga, F. A., Osorio, J., Calderón-Jofré, R., and Pedreros, A. (2018). Hemoconcentration during maximum exercise in miners with chronic intermittent exposure to hypobaric hypoxia (3800 m). *High Alt. Med. Biol.* 19. doi:10.1089/ham.2017.0011

Moraga, F. A., Jiménez, D., Richalet, J. P., Vargas, M., and Osorio, J. (2014). Periodic breathing and oxygen supplementation in Chilean miners at high altitude (4200 m). *Respir. Physiol. Neurobiol.* 203, 109–115. doi: 10.1016/j.resp.2014.09.001

Mortola, J. P. (2017). Gender and the circadian pattern of body temperature in normoxia and hypoxia. *Respir. Physiol. Neurobiol.* 245, 4–12. doi: 10.1016/j.resp.2016.11.002

Oh, J. H., Yoo, H., Park, H. K., and Do, Y. R. (2015). Analysis of circadian properties and healthy levels of blue light from smartphones at night. *Sci. Rep.* 5:11325. doi: 10.1038/srep11325

Pedreros-Lobos, A., Calderón-Jofré, R., Moraga, D., and Moraga, F. A. (2021). Cardiovascular risk is increased in miner's chronic intermittent hypobaric hypoxia exposure from 0 to 2,500 m? *Front. Physiol* 12:647976. doi: 10.3389/fphys.2021.647976

Peschke, E., Bähr, I., and Mühlbauer, E. (2013). Melatonin and pancreatic islets: interrelationships between melatonin, insulin and glucagon. *Int. J. Mol. Sci.* 14, 6981–7015. doi: 10.3390/IJMS14046981

Pires-Lapa, M. A., Carvalho-Sousa, C. E., Cecon, E., Fernandes, P. A., and Markus, R. P. (2018). β-Adrenoceptors trigger melatonin synthesis in phagocytes. *Int. J. Mol. Sci.* 19:2182. doi: 10.3390/ijms19082182

Richalet, J. P., Donoso, M. V., Jiménez, D., Antezana, A. M., Hudson, C., Cortès, G., et al. (2002). Chilean miners commuting from sea level to 4500 m: a prospective study. *High Alt. Med. Biol.* 3, 159–166. doi: 10.1089/15270290260131894

Silva-Urra, J. A., Núñez-Espinosa, C. A., Niño-Mendez, O. A., Gaitán-Peñas, H., Altavilla, C., Toro-Salinas, A., et al. (2015). Circadian and sex differences after acute high-altitude exposure: are early acclimation responses improved by blue light? *Wilderness Environ. Med.* 26, 459–471. doi: 10.1016/j.wem.2015.06.009

Spiegel, R. (1984). Sleep disorders in the aged. *Internist (Berl).* 25, 552–555.

Tan, D. X., Manchester, L. C., Liu, X., Rosales-Corral, S. A., Acuna-Castroviejo, D., and Reiter, R. J. (2013). Mitochondria and chloroplasts as the original sites of melatonin synthesis: a hypothesis related to melatonin's primary function and evolution in eukaryotes. *J. Pineal Res.* 54, 127–138. doi: 10.1111/JPI.12026

Tan, D.-X., Chen, L. D., Poeggeler, B., Manchester, L. C., and Reiter, R. (1993). Melatonin: a potent endogenous hydroxyl radical scavenger. *Endocr. J.* 1, 57–60.

Tapia, M., Wulff-Zottele, C., De Gregorio, N., Lang, M., Varela, H., Serón-Ferré, M. J., et al. (2018). Melatonin relations with respiratory quotient weaken on acute exposure to high altitude. *Front. Physiol* 9:798. doi: 10.3389/FPHYS.2018.00798

Vargas, M., Jiménez, D., León-Velarde, F., Osorio, J., and Mortola, J. P. (2001). Circadian patterns in men acclimatized to intermittent hypoxia. *Respir. Physiol.* 126, 233–243. doi: 10.1016/S0034-5687(01)00226-2

Vearrier, D., and Greenberg, M. I. (2011). Occupational health of miners at altitude: adverse health effects, toxic exposures, pre-placement screening, acclimatization, and worker surveillance. *Clin. Toxicol.* 49, 629–640. doi: 10.3109/15563650.2011.607169

Vinnikov, D., Brimkulov, N., and Redding-Jones, R. (2011). Four-year prospective study of lung function in workers in a high altitude (4000 m) mine. *High Alt. Med. Biol.* 12, 65–69. doi: 10.1089/ham.2010.1033

Viscor, G., Torrella, J. R., Corral, L., Ricart, A., Javierre, C., Pages, T., et al. (2018). Physiological and biological responses to short-term intermittent hypobaric hypoxia exposure: from sports and mountain medicine to new biomedical applications. *Front. Physiol.* 9:814. doi: 10.3389/fphys.2018.00814

Waggener, T. B., Brusil, P. J., Kronauer, R. E., Gabel, R. A., and Inbar, G. F. (1984). Strength and cycle time of high-altitude ventilatory patterns in unacclimatized humans. *J. Appl. Physiol. Respir. Environ. Exerc. Physiol.* 56, 576–581. doi: 10.1152/jappl.1984.56.3.576

Wehr, T. A. (1991). The durations of human melatonin secretion and sleep respond to changes in daylength (photoperiod). *J. Clin. Endocrinol. Metab.* 73, 1276–1280. doi: 10.1210/jcem-73-6-1276

West, J. B., Peters, R. M., Aksnes, G., Maret, K. H., Milledge, J. S., and Schoene, R. B. (1986). Nocturnal periodic breathing at altitudes of 6,300 and 8,050 m. *J. Appl. Physiol.* 61, 280–287. doi: 10.1152/jappl.1986.61.1.280

Xie, S., Deng, Y., Pan, Y. Y., Wang, Z. H., Ren, J., Guo, X. L., et al. (2015). Melatonin protects against chronic intermittent hypoxia-induced cardiac hypertrophy by modulating autophagy through the 5' adenosine monophosphate-activated protein kinase pathway. *Biochem. Biophys. Res. Commun.* 464, 975–981. doi: 10.1016/j.bbrc.2015.06.149

Yasukouchi, A., Maeda, T., Hara, K., and Furuune, H. (2019). Non-visual effects of diurnal exposure to an artificial skylight, including nocturnal melatonin suppression. *J. Physiol. Anthropol.* 38:10. doi: 10.1186/S40101-019-0203-4

11

Experimental Evidence of A_{2A}–D_2 Receptor–Receptor Interactions in the Rat and Human Carotid Body

Elena Stocco[1], Maria Martina Sfriso[1], Giulia Borile[2,3], Martina Contran[1], Silvia Barbon[1], Filippo Romanato[2,3], Veronica Macchi[1], Diego Guidolin[1], Raffaele De Caro[1] and Andrea Porzionato[1]*

[1] Department of Neuroscience, Institute of Human Anatomy, University of Padova, Padua, Italy, [2] Department of Physics and Astronomy "G. Galilei," University of Padova, Padua, Italy, [3] Institute of Pediatric Research Città della Speranza, Padua, Italy

***Correspondence:**
Raffaele De Caro
raffaele.decaro@unipd.it

Adenosine A^{2A} receptors ($A_{2A}R$) and dopamine D_2 receptors (D_2R) are known to be involved in the physiological response to hypoxia, and their expression/activity may be modulated by chronic sustained or intermittent hypoxia. To date, $A_{2A}R$ and D_2R can form transient physical receptor–receptor interactions (RRIs) giving rise to a dynamic equilibrium able to influence ligand binding and signaling, as demonstrated in different native tissues and transfected mammalian cell systems. Given the presence of $A_{2A}R$ and D_2R in type I cells, type II cells, and afferent nerve terminals of the carotid body (CB), the aim of this work was to demonstrate here, for the first time, the existence of $A_{2A}R$–D_2R heterodimers by *in situ* proximity ligation assay (PLA). Our data by PLA analysis and tyrosine hydroxylase/S100 colocalization indicated the formation of $A_{2A}R$–D_2R heterodimers in type I and II cells of the CB; the presence of $A_{2A}R$–D_2R heterodimers also in afferent terminals is also suggested by PLA signal distribution. RRIs could play a role in CB dynamic modifications and plasticity in response to development/aging and environmental stimuli, including chronic intermittent/sustained hypoxia. Exploring other RRIs will allow for a broad comprehension of the regulative mechanisms these interactions preside over, with also possible clinical implications.

Keywords: carotid body, type I cells, adenosine A_{2A} receptors, dopamine D_2 receptors, heterodimes, *in situ* PLA

INTRODUCTION

In mammals and humans, the carotid bodies (CBs) are chemosensory organs located at the bifurcations of the common carotid arteries with a critical role in maintaining homeostasis during both development/aging (Di Giulio, 2018; Sacramento et al., 2019) and environmental variations (e.g., levels of O_2, CO_2, and arterial blood pH) (Iturriaga and Alcayaga, 2004; Iturriaga et al., 2016; Prabhakar and Peng, 2017; Di Giulio, 2018; Iturriaga, 2018) with also a sensing function with respect to metabolic factors (Porzionato et al., 2011; Conde et al., 2018; Cunha-Guimaraes et al., 2020; Sacramento et al., 2020).

The CB regulatory function is strictly related to its specific organization. Morphologically, in the CB parenchyma two types of cells can be distinguished: "neuron-like" chemosensitive type I cells, positive for tyrosine hydroxylase (TH), and "glial-like" supportive type II cells, positive for glial fibrillary acidic protein (GFAP) (Pardal et al., 2007; Tse et al., 2012). Sensitive innervation of the CB is mainly mediated by afferent terminals of the carotid sinus nerve, branch of the glossopharyngeal nerve, arising from neurons located in the petrosal ganglion (PG).

Neurotransmission in the CB involves a complex interplay of excitatory and inhibitory signals (Iturriaga and Alcayaga, 2004; Nurse, 2005; Fitzgerald et al., 2009; Porzionato et al., 2018; Stocco et al., 2020). Type I cells produce several neurotransmitters [e.g., dopamine, noradrenaline, adrenaline, acetylcholine, serotonin, adenosine, adenosine 5′-triphosphate (ATP)] and neuromodulators (e.g., enkephalins, neuropeptide Y, calcitonin gene-related peptide, galanin, endothelins, bombesin, adrenomedullin, kisspeptins, leptin) (Varas et al., 2003; Iturriaga and Alcayaga, 2004; Porzionato et al., 2008), in turn acting in an autocrine/paracrine manner on a broad spectrum of different ionotropic/metabotropic receptors located in afferent nerve fibers, type I cells, and type II cells, these latter also showing a role in the coordination of chemosensory transduction (Nurse, 2014; Porzionato et al., 2018; Stocco et al., 2020). Among these receptors, some metabotropic G protein-coupled receptors (GPCRs) (e.g., A_{2A}, $D_{1/2}$, $H_{1/2/3}$, $M_{1/2}$, 5-HT_{2A}, and others) are also involved; in particular, A_{2A} and D_2 have attracted the attention of many researchers, resulting among the most studied GPCRs (Aldossary et al., 2020).

The presence of $A_{2A}R$ was verified in rat (Gauda, 2000; Kobayashi et al., 2000; Xu et al., 2006; Bairam et al., 2009) and human (Fagerlund et al., 2010) CB specimens, where it showed to be expressed in type I cells, colocalizing with tyrosine-hydroxylase (TH) (Gauda, 2000; Gauda et al., 2000; Kobayashi et al., 2000; Bairam et al., 2009) or β-III-tubulin (Fagerlund et al., 2010). Considering the methodological approaches, different techniques were adopted, including *in situ* hybridization analysis (Gauda, 2000), immunohistochemistry (Kobayashi et al., 2000; Fagerlund et al., 2010), Western blot analysis (Bairam et al., 2009), and Ca^{2+} imaging technique (Xu et al., 2006). Also, D_2R presence was reported in CB type I cells in rats (Czyzyk-Krzeska et al., 1992; Holgert et al., 1995; Gauda et al., 1996, 2001; Bairam and Khandjian, 1997; Gauda, 2000; Kinkead et al., 2005; Wakai et al., 2015), rabbits (Bairam et al., 1996b; Bairam and Khandjian, 1997; Bairam et al., 2003), cats (Bairam and Khandjian, 1997), and humans (Fagerlund et al., 2010). CB specimens were analyzed through *in situ* hybridization (Czyzyk-Krzeska et al., 1992; Holgert et al., 1995; Gauda, 2000), RT-PCR (Bairam et al., 1996b, 2003; Bairam and Khandjian, 1997; Kinkead et al., 2005), and immunofluorescence (Wakai et al., 2015).

Apart from type I cells, some data support the expression of $A_{2A}R$ and D_2R also in type II cells (Kaelin-Lang et al., 1998; Leonard and Nurse, 2020). Additionally, $A_{2A}R$ (Gauda, 2000; Gauda et al., 2000; Conde et al., 2006, 2017, 2012; Zhang et al., 2018; Sacramento et al., 2019) and D_2R (Czyzyk-Krzeska et al., 1992; Schamel and Verna, 1993; Bairam et al., 1996a,b) were also demonstrated in PG neurons and afferent fibers in the CB.

As demonstrated for transfected mammalian cell systems and different native tissues (i.e., central nervous system, mammary gland, liver, cancer tissues), $A_{2A}R$ and D_2R can establish transient physical receptor–receptor interactions (RRIs) giving rise to a dynamic equilibrium between their specific monomeric form and homo/heterocomplexes (dimers or receptor mosaics) (Ferré et al., 2014; Guidolin et al., 2015). Such RRIs, in turn, likely modulate ligand binding and signaling, thus affecting the physio-pathological features but also the pharmacology of the nervous system.

Despite that the presence of $A_{2A}R$ and D_2R has been broadly recognized in the CB, the possible existence of $A_{2A}R$–D_2R heterodimers was never verified before, but only hypothesized in a previous work (Porzionato et al., 2018). Thus, in this study, rat and human CB specimens were investigated by proximity ligation assay (PLA) technique to assess the eventual interaction between $A_{2A}R$ and D_2R, thus corroborating the above working hypothesis and possibly opening the doors to the analysis of further possible RRIs in the CB.

MATERIALS AND METHODS

Tissue Collection

The animal study was reviewed and approved by the ethical committee of Padua University, in agreement with the Italian Department of Health guidelines (Authorization No. 702/2016-PR of July 15, 2016). Human tissues were managed by the Body Donation Program of the Section of Human Anatomy, University of Padova (Macchi et al., 2011; Porzionato et al., 2012), according to European, Italian, and Regional guidelines (De Caro et al., 2009; Riederer et al., 2012). Excision was further authorized by the Italian law No. 10 of February 10, 2020, entitled "Rules regarding the disposition of one's body and post-mortem tissues for study, training, and scientific research purposes" (Boscolo-Berto et al., 2020). Donors' written informed consent was signed upon joining the Body Donation Program; here, Donor's authorization expressly allowed to use Body and Body Parts also for research purposes, after donation.

Rat CBs were excised from 5 adult Sprague-Dawley rats; tissue isolation occurred immediately after euthanasia. Human CBs were obtained at autopsy from 5 adult subjects [3 males, 2 females; mean age 46 years, standard deviation (SD) ± 3.6] with no clinical sign of chronic pulmonary and/or cardiovascular diseases. Eventual pharmacological therapies that could have influenced the CB plasticity constituted a further exclusion criterion. Autopsies occurred within 30 h after death, according to Italian Law. On the basis of our previous experience (Porzionato et al., 2005, 2006, 2011), the tissues are viable and adequate for immunohistochemistry/immunofluorescence studies after this death–autopsy interval.

According to routine protocols, once isolated, the CBs were promptly fixed in 10% phosphate-buffered formalin for 72 h, dehydrated through ascending alcohols and xylene, clarified through xylene, and paraffin embedded.

Immunohistochemical Analysis

Preliminarily, the primary antibodies used were tested by immunohistochemistry; this is an important step before PLA assay, whose performance critically depends on the antibodies' quality as the GPCR antibodies are notoriously problematic (Michel et al., 2009; Trifilieff et al., 2011).

Longitudinal serial sections of the whole fixed carotid bifurcation (5 μm in thickness) were prepared, dewaxed according to routine protocols, and immunostained by anti-$A_{2A}R$ antibody (monoclonal mouse antibody; ab79714, Abcam, United Kingdom) and anti-D_2R antibody (polyclonal rabbit antibody; ab150532, Abcam). The anti-$A_{2A}R$ antibody and the anti-D_2R antibody were used with a dilution of 1:100 and 1:200, respectively; antigen retrieval occurred before both staining with high pH (EnVision^{TM} FLEX, High pH, K8012) and low pH (EnVision^{TM} FLEX, Low pH, K8005) buffer. The sections were incubated using the DAKO Autostainer Plus Staining System (EnVision^{TM} FLEX, High pH). Immunostaining specificity was confirmed by sections incubated without primary antibody, which did not show immunoreactivity.

Proximity-Ligation Assay (PLA)

PLA technology allows easy visualization of endogenous protein–protein interactions at the single-molecule level. The method relies on the use of combinations of antibodies coupled to complementary oligonucleotides that are amplified and revealed with a fluorescent probe. Each single protein–protein interaction is visualized as a fluorescent spot.

In situ PLA was performed according to the manufacturer's instructions on 5-μm rat and human CB slices using the following: mouse anti-A_{2A} primary antibody (dilution: 1:100); rabbit anti-D_2R primary antibody (dilution: 1:200); Duolink® *in situ* PLA detection kit (DUO92014, Sigma-Aldrich, St Louis, MO, United States); Duolink® anti-rabbit PLUS probe (DUO92002, Sigma-Aldrich); and Duolink® anti-mouse MINUS probe (DUO82040, Sigma-Aldrich). Briefly, the slices were blocked with Duolink® blocking solution, in a humid chamber for 60 min at 37°C and then incubated with the primary antibodies (anti-$A_{2A}R$ and anti-D_2R) solution prepared in the antibody diluent solution; incubation occurred in a humid chamber for 1 h at room temperature (RT). Thereafter, the primary antibody solution was tapped off and the slices were washed with wash buffer at RT, before incubation with the anti-rabbit and anti-mouse secondary antibody-conjugated PLA probes in a preheated humidity chamber, for 1 h at 37°C. After hybridization, ligation and amplification steps were performed. For TH and S100 colocalization analysis, after the amplification step, the slices were rinsed in wash buffer and (a) incubated with anti-TH (1:6,000) in Antibody Diluent solution (Dako) or (b) incubated with anti-S100 (1:7,000) in a humid chamber at 4°C, overnight. Subsequently, after a wash in PBS, incubation was performed using mouse Alexa Fluor-488 (1:100; 1 h at RT) for TH or rabbit Alexa Fluor-488 (1:500; 1 h at RT) for S100. Thereafter, the sections were rinsed in PBS and mounted with Vectashield mounting medium for fluorescence with DAPI (Vector Laboratories, Burlingame, CA, United States) for 15 min at RT.

Immunofluorescence and PLA signals were analyzed and acquired with Zeiss800 confocal microscope equipped with 63× oil objective (NA = 1.4). For each field of view, z-stacks were acquired for a total thickness of 10 μm. Images were acquired enabling the identification of the $A_{2A}R$–D_2R heterodimers at confocal microscopy as red dots. In order to better detail the localization of the red dots with reference to nuclei and membranes of different cell types, images were analyzed with the help of z projections and 3D volume rendering through different perspectives. This permitted to better localize the red dots without bias due to plane overlapping. In particular, Z-stacks were acquired and exported with ZenBlue software. For image visualization in 2D, z projections were performed with FIJI software, while 3D volume rendering was reconstructed with IMARIS software.

Negative control experiments were performed avoiding the conjugation of the primary antibodies with the Duolink® Probes; in turn, no positive reaction occurred, and no red dots were visualized. The specificity of the double immunolabeling was verified by replacing the primary antibodies with PBS.

Quantification of the PLA signal was performed on z-stack images, and the number of red dots was manually counted with ImageJ, using the cell counter plugin. The average data referring to the density of positive PLA elements ± SD are related to images acquired from at least 3 randomly chosen fields from three slides of each animal/patient. The percentages of colocalization of red dots with TH and S100 immunostainings were also calculated.

RESULTS

$A_{2A}R$ and D_2R by Immunohistochemistry

Adenosine $A_{2A}R$ and dopamine D_2R were identified through immunohistochemistry in both rat and human CBs (**Figure 1**). Considering 3′-diaminobenzidine tetrahydrochloride (DAB) distribution, $A_{2A}R$- and D_2R-positive elements were mainly localized in correspondence of type I cells, being similarly arranged in clusters. However, partial immunostaining of $A_{2A}R$ and D_2R also in type II cells and PG nerve terminals cannot be excluded.

Detection of the $A_{2A}R$–D_2R Heterodimers by PLA

PLA is an antibody-based method to detect biomolecules in physical proximity, and thus, it is recognized as an important experimental approach to demonstrate physical RRIs when native molecules are localized within a radius of 0–16 nm, a distance considered crucial for heteromer formation. Only in case of physical closeness of proteins will a signal be produced. Here, possible heterodimerization between $A_{2A}R$ and D_2R was verified through PLA. Under a confocal microscope, in both rat and human CBs, most red dots were recognized close to the DAPI-stained nuclei but not inside them, supporting location at the plasma membrane level; 3D visualization of the tissues allowed for a better topographical analysis (**Figures 2**, **3**). As it regards the few red dots which were far away from the nuclei, we cannot exclude a localization in afferent terminals from the carotid sinus nerve. A homogeneous distribution of heterodimers was observed in all specimens with a mean density (± standard deviation) of $(3.5 \pm 0.67) \times 10^{-3}$ heterodimers/μm^2 and $(5.9 \pm 1.4) \times 10^{-3}$ heterodimers/μm^2 in rat and human samples, respectively.

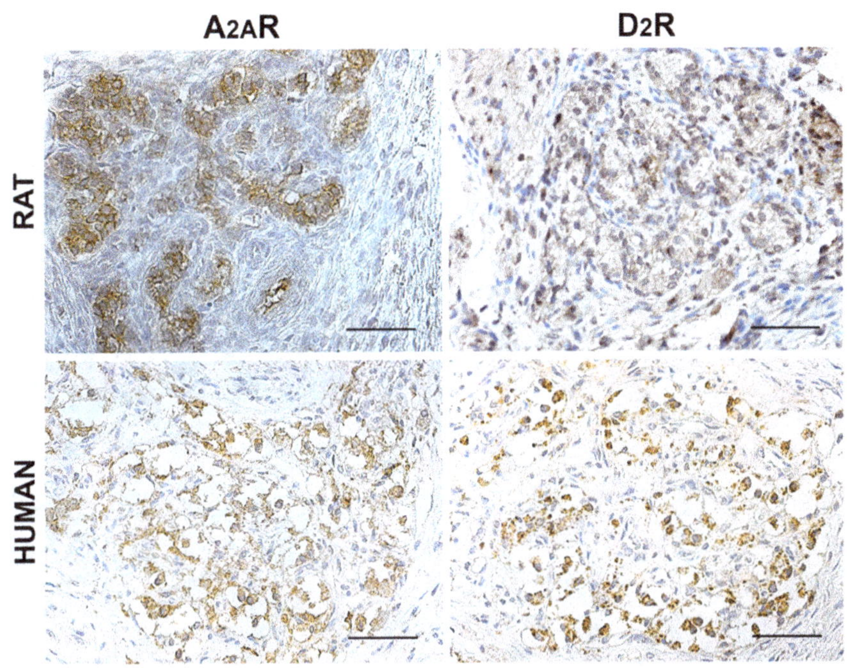

FIGURE 1 | Distribution of adenosine $A_{2A}R$ and dopamine D_2R in rat and human CB. Positive immunostaining in clusters of roundish cells is consistent with type I cells, although some positive elongated cells may be considered as type II cells. Scale bar: 50 μm.

After PLA, specific TH and S100 immunostaining was also performed to distinguish type I and type II cells. This methodological approach allowed to assess by confocal microscopy the localization of the $A_{2A}R$–D_2R heterodimers with respect to the CB constituent cells. In all stained specimens, S100-immunopositive cells, corresponding to type II cells, were specifically visualized as yellow elements; TH immunoreactivity was observed in the cytoplasm of CB type I cells and visualized in green (**Figure 4**). We cannot exclude possible visualization of TH-positive afferent nerve fibers, as also PG terminals may be TH immunoreactive (Katz et al., 1983; Katz and Black, 1986).

In rats, the percentages of TH and S100 colocalizations of red dots were 51.49 ± 5.97 and 55.84 ± 3.63, respectively. In human samples, the percentages of TH and S100 colocalizations of red dots were 60.65 ± 8.49 and 50.75 ± 6.30, respectively. Significant differences were not found between TH and S100 colocalizations in the two different species.

As previously stated, the presence of red dots far away from nuclei and possibly positive for TH may be interpreted as localization of $A_{2A}R$–D_2R heterodimers in PG terminals, as they may express $A_{2A}R$ (Gauda, 2000; Gauda et al., 2000; Conde et al., 2012; Zhang et al., 2018; Sacramento et al., 2019) and D_2R (Czyzyk-Krzeska et al., 1992; Schamel and Verna, 1993; Bairam et al., 1996a,b).

DISCUSSION

Type I CB cells release many different neurotransmitters (i.e., acetylcholine, adenosine, ATP, dopamine) with excitatory or inhibitory effects (Iturriaga and Alcayaga, 2004). Among the main receptors mediating adenosine and dopamine function in the CB, $A_{2A}R$, and D_2R are included. Experimental data support the presence of $A_{2A}R$ (Gauda, 2000; Gauda et al., 2000; Kobayashi et al., 2000; Xu et al., 2006; Bairam et al., 2009; Fagerlund et al., 2010) and D_2R (Czyzyk-Krzeska et al., 1992; Holgert et al., 1995; Gauda et al., 1996, 2001; Bairam et al., 1996b, 2003; Bairam and Khandjian, 1997; Gauda, 2000; Kinkead et al., 2005; Fagerlund et al., 2010; Wakai et al., 2015) in CB type I cells. Kaelin-Lang et al. (1998) also recognized, by *in situ* hybridization on rats, $A_{2A}R$-positive elements likely attributable to type II cells. Even referring to D_2R, a recent paper by Leonard and Nurse (2020), considering the possible inhibitory role of dopamine on type II cell function, suggests D_2R localization in type II cells. Our data indicated the presence of $A_{2A}R$–D_2R heterodimers both in type I and II cells of rats and humans.

PG neurons and terminals are known to express $A_{2A}R$ (Gauda, 2000; Gauda et al., 2000; Conde et al., 2012; Zhang et al., 2018; Sacramento et al., 2019) and D_2R (Czyzyk-Krzeska et al., 1992; Schamel and Verna, 1993; Bairam et al., 1996a,b). Moreover, afferent terminals in the CB may also express TH (Katz et al., 1983; Katz and Black, 1986). Thus, red dots far away from nuclei and colocalizing with faint fluorescent staining may be interpreted as nerve localization of $A_{2A}R$–D_2R heterodimers.

Typically, $A_{2A}Rs$ are coupled to G_s protein, whose activation increases the cAMP levels, promoting an excitatory behavior (Weaver, 1993; Lahiri et al., 2007; De Caro et al., 2013). In the CB, the increase of adenosine levels determined by hypoxia induces the increase in intracellular cAMP through stimulation of $A_{2A}R$ (Lahiri et al., 2007). Adenosine activation of $A_{2A}R$ also triggers

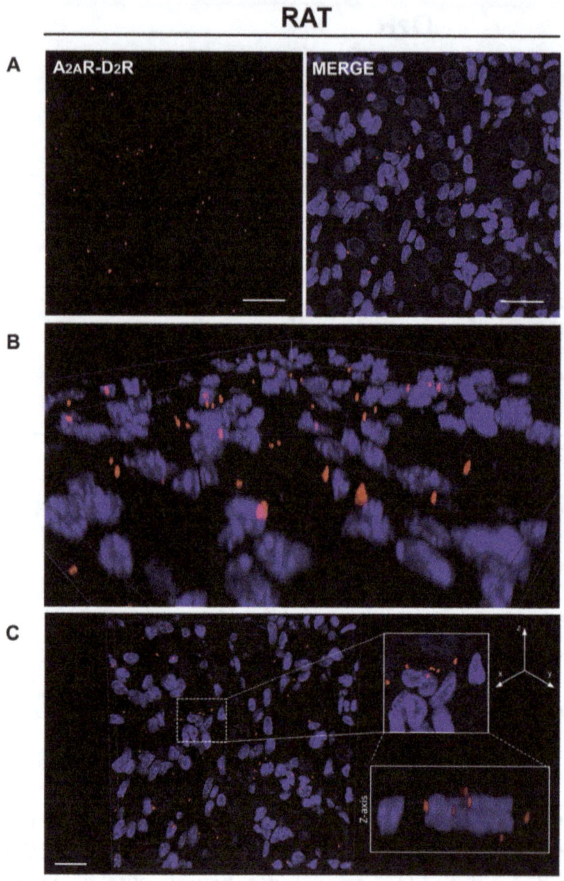

FIGURE 2 | (A) Evidence for the existence of $A_{2A}R$–D_2R heterodimers in rat CB samples by PLA. Red dots showed the proximity of adenosine $A_{2A}R$ and dopamine D_2R, indicating $A_{2A}R$–D_2R heterodimerization. The merged images highlighted the $A_{2A}R$–D_2R localization with respect to the cell nuclei (blue-fluorescent DAPI). Scale bar: 25 μm. **(B)** Representative 3D volume rendering of a sample area from **(A)** allowing assessment of red dot localization with respect to the cell nuclei. **(C)** Representative image of nuclei/red dots apparently appearing as superimposed (white dotted square in the image; corresponding magnification on the right side insert) and visualized in detail through z projection (lower right insert), thus showing a localization adjacent to the nucleus, but not inside it. Scale bar: 20 μm.

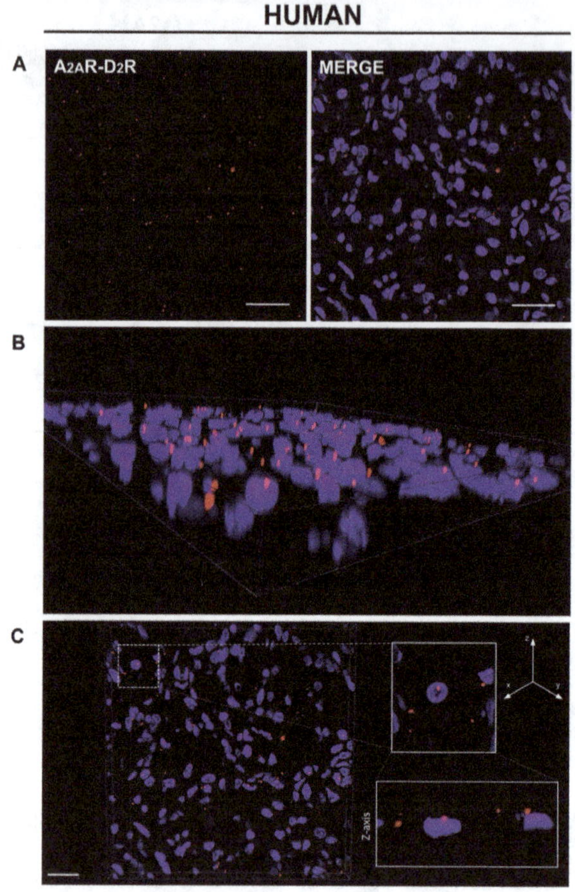

FIGURE 3 | (A) Evidence for the existence of $A_{2A}R$–D_2R heterodimers in human CB samples by PLA. Red dots showed the proximity of adenosine $A_{2A}R$ and dopamine D_2R, indicating $A_{2A}R$–D_2R heterodimerization. The merged images highlighted the $A_{2A}R$–D_2R localization with respect to the cell nuclei (blue-fluorescent DAPI). Scale bar: 25 μm. **(B)** Representative 3D volume rendering of a sample area from **(A)** allowing assessment of red dot localization with respect to the cell nuclei. **(C)** Representative image of nuclei/red dots apparently appearing as superimposed (white dotted square in the image; corresponding magnification on the right side insert) and visualized in detail through z projection (lower right insert), thus showing a localization adjacent to the nucleus, but not inside it. Scale bar: 20 μm.

Ca^{2+} rise during hypoxia (Kobayashi et al., 2000; Tse et al., 2012). Similarly, $A_{2A}Rs$ also mediate the effect of hypercapnia (Sacramento et al., 2018). Conversely, D_2Rs are coupled to inhibitory G_1/G_0 proteins and their activation decreases cAMP levels with the onset of an autocrine/paracrine inhibitory signal (Zeng et al., 2007; Wakai et al., 2015; Zhang et al., 2018). Hypoxia is also responsible for dopamine release from CB type I cells and activation of postsynaptic D_2R (Prieto-Lloret et al., 2007) and D_2R activation exerting inhibitory effects (Gonzalez et al., 1994) on ventilation, both during rest (Zapata and Zuazo, 1980) and hypoxic exposure (Nishino and Lahiri, 1981), although direct activation of D_2R in PG terminals could also have a modulatory (Alcayaga et al., 1999; Alcayaga et al., 2003) or even excitatory effect (Alcayaga et al., 2006; Iturriaga et al., 2009), depending on species involved.

Another possible regulative mechanism exists for these receptors, based on direct reciprocal interactions. The formation of $A_{2A}R$–D_2R complexes was highlighted in transfected cells, including SH-SY5Y (Hillion et al., 2002; Xie et al., 2010) and HEK-293T cells (Navarro et al., 2014), neuronal primary cultures of rat striatum (Navarro et al., 2014) and enkephalin-containing GABAergic neurons from the mammal striatum (Fink et al., 1992; Fuxe et al., 1998; Trifilieff et al., 2011). $A_{2A}R$–D_2R heterodimers are key modulators of striatal neuronal function (Taura et al., 2018); here, heterodimerization showed to modulate GABAergic striato-pallidal neuronal activity. Reciprocal antagonistic interactions occur within the $A_{2A}R$–D_2R heterodimer (Fuxe et al., 2005). In particular, $A_{2A}R$ ligands decrease both the affinity and the signal intensity of D_2R ligands (Ferré et al., 2016), determining the increased

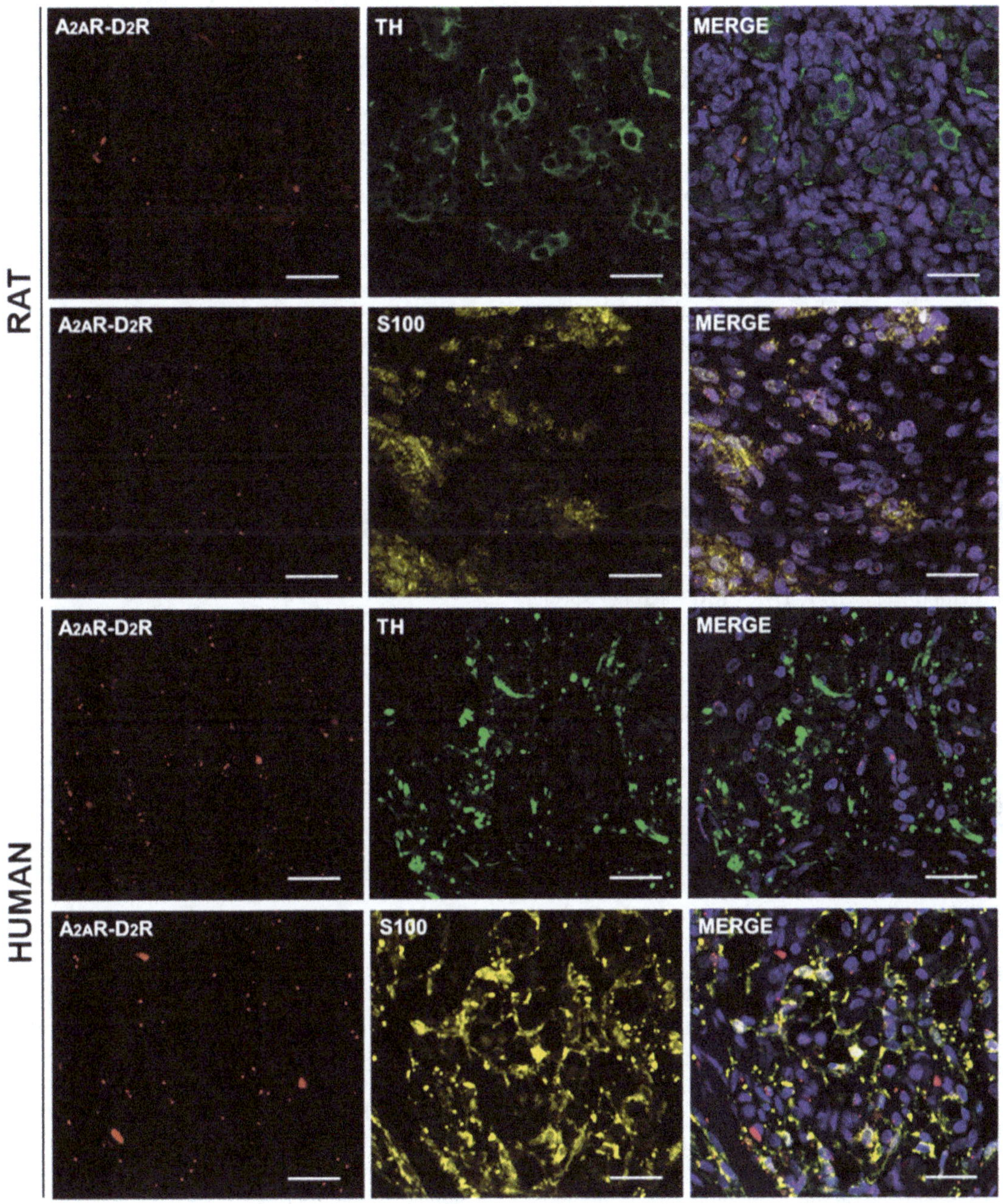

FIGURE 4 | TH and S100 immunofluorescence in representative rat and human CB samples after $A_{2A}R$–D_2R PLA. Red dots showed A_{2A}–D_2 receptors heterodimers; anti-TH (visualized in green) and anti-S100 (visualized in yellow) staining allowed to distinguish type I and type II cells, respectively. Cell nuclei were recognizable after DAPI staining (visualized in blue) in the merge images. Scale bar: 25 μm.

excitatory activity of adenosine, while D_2R agonists decrease the binding of $A_{2A}R$ ligands (Fernández-Dueñas et al., 2018), causing increased inhibitory activity of dopamine. For instance, after incubation of striatal membrane preparations with the $A_{2A}R$ agonist CGS21680, the affinity of the high-affinity D_2R agonist-binding site decreases (Fuxe et al., 1998; Guidolin et al., 2018). $A_{2A}R$–D_2R interactions may be modulated by different drugs (some of which with well-known effects on the CB); for instance, the psychostimulant effects of caffeine are also mediated by the blockage of the allosteric modulation within the $A_{2A}R$–D_2R heterodimer, by which adenosine decreases the affinity and intrinsic efficacy of dopamine at the D_2R (Bonaventura et al., 2015).

Existence of RRI (A_{2B}–D_2) in CB chemoreceptors was first postulated by Conde et al. (2008) to explain the possible mechanism involved in catecholamine release by the CB. Thereafter, due to the glomic expression of a huge amount of different G protein-coupled receptors, our group hypothesized a possible heterodimerization between many other different receptors in the CB (Porzionato et al., 2018). Thus, the aim of this experimental work was to verify the existence of RRIs in the CB, suggesting a possible experimental strategy for its future characterization but also a new interpretive key for a broad comprehension of the regulative mechanisms it presides over.

To date, many biochemical and/or biophysical methods are available to demonstrate receptor colocalization. Among them, the PLA technique allows easy visualization of endogenous protein–protein interactions at the single molecule level (Ristic et al., 2016). Our data by PLA analysis confirmed the existence of $A_{2A}R$–D_2R heterodimers in both type I and type II cells of the CB, indicating that RRI may have a role in the functional modulation of these cells.

The identification of $A_{2A}R$–D_2R RRI in type II cells further supports a role for these cells in chemosensory modulation, in accordance with other authors (Kaelin-Lang et al., 1998; Tse et al., 2012; Leonard and Nurse, 2020). This finding, to be further detailed, could be particularly intriguing as $A_{2A}R$–D_2R heterodimers have also been identified in astrocytes (Cervetto et al., 2017, 2018; Pelassa et al., 2019; Guidolin et al., 2020).

The confirmation of $A_{2A}R$–D_2R RRI across species strengthens the idea on their contributory role in physiological events mediated by the CB. The differences between rats and humans in terms of amount and distribution of $A_{2A}R$–D_2R RRI may conversely be ascribed to species-specific differences and/or to potential exposure to different stimuli. The CB is known to undergo plastic changes in response to development/aging and various environmental stimuli, including chronic intermittent/sustained hypoxia. Its function is strictly related to these dynamic modifications (Iturriaga et al., 2006; López-Barneo et al., 2009; Dmitrieff et al., 2011; Kumar and Prabhakar, 2012; Bavis et al., 2013; Del Rio et al., 2014; Pulgar-Sepúlveda et al., 2018; Bavis et al., 2019; Liu et al., 2019), which can be also ascribed to the specific receptor behavior.

Various environmental stimuli could potentially modulate $A_{2A}R$–D_2R RRI. For instance, $A_{2A}R$ can be present intracellularly and migrate to the cell membrane upon stimulation (Arslan et al., 2002; Milojević et al., 2006; Yu et al., 2006; Sacramento et al., 2015). In this sense, hypoxic effects on RRI will be surely to be evaluated, as hypoxia exerts an increase in adenosine and dopamine release from CB chemoreceptors (Conde et al., 2012), likely inducing a receptor-level modulation, as shown in rabbits by Bairam et al. (2003). Chronic caffeine treatment induces an increase in both adenosine and dopamine (Conde et al., 2012), and neonatal caffeine treatment increases the mRNA levels encoding for $A_{2A}R$ (Montandon et al., 2008; Bairam et al., 2009) and D_2 in male rats CB (not in female) (Montandon et al., 2008). Moreover, $A_{2A}R$ and D_2R expressions are also modulated by age. D_2R mRNA increases with maturation (Gauda et al., 2000, 2001; Gauda, 2000; Gauda and Lawson, 2000), whereas $A_{2A}R$ mRNA decreases (Gauda, 2000; Gauda and Lawson, 2000). Thus, further analyses will also have to address possible changes in $A_{2A}R$–D_2R RRI in response to development/age, hypoxic stimuli, or possible effects by other factors (drugs, metabolism, and others), allowing for a broad comparative study in different pathophysiological conditions.

Moreover, future perspectives of the work will include the involvement of other methods to better detail RRI, such as biophysical (e.g., bioluminescence- and fluorescence-resonance energy transfer; specialized microscopic techniques; X-ray crystallography) and biochemical analyses.

ETHICS STATEMENT

The studies involving human participants were reviewed and approved by the Body Donation Program of the Section of Human Anatomy, University of Padova, according to European, Italian and regional guidelines. Excision was furtherly authorized by the Italian law No. 10 of February 10, 2020, entitled "Rules regarding the disposition of one's body and post-mortem tissues for study, training, and scientific research purposes." The patients/participants provided their written informed consent to participate in this study. The animal study was reviewed and approved by the Ethical Committee of Padua University, in accordance with the Italian Department of Health Guidelines.

AUTHOR CONTRIBUTIONS

AP, RD, VM, ES, and MS designed the study. MS and ES performed the experiments. MC and SB supported the experiments. GB and FR performed the confocal microscopy analyses. AP, RD, ES, MS, DG, and VM interpreted the data. ES and AP wrote the manuscript. RD and AP supervised the final manuscript. All authors have read and agreed to the published version of the manuscript.

REFERENCES

Alcayaga, J., Retamal, M., Cerpa, V., Arroyo, J., and Zapata, P. (2003). Dopamine inhibits ATP-induced responses in the cat petrosal ganglion in vitro. *Brain Res.* 966, 283–287. doi: 10.1016/s0006-8993(02)04215-4

Alcayaga, J., Soto, C. R., Vargas, R. V., Ortiz, F. C., Arroyo, J., and Iturriaga, R. (2006). Carotid body transmitters actions on rabbit petrosal ganglion in vitro. *Adv. Exp. Med. Biol.* 580, 331–337. doi: 10.1007/0-387-31311-7_51

Alcayaga, J., Varas, R., Arroyo, J., Iturriaga, R., and Zapata, P. (1999). Dopamine modulates carotid nerve responses induced by acetylcholine on the cat petrosal ganglion in vitro. *Brain Res.* 831, 97–103. doi: 10.1016/s0006-8993(99)01402-x

Aldossary, H. S., Alzahrani, A. A., Nathanael, D., Alhuthail, E. A., Ray, C. J., Batis, N., et al. (2020). G-Protein-Coupled Receptor (GPCR) Signaling in the Carotid Body: roles in Hypoxia and Cardiovascular and Respiratory Disease. *Int. J. Mol. Sci.* 21:6012. doi: 10.3390/ijms21176012

Arslan, G., Kull, B., and Fredholm, B. B. (2002). Anoxia redistributes adenosine A(2A) receptors in PC12 cells and increases receptor-mediated formation of cAMP. *Naunyn Schmiedebergs Arch. Pharmacol.* 365, 150–157. doi: 10.1007/s002100100456

Bairam, A., Carroll, J. L., Labelle, Y., and Khandjian, E. W. (2003). Differential changes in dopamine D2- and D1-receptor mRNA levels induced by hypoxia in the arterial chemoreflex pathway organs in one-day-old and adult rabbits. *Biol. Neonate* 84, 222–231. doi: 10.1159/000072306

Bairam, A., Dauphin, C., Rousseau, F., and Khandjian, E. W. (1996a). Dopamine D2 receptor mRNA isoforms expression in the carotid body and petrosal ganglion of developing rabbits. *Adv. Exp. Med. Biol.* 410, 285–289. doi: 10.1007/978-1-4615-5891-0_43

Bairam, A., Dauphin, C., Rousseau, F., and Khandjian, E. W. (1996b). Expression of dopamine D2-receptor mRNA isoforms at the peripheral chemoreflex afferent pathway in developing rabbits. *Am. J. Respir. Cell Mol. Biol.* 15, 374–381. doi: 10.1165/ajrcmb.15.3.8810642

Bairam, A., Joseph, V., Lajeunesse, Y., and Kinkead, R. (2009). Altered expression of adenosine A1 and A2A receptors in the carotid body and nucleus tractus solitarius of adult male and female rats following neonatal caffeine treatment. *Brain Res.* 1287, 74–83. doi: 10.1016/j.brainres.2009.06.064

Bairam, A., and Khandjian, E. W. (1997). Expression of dopamine D2 receptor mRNA isoforms in the carotid body of rat, cat and rabbit. *Brain Res.* 760, 287–289.

Bavis, R. W., Fallon, S. C., and Dmitrieff, E. F. (2013). Chronic hyperoxia and the development of the carotid body. *Respir. Physiol. Neurobiol.* 185, 94–104. doi: 10.1016/j.resp.2012.05.019

Bavis, R. W., Millström, A. H., Kim, S. M., MacDonald, C. A., O'Toole, C. A., Asklof, K., et al. (2019). Combined effects of intermittent hyperoxia and intermittent hypercapnic hypoxia on respiratory control in neonatal rats. *Respir. Physiol. Neurobiol.* 260, 70–81. doi: 10.1016/j.resp.2018.11.002

Bonaventura, J., Navarro, G., Casadó-Anguera, V., Azdad, K., Rea, W., Moreno, E., et al. (2015). Allosteric interactions between agonists and antagonists within the adenosine A_{2A} receptor-dopamine D_2 receptor heterotetramer. *Proc. Natl. Acad. Sci. U. S. A.* 112, E3609–E3618. doi: 10.1073/pnas.1507704112

Boscolo-Berto, R., Porzionato, A., Stecco, C., Macchi, V., and De Caro, R. (2020). Body donation in Italy: lights and shadows of law No. 10/2020. *Clin. Anat.* 33, 950–959. doi: 10.1002/ca.23623

Cervetto, C., Venturini, A., Guidolin, D., Maura, G., Passalacqua, M., Tacchetti, C., et al. (2018). Homocysteine and A2A-D2 Receptor-Receptor Interaction at Striatal Astrocyte Processes. *J. Mol. Neurosci.* 65, 456–466. doi: 10.1007/s12031-018-1120-4

Cervetto, C., Venturini, A., Passalacqua, M., Guidolin, D., Genedani, S., Fuxe, K., et al. (2017). A2A-D2 receptor-receptor interaction modulates gliotransmitter release from striatal astrocyte processes. *J. Neurochem.* 140, 268–279. doi: 10.1111/jnc.13885

Conde, S. V., Gonzalez, C., Batuca, J. R., Monteiro, E. C., and Obeso, A. (2008). An antagonistic interaction between A2B adenosine and D2 dopamine receptors modulates the function of rat carotid body chemoreceptor cells. *J. Neurochem.* 107, 1369–1381. doi: 10.1111/j.1471-4159.2008.05704.x

Conde, S. V., Monteiro, E. C., and Sacramento, J. F. (2017). Purines and Carotid Body: new Roles in Pathological Conditions. *Front. Pharmacol.* 8:913. doi: 10.3389/fphar.2017.00913

Conde, S. V., Obeso, A., Vicario, I., Rigual, R., Rocher, A., and Gonzalez, C. (2006). Caffeine inhibition of rat carotid body chemoreceptors is mediated by A2A and A2B adenosine receptors. *J. Neurochem.* 98, 616–628. doi: 10.1111/j.1471-4159.2006.03912.x

Conde, S. V., Ribeiro, M. J., Obeso, A., Rigual, R., Monteiro, E. C., and Gonzalez, C. (2012). Chronic caffeine intake in adult rat inhibits carotid body sensitization produced by chronic sustained hypoxia but maintains intact chemoreflex output. *Mol. Pharmacol.* 82, 1056–1065. doi: 10.1124/mol.112.081216

Conde, S. V., Sacramento, J. F., and Guarino, M. P. (2018). Carotid body: a metabolic sensor implicated in insulin resistance. *Physiol. Genomics.* 50, 208–214. doi: 10.1152/physiolgenomics.00121.2017

Cunha-Guimaraes, J. P., Guarino, M. P., Timóteo, A. T., Caires, I., Sacramento, J. F., Ribeiro, M. J., et al. (2020). Carotid body chemosensitivity: early biomarker of dysmetabolism in humans. *Eur. J. Endocrinol.* 182, 549–557. doi: 10.1530/EJE-19-0976

Czyzyk-Krzeska, M. F., Lawson, E. E., and Millhorn, D. E. (1992). Expression of D_2 dopamine receptor mRNA in the arterial chemoreceptor afferent pathway. *J. Auton. Nerv. Syst.* 41, 31–39. doi: 10.1016/0165-1838(92)90124-y

De Caro, R., Macchi, V., and Porzionato, A. (2009). Promotion of body donation and use of cadavers in anatomical education at the University of Padova. *Anat. Sci. Educ.* 2, 91–92. doi: 10.1002/ase.69

De Caro, R., Macchi, V., Sfriso, M. M., and Porzionato, A. (2013). Structural and neurochemical changes in the maturation of the carotid body. *Respir. Physiol. Neurobiol.* 185, 9–19. doi: 10.1016/j.resp.2012.06.012

Del Rio, R., Moya, E. A., and Iturriaga, R. (2014). Carotid body potentiation during chronic intermittent hypoxia: implication for hypertension. *Front. Physiol.* 5:434. doi: 10.3389/fphys.2014.00434

Di Giulio, C. (2018). Ageing of the carotid body. *J. Physiol.* 596, 3021–3027. doi: 10.1113/JP275300

Dmitrieff, E. F., Wilson, J. T., Dunmire, K. B., and Bavis, R. W. (2011). Chronic hyperoxia alters the expression of neurotrophic factors in the carotid body of neonatal rats. *Respir. Physiol. Neurobiol.* 175, 220–227. doi: 10.1016/j.resp.2010.11.007

Fagerlund, M. J., Kåhlin, J., Ebberyd, A., Schulte, G., Mkrtchian, S., and Eriksson, L. I. (2010). The human carotid body: expression of oxygen sensing and signaling genes of relevance for anesthesia. *Anesthesiology* 113, 1270–1279. doi: 10.1097/ALN.0b013e3181fac061

Fernández-Dueñas, V., Ferré, S., and Ciruela, F. (2018). Adenosine A2A-dopamine D2 receptor heteromers operate striatal function: impact on Parkinson's disease pharmacotherapeutics. *Neural Regen. Res.* 13, 241–243. doi: 10.4103/1673-5374.226388

Ferré, S., Bonaventura, J., Tomasi, D., Navarro, G., Moreno, E., Cortés, A., et al. (2016). Allosteric mechanisms within the adenosine A2A-dopamine D2 receptor heterotetramer. *Neuropharmacology* 104, 154–160. doi: 10.1016/j.neuropharm.2015.05.028

Ferré, S., Casado, V., Devi, L. A., Filizola, M., Jockers, R., Lohse, M. J., et al. (2014). G protein-coupled receptor oligomerization revisited: functional and pharmacological perspectives. *Pharmacol. Rev.* 66, 413–434. doi: 10.1124/pr.113.008052

Fink, J. S., Weaver, D. R., Rivkees, S. A., Peterfreund, R. A., Pollack, A. E., Adler, E. M., et al. (1992). Molecular cloning of the rat A2 adenosine receptor: selective co-expression with D2 dopamine receptors in rat striatum. *Brain Res. Mol. Brain Res.* 14, 186–195. doi: 10.1016/0169-328x(92)90173-9

Fitzgerald, R. S., Eyzaguirre, C., and Zapata, P. (2009). Fifty years of progress in carotid body physiology – invited article. *Adv. Exp. Med. Biol.* 648, 19–28. doi: 10.1007/978-90-481-2259-2_2

Fuxe, K., Ferré, S., Canals, M., Torvinen, M., Terasmaa, A., Marcellino, D., et al. (2005). Adenosine A2A and dopamine D2 heteromeric receptor complexes and their function. *J. Mol. Neurosci.* 26, 209–219. doi: 10.1385/JMN:26:2-3:209

Fuxe, K., Ferré, S., Zoli, M., and Agnati, L. F. I. (1998).). Integrated events in central dopamine transmission as analyzed at multiple levels. Evidence for intramembrane adenosine A2A/dopamine D2 and adenosine A1/dopamine D1 receptor interactions in the basal ganglia. *Brain Res. Rev.* 26, 258–273. doi: 10.1016/s0165-0173(97)00049-0

Gauda, E. B. (2000). Expression and localization of A2a and A1-adenosine receptor genes in the rat carotid body and petrosal ganglia. A2a and A1-adenosine receptor mRNAs in the rat carotid body. *Adv. Exp. Med. Biol.* 475, 549–558.

Gauda, E. B., Bamford, O., and Gerfen, C. R. (1996). Developmental expression of tyrosine hydroxylase, D2-dopamine receptor and substance P genes in the carotid body of the rat. *Neuroscience* 75, 969–977. doi: 10.1016/0306-4522(96)00312-0

Gauda, E. B., Cooper, R., Akins, P. K., and Wu, G. (2001). Prenatal nicotine affects catecholamine gene expression in newborn rat carotid body and petrosal ganglion. *J. Appl. Physiol.* 91, 2157–2165. doi: 10.1152/jappl.2001.91.5.2157

Gauda, E. B., and Lawson, E. E. (2000). Developmental influences on carotid body responses to hypoxia. *Respir. Physiol.* 121, 199–208. doi: 10.1016/s0034-5687(00)00128-6

Gauda, E. B., Northington, F. J., Linden, J., and Rosin, D. L. (2000). Differential expression of a(2a), A(1)-adenosine and D(2)-dopamine receptor genes in rat peripheral arterial chemoreceptors during postnatal development. *Brain Res.* 872, 1–10. doi: 10.1016/s0006-8993(00)02314-3

Gonzalez, C., Almaraz, L., Obeso, A., and Rigual, R. (1994). Carotid body chemoreceptors: from natural stimuli to sensory discharges. *Physiol. Rev.* 74, 829–898. doi: 10.1152/physrev.1994.74.4.829

Guidolin, D., Agnati, L. F., Marcoli, M., Borroto-Escuela, D., and Fuxe, K. (2015). G-protein-coupled receptor type A heteromers as an emerging therapeutic target. *Expert Opin. Ther. Targets* 19, 265–283. doi: 10.1517/14728222.2014.981155

Guidolin, D., Marcoli, M., Tortorella, C., Maura, G., and Agnati, L. F. (2018). G protein-coupled receptor-receptor interactions give integrative dynamics to intercellular communication. *Rev. Neurosci.* 29, 703–726. doi: 10.1515/revneuro-2017-0087

Guidolin, D., Marcoli, M., Tortorella, C., Maura, G., and Agnati, L. F. (2020). Adenosine A2A-dopamine D2 receptor-receptor interaction in neurons and astrocytes: evidence and perspectives. *Prog. Med. Biol. Transl. Sci.* 169, 247–277. doi: 10.1016/bs.pmbts.2019.11.004

Hillion, J., Canals, M., Torvinen, M., Casadó, V., Scott, R., Terasmaa, A., et al. (2002). Coaggregation, cointernalization, and codesensitization of adenosine A2A receptors and dopamine D2 receptors. *J. Biol. Chem.* 277, 18091–18097. doi: 10.1074/jbc.M107731200

Holgert, H., Hökfelt, T., Hertzberg, T., and Lagercrantz, H. (1995). Functional and developmental studies of the peripheral arterial chemoreceptors in rat: effects of nicotine and possible relation to sudden infant death syndrome. *Proc. Natl. Acad. Sci. U. S. A.* 92, 7575–7579. doi: 10.1073/pnas.92.16.7575

Iturriaga, R. (2018). Translating carotid body function into clinical medicine. *J. Physiol.* 596, 3067–3077. doi: 10.1113/JP275335

Iturriaga, R., and Alcayaga, J. (2004). Neurotransmission in the carotid body: transmitters and modulators between glomus cells and petrosal ganglion nerve terminals. *Brain Res. Brain Res. Rev.* 47, 46–53. doi: 10.1016/j.brainresrev.2004.05.007

Iturriaga, R., Alcayaga, J., and Gonzalez, C. (2009). Neurotransmitters in carotid body function: the case of dopamine–invited article. *Adv. Exp. Med. Biol.* 648, 137–143. doi: 10.1007/978-90-481-2259-2_16

Iturriaga, R., Del Rio, R., Idiaquez, J., and Somers, V. K. (2016). Carotid body chemoreceptors, sympathetic neural activation, and cardiometabolic disease. *Biol. Res.* 49:13. doi: 10.1186/s40659-016-0073-8

Iturriaga, R., Rey, S., Alcayaga, J., and Del Rio, R. (2006). Chronic intermittent hypoxia enhances carotid body chemosensory responses to acute hypoxia. *Adv. Exp. Med. Biol.* 580, 227–232. doi: 10.1007/0-387-31311-7_35

Kaelin-Lang, A., Lauterburg, T., and Burgunder, J. M. (1998). Expression of adenosine A2a receptor gene in rat dorsal root and autonomic ganglia. *Neurosci. Lett.* 246, 21–24. doi: 10.1016/s0304-3940(98)00216-x

Katz, D. M., and Black, I. B. (1986). Expression and regulation of catecholaminergic traits in primary sensory neurons: relationship to target innervation in vivo. *J. Neurosci.* 6, 983–989. doi: 10.1523/JNEUROSCI.06-04-00983.1986

Katz, D. M., Markey, K. A., Goldstein, M., and Black, I. B. (1983). Expression of catecholaminergic characteristics by primary sensory neurons in the normal adult rat in vivo. *Proc. Natl. Acad. Sci. U. S. A.* 80, 3526–3530. doi: 10.1073/pnas.80.11.3526

Kinkead, R., Joseph, V., Lajeunesse, Y., and Bairam, A. (2005). Neonatal maternal separation enhances dopamine D(2)-receptor and tyrosine hydroxylase mRNA expression levels in carotid body of rats. *Can. J. Physiol. Pharmacol.* 83, 76–84. doi: 10.1139/y04-106

Kobayashi, S., Conforti, L., and Millhorn, D. E. (2000). Gene expression and function of adenosine A(2A) receptor in the rat carotid body. *Am. J. Physiol. Lung Cell. Mol. Physiol.* 279, L273–L282. doi: 10.1152/ajplung.2000.279.2.L273

Kumar, P., and Prabhakar, N. R. (2012). Peripheral chemoreceptors: function and plasticity of the carotid body. *Compr. Physiol.* 2, 141–219. doi: 10.1002/cphy.c100069

Lahiri, S., Mitchell, C. H., Reigada, D., Roy, A., and Cherniack, N. S. (2007). Purines, the carotid body and respiration. *Respir. Physiol. Neurobiol.* 157, 123–129. doi: 10.1016/j.resp.2007.02.015

Leonard, E. M., and Nurse, C. A. (2020). Expanding Role of Dopaminergic Inhibition in Hypercapnic Responses of Cultured Rat Carotid Body Cells: involvement of Type II Glial Cells. *Int. J. Mol. Sci.* 21:5434. doi: 10.3390/ijms21155434

Liu, P., Zhang, H. M., Hu, K., Zhou, X. F., and Tang, S. (2019). Sensory plasticity of carotid body is correlated with oxidative stress in paraventricular nucleus during chronic intermittent hypoxia. *J. Cell Physiol.* 234, 13534–13543. doi: 10.1002/jcp.28031

López-Barneo, J., Ortega-Sáenz, P., Pardal, R., Pascual, A., Piruat, J. I., Durán, R., et al. (2009). Oxygen sensing in the carotid body. *Ann. N. Y. Acad. Sci.* 1177, 119–131. doi: 10.1111/j.1749-6632.2009.05033.x

Macchi, V., Porzionato, A., Stecco, C., Tiengo, C., Parenti, A., Cestrone, A., et al. (2011). Body parts removed during surgery: a useful training source. *Anat. Sci. Educ.* 4, 151–156. doi: 10.1002/ase.218

Michel, M. C., Wieland, T., and Tsujimoto, G. (2009). How reliable are G-protein-coupled receptor antibodies? *Naunyn Schmiedebergs Arch. Pharmacol.* 379, 385–388. doi: 10.1007/s00210-009-0395-y

Milojević, T., Reiterer, V., Stefan, E., Korkhov, V. M., Dorostkar, M. M., Ducza, E., et al. (2006). The ubiquitin-specific protease Usp4 regulates the cell surface level of the A2A receptor. *Mol. Pharmacol.* 69, 1083–1094. doi: 10.1124/mol.105.015818

Montandon, G., Bairam, A., and Kinkead, R. (2008). Neonatal caffeine induces sex-specific developmental plasticity of the hypoxic respiratory chemoreflex in adult rats. *Am. J. Physiol. Regul. Integr. Comp. Physiol.* 295, R922–R934. doi: 10.1152/ajpregu.00059.2008

Navarro, G., Aguinaga, D., Moreno, E., Hradsky, J., Reddy, P. P., Cortés, A., et al. (2014). Intracellular calcium levels determine differential modulation of allosteric interactions within G protein-coupled receptor heteromers. *Chem. Biol.* 21, 1546–1566. doi: 10.1016/j.chembiol.2014.10.004

Nishino, T., and Lahiri, S. (1981). Effects of dopamine on chemoreflexes in breathing. *J. Appl. Physiol.* 50, 892–897. doi: 10.1152/jappl.1981.50.4.892

Nurse, C. A. (2005). Neurotransmission and neuromodulation in the chemosensory carotid body. *Auton. Neurosci.* 120, 1–9. doi: 10.1016/j.autneu.2005.04.008

Nurse, C. A. (2014). Synaptic and paracrine mechanisms at carotid body arterial chemoreceptors. *J. Physiol.* 592, 3419–3426. doi: 10.1113/jphysiol.2013.269829

Pardal, R., Ortega-Sáenz, P., Durán, R., and López-Barneo, J. (2007). Glia-like stem cells sustain physiologic neurogenesis in the adult mammalian carotid body. *Cell* 131, 364–377. doi: 10.1016/j.cell.2007.07.043

Pelassa, S., Guidolin, D., Venturini, A., Averna, M., Frumento, G., Campanini, L., et al. (2019). A2A-D2 Heteromers on Striatal Astrocytes: biochemical and Biophysical Evidence. *Int. J. Mol. Sci.* 20:2457. doi: 10.3390/ijms20102457

Porzionato, A., Macchi, V., Belloni, A. S., Parenti, A., and De Caro, R. (2006). Adrenomedullin immunoreactivity in the human carotid body. *Peptides* 27, 69–73. doi: 10.1016/j.peptides.2005.07.017

Porzionato, A., Macchi, V., Guidolin, D., Parenti, A., Ferrara, S. D., and De Caro, R. (2005). Histopathology of carotid body in heroin addiction. Possible chemosensitive impairment. *Histopathology* 46, 296–306. doi: 10.1111/j.1365-2559.2005.02060

Porzionato, A., Macchi, V., Parenti, A., and De Caro, R. (2008). Trophic factors in the carotid body. *Int. Rev. Cell Mol. Biol.* 269, 1–58. doi: 10.1016/S1937-6448(08)01001-0

Porzionato, A., Macchi, V., Stecco, C., Mazzi, A., Rambaldo, A., Sarasin, G., et al. (2012). Quality management of Body Donation Program at the University of Padova. *Anat. Sci. Educ.* 5, 264–272. doi: 10.1002/ase.1285

Porzionato, A., Rucinski, M., Macchi, V., Stecco, C., Castagliuolo, I., Malendowicz, L. K., et al. (2011). Expression of leptin and leptin receptor isoforms in the rat and human carotid body. *Brain Res.* 1385, 56–67. doi: 10.1016/j.brainres.2011.02.028

Porzionato, A., Stocco, E., Guidolin, D., Agnati, L., Macchi, V., and De Caro, R. (2018). Receptor-Receptor Interactions of G Protein-Coupled Receptors in the Carotid Body: a Working Hypothesis. *Front. Physiol.* 9:697. doi: 10.3389/fphys.2018.00697

Prabhakar, N. R., and Peng, Y. J. (2017). Oxygen Sensing by the Carotid Body: past and Present. *Adv. Exp. Med. Biol.* 977, 3–8. doi: 10.1007/978-3-319-55231-6_1

Prieto-Lloret, J., Donnelly, D. F., Rico, A. J., Moratalla, R., González, C., and Rigual, R. J. (2007). Hypoxia transduction by carotid body chemoreceptors in mice lacking dopamine D(2) receptors. *J. Appl. Physiol.* 103, 1269–1275. doi: 10.1152/japplphysiol.00391.2007

Pulgar-Sepúlveda, R., Varas, R., Iturriaga, R., Del Rio, R., and Ortiz, F. C. (2018). Carotid Body Type-I Cells Under Chronic Sustained Hypoxia: focus on Metabolism and Membrane Excitability. *Front. Physiol.* 9:1282. doi: 10.3389/fphys.2018.01282

Riederer, B. M., Bolt, S., Brenner, E., Bueno-Lopez, J. L., Circulescu, A. R. M., Davies, D. C., et al. (2012). The legal and ethical framework governing Body Donation in Europe-1st update on current practice. *Eur. J. Anat.* 16, 1–21.

Ristic, M., Brockly, F., Piechaczyk, M., and Bossis, G. (2016). Detection of Protein–Protein Interactions and Posttranslational Modifications Using the Proximity Ligation Assay: application to the Study of the SUMO Pathway. *Methods Mol. Biol.* 1449, 279–290. doi: 10.1007/978-1-4939-3756-1_17

Sacramento, J. F., Andrzejewski, K., Melo, B. F., Ribeiro, M. J., Obeso, A., and Conde, S. V. (2020). Exploring the Mediators that Promote Carotid Body Dysfunction in Type 2 Diabetes and Obesity Related Syndromes. *Int. J. Mol. Sci.* 21:5545. doi: 10.3390/ijms21155545

Sacramento, J. F., Melo, B. F., and Conde, S. V. (2018). Adenosine Mediates Hypercapnic Response in the Rat Carotid Body via A2A and A2B Receptors. *Adv. Exp. Med. Biol.* 1071, 89–93. doi: 10.1007/978-3-319-91137-3_11

Sacramento, J. F., Olea, E., Ribeiro, M. J., Prieto-Lloret, J., Melo, B. F., Gonzalez, C., et al. (2019). Contribution of adenosine and ATP to the carotid body chemosensory activity in ageing. *J. Physiol.* 597, 4991–5008. doi: 10.1113/JP274179

Sacramento, J. F., Ribeiro, M. J., Yubero, S., Melo, B. F., Obeso, A., Guarino, M. P., et al. (2015). Disclosing caffeine action on insulin sensitivity: effects on rat skeletal muscle. *Eur. J. Pharm. Sci.* 70, 107–116. doi: 10.1016/j.ejps.2015.01.011

Schamel, A., and Verna, A. (1993). Localization of dopamine D2 receptor mRNA in the rabbit carotid body and petrosal ganglion by in situ hybridization. *Adv. Exp. Med. Biol.* 337, 85–91. doi: 10.1007/978-1-4615-2966-8_13

Stocco, E., Barbon, S., Tortorella, C., Macchi, V., De Caro, R., and Porzionato, A. (2020). Growth Factors in the Carotid Body-An Update. *Int. J. Mol. Sci.* 21:7267. doi: 10.3390/ijms21197267

Taura, J., Valle-León, M., Sahlholm, K., Watanabe, M., Van Craenenbroeck, K., Fernández-Dueñas, V., et al. (2018). Behavioral control by striatal adenosine A2A -dopamine D2 receptor heteromers. *Genes Brain Behav.* 17:e12432. doi: 10.1111/gbb.12432

Trifilieff, P., Rives, M. L., Urizar, E., Piskorowski, R. A., Vishwasrao, H. D., Castrillon, J., et al. (2011). Detection of antigen interactions ex vivo by proximity ligation assay: endogenous dopamine D2-adenosine A2A receptor complexes in the striatum. *Biotechniques* 51, 111–118. doi: 10.2144/000113719

Tse, A., Yan, L., Lee, A. K., and Tse, F. W. (2012). Autocrine and paracrine actions of ATP in rat carotid body. *Can. J. Physiol. Pharmacol.* 90, 705–711. doi: 10.1139/y2012-054

Varas, R., Alcayaga, J., and Iturriaga, R. (2003). ACh and ATP mediate excitatory transmission in cat carotid identified chemoreceptor units in vitro. *Brain Res.* 988, 154–163. doi: 10.1016/s0006-8993(03)03366-3

Wakai, J., Takayama, A., Yokoyama, T., Nakamuta, N., Kusakabe, T., and Yamamoto, Y. (2015). Immunohistochemical localization of dopamine D2 receptor in the rat carotid body. *Acta Histochem.* 117, 784–789. doi: 10.1016/j.acthis.2015.07.007

Weaver, D. R. (1993). A2a adenosine receptor gene expression in developing rat brain. *Brain Res. Mol. Brain Res.* 20, 313–327. doi: 10.1016/0169-328x(93)90058-w

Xie, H., Hu, L., and Li, G. (2010). SH-SY5Y human neuroblastoma cell line: in vitro cell model of dopaminergic neurons in Parkinson's disease. *Chin. Med. J.* 123, 1086–1092.

Xu, F., Xu, J., Tse, F. W., and Tse, A. (2006). Adenosine stimulates depolarization and rise in cytoplasmic [Ca2+] in type I cells of rat carotid bodies. *Am. J. Physiol. Cell Physiol.* 290, C1592–C1598. doi: 10.1152/ajpcell.00546.2005

Yu, W., Zacharia, L. C., Jackson, E. K., and Apodaca, G. (2006). Adenosine receptor expression and function in bladder uroepithelium. *Am. J. Physiol. Cell. Physiol.* 291, C254–C265. doi: 10.1152/ajpcell.00025.2006

Zapata, P., and Zuazo, A. (1980). Respiratory effects of dopamine-induced inhibition of chemosensory inflow. *Respir. Physiol.* 40, 79–92. doi: 10.1016/0034-5687(80)90006-7

Zeng, C., Zhang, M., Asico, L. D., Eisner, G. M., and Jose, P. A. (2007). The dopaminergic system in hypertension. *Clin. Sci.* 112, 583–597. doi: 10.1042/CS20070018

Zhang, M., Vollmer, C., and Nurse, C. A. (2018). Adenosine and dopamine oppositely modulate a hyperpolarization-activated current I h in chemosensory neurons of the rat carotid body in co-culture. *J. Physiol.* 596, 3101–3117. doi: 10.1113/JP274743

12

Effect of Nocturnal Oxygen Therapy on Daytime Pulmonary Hemodynamics in Patients with Chronic Obstructive Pulmonary Disease Traveling to Altitude

Mona Lichtblau, Tsogyal D. Latshang, Sayaka S. Aeschbacher, Fabienne Huber, Philipp M. Scheiwiller, Stefanie Ulrich, Simon R. Schneider, Elisabeth D. Hasler, Michael Furian, Konrad E. Bloch, Stéphanie Saxer† *and Silvia Ulrich**†

Department of Pulmonology, University Hospital Zurich, Zurich, Switzerland

***Correspondence:**
Silvia Ulrich
silvia.ulrich@usz.ch

† These authors have contributed equally to this work

Introduction: We investigated whether nocturnal oxygen therapy (NOT) mitigates the increase of pulmonary artery pressure in patients during daytime with chronic obstructive pulmonary disease (COPD) traveling to altitude.

Methods: Patients with COPD living below 800 m underwent examinations at 490 m and during two sojourns at 2,048 m (with a washout period of 2 weeks < 800 m between altitude sojourns). During nights at altitude, patients received either NOT (3 L/min) or placebo (ambient air 3 L/min) via nasal cannula according to a randomized crossover design. The main outcomes were the tricuspid regurgitation pressure gradient (TRPG) measured by echocardiography on the second day at altitude (under ambient air) and various other echocardiographic measures of the right and left heart function. Patients fulfilling predefined safety criteria were withdrawn from the study.

Results: Twenty-three COPD patients [70% Global Initiative for Chronic Obstructive Lung Disease (GOLD) II/30% GOLD III, mean ± SD age 66 ± 5 years, FEV_1 54% ± 13% predicted] were included in the per-protocol analysis. TRPG significantly increased when patients traveled to altitude (from low altitude 21.7 ± 5.2 mmHg to 2,048 m placebo 27.4 ± 7.3 mmHg and 2,048 m NOT 27.8 ± 8.3 mmHg) difference between interventions (mean difference 0.4 mmHg, 95% CI −2.1 to 3.0, $p = 0.736$). The tricuspid annular plane systolic excursion was significantly higher after NOT vs. placebo [2.6 ± 0.6 vs. 2.3 ± 0.4 cm, mean difference (95% confidence interval) 0.3 (0.1 – 0.5) cm, $p = 0.005$]. During visits to 2,048 m until 24 h after descent, eight patients (26%) using placebo and one (4%) using

NOT had to be withdrawn because of altitude-related adverse health effects ($p < 0.001$).

Conclusion: In lowlanders with COPD remaining free of clinically relevant altitude-related adverse health effects, changes in daytime pulmonary hemodynamics during a stay at high altitude were trivial and not modified by NOT.

Keywords: chronic obstructive pulmonary disease, altitude, oxygen, echocardiography, right heart function

INTRODUCTION

Chronic obstructive pulmonary disease (COPD) is a highly prevalent disease and according to the World Health Organization one of the three leading causes of death worldwide (Rhodes et al., 1991). Inhaled noxious particles, mainly cigarette smoke and indoor air pollution, cause chronic inflammation leading to increased collapsibility and narrowing of the airways reflected by a decreased forced expiratory volume in 1 s (FEV_1) (Global Initiative for Chronic Obstructive Lung Disease, 2019). It is known that patients with COPD frequently suffer from right heart dysfunction due to progressive pulmonary hypertension (PH) especially during exercise and in the presence of frequent comorbidities, such as obstructive sleep apnea or nocturnal hypoxemia (Macnee, 2010; Ulrich et al., 2010; Fossati et al., 2014; Global Initiative for Chronic Obstructive Lung Disease, 2019). It has been shown that COPD patients with an elevated pulmonary artery pressure (PAP) have a worse survival than those with a normal PAP (Macnee, 2010).

The current Global Initiative for Chronic Obstructive Lung Disease (GOLD) guidelines include recommendations for the use of long-term oxygen therapy (>15 h/day) in hypoxemic patients as well as the use of short-term oxygen therapy during air travel (Johnson, 2010). During flights, a partial pressure of oxygen (PaO_2) of at least 50 mmHg should be maintained, and patients with an oxygen saturation (SpO_2) above 95% at rest and $SpO_2 > 84\%$ during the 6-min walking test at sea level are usually able to travel without supplemental oxygen. Recommendations for altitude sojourns in COPD patients are lacking; meanwhile, several studies on COPD patients and altitude travel have been conducted (Furian et al., 2018b,c, 2019; Muralt et al., 2018; Latshang et al., 2019; Lichtblau et al., 2019a,b, 2020; Schwarz et al., 2019; Tan et al., 2020; Carta et al., 2021). It is known that patients with COPD may suffer from hypoxemia when traveling to altitude and that altitude travel increases PAP, induces the occurrence of intracardiac and intrapulmonary right-to-left shunts, and reduces exercise capacity (Furian et al., 2018a,b; Lichtblau et al., 2018, 2019b, 2020; Latshang et al., 2019; Schwarz et al., 2019).

Nocturnal oxygen therapy (NOT) has been shown to improve hypoxemia, sleep apnea, and subjective sleep quality in patients with COPD traveling to altitude (Tan et al., 2020). Whether NOT positively affects the altitude-induced increase of the PAP is unknown. Thus, the aim of the current study was to investigate whether NOT could mitigate the effect of altitude on PAP in stable COPD patients traveling to 2,048 m.

MATERIALS AND METHODS

Study Design

This randomized, placebo-controlled, crossover trial in patients with COPD living below 800 m was performed between January 1 and October 31, 2014 within the scope of a project evaluating effects of oxygen on various outcomes in COPD patients staying at high altitude. Baseline characteristics and data on nocturnal oxygenation, sleep apnea, and altitude-related adverse health effects have been reported (Tan et al., 2020); but data on echocardiographic findings, the focus of the current study, have not been published. Patients were assessed at low altitude (Zurich, 490 m); and during two altitude sojourns for 2 days at 2,048 m (St. Moritz), where they either received NOT or placebo (ambient air) during nights, in a randomized order, echocardiography was performed in the morning after the first night at altitude. Between the altitude sojourns, they had a 2-weeks washout period < 800 m. The protocol was approved by the cantonal ethics committee of Zurich (KEK 2013-0088), and all patients gave written informed consent.

Patients

Adult patients (18–75 years) diagnosed with COPD GOLD grades 2–3 permanently living < 800 m were included. Exclusion criteria were hypoxemia defined as oxygen saturation by pulse oximetry (SpO_2) lower than 92% at 490 m, home oxygen or continuous positive airway pressure (CPAP) therapy, any uncontrolled cardiovascular disease, or history of obstructive sleep syndrome (Tan et al., 2020).

Randomization, Intervention, Blinding, and Sample Size

Patients were randomly assigned by blocks of four: (1) 490 m, placebo 2,048 m, NOT 2,048 m; (2) 490 m, NOT 2,048 m, placebo 2,048 m; (3) placebo 2,048 m, NOT 2,048 m, 490 m; and (4) NOT 2,048 m, placebo 2,048 m, 490 m. Patients traveled from 490 to 2,048 m by train and car within 3 h. During nights at altitude, patients received either 3 L/min NOT or placebo (ambient air) provided by an identical-looking oxygen concentrator (EverFlo, Philips Respironics, Zofingen, Switzerland) via nasal cannula.

Patients were monitored with an online sleep study with camera view during the night, ensuring compliance. Patients and assessors of echocardiography were blinded to the gas mixture.

A total of 18 participants were required for a minimal detectable change of tricuspid regurgitation pressure gradient (TRPG) of 5 (SD ± 5 mmHg) with a power of 0.8 and a significance level of 0.05.

Assessments

Echocardiography was performed at 490 m and on the second day at 2,048 m (after the first night with NOT/placebo) during ambient air breathing as described before (Lichtblau et al., 2019b). Echocardiographic recordings were performed with a real-time, phased array sector scanner (CX 50, Philips, Philips Respironics, Zofingen, Switzerland) with an integrated color Doppler system and a transducer containing crystal sets for imaging (1–5 MHz) and for continuous-wave Doppler. Measurements were carried out according to guidelines of the European Association of Echocardiography (Galderisi et al., 2017). Systolic PAP (sPAP) was calculated by summing up the TRPG (calculated with the Bernoulli equation from the peak velocity of the tricuspid regurgitation $\Delta P = 4 \times V^2{}_{max}$) and the right atrial pressure (RAP; estimated on the basis of the inferior vena cava diameter and collapse) (Rudski et al., 2010; Lichtblau et al., 2019b). The right atrium and ventricle were manually traced, and fractional area change (FAC) calculated (% systolic/diastolic right ventricular area). Tricuspid annular plane systolic excursion (TAPSE) was measured by M-mode and the right ventricular free wall velocity by tissue Doppler imaging. Mean PAP (mPAP) was calculated from sPAP with the following formula: mPAP = sPAP × 0.61 + 2 (Chemla et al., 2004). Pulmonary artery wedge pressure (PAWP) was calculated as 1.24 × (E/e′) + 1.9 (Doutreleau et al., 2016). Cardiac output was calculated using the left ventricular (LV) outflow tract velocity time integral. Pulmonary vascular resistance (PVR) was calculated with the following formula: PVR = (mPAP − PAWP)/cardiac output, and left heart function was assessed according to the current guidelines (Galderisi et al., 2017). Pressure/flow relation was calculated with mPAP/cardiac output, and right ventricular arterial coupling was calculated with TAPSE/sPAP (Tello et al., 2019).

Arterial blood gas analysis was performed on radial artery blood sample and was drawn in the morning during ambient air breathing (RapidPoint 405, Siemens Healthcare Diagnostics AG, Zurich, Switzerland).

Outcomes

Primary outcome was the differences in TRPG between NOT and placebo treatment. Secondary outcomes were additional echocardiographic variables of the right and left heart.

Patients who suffered from an altitude-related adverse health effects were excluded from the study, according to the following predefined safety criteria (Tan et al., 2020):

- severe hypoxemia ($SpO_2 < 75\%$ for > 30 min at any time while at high altitude),
- intercurrent illness (e.g., exacerbation of COPD, cardiovascular disease, infection, or new diseases),
- AMS (Environmental Symptoms Questionnaire Cerebral score ≥ 0.7; Sampson et al., 1983), and
- any other conditions that required therapy.

Statistical Analysis

Analysis was performed per protocol including patients who underwent all three sessions; missing values were not replaced. The data are summarized as mean and SD. Mean differences and 95% confidence intervals (95% CIs) between measures at 490 m and at 2,048 m with NOT or placebo were calculated. All outcomes were computed using linear mixed models with outcomes as dependent variables and altitude and intervention as independent variables. We herewith included all time points in one model and assumed that data are normally distributed ($n > 30$). Statistical significance was assumed when 95% CIs of mean differences did not overlap zero or $p < 0.05$. Statistical analysis was performed with Stata version 15.1 (StataCorp, College Station, TX, United States).

RESULTS

The patient flow is shown in **Figure 1**. Five patients were excluded from the analysis because they received oxygen therapy at night in the placebo phase due to hypoxemia during sleep, according to predefined safety criteria. Two patients dropped out due to COPD exacerbations, and another two patients due to acute onset of cardiovascular disease. A total of 23 patients were included in the per-protocol analysis.

Patients were on average 66 ± 5 years old (10 males and 13 females, FEV_1 53.7% ± 12.8% predicted), and baseline characteristics including medications are listed in **Table 1**. Patients were mostly classified as COPD GOLD II (70%) and the remaining as GOLD III.

At 2,048 m, patients revealed a significantly higher heart rate (72 ± 9 bpm at low altitude vs. 79 ± 9 bpm at 2,048 m placebo and 78 ± 11 bpm at 2,048 m NOT), along with a significant lower oxygen saturation (95.3% ± 1.6% vs. 90.6% ± 2.8% with placebo and 91.3% ± 3.3% with NOT) and a lower PaO_2 (67.7 ± 6.6 vs. 59.3 ± 6.0 mmHg with placebo and 58.7 ± 7.2 mmHg with NOT) and $PaCO_2$ (36.9 ± 3.0 vs. 34.2 ± 3.8 mmHg with placebo, 34.1 ± 4.1 mmHg with NOT) compared with low altitude (**Table 2**). Hematocrit did significantly differ from 490 to 2,048 m with NOT (41.2% ± 3.2% vs. 42.5% ± 3.6% with placebo, $p = 0.078$ and 42.9% ± 3.9% with NOT, $p = 0.037$) and hemoglobin with both placebo and NOT (14.1 ± 1.2 vs. 14.5 ± 1.2 g/L, $p = 0.031$ and 14.6 ± 1.3 g/L with NOT, $p = 0.016$) (**Table 2**). No relevant differences between placebo and NOT treatment were found.

Table 3 displays echocardiography measurements of the participants at low altitude and at high altitude with and without NOT. COPD patients significantly increased their TRPG from 490 to 2,048 m (490 m 21.7 ± 5.2 mmHg vs. 2,048 m 27.4 ± 7.3 mmHg with placebo and 2,048 m 27.8 ± 8.3 mmHg

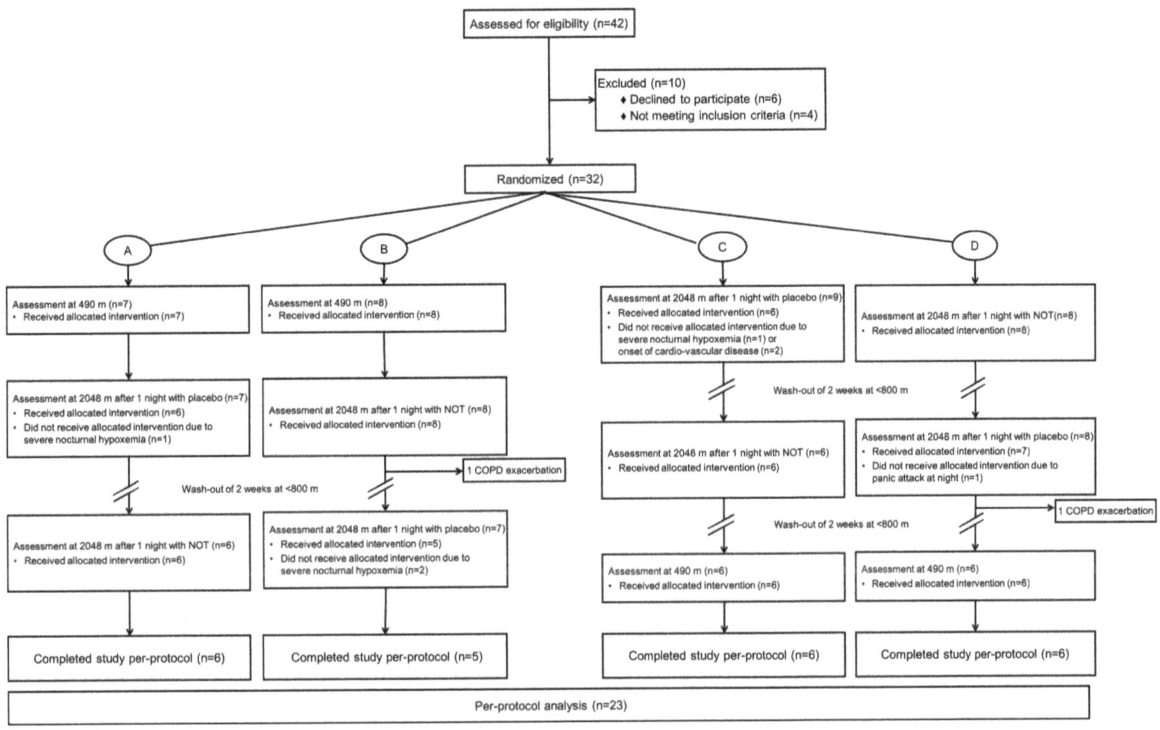

FIGURE 1 | Patient flow.

with NOT) and consequently the sPAP and mPAP with no significant difference between treatments (**Figure 2**).

TAPSE was higher after NOT vs. placebo [2.5 ± 0.5 vs. 2.3 ± 0.4 cm with placebo and 2.6 ± 0.6 cm with NOT, mean differences (95% CI) 0.3 (0.1 –0.5), $p = 0.005$], whereas the right ventricular anterior wall diameter was measured slightly higher under NOT vs. placebo [0.6 ± 0.2 vs. 0.5 ± 0.3 cm with placebo and 0.6 ± 0.3 cm with NOT, mean difference (95% CI) 0.1 (0.0–0.2), $p = 0.046$].

Right ventricular arterial coupling was decreased and PVR elevated at 2,048 m with no difference between treatments [coupling: 490 m 1.1 ± 0.3 mm/mmHg vs. 2,048 m 0.8 ± 0.2 mm/mmHg with placebo and 0.8 ± 0.2 mm/mmHg with NOT, both $p < 0.05$; PVR: 490 m 1.2 ± 0.6 Wood units (WU) vs. 2,048 m 2.1 ± 1.1 WU with placebo and 1.8 ± 1.1 WU with NOT, both $p < 0.05$] (**Table 3**).

DISCUSSION

This is the first randomized controlled trial investigating the effect of NOT on the PAP in patients with COPD traveling to altitude. NOT did not mitigate the effect of hypoxia-induced increase of the TRPG measured on ambient air the second day in lowlanders with COPD traveling to 2,048 m compared with placebo.

At low altitude, TRPG of the presently investigated COPD patients was 21.7 ± 5.2 mmHg and thus within a normal range and comparable with that of healthy subjects, where a tricuspid regurgitation velocity of 2.55 m/s, corresponding to a TRPG of 26 mmHg, is defined as the upper limit of normal (Marra et al., 2018).

The altitude-induced increase of TRPG was less pronounced than in a study published previously (Lichtblau et al., 2019b), where COPD patients increased their TRPG from 23 (19; 29) mmHg to 32 (25; 41) mmHg during a sojourn to 2,590 m in comparison to the increase to 27.4 ± 7.3 mmHg with placebo and to 27.8 ± 8.3 mmHg NOT at an altitude of 2,048 m in the current study. The difference in altitude can be one of the reasons for this less pronounced PAP increase or the fact that in the current study patients with altitude-related adverse health effects were excluded. At an altitude of 3,100 m, even higher values were obtained (from 20 ± 4 mmHg at lowland to 31 ± 9 mmHg at highland) in COPD patients with milder disease severity (GOLD 1 and 2 only) (Lichtblau et al., 2019a,b). In another study, lifelong altitude residents with COPD showed a significantly higher mPAP than did lowlanders with COPD (lowlanders 26.8 ± 11.1 mmHg and highlanders 36.1 ± 10.2 mmHg) and also comparably higher with our results (mPAP 16 ± 4 mmHg at lowland, 21 ± 4 mmHg at altitude with placebo, and 22 ± 5 mmHg with NOT). However, while mPAP in the current study was derived from sPAP, Guvenc et al. (2013) estimated mPAP from pulmonary acceleration time, and therefore, the comparison of the studies is difficult.

Likewise to TRPG, for heart rate and FAC, similar changes in patients with COPD at increasing altitudes were found (Lichtblau et al., 2019b).

TABLE 1 | Baseline characteristics.

Age, years	66.0 ± 5.1
Sex, males/females	10/13
Body mass index, kg/m^2	25.3 ± 3.9
Pack years, years	38.2 ± 31.5
COPD GOLD	
II	16 (70)
III	7 (30)
FEV_1,% predicted	53.7 ± 12.8
FVC,% predicted	90.3 ± 11.5
FEV_1/FVC	54.3 ± 11.8
TLco adjusted for hemoglobin,% predicted	71.4 ± 20.2
6-min walking distance, m	543 ± 89
SpO_2 at end of 6-min walking distance,%	92.5 ± 3.9
Medication	
Inhaled glucocorticosteroids	2 (9)
Inhaled β-adrenergics	17 (74)
Inhaled anticholinergics	18 (78)
Diuretics	2 (9)
Antihypertensive medication	12 (52)
Antidiabetics	3 (13)
Antidepressants	3 (13)

Values are presented as mean ± SD or numbers and proportions.
COPD, chronic obstructive pulmonary disease; GOLD, Global Initiative for Chronic Obstructive Lung Disease; FEV_1, forced expiratory volume in the first second of expiration; FVC, forced vital capacity; TLco, diffusing capacity for carbon monoxide; SpO_2, oxygen saturation.

There were two significant differences between treatments, namely, the TAPSE [0.3 (0.1–0.5)] and the PAWP [1.9 (0.4–3.4)]. The difference of the PAWP is difficult to interpret since this variable is prone to measurement inaccuracy, and we therefore caution to overinterpret this result. TAPSE as a measure of right heart function was better after NOT, potentially indicating a beneficial effect of NOT or showing an increase in right heart contractility as a reaction to the acute drop in oxygen levels after the night on NOT.

Exposure to altitude induced an increase in PVR in both treatment arms, with a tendency toward a lesser increase with NOT but no relevant difference between the groups with a mean difference of −0.33 (−0.76–0.10) WU. In a previous study with 95 COPD patients exposed to 3,100 m, preventive treatment with dexamethasone showed a significant mitigating effect with a mean difference of −0.5 (−0.9 to −0.1) WU between the placebo and the treatment group (Lichtblau et al., 2019a). The less pronounced and non-significant effect of NOT in the current study might be explained by the fact, that in this study, all measurements were performed on ambient air at 2,048 m after the night with NOT; and thus, a potential vasodilator effect of oxygen may not have persisted anymore, which was already shown in the arterial blood gas analysis published in the main paper where no difference was found between NOT and placebo at 2,048 m (Tan et al., 2020). Looking more closely at the course of PAP and PVR during acute exposure to hypoxia reveals that an excess increase occurs within the acute phase (<180 min) as described *in vitro* and *in vivo*, followed by a dip and a steady increase over the next hours (Sommer et al., 2016). In the current study, echocardiography was performed only few hours after receiving either oxygen or ambient air, and therefore, patients receiving NOT were potentially still in the overcompensating phase. Two studies in patients with PH have shown reduction in mPAP during acute exposure with oxygen therapy. The first study in 104 PH patients revealed a reduction of mPAP from 46.4 ± 1.3 to 42.2. ± 1.3 mmHg with 5 L/min oxygen therapy via nasal cannula (Leuchte et al., 2013), and the second study in 28 PH patients has shown that acute hyperoxia with 100% FiO_2 lowers mPAP by 4 (2-6) mmHg (Groth et al., 2018). Hemodynamics after oxygen withdrawal have not been studied; however, Leuchte et al. (2013) found that the effect of oxygen on invasively measured hemodynamics disappeared 15 min after stopping supplemental oxygen. We can only speculate that patients in the current study had a mitigating effect on PAP while receiving NOT during the nights; however, potential beneficial effects seem not to be sustainable during the following morning when echocardiography was performed, and whether NOT given for several nights would be beneficial during longer altitude sojourns remains unclear. At lowland, a study in COPD patients did not show a significant benefit after 2 years with NOT on PAP (control group 19.8 ± 5.6–20.5 ± 6.5 mmHg and NOT 18.3 ± 4.7 –19.5 ± 5.3 mmHg, $p = 0.79$). A recent trial was stopped prematurely because of recruitment and retention difficulties, showing—in this underpowered analysis—no clear positive or negative effect on survival or progression to long-term oxygen therapy in COPD patients (Lacasse et al., 2020) and therefore emphasizing again the need of efficiently powered trials to study the long-term effect of NOT in patients with COPD. However, according to our previous publication from the current trial, NOT had a positive effect on various sleep measures, but not on daytime exercise capacity, blood gases, or cognitive performance compared with placebo at altitude (Tan et al., 2020). Echocardiographic right-to-left shunt measurements were not performed during this study, but from previous trials, it is known that hypobaric hypoxia induces a higher prevalence of intracardiac and intrapulmonary right-to-left shunts in lowlander COPD patients traveling to altitude (Lichtblau et al., 2020); and therefore, patients with COPD and right-to-left shunt might even less profit from supplemental oxygen. On the contrary, Lovering et al. (2008) have demonstrated prevention of exercise-induced intrapulmonary shunts in healthy humans with high levels of hyperoxia (100% FiO_2).

Limitations

According to the safety criteria of the current study protocol, patients who experienced altitude-related adverse health effects received oxygen and were excluded from this analysis, which biased our results toward no between-group difference, as the proportion of excluded patients in the group receiving placebo was much higher than that in those who received NOT. However, performing an echocardiography immediately during the night when patients under placebo got hypoxemic was not feasible, and performing an echocardiography under oxygen therapy in these patients would also have biased the results. We chose the time point of echocardiography after the first night at altitude

TABLE 2 | Vital signs and blood gases.

	490 m baseline	2,048 m placebo	2,048 m NOT	2,048 m NOT vs. placebo	*p*-value
Heart rate, bpm	72 ± 9	79 ± 9[a]	78 ± 11[a]	−1 (−4 to 2)	0.544
Diastolic blood pressure, mmHg	73 ± 10	78 ± 10	78 ± 9	1(−3 to 5)	0.697
Systolic blood pressure, mmHg	129 ± 19	133 ± 14	130 ± 19	−3 (−9 to 2)	0.252
SpO_2,%	95.3 ± 1.6	90.6 ± 2.8[a]	91.3 ± 3.3[a]	0.7 (−0.5 to 1.9)	0.250
PaO_2, mmHg	67.7 ± 6.6	59.3 ± 6.0[a]	58.7 ± 7.2[a]	−0.6 (−2.6 to 1.3)	0.519
$PaCO_2$, mmHg	36.9 ± 3.0	34.2 ± 3.8[a]	34.1 ± 4.1[a]	0.2 (−1.1 to 1.5)	0.758
Hematocrit,%	41.2 ± 3.2	42.5 ± 3.6	42.9 ± 3.9[a]	0.1 (−0.5 to 0.8)	0.708
Hemoglobin, g/dl	14.1 ± 1.2	14.5 ± 1.2[a]	14.6 ± 1.3[a]	0.0 (−0.2 to 0.3)	0.761

Data are presented as mean ± SD.
SpO_2, oxygen saturation by pulse oximetry; PaO_2, partial pressure of arterial oxygen; $PaCO_2$, partial pressure of arterial carbon dioxide.
[a]$p < 0.05$ vs. 490 m.

TABLE 3 | Echocardiographic measurements.

	490 m baseline	2,048 m placebo	2,048 m NOT	2,048 m NOT vs. placebo	*p*-value
TRPG, mmHg	21.7 ± 5.2	27.4 ± 7.3[a]	27.8 ± 8.3[a]	0.4 (−2.1 to 3.0)	0.736
sPAP, mmHg	24.7 ± 5.2	31.3 ± 7.2[a]	32.1 ± 8.9[a]	0.9 (−2.1 to 3.9)	0.517
mPAP, mmHg	16.4 ± 4.4	21.1 ± 4.4[a]	21.6 ± 5.4[a]	0.5 (−1.3 to 2.4)	0.560
RAP, mmHg	3.0 ± 0.0	3.9 ± 1.9	4.3 ± 2.2[a]	0.4 (−0.5 to 1.4)	0.350
RA area, cm^2	12.6 ± 2.3	12.9 ± 3.5	13.8 ± 4.2[a]	0.9 (−0.2 to 2.0)	0.123
RVEDA, cm^2	14.4 ± 4.0	13.5 ± 3.8	13.2 ± 3.5	−0.3 (−1.6 to 1.0)	0.682
RVESA, cm^2	8.6 ± 3.0	8.3 ± 2.8	8.2 ± 2.9	−0.1 (−1.0 to 0.8)	0.809
FAC,%	41.0 ± 8.7	38.6 ± 6.6	38.0 ± 10.2	−0.7 (−5.2 to 3.9)	0.772
TAPSE, cm	2.5 ± 0.5	2.3 ± 0.4	2.6 ± 0.6	0.3 (0.1 to 0.5)	0.005
Eccentricity index end-diastolic	1.1 ± 0.1	1.1 ± 0.1	1.1 ± 0.1	0.0 (−0.0 to 0.1)	0.288
Eccentricity index end-systolic	1.0 ± 0.1	1.1 ± 0.1	1.1 ± 0.1[a]	0.0 (−0.0 to 0.7)	0.293
RV anterior wall diameter, cm	0.6 ± 0.2	0.5 ± 0.1	0.6 ± 0.3	0.1 (0.0 to 0.2)[b]	0.046
RV diameter end-diastolic, cm	2.9 ± 0.5	2.7 ± 0.7	2.8 ± 0.5	0.2 (−0.1 to 0.4)	0.317
TDI tricuspid annular systolic velocity, cm/s	14.6 ± 2.9	15.9 ± 2.9	16.7 ± 4.5[a]	0.9 (−0.6 to 2.3)	0.237
Stroke volume, ml	82.4 ± 18.0	83.6 ± 18.0	90.6 ± 22.7	6.8 (−3.4 to 16.9)	0.194
Cardiac output, L/min	6.0 ± 1.6	6.5 ± 1.6	6.9 ± 1.7[a]	0.4 (−0.4 to 1.2)	0.357
Cardiac index, L/min/m^2	3.4 ± 0.9	3.6 ± 0.8	3.9 ± 0.9[a]	0.2 (−0.2 to 0.7)	0.329
mPAP/cardiac output	3.0 ± 0.9	3.5 ± 1.1[a]	3.4 ± 1.1	−0.1 (−0.6 to 0.4)	0.764
TAPSE/sPAP, mm/mmHg	1.1 ± 0.3	0.8 ± 0.2[a]	0.8 ± 0.2[a]	0.1 (−0.0 to 0.2)	0.209
PAWP, mmHg	10.3 ± 2.3	9.0 ± 2.2	10.9 ± 4.5	1.9 (0.4 to 3.4)	0.011
PVR, WU	1.2 ± 0.6	2.1 ± 1.1[a]	1.8 ± 1.1[a]	−0.3 (−0.8 to 0.1)	0.134
PVR corrected for hematocrit	1.4 ± 0.8	2.3 ± 1.2[a]	2.2 ± 1.9[a]	−0.1 (−0.8 to 0.6)	0.785
Ejection fraction (biplan),%	63.5 ± 6.9	67.1 ± 6.5[a]	66.5 ± 7.3	−0.5 (−3.8 to 2.7)	0.750
LV internal dimension end-diastolic, cm	4.2 ± 0.9	4.1 ± 0.6	4.1 ± 0.4	−0.0 (−0.3 to 0.3)	0.969
LV internal dimension end-systolic, cm	2.8 ± 0.6	2.7 ± 0.5	2.8 ± 0.5	0.2 (−0.1 to 0.4)	0.249
LV posterior wall end-diastolic, cm	1.0 ± 0.6	0.8 ± 0.1[a]	0.9 ± 0.1	0.0 (−0.1 to 0.2)	0.633
MV E/A	1.0 ± 0.4	0.8 ± 0.3[a]	0.9 ± 0.3[a]	0.1 (−0.0 to 0.2)	0.189

Data are presented as mean ± SD.
TRPG, tricuspid regurgitation pressure gradient; sPAP, systolic pulmonary artery pressure; mPAP, mean pulmonary artery pressure; PAWP, pulmonary arterial wedge pressure; RAP, right atrial pressure; RA, right atrium; RVEDA, right ventricle end-diastolic area; RVESA, right ventricle end-systolic area; FAC, fractional area change; TAPSE, tricuspid annular plane systolic excursion; RV, right ventricle; TDI, tissue Doppler imaging; PVR, pulmonary vascular resistance; LV, left ventricle; MV, mitral valve; Peak E, early mitral inflow velocity; Peak A, peak atrial filling velocity; E/A, ratio of transmitral early diastolic to late diastolic velocity.
[a]$p < 0.05$ vs. 490 m.

on NOT vs. placebo in order to see whether NOT would have a prolonged effect on pulmonary hemodynamics even after several hours on ambient air. Whether long-term treatment with oxygen at altitude or a longer treatment with NOT would have had a beneficial effect on pulmonary hemodynamics remains to be investigated. The sample size of our study was relatively small, but estimation for a minimal detectable change of a TRPG 5 ± 5 mmHg with a power of 0.8 and a significance level of 0.05 would have required 18 participants, a number that was met by the 23 patients who completed the study. We included COPD

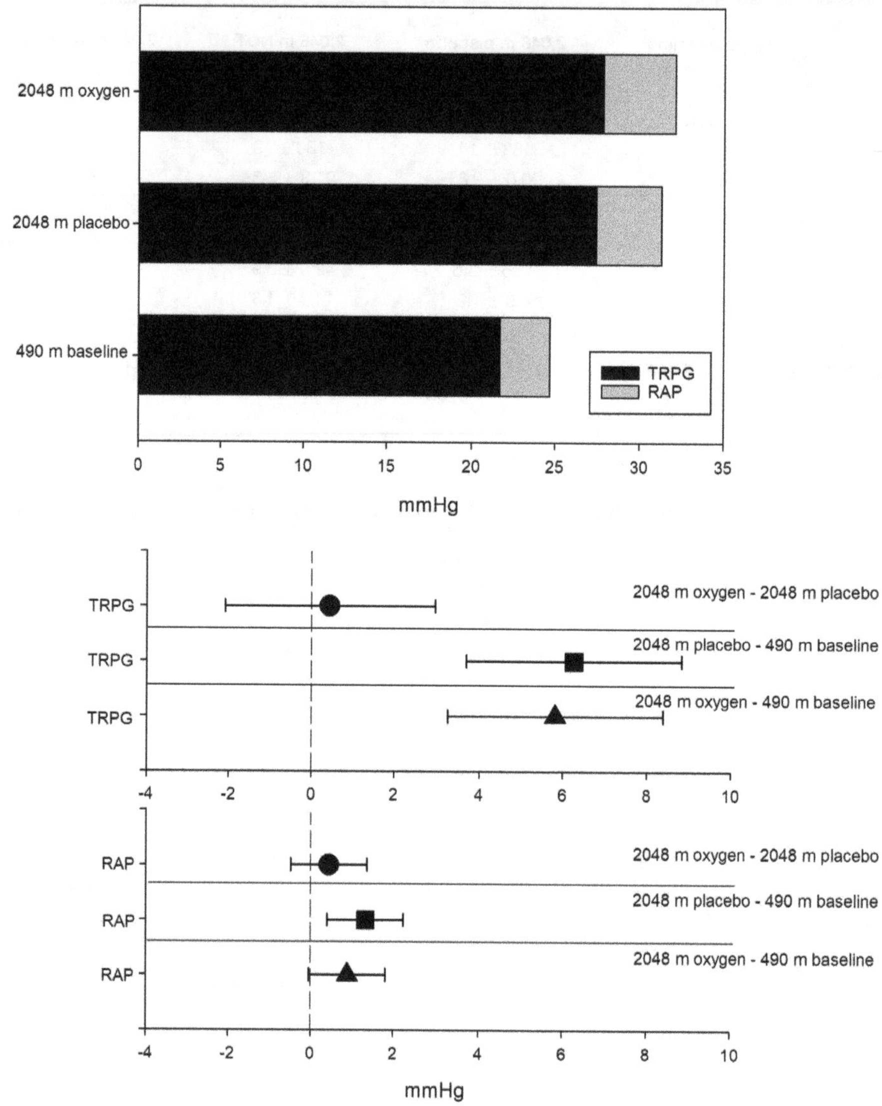

FIGURE 2 | Systolic pulmonary artery pressure displayed as sum of the tricuspid regurgitation pressure gradient (TRPG) and the right atrial pressure (RAP) at 490 and 2,048 m [with placebo and nocturnal oxygen therapy (NOT), respectively]. The lower part shows the differences of the TRPG and the RAP for ●, 2,048 m oxygen, 2,048 m placebo; ■, 2,048 m placebo, 490 m baseline; and ▲, 2,048 m oxygen, 490 m baseline.

GOLD 2 and 3, and our data cannot be extrapolated for more or less severe COPD patients.

CONCLUSION

In lowlanders with COPD remaining free of clinically relevant altitude-related adverse health effects, changes in daytime pulmonary hemodynamics during a stay at high altitude were trivial and not modified by NOT.

ETHICS STATEMENT

The studies involving human participants were reviewed and approved by the Ethics Committee of Zurich. The patients/participants provided their written informed consent to participate in this study.

AUTHOR CONTRIBUTIONS

SiU was the guarantor and took responsibility for the content of the manuscript, including the data and analysis. ML, SiU, and SS contributed to acquiring, analyzing, and interpreting the data, writing and revising the article critically for important intellectual content, and providing final approval of the version to be published. SA, FH, PS, StU, SRS, EH, and MF contributed to data collection, analysis, and revising the article critically for important intellectual content. SiU, TL, and KB conceived the project and contributed to data collection, analysis and interpretation, writing the manuscript, revising the article critically for important intellectual content, and providing final approval of the version to be published. All authors were took responsibility for all aspects of the reliability and freedom from bias of the data presented and their discussed interpretation.

REFERENCES

Carta, A. F., Bitos, K., Furian, M., Mademilov, M., Sheraliev, U., Marazhapov, N. H., et al. (2021). ECG changes at rest and during exercise in lowlanders with COPD travelling to 3100 m. *Int. J. Cardiol.* 324, 173–179. doi: 10.1016/j.ijcard.2020.09.055

Chemla, D., Castelain, V., Humbert, M., Hebert, J. L., Simonneau, G., Lecarpentier, Y., et al. (2004). New formula for predicting mean pulmonary artery pressure using systolic pulmonary artery pressure. *Chest* 126, 1313–1317. doi: 10.1378/chest.126.4.1313

Doutreleau, S., Canuet, M., Enache, I., Di Marco, P., Lonsdorfer, E., Oswald-Mammoser, M., et al. (2016). Right heart hemodynamics in pulmonary hypertension- an echocardiography and catheterization study. *Circ. J.* 80, 2019–2025. doi: 10.1253/circj.cj-16-0206

Fossati, L., Muller-Mottet, S., Hasler, E., Speich, R., Bloch, K. E., Huber, L. C., et al. (2014). Long-term effect of vasodilator therapy in pulmonary hypertension due to COPD: a retrospective analysis. *Lung* 192, 987–995. doi: 10.1007/s00408-014-9650-1

Furian, M., Flueck, D., Latshang, T. D., Scheiwiller, P. M., Segitz, S. D., Mueller-Mottet, S., et al. (2018a). Exercise performance and symptoms in lowlanders with COPD ascending to moderate altitude: randomized trial. *Int. J. Chron. Obstruct. Pulmon. Dis.* 13, 3529–3538. doi: 10.2147/copd.s173039

Furian, M., Hartmann, S. E., Latshang, T. D., Flueck, D., Murer, C., Scheiwiller, P. M., et al. (2018b). Exercise performance of lowlanders with COPD at 2,590 m: data from a randomized trial. *Respiration* 95, 422–432. doi: 10.1159/000486450

Furian, M., Lichtblau, M., Aeschbacher, S. S., Estebesova, B., Emilov, B., Sheraliev, U., et al. (2018c). Efficacy of dexamethasone in preventing acute mountain sickness in COPD patients: randomized trial. *Chest* 154, 788–797. doi: 10.1016/j.chest.2018.06.006

Furian, M., Lichtblau, M., Aeschbacher, S. S., Estebesova, B., Emilov, B., Sheraliev, U., et al. (2019). Effect of dexamethasone on nocturnal oxygenation in lowlanders with chronic obstructive pulmonary disease traveling to 3100 meters: a randomized clinical trial. *JAMA Netw. Open* 2:e190067. doi: 10.1001/jamanetworkopen.2019.0067

Galderisi, M., Cosyns, B., Edvardsen, T., Cardim, N., Delgado, V., Di Salvo, G., et al. (2017). Standardization of adult transthoracic echocardiography reporting in agreement with recent chamber quantification, diastolic function, and heart valve disease recommendations: an expert consensus document of the European Association of Cardiovascular Imaging. *Eur. Heart J. Cardiovasc. Imaging* 18, 1301–1310. doi: 10.1093/ehjci/jex244

Global Initiative for Chronic Obstructive Lung Disease (2019). *Global Strategy for the Diagnosis, Management, and Prevention of Chronic Obstructive Pulmonary Disease.* Available online at: https://goldcopd.org/wp-content/uploads/2018/11/GOLD-2019-v1.7-FINAL-14Nov2018-WMS.pdf (accessed July 11, 2019).

Groth, A., Saxer, S., Bader, P. R., Lichtblau, M., Furian, M., Schneider, S. R., et al. (2018). Acute hemodynamic changes by breathing hypoxic and hyperoxic gas mixtures in pulmonary arterial and chronic thromboembolic pulmonary hypertension. *Int. J. Cardiol.* 270, 262–267. doi: 10.1016/j.ijcard.2018.05.127

Guvenc, T. S., Erer, H. B., Kul, S., Perincek, G., Ilhan, S., Sayar, N., et al. (2013). Right ventricular morphology and function in chronic obstructive pulmonary disease patients living at high altitude. *Heart Lung Circ.* 22, 31–37. doi: 10.1016/j.hlc.2012.08.004

Johnson, D. C. (2010). Association of chronic mountain sickness with abnormal pulmonary microcirculation: importance of adjusting predicted diffusing capacity of the lung for carbon monoxide for altitude, hemoglobin, and lung volume. *Chest* 138, 757–758; author reply 758.

Lacasse, Y., Series, F., Corbeil, F., Baltzan, M., Paradis, B., Simao, P., et al. (2020). Randomized trial of nocturnal oxygen in chronic obstructive pulmonary disease. *N. Engl. J. Med.* 383, 1129–1138.

Latshang, T. D., Tardent, R. P. M., Furian, M., Flueck, D., Segitz, S. D., Mueller-Mottet, S., et al. (2019). Sleep and breathing disturbances in patients with chronic obstructive pulmonary disease traveling to altitude: a randomized trial. *Sleep* 42, 1–10.

Leuchte, H. H., Baezner, C. J., Baumgartner, R. A., Mernitz, P., Neurohr, C., and Behr, J. (2013). Acute hemodynamic responses to supplemental oxygen and their prognostic implications in pulmonary hypertension. *Respiration* 85, 400–407. doi: 10.1159/000340009

Lichtblau, M., Furian, M., Aeschbacher, S. S., Bisang, M., Sheraliev, U., Mademilov, M., et al. (2020). Right-to-left shunts in lowlanders with COPD traveling to altitude: a randomized controlled trial with dexamethasone. *J. Appl. Physiol.* 128, 117–126. doi: 10.1152/japplphysiol.00548.2019

Lichtblau, M., Furian, M., Aeschbacher, S. S., Bisang, M., Ulrich, S., Saxer, S., et al. (2018). Dexamethasone improves pulmonary hemodynamics in COPD-patients going to altitude: a randomized trial. *Int. J. Cardiol.* 283, 159–164. doi: 10.1016/j.ijcard.2018.12.052

Lichtblau, M., Furian, M., Aeschbacher, S. S., Bisang, M., Ulrich, S., Saxer, S., et al. (2019a). Dexamethasone improves pulmonary hemodynamics in COPD-patients going to altitude: a randomized trial. *Int. J. Cardiol.* 283, 159–164.

Lichtblau, M., Latshang, T. D., Furian, M., Muller-Mottet, S., Kuest, S., Tanner, F., et al. (2019b). Right and left heart function in lowlanders with COPD at altitude: data from a randomized study. *Respiration* 97, 125–134. doi: 10.1159/000492898

Lovering, A. T., Stickland, M. K., Amann, M., Murphy, J. C., O'brien, M. J., Hokanson, J. S., et al. (2008). Hyperoxia prevents exercise-induced intrapulmonary arteriovenous shunt in healthy humans. *J. Physiol.* 586, 4559–4565. doi: 10.1113/jphysiol.2008.159350

Macnee, W. (2010). Right heart function in COPD. *Semin. Respir. Crit. Care Med.* 31, 295–312. doi: 10.1055/s-0030-1254070

Marra, A. M., Naeije, R., Ferrara, F., Vriz, O., Stanziola, A. A., D'alto, M., et al. (2018). Reference ranges and determinants of tricuspid regurgitation velocity in healthy adults assessed by two-dimensional doppler-echocardiography. *Respiration* 96, 425–433. doi: 10.1159/000490191

Muralt, L., Furian, M., Lichtblau, M., Aeschbacher, S. S., Clark, R. A., Estebesova, B., et al. (2018). Postural control in lowlanders with COPD traveling to 3100 m: data from a randomized trial evaluating the effect of preventive dexamethasone treatment. *Front. Physiol.* 9:752. doi: 10.3389/fphys.2018.00752

Rhodes, J., Barst, R. J., Garofano, R. P., Thoele, D. G., and Gersony, W. M. (1991). Hemodynamic correlates of exercise function in patients with primary pulmonary hypertension. *J. Am. Coll. Cardiol.* 18, 1738–1744. doi: 10.1016/0735-1097(91)90513-9

Rudski, L. G., Lai, W. W., Afilalo, J., Hua, L., Handschumacher, M. D., Chandrasekaran, K., et al. (2010). Guidelines for the echocardiographic assessment of the right heart in adults: a report from the American Society of Echocardiography endorsed by the European Association of Echocardiography, a registered branch of the European Society of Cardiology, and the Canadian Society of Echocardiography. *J. Am. Soc. Echocardiogr.* 23, 685–713; quiz 786–688.

Sampson, J. B., Cymerman, A., Burse, R. L., Maher, J. T., and Rock, P. B. (1983). Procedures for the measurement of acute mountain sickness. *Aviat. Space Environ. Med.* 54, 1063–1073.

Schwarz, E. I., Latshang, T. D., Furian, M., Fluck, D., Segitz, S., Muller-Mottet, S., et al. (2019). Blood pressure response to exposure to moderate altitude in patients with COPD. *Int. J. Chron. Obstruct. Pulmon. Dis.* 14, 659–666. doi: 10.2147/copd.s194426

Sommer, N., Strielkov, I., Pak, O., and Weissmann, N. (2016). Oxygen sensing and signal transduction in hypoxic pulmonary vasoconstriction. *Eur. Respir. J.* 47, 288–303. doi: 10.1183/13993003.00945-2015

Tan, L., Latshang, T. D., Aeschbacher, S. S., Huber, F., Flueck, D., Lichtblau, M., et al. (2020). Effect of nocturnal oxygen therapy on nocturnal hypoxemia and sleep apnea among patients with chronic obstructive pulmonary disease traveling to 2048 meters: a randomized clinical trial.

JAMA Netw. Open 3:e207940. doi: 10.1001/jamanetworkopen.2020.7940

Tello, K., Wan, J., Dalmer, A., Vanderpool, R., Ghofrani, H. A., Naeije, R., et al. (2019). Validation of the tricuspid annular plane systolic excursion/systolic pulmonary artery pressure ratio for the assessment of right ventricular-arterial coupling in severe pulmonary hypertension. *Circ. Cardiovasc. Imaging* 12:e009047.

Ulrich, S., Hersberger, M., Fischler, M., Nussbaumer-Ochsner, Y., Treder, U., Russi, E. W., et al. (2010). Genetic polymorphisms of the serotonin transporter, but not the 2a receptor or nitric oxide synthetase, are associated with pulmonary hypertension in chronic obstructive pulmonary disease. *Respiration* 79, 288–295. doi: 10.1159/000226243

13

Inside the Alterations of Circulating Metabolome in Antarctica: The Adaptation to Chronic Hypoxia

Michele Dei Cas[1], Camillo Morano[1], Sara Ottolenghi[1,2], Roberto Dicasillati[3], Gabriella Roda[4], Michele Samaja[1,5†] and Rita Paroni[1†]*

[1]Department of Health Sciences, Università degli Studi di Milano, Milan, Italy, [2]Department of Medicine and Surgery, Università degli Studi di Milano-Bicocca, Milan, Italy, [3]Department of General Surgery, ASST Santi Paolo e Carlo, San Paolo Hospital, Milan, Italy, [4]Department of Pharmaceutical Sciences, Università degli Studi di Milano, Milan, Italy, [5]MAGI Group, Brescia, Italy

***Correspondence:**
Michele Samaja
michele.samaja@unimi.it

[†]These authors have contributed equally to this work

Although the human body may dynamically adapt to mild and brief oxygen shortages, there is a growing interest in understanding how the metabolic pathways are modified during sustained exposure to chronic hypoxia. Located at an equivalent altitude of approximately 3,800 m asl, the Concordia Station in Antarctica represents an opportunity to study the course of human adaption to mild hypoxia with reduced impact of potentially disturbing variables else than oxygen deprivation. We recruited seven healthy subjects who spent 10 months in the Concordia Station, and collected plasma samples at sea level before departure, and 90 days, 6 months, and 10 months during hypoxia. Samples were analyzed by untargeted liquid chromatography high resolution mass spectrometry to unravel how the non-polar and polar metabolomes are affected. Statistical analyses were performed by clustering the subjects into four groups according to the duration of hypoxia exposure. The non-polar metabolome revealed a modest decrease in the concentration of all the major lipid classes. By contrast, the polar metabolome showed marked alterations in several metabolic pathways, especially those related to amino acids metabolism, with a particular concern of arginine, glutamine, phenylalanine, tryptophan, and tyrosine. Remarkably, all the changes were evident since the first time point and remained unaffected by hypoxia duration (with the exception of a slight return of the non-polar metabolome after 6 months), highlighting a relative inability of the body to compensate them. Finally, we identified a few metabolic pathways that emerged as the main targets of chronic hypoxia.

Keywords: chronic hypoxia, adaptation, Antarctica, metabolites, metabolomics, lipidomics

INTRODUCTION

About 83 million people permanently reside above 2,500 m asl (Beall, 2014) and numberless people are exposed to moderate or high altitudes for touristic and job-related reasons worldwide, yet sojourning at altitude still represents a challenge because of systemic hypoxia, i.e., lower oxygen supply with respect to the body's need. Although humans can adapt, at least partially, to mild and brief oxygen shortages, hypoxia still remains a potentially lethal situation that represents a great burden in terms of lost lives and social costs for care and rehabilitation, especially for children in low- and middle-income countries (Lam et al., 2020). Nevertheless, despite a plethora of studies (10,194 articles with the term "hypoxia" in the title have been published in PubMed in 2020, compared to 5,610 in 2010 and 2,670 in 2000), systemic hypoxia has not yet been examined to a sufficient detail to grant adequate and safe therapeutic countermeasures. This issue is further aggravated by the occurrence of adaptive patterns that may potentially lead to pathological conditions.

Long-term adaptation of sea-level dwellers to hypoxia involves metabolic, respiratory, circulatory, and genetic mechanisms (Julian, 1985; Moore, 1985; Storz, 2021). Among these, the mechanisms related to respiratory adaptation are particularly suitable to monitor hypoxia adaptation. Yet the comprehension of these mechanisms requires the availability of experimental models wherein altitude hypoxia represents the unique major variable, with exclusion of poorly controllable factors, such as strenuous exercise, psychological stress, excessive temperature fluctuations, altitude changes, irregular feeding, and liquids assumption. The French-Italian Concordia Station in the Antarctica represents an opportunity to study the progress of human adaptation to hypoxia. The station is located at 3,233 m asl, but high latitude reduces the local barometric pressure and the amount of oxygen in breathed air mimics an approximate altitude of 3,800 m asl that leads to arterial oxygen saturation in the 91–94% range (Porcelli et al., 2017). As this condition is to be classified as mild hypoxia (Jahan et al., 2014), it represents a non-dangerous situation to whom healthy humans are predicted to adapt. As the subjects who winter-over at the Concordia Station do not have any possibility to change altitude for up to 10 months, this provided the chance to get an insight into the effects of mild hypoxia in the absence of disturbing factors.

In this study, we report the non-polar and polar metabolomes in plasma samples obtained from subjects exposed to mild hypoxia in the search of signs of long-term adaptation or return to baseline conditions. The non-polar and polar metabolomes were investigated by an up-to-date liquid chromatography high resolution mass spectrometry (LC-HR-MS) platform looking for metabolic pathways with impact on the human body response to hypoxia. The working hypothesis is that the absence of confounding factors and the lack of observable distressful outcomes would enable to focus into the physiological mechanisms underlying the body adaptation to mild hypoxia, a stressing condition that is more common than moderate and extreme hypoxia.

Abbreviations: AMS, Acute Mountain Sickness; Car, Carnitines; CASE, Campesterol Esters; CE, Cholesterol Esters; Cer, Ceramides; COA, Coenzyme A; DHCer, Dihydro Ceramides; DG, Diacylglycerols; EtherDG, Ether-linked Diacylglycerols; EtherLPC, Ether-linked Lysophosphatidylcholines; EtherLPE, Ether-linked Lysophosphatidylethanolamines; EtherPC, Ether-linked Phosphatidylcholines; EtherPE, Ether-linked Phosphatidylethanolamines; EtherTG, Ether-linked Triacylglycerols; LacCer, Lactosyl-Ceramides; Gb3, Globosides; LPC, Lysophosphatidylcholines; LPE, Lysophosphatidylethanolamines; MG, Monoacylglycerols; NAE, N-acylethanolamines; OxTG, Oxidized Triacylglycerols; PC, Phosphatidylcholines; PE, Phosphatidylethanolamines; PI, Phosphatidylinositols; PLS-DA, Partial Least Squares Discriminant Analysis; SM, Sphingomyelins; TG, Triacylglycerols; vitE, Tocopherols.

MATERIALS AND METHODS

Subjects

Seven healthy crew members in the Concordia Station (all men, aged 25–55, mean 41 years old) participated in this study. All enrolled subjects signed a declaration whereby they were informed of the risks of the study and agreed in performing the planned measurements for the full duration of the study. This study, that was approved by the Ethical Committee of the San Paolo Hospital in Milan, was conducted within the framework of the European Space Agency's Life Science campaign at the Concordia Station.

Study Design

The data reported in this study were obtained during the winter-over campaign in 2019. Baseline measurements (Group 0) were performed before the start of the mission at the European Space Agency Centre in Cologne (Germany, 91 m asl). Then, subjects were studied at three time points: 90 days (Group 90) after reaching the Concordia Station, 150–180 days (Mid-Winter, Group MW), and at the end of the winter-over campaign, immediately before leaving, 300 days after their arrival (Group END). The temperature inside the Concordia Station, a French-Italian research facility located at Dome C on the Antarctic Plateau, was permanently 22 ± 2°C despite the average air temperature, humidity and wind speed outside the Station were −58 ± 9°C, 41 ± 10%, and 2.8 m/s, respectively. Located at a geographical altitude of 3,233 m asl, the mean barometric pressure during the winter-over (478 mmHg) corresponds to an altitude of approximately 3,800 m asl in the rest of the world, a value slightly lower than that reported elsewhere (Venemans-Jellema et al., 2014), probably because the oxygen fraction in the Antarctica air (20.82–20.90%) is lower than that in the rest of the world (Kanwisher, 1957). However, all subjects were examined weekly by a staff physician for assessment of the Acute Mountain Sickness (AMS) score according to the Lake Louise symptom scale (Ferrazzini et al., 1987).

At all time points, blood samples were obtained from the antecubital vein in K_2 EDTA vacuum tubes while fasting in the morning, centrifuged (2,500 rpm, 15 min) and plasma was stored at −80°C until analyses performed in the laboratory in Milan.

Chemicals and Reagents

The chemicals acetonitrile, 2-propanol, methanol, ethanol, chloroform, formic acid, ammonium acetate, and ammonium formate were all at analytical grade and purchased by Sigma-Aldrich (St. Louis, MO, United States). All aqueous solutions were prepared using purified water at a Milli-Q grade (Burlington, MA, United States).

Creation of an In-House Metabolites Library

The Mass Spectrometry Metabolite Library (Supplied by IROA Technologies; Gonzalez-Ruiz et al., 2017; Pezzatti et al., 2019) was purchased by Sigma-Aldrich (St. Louis, MO, United States) and includes 603 unique metabolites divided in seven plates: five with polar metabolites and two with lipid-related molecules (for the composition of the plates, see **Supplementary Table S1**). Stock solutions of the analytes were prepared at the concentration of 25 µg/ml according to the manufacturer's instructions by using 5% methanol in water for plates 1–5 and methanol/chloroform (1:1, v/v) for lipids. Each plate was shaken on an oscillator thermo-mixer for 30 min at 1,000 rpm at 5°C. Twenty-nine pools were prepared, so that each one contained a maximum of 22 standards with distinct exact masses; isomers were never mixed in the same vial. The different mixes' final concentration was about 1.25 µg/ml (for the composition of each pool, see **Supplementary Table S2**). Five µl of each vial was directly injected in LC–MS/MS (see "Analysis by LC-HR-MS").

After LC–MS analysis of the standard pools, data were manually processed by MS-DIAL (ver 4.0) or semi-automatically by MSLDiscovery (ver. 3.1B.15), checking for the most prominent adducts for each analyte in both polarities (Simon-Manso et al., 2013; see "LC-HR-MS Data Processing"). The retention time (Rt), intensity, three prevalent MS/MS fragments, and S/N for each standard peak were annotated only when at least one of the accurate masses of the adducts was in accordance with those reported in MSLDiscovery Database (m/z ± 0.02 Da, <30 ppm). Final curation of the "in-house" attained Database, and compounds validation, was then made on the basis of isotopic distribution, the number of recognized adducts, and MS/MS spectra. The in-house Database comprised at the end 506 metabolites (see **Supplementary Table S3**).

Plasma Extraction Procedures

Non-polar Metabolites

Plasma (25 µl) was diluted with water (75 µl) and added with cold methanol/chloroform mixture (850 µl, 2:1, v/v). They were ice-sonicated and extracted with an oscillator thermo-mixer (30 min 5°C, 1,000 rpm). After centrifugation (15 min at 13,400 rpm), the organic phase was evaporated under a stream of nitrogen. The residues were dissolved in 100 µl of isopropanol/acetonitrile (2:1, v/v) + 0.1 mm BHT and withdrawn in a glass vial (Dei Cas et al., 2020).

Polar Metabolites

Plasma (50 µl) was diluted with water (50 µl) and added with cold methanol/ethanol mixture (400 µl, 1:1, v/v). They were ice-sonicated and extracted with an oscillator thermo-mixer (30 min 5°C, 1,000 rpm). After centrifugation (15 min at 13,400 rpm), the protein debris was discharged, and the clean supernatant was evaporated under a stream of nitrogen. The residues were dissolved in 50 µl of water and withdrawn in a vial (Wawrzyniak et al., 2018).

Analysis by LC-HR-MS

The instrument consisted of a Shimadzu UPLC coupled with a Triple TOF 6600 Sciex (Concord, Canada) equipped with Turbo Spray IonDrive. All samples were analyzed in duplicate in both positive and negative mode with electrospray ionization.

Untargeted Lipidomics

The instrument settings were as follows: CUR = 35, GS1 = 55, GS2 = 65, capillary voltage ±5.5 kV, and source temperature 350°C. Spectra were contemporarily acquired by full-mass scan from *m/z* 200 to 1,500 (100 ms accumulation time) and data-dependent acquisition from *m/z* 50 to 1,500 (40 ms accumulation time, top-20 spectra per cycle 0.8 s). Declustering potential (DP) was fixed to 50 eV, and the collision energy (CE) was 35 ± 15 eV. The chromatographic separation was reached on a reverse-phase Acquity CSH C18 column 1.7 µm, 2.1 × 100 mm (Waters, MA, United States) equipped with a pre-column by using, as mobile phase (A) water/acetonitrile (60:40) and, as mobile phase (B) 2-propanol/acetonitrile (90:10), both containing 10-mm ammonium acetate and 0.1% of formic acid (Dei Cas et al., 2020). The flow rate was 0.4 ml/min, and the column temperature was 55°C. The elution gradient (%B) was set as below: 0–2.0 min (40%), 2.0–2.5 min (40–50%), 2.5–12.5 min (50–55%), 12.5–13.0 min (55–70%), 13.0–19.0 min (70–99%), 19.0–24.0 min (99%), and 24.0–24.2 (99–40%) and kept constant until 30 min. Five µl of clear organic supernatant was directly injected in the LC–MS/MS.

Untargeted Metabolomics

The instrument settings were as follows: CUR = 35, GS1 = 40, GS2 = 40, capillary voltage ±5.5 kV, and source temperature 500°C. Spectra were contemporarily acquired by full-mass scan from *m/z* 50 to 1,000 (100 ms accumulation time) and data-dependent acquisition from *m/z* 40 to 1,000 (40 ms accumulation time, top-20 spectra per cycle 0.8 s). Declustering potential (DP) was fixed to 60 eV, and collision energy (CE) was 30 ± 15 eV. Chromatographic separation was achieved on a reverse-phase Acquity HSS T3 column 1.7 µm, 2.1 × 100 mm (Waters, MA, United States) equipped with pre-column using as mobile phase (A) water and as mobile phase (B) methanol both containing 0.1% of formic acid (Want et al., 2013). The flow rate was 0.4 ml/min and the column temperature was 40°C. The elution gradient (%B) was set as below: 0–2.0 min (1%), 2.0–6.0 min (1–25%), 6.0–10.0 min (25–80%), 10.0–12.0 min (80–90%), 12.0–21.0 min (90–99%), 21.0–23.0 min (99–99%), and 23.0–23.2 min (99–1%) held until 30 min. Five µl of clear aqueous supernatant was directly injected in LC–MS/MS.

LC-HR-MS Data Processing

The spectra deconvolution, peak alignment, and sample normalization were attained using MS-DIAL (ver. 4.0; Tsugawa et al., 2015; Cajka et al., 2017; Huan et al., 2017). MS and MS/MS tolerance for peak profile were set to 0.01 and 0.05 Da, respectively. Identification was achieved matching molecular (*m/z* ± 0.02) and MS/MS experimental spectra (*m/z* ± 0.05) with (Beall, 2014) the Fiehn Hilic library for metabolomics or (Lam et al., 2020) the LipidBlast library for lipidomics. MS-DIAL post-identification was completed by the in-house library, which also considered analytes retention times. Features that met the following criteria were extracted and used for further analysis: (Beall, 2014) the CV% of the feature in the QC sample, repeatedly injected all along with the batch, should be <30%, and (Lam et al., 2020) the value of the feature peak was more than 10-fold the value of the same feature in the blank. Intensities of the remained metabolites were normalized by Lowess algorithm.

Statistical Analysis

Multivariate analysis was achieved with MetaboAnalyst 5.0, after data log-transformation and auto-scaling. Partial least squares discriminant analysis (PLS-DA) was performed to increase the group separation and to identify the variables with high Variance Importance in Projection score (VIP), assuming a cut-off value of 1.0 to disclose the discriminating variables. In PLS-DA, the dimension of a dataset is reduced while retaining as much information as possible; particularly, all the data acquired from a sample are condensed in a single dot, characterized by two dimensions. To further corroborate data, univariate statistical analysis was performed by GraphPad Prism 9.0 (GraphPad Software, Inc., La Jolla, California, United States) using one-way ANOVA followed by the Dunnett *post-hoc* test to compare metabolites against baseline (time 0) for each subject.

To confirm the relevance of the identified metabolites in precise metabolic pathways affected by hypoxia, the pathway analysis was performed based on *Homo sapiens* KEGG pathway networks (release 99, 2021/07). The value of p was corrected for the false discovery rate. Visualization of the results was attained using GraphPad Prism 9.0 (GraphPad Software, Inc., La Jolla, California, United States). In all tests, $p < 0.05$ was considered statistically significant.

RESULTS

The environmental conditions at the Concordia Station were predicted to cause some degree of emotional stress (Caputo et al., 2020), but all subjects remained in good health for the whole duration of the study and never experienced signs of high-altitude illness (AMS score < 1).

Non-polar Metabolome

By processing the LC-HR-MS data as described in "LC-HR-MS Data Processing", we identified ~1,000 lipid species in the plasma of each subject. The discriminant analysis (PLS-DA), useful to highlight the changes in the lipidome along the chronic hypoxia exposure period, showed a separation of 28.1% on principal component (PC1). The analysis showed a remarkable separation between the lipidome gathered at sea level before departure (time 0), and all the other observation times during hypoxia (**Figure 1A**).

To rank the discriminating features alongside the exposure to hypoxia, we used the VIP scores derived from the PLS-DA, assuming 1.0 as cut-off value. With this process, we selected 220 discriminant lipid species with VIP > 1.0 that emerged as markers of the differences among the plasma samples gathered at the four time points. They were then ordered and grouped according to their classes and visualized as a heat map after transformation to values of z (**Figures 1B,C** and **Supplementary Figure S1**). To detect those metabolites that were changed ($p < 0.05$) in at least one time point with respect to baseline, we employed univariate ANOVA. Apart from the 90-day time point, which often showed mild non-significant changes in some lipid species, the trend depicted a decrease in nine plasma lipid species along with hypoxia time, while Vitamin E levels resulted increased (**Figure 1B**). Although the data points taken in hypoxia appear consistently different from baseline at any time, a slight but significant ($p < 0.01$) change was observed between MW and END along PC1, highlighting a possible normalization of the non-polar metabolome after 6-month hypoxia. Such change, however, was not observed along neither PC2 nor PC3.

Polar Metabolome

After applying to LC-HR-MS data the same processing procedure described in paragraph "LC-HR-MS Data Processing", we identified $n = 146$ polar metabolites in the plasma of each subject (**Supplementary Table S4**). PLS-DA on polar metabolites showed a more remarkable separation than lipids between non-hypoxic and hypoxic conditions (PC1 = 41.2% vs. 28.3%; **Figure 2A**). The PLS-DA performed on these metabolites helped identifying $n = 69$ metabolites with VIP > 1 that are related with hypoxia (**Figure 2B**). **Figure 2C** shows as the heat map of the metabolites that satisfy two conditions: VIP > 1 and $p < 0.05$ at least at one time point during the observation period ($n = 65$). Whereas PLS-DA component 1 describes the immediate responses to environment changes, component 2 shows the progressive change of the polar metabolome during hypoxia exposure. The VIP metabolites calculated on both PC1 and PC2 are listed in **Supplementary Table S5**. Particularly, the results from this analysis appear consistent with the previous ones, as most of the metabolites are found in both VIP groups, such as ornithine, nicotinamide, and N-acetylputrescine. By contrast, other molecules, such as, for instance, propionylcarnitine, are VIP metabolites following PC2 only.

Pathway Analysis

To discover the metabolic pathways mostly involved during hypoxia adaptation, we performed three different pathway analyses comparing the metabolomes of the three time points during hypoxia with the baseline one. The bubble graph in **Figure 3** shows schematically the modulation of the pathways. For each metabolism pathway, the coverage is represented by the size of the circles, while the position on the X-axis indicates the impact in a scale from 0 to 1 and the bubble color the value of p. All the pathways indicated therein have an impact of at least 0.3. Most of the pathways implicated in chronic hypoxia seem to be linked to the metabolism of amino acids. More specifically, the pathways with higher impact and coverage resulted to be associated to the biosynthesis of phenylalanine, tyrosine, and tryptophan (map 00040 in KEGG). **Figure 4** displays, instead, the relation of each metabolite to the modulated pathway itself and their levels across the groups. For each of the pathways represented as a bubble in **Figure 3**, all the

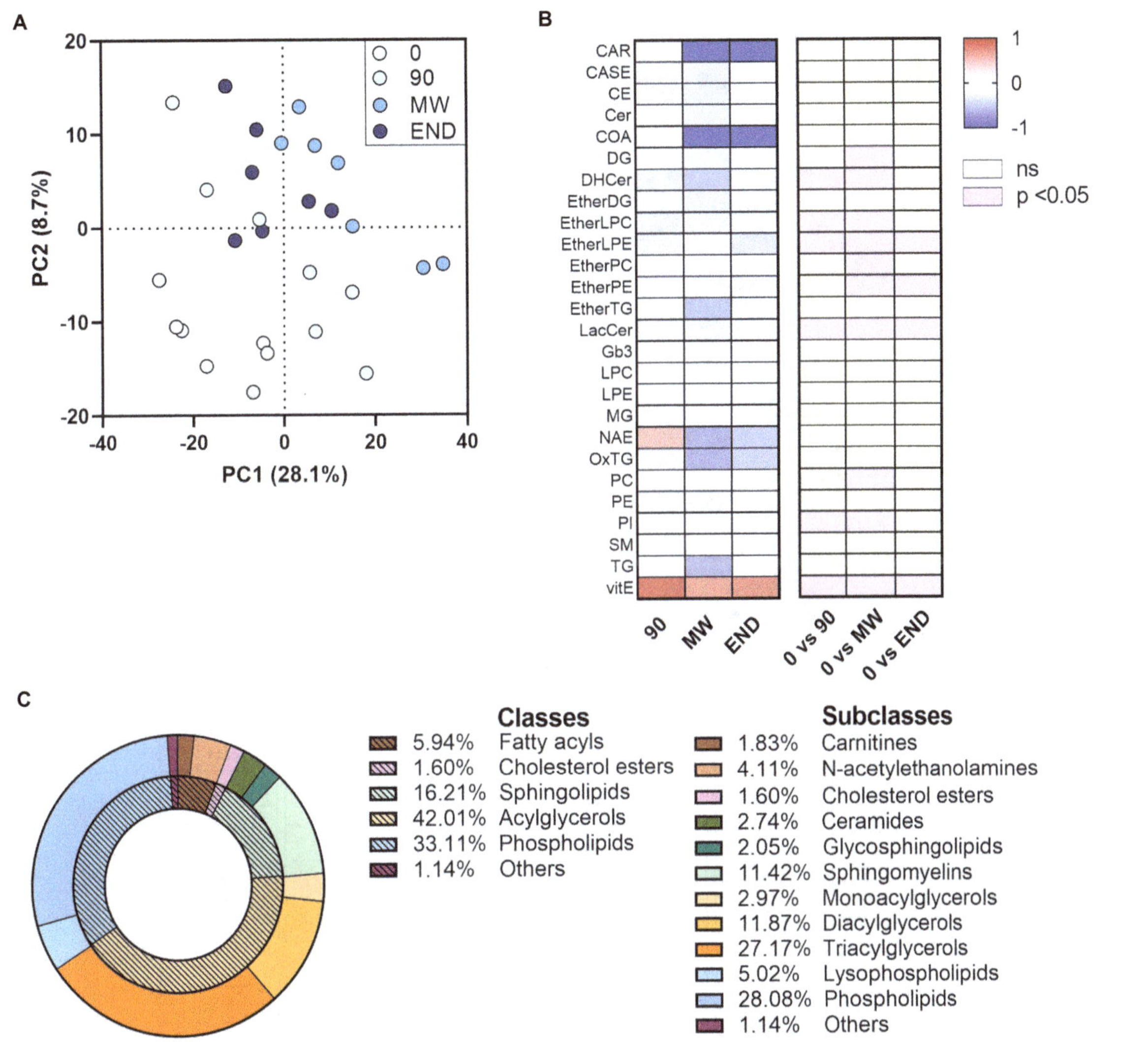

FIGURE 1 | Alterations in circulating lipidome during 10 months of chronic hypoxia in the Antarctica. **(A)** Multivariate analysis visualized as principal discriminant analysis of lipids in plasma after 0, 90, 150–180 (MW), and 300 days (END) in the Antarctica. **(B)** Discriminant lipids were chosen between those with a VIP > 1.0, then ordered and summed according to their class, and finally visualized as a heat map after transformation to values of *z*. Data are shown as log-fold change of each time points (90, MW, END) over baseline values. The three columns on the right show the significance of the difference vs. time 0 by one-way ANOVA and the Dunnett *post-hoc* test. **(C)** Discriminant (VIP) lipids grouped in their classes and subclasses as a donut chart graph.

detected metabolites are annotated from the *H. sapiens* KEGG pathway networks, their variation over time and the significance of the variation.

DISCUSSION

When the effects of chronic hypoxia in humans are investigated at altitude, many disturbing factors may interfere with the measurement of metabolic and physiological variables. These may include exposure to cold, development of anxiety, heavy exercise, abrupt altitude changes, environmental-born stress, food ingestion irregularities, or even starving. By contrast, the logistics of the Concordia Station, with reduced fluctuations in temperature and humidity, comforting environment, regular feeding, and drinking, impossibility to change altitude and relatively controlled psychological stress should reduce, or even prevent, the occurrence of disturbing factors. Specifically, although cold exposure during outdoor activities may affect the lipidome profile (Lynes et al., 2018; Coolbaugh et al., 2019), we exclude this as a potential confounding factor in this study, due to the low exposure volume and the great preventive attention paid by the subjects. It is known that the lack of natural sunlight may alter the fasting plasma metabolome in healthy subjects (Noordam et al., 2019). Therefore, it is possible that the rupture in the circadian rhythms in the subjects studied here may represent a confounding factor because the MW time point corresponds to day-long lightless conditions in contrast to the 90 and END points. Although indoor light tended to preserve in part the day-night light cycle, this

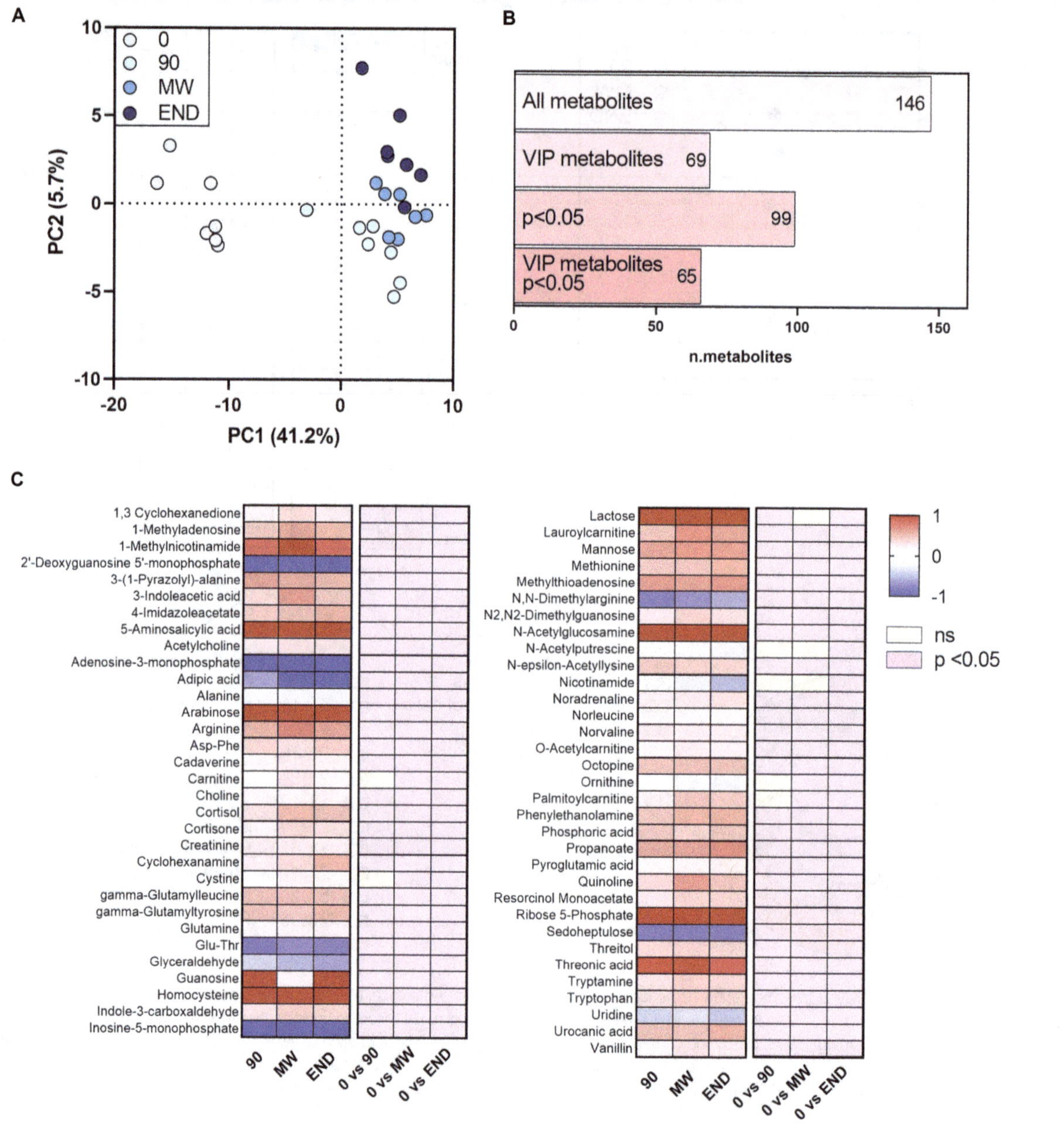

FIGURE 2 | Alterations in the circulating polar metabolome during 10 months of chronic hypoxia in the Antarctica. **(A)** Multivariate analysis visualized as principal discriminant analysis of polar metabolites in plasma after 0, 90, 150–180 (MW), and 300 days (END) in Antarctica. **(B)** Number of identified metabolites in each subgroup: VIP, metabolites with $p < 0.05$ and VIP with $p < 0.05$. **(C)** Heat map of discriminant metabolites with VIP > 1.0, and at least one time point with $p < 0.05$ vs. time 0 after transformation to values of *z*. Data are shown as log-fold change of each time points (90, MW, END) over baseline. The three columns on the right show the significance of the difference vs. time 0 by one-way ANOVA and the Dunnett *post-hoc* test.

confounding factor should be taken as a potential limit of this study.

Therefore, in this study, hypoxia may be considered the only variable that influenced the measurements. The duration of the subjects' sojourn at altitude (10 months) enables focusing into relatively long-term adaptation to hypoxia. The degree of hypoxia at the Concordia Station, equivalent to approximately 3,800 m asl, is compatible with the body's need to adapt, yet it is not extreme, with the risk to conflict with altitude sickness. Indeed, the blood gas values at the Concordia Station revealed decreased pCO_2 with alkalemia resulting from moderate increase of the breathing rate to balance hypoxia (Porcelli et al., 2017). The inadequate renal compensation to cope with increased CO_2 washout in the lungs nevertheless produced a persistent base excess of −4 mEq/l, to be compared with −6 mEq/l found at 6,450 m asl (Samaja et al., 1997).

Today LC-HR-MS represents a powerful approach to address the metabolome changes in response to hypoxia. Despite the

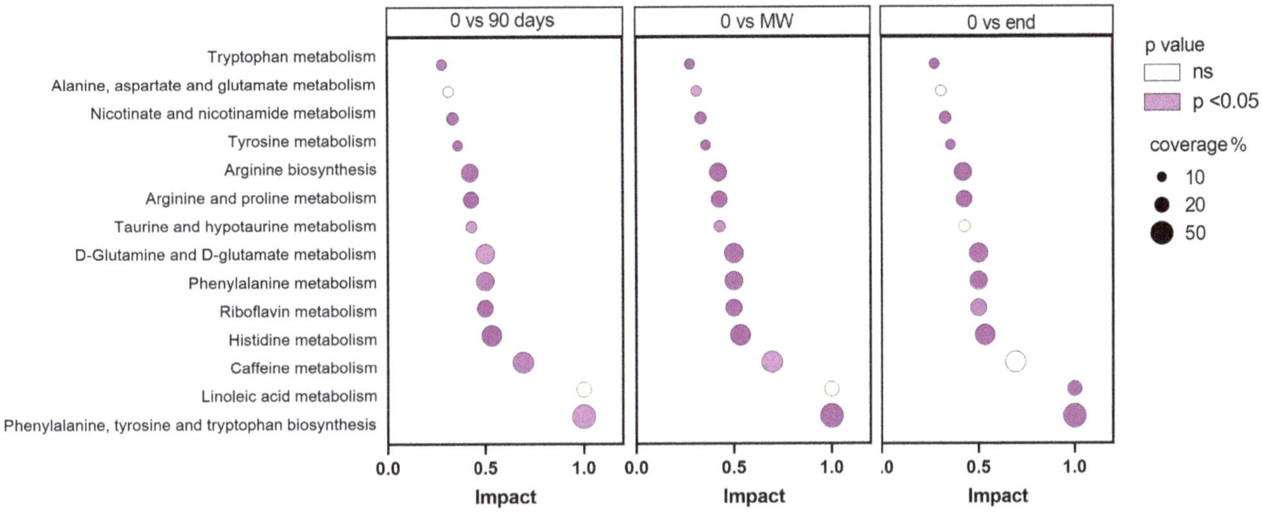

FIGURE 3 | Schematic diagram of the most altered metabolic pathways after 90 days, MW and 9 months in Antarctica with respect to baseline. Values of *p* were corrected for false discovery rate. Enrichment pathway analysis was performed based on *Homo sapiens* KEGG pathway networks. In purple, are reported those significantly modulated by performing one-way ANOVA and the Dunnett *post-hoc* test; in yellow, those not modulated. For each metabolism pathway, the coverage is represented by the size of the circles, while the position on the X-axis indicates the impact in a scale from 0 to 1.

low number of subjects, most of the metabolome changes were statistically consistent and visible since $t = 90$ days. Because they remained independent of the hypoxia duration until $t = 300$ days, this highlights human inability to compensate the observed changes with return to baseline values. This feature might be interpreted as lack of adaptation to hypoxia, in the same way as it has been previously observed as for the changes induced by hypoxia on the acid–base status and on the erythropoietic stimulus (Porcelli et al., 2017).

Whereas some of the observed changes appear occasional and perhaps dependent on the individual diet (e.g., caffeine, 1,7-dimethyluric acid, and Vitamin E), other changes may be referred to as part of one or more mechanisms of hypoxia adaptation, with special concern of the metabolism of amino acids. Exposure to altitude hypoxia is well known to increase protein catabolism (Pasiakos et al., 2017). However, the finding that the whole pool of proteogenic amino acid is not altered by hypoxia nor to vary with time (**Supplementary Figure S2**) suggests the lack of significant hypoxia-induced protein catabolism. Most likely, the living conditions at the Concordia Station exclude this potentially confounding variable (Rathor et al., 2021); thus, the variations of individual amino acids may be attributed solely to selective recruitment of hypoxia-linked metabolic pathways (see also **Supplementary Figure S3**).

The increase in the plasma levels of some amino acids agrees with a study performed in 34 volunteers ascending progressively to 6,885 m asl in 19 days, that showed altitude-related increases in tryptophan, serotonin, and peroxidation-sensitive lipids, together with enhanced oxidative stress (Pichler Hefti et al., 2013). In an attempt to associate the variations of single amino acids to hypoxia-linked pathways, we focused into those species that displayed marked (>0.5) and significant ($p < 0.05$) changes over the three time points.

High glutamine may be related to the disruption of the ammonia vs. glutamate balance with potential to affect negatively the brain cognitive function (Dos Santos et al., 2020), while depleted levels of the excitatory neurotransmitter glutamate may be associated to increased brain uptake of glutamate to stimulate ventilation in an attempt to compensate lower oxygen saturation (Honda et al., 1985). The disruption of the ammonia vs. glutamate balance is likely related to altered nitrogen metabolism and supported by the decreases in N-acetylputrescine, spermine, and ornithine, polyamines with relevant physiological roles on angiogenesis and reproductive physiology (Lenis et al., 2017; **Supplementary Figure S4**).

Higher plasma tryptophan may highlight lower activity of the tryptophan hydroxylase reaction, the rate-limiting enzyme in serotonin synthesis because it requires molecular oxygen (Fitzpatrick, 1999). Enhanced hypoxia vulnerability of this enzyme (Vaccari et al., 1978) is expected to lower brain serotonin synthesis, which results in depression, reduced appetite and motivation, and disruption of sleep patterns (Katz, 1982), as commonly found in altitude residents (Maa, 2010; DelMastro et al., 2011). Likewise, higher tryptophan may also recruit the kynurenine pathway. Untargeted metabolomic analysis already revealed that these pathways are upregulated in a model of perinatal asphyxia and neonatal hypoxia-ischemia encephalopathy (Denihan et al., 2019). Furthermore, enhanced activity of the kynurenine pathway is a common finding in umbilical cord blood and placental samples in normal and fetal growth restriction pregnancies, as well as in the media of placental explants incubated with 5–8% oxygen (Murthi et al., 2017).

The kynurenine pathway is also linked to the nicotinamide pathway to account for the increased levels of 1-methylnicotinamide observed in this study. The observed decrease in nicotinamide may be related to its higher use in

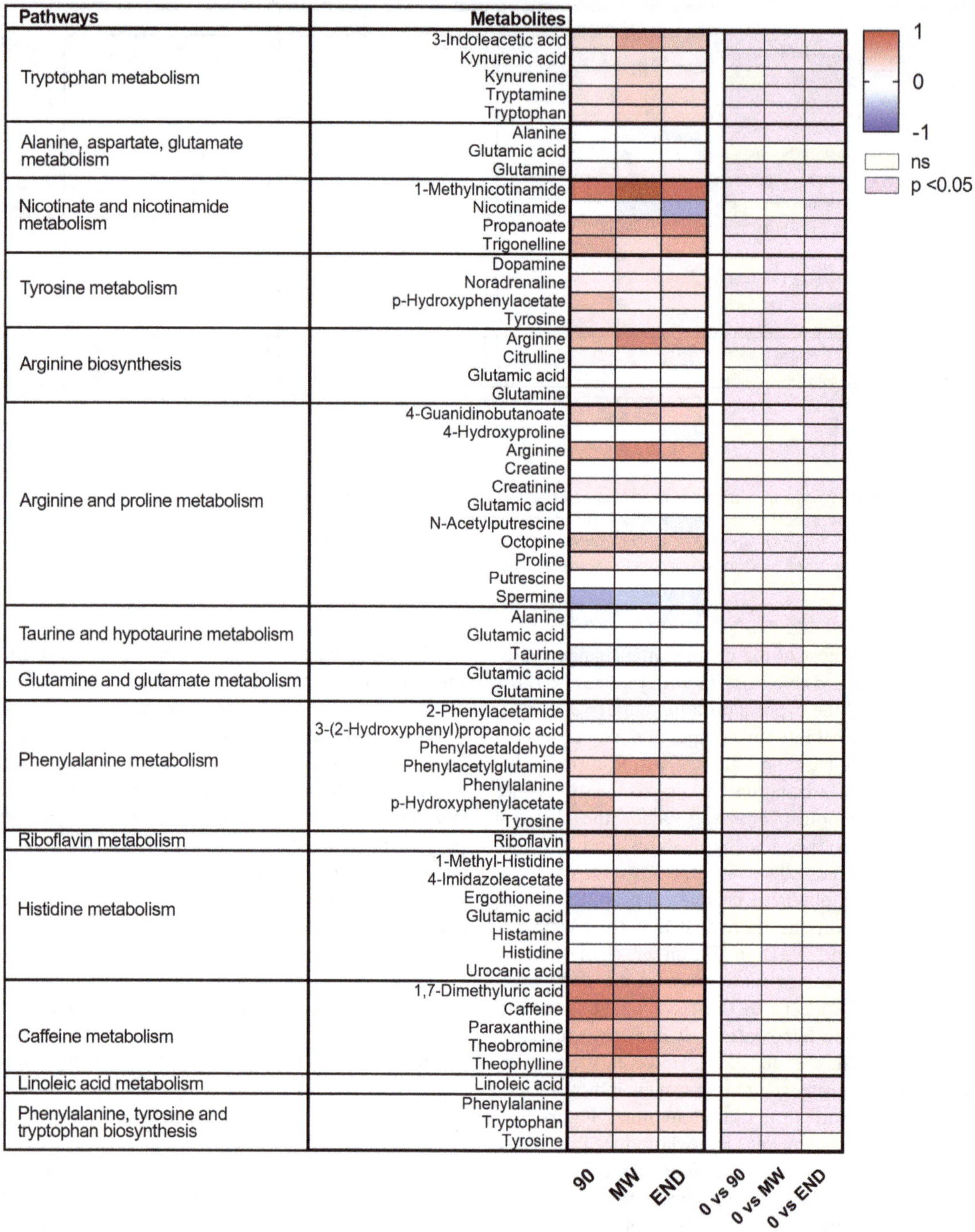

FIGURE 4 | Heat map of the metabolites included in the pathways significantly affected by hypoxia for every time point. On the right, are indicated in violet those significantly modulated by performing one-way ANOVA and the Dunnett *post-hoc* test; in yellow, those not modulated.

the nicotinamide phosphoribosyltransferase reaction that promotes pulmonary vascular remodeling in the development of pulmonary arterial hypertension (Chen et al., 2017), a common finding in chronic hypoxia (Ottolenghi et al., 2020; Gassmann et al., 2021). As a matter of facts, either nicotinamide (Sztormowska-Achranowicz et al., 2020) or niacin (or nicotinic acid; Jia et al., 2020) are being investigated as drugs to ameliorate progression of hypoxia-induced pulmonary hypertension.

A precursor of NO, arginine is often used as a vasodilator drug in several human diseases, but the effect of hypoxia on NO bioavailability is still debated. In a most recent view, improved NO bioavailability appears to favor human adaptation to altitude (Beall et al., 2012) and underlies the Tibetans' response to altitude hypoxia (Erzurum et al., 2007). This is compatible with either the increased plasma arginine observed in this study, and the beneficial effects of supplementing arginine (Schneider et al., 2001) or sildenafil (Xu et al., 2014) at altitude.

Finally, octopin, a derivative of alanine and arginine that may function as an analog of lactic acid in invertebrate muscles (Hochachka et al., 1977), was found to be increased in marine animals exposed to 50% oxygen shortage without changes in protein turnover (Capaz et al., 2017).

Comparing the reported findings with the literature *-omics* data may be of limited value due to extremely different materials and hypoxia administration protocols. A first cohort of studies concerns LC-HR-MS analyses performed in contexts related to acute hypoxia. A study aimed at identifying plasma metabolites predictive of AMS insurgence in 60 subjects after 4 days at 5,300 m asl revealed variations in up to 44 metabolites of the pathways related to inflammation, energy consumption (e.g., TCA, fatty acids, and amino acids), bile acids, and hemoglobin metabolism (Liao et al., 2016). Another study of the red blood cell metabolome after 1–16 days at 5,000 m asl highlighted promoted glycolysis and deregulated pentose phosphate pathway, purine catabolism, glutathione homeostasis, arginine/NO, and sulfur/H_2S (D'Alessandro et al., 2016). A third study performed in four subjects exposed for 2 days at 4,559 m asl revealed subject-dependent redox-changes (Cumpstey et al., 2019). Finally, a study in eight subjects exercising in a hypobaric chamber at an equivalent altitude of 4,300 m asl for 8 h revealed increased glycolysis and TCA cycle activity, amino acid breakdown, oxidative stress, fatty acid storage, and decreased fatty acid mobilization (Margolis et al., 2021). The last findings are compatible with acute onset of hypoxia-mediated peripheral insulin resistance, which is to be compared with the increased levels of some amino acids observed in the present report, along with depressed pool of lipids, cofactors, and vitamins. Thus, despite some analogies, comparing the data reported here with those obtained in acute hypoxia appears difficult.

Another cohort of *-omics* studies compared gene analysis of altitude vs. sea-level populations in the search of changes in the evolutionary processes that have tinkered differently on the various altitude populations across the world, who followed different routes of hypoxia adaptation (Beall, 2007). Such gene changes are expected to impact the metabolome. The genic differences between Andeans and Tibetans, presumably a paradigm of human generational hypoxia adaptation, as from the occurrence of Chronic Mountain Sickness, highlighted a panel of approximately 120 genes that responded differentially to hypoxia and are related to the development of the nervous, lymphoid, cardiovascular, and erythropoietic systems (Azad et al., 2017). Likewise, a gene expression study in acclimatized altitude populations revealed reduced oxidative capacity, decreased oxidation of fatty acids, and decreased ATP turnover with respect to lowlanders (Murray et al., 2018). Other genome-wide scans of high-altitude populations identified the oxygen-sensing machinery as responsible for phenotypic adjustments leading to adaptation (Storz, 2021). Certainly, genetic signals eventually impact differentially the metabolic adaptation to hypoxia but as a matter of facts studies performed in populations residing at altitude could not yet distinguish the roles played by genes, Darwinian evolution and environmental factors.

A further cohort of studies potentially useful to compare the reported data concerns the *-omics* in patients affected by pathological hypoxia secondary to pulmonary diseases as Acute respiratory distress syndrome (ARDS), Chronic obstructive pulmonary disease, and perhaps asthma. NMR-based metabolome in ARDS patients grouped by disease severity identified major involvement of amino acid-linked pathways, especially glutamate, threonine, taurine, lysine, arginine, and proline (Viswan et al., 2017). Other studies in asthma patients reviewed in (Kelly et al., 2017) revealed a wide range of affected variables. A recent review extended to all *-omics* techniques confirmed these features (Sim et al., 2021). It is therefore likely that the pulmonary pathologies that lead to chronic hypoxemia involve more pathways than those triggered by physiological hypoxia only, e.g., inflammation, iron handling dysfunction, and redox imbalance (Duca et al., 2021), thereby making it difficult to compare pathological with physiological hypoxia.

Limits of the Study

Although data reported here were obtained under conditions of month-long hypoxia of mild intensity, it remains to be clarified whether longer or more severe challenges would enable better insight into the mechanisms underlying human adaptation to hypoxia. However, the present study, which compares the same subjects at sea level before departure and at three time points during hypoxia, may help to enucleate the effects of hypoxia as a single factor, keeping to a minimum the incidence of hypoxia-associated disturbing variables.

In the present investigation, we identified a panel of polar and non-polar metabolites that are systematically altered by chronic hypoxia. Yet, despite the statistical significance obtained using the most conservative tests, the size limit of the recruited population necessarily prevents expanding these findings to the general population facing a mild hypoxia challenge. Furthermore, the existing literature is not yet sufficiently developed to determine whether the changes described in the present report represent spurious findings or reflect the substantial heterogeneity and limited statistical power. Therefore, this study necessarily represents a preliminary report that needs validation from further larger size studies, possibly including gene correlations. Further studies should use standardized methods and – perhaps most important – reduce to a reasonable minimum the population's background noise, i.e., not simply the usual macroscopic variables as smoking, alcohol/drug assumption, and diseases, but also abrupt changes in altitude, environment temperature/humidity, activity, and feeding and life behavior.

Both the polar and the non-polar metabolomes were characterized by relevant adjustments within 90-day hypoxia. While the polar metabolome did not change further until at least 300-day hypoxia, the non-polar metabolome apparently displayed a slight but statistically significant return toward the baseline situation after MW to be evaluated in future studies. Nevertheless, these observations highlight the completion of the metabolome response within 90-day hypoxia, accompanied by the human body's inability to perform longer term adjustments.

Finally, the rupture of the circadian rhythms due to extremely variable light conditions during the year may be a point of concern to be examined in further studies. Likewise, even the contribute of a regular exercise program, which was not accounted for in the present investigation, to both the polar and non-polar metabolome changes, does merit future *ad-hoc* studies.

CONCLUSION

The analysis of non-polar and polar metabolome patterns in the plasma from humans exposed to mild hypoxia (barometric pressure of 478 mmHg, equivalent to 3,800 m asl) revealed minor changes in the lipidome as compared to marked changes in the polar metabolite pattern. Remarkably, such changes occur within 90 days after the start of hypoxia and were constant over time for at least 300 days (with the exception of a slight return of the non-polar metabolome after 6 months), thus highlighting either a relatively acute response or the inability of the human body to further adjust the metabolism after the initial phase. KEGG analysis enabled identifying, among the pathways affected by hypoxia, the metabolism of some amino acids, chiefly arginine, glutamine, phenylalanine, tryptophan, and tyrosine, as major candidates that presumably drive the human response, perhaps adaptation, to a potentially lethal situation that challenge an intolerably high number of patients affected by pulmonary and circulatory diseases worldwide.

ETHICS STATEMENT

The studies involving human participants were reviewed and approved by Ethical Committee of the San Paolo Hospital in Milan (154/ST/ 2014). The patients/participants provided their written informed consent to participate in this study.

AUTHOR CONTRIBUTIONS

All authors contributed extensively to the work presented in this manuscript and approved the submitted version. MD, RP, SO, and MS: conceptualization. MD and CM: investigation and formal analysis. MD and SO: visualization. RD, GR, SO, and MS: resources. RD, GR, MS, and RP: supervision. MD, SO, and CM: writing—original draft. RP, MS, and SO: writing—review and editing.

ACKNOWLEDGMENTS

This study has been made possible by the contribution of several people and organizations. First, we are deeply indebted with the Members of the crew who sojourned for 10 months at the Concordia Station, donated their blood, and always collaborated constructively for the success of this study. We are also indebted to ENEA for the logistic support and for materials shipping to and from Antarctica. Part of this work was carried out in OMICs, an advanced Mass Spectrometry platform established at the University of Milan, Italy. Professor. Michele Maffia, University of Salento, Lecce, Italy, and Dr. Maria Rosaria Coscia, Institute of Biochemistry and Cell Biology, National Research Council, Naples, Italy, for kindly providing the samples used for the reported analyses.

REFERENCES

Azad, P., Stobdan, T., Zhou, D., Hartley, I., Akbari, A., Bafna, V., et al. (2017). High-altitude adaptation in humans: from genomics to integrative physiology. *J. Mol. Med.* 95, 1269–1282. doi: 10.1007/s00109-017-1584-7

Beall, C. M. (2007). Two routes to functional adaptation: Tibetan and Andean high-altitude natives. *Proc. Natl. Acad. Sci. U. S. A.* 104, 8655–8660. doi: 10.1073/pnas.0701985104

Beall, C. M. (2014). Adaptation to high altitude: phenotypes and genotypes. *Annu. Rev. Anthropol.* 43, 251–272. doi: 10.1146/annurev-anthro-102313-030000

Beall, C. M., Laskowski, D., and Erzurum, S. C. (2012). Nitric oxide in adaptation to altitude. *Free Radic. Biol. Med.* 52, 1123–1134. doi: 10.1016/j.freeradbiomed.2011.12.028

Cajka, T., Smilowitz, J. T., and Fiehn, O. (2017). Validating quantitative untargeted lipidomics across nine liquid chromatography-high-resolution mass spectrometry platforms. *Anal. Chem.* 89, 12360–12368. doi: 10.1021/acs.analchem.7b03404

Capaz, J. C., Tunnah, L., MacCormack, T. J., Lamarre, S. G., Sykes, A. V., and Driedzic, W. R. (2017). Hypoxic induced decrease in oxygen consumption in cuttlefish (*Sepia officinalis*) is associated with minor increases in mantle octopine but no changes in markers of protein turnover. *Front. Physiol.* 8:344. doi: 10.3389/fphys.2017.00344

Caputo, V., Pacilli, M. G., Arisi, I., Mazza, T., Brandi, R., Traversa, A., et al. (2020). Genomic and physiological resilience in extreme environments are associated with a secure attachment style. *Transl. Psychiatry* 10, 1–11. doi: 10.1038/s41398-020-00869-4

Chen, J., Sysol, J. R., Singla, S., Zhao, S., Yamamura, A., Valdez-Jasso, D., et al. (2017). Nicotinamide phosphoribosyltransferase promotes pulmonary vascular remodeling and is a therapeutic target in pulmonary arterial hypertension. *Circulation* 135, 1532–1546. doi: 10.1161/CIRCULATIONAHA.116.024557

Coolbaugh, C. L., Damon, B. M., Bush, E. C., Welch, E. B., and Towse, T. F. (2019). Cold exposure induces dynamic, heterogeneous alterations in human brown adipose tissue lipid content. *Sci. Rep.* 9:13600. doi: 10.1038/s41598-019-49936-x

Cumpstey, A. F., Minnion, M., Fernandez, B. O., Mikus-Lelinska, M., Mitchell, K., Martin, D. S., et al. (2019). Pushing arterial-venous plasma biomarkers to new heights: a model for personalised redox metabolomics? *Redox Biol.* 21:101113. doi: 10.1016/j.redox.2019.101113

D'Alessandro, A., Nemkov, T., Sun, K., Liu, H., Song, A., Monte, A. A., et al. (2016). AltitudeOmics: red blood cell metabolic adaptation to high altitude hypoxia. *J. Proteome Res.* 15, 3883–3895. doi: 10.1021/acs.jproteome.6b00733

Dei Cas, M., Zulueta, A., Mingione, A., Caretti, A., Ghidoni, R., Signorelli, P., et al. (2020). An innovative lipidomic workflow to investigate the lipid profile in a cystic fibrosis cell line. *Cell* 9:1197. doi: 10.3390/cells9051197

DelMastro, K., Hellem, T., Kim, N., Kondo, D., Sung, Y. H., and Renshaw, P. F. (2011). Incidence of major depressive episode correlates with elevation of substate region of residence. *J. Affect. Disord.* 129, 376–379. doi: 10.1016/j.jad.2010.10.001

Denihan, N. M., Kirwan, J. A., Walsh, B. H., Dunn, W. B., Broadhurst, D. I., Boylan, G. B., et al. (2019). Untargeted metabolomic analysis and pathway discovery in perinatal asphyxia and hypoxic-ischaemic encephalopathy. *J. Cereb. Blood Flow Metab.* 39, 147–162. doi: 10.1177/0271678X17726502

Dos Santos, Q. M., Souza, W., Lemos, V. A., Caris, A. V., and Thomatieli-Santos, R. V. (2020). The possible importance of glutamine supplementation to mood and cognition in hypoxia from high altitude. *Nutrients* 12:3627. doi: 10.3390/nu12123627

Duca, L., Ottolenghi, S., Coppola, S., Rinaldo, R., Dei Cas, M., Rubino, F. M., et al. (2021). Differential redox state and iron regulation in chronic obstructive pulmonary disease, acute respiratory distress syndrome and coronavirus disease 2019. *Antioxidants* 10:1460. doi: 10.3390/antiox10091460

Erzurum, S. C., Ghosh, S., Janocha, A. J., Xu, W., Bauer, S., Bryan, N. S., et al. (2007). Higher blood flow and circulating NO products offset high-altitude hypoxia among Tibetans. *Proc. Natl. Acad. Sci. U. S. A.* 104, 17593–17598. doi: 10.1073/pnas.0707462104

Ferrazzini, G., Maggiorini, M., Kriemler, S., Bärtsch, P., and Oelz, O. (1987). Successful treatment of acute mountain sickness with dexamethasone. *Br. Med. J.* 294, 1380–1382. doi: 10.1136/bmj.294.6584.1380

Fitzpatrick, P. F. (1999). Tetrahydropterin-dependent amino acid hydroxylases. *Annu. Rev. Biochem.* 68, 355–381. doi: 10.1146/annurev.biochem.68.1.355

Gassmann, M., Cowburn, A., Gu, H., Li, J., Rodriguez, M., Babicheva, A., et al. (2021). Hypoxia-induced pulmonary hypertension-utilizing experiments of nature. *Br. J. Pharmacol.* 178, 121–131. doi: 10.1111/bph.15144

Gonzalez-Ruiz, V., Pezzatti, J., Roux, A., Stoppini, L., Boccard, J., and Rudaz, S. (2017). Unravelling the effects of multiple experimental factors in metabolomics, analysis of human neural cells with hydrophilic interaction liquid chromatography hyphenated to high resolution mass spectrometry. *J. Chromatogr. A* 1527, 53–60. doi: 10.1016/j.chroma.2017.10.055

Hochachka, P. W., Hartline, P. H., and Fields, J. H. (1977). Octopine as an end product of anaerobic glycolysis in the chambered nautilus. *Science* 195, 72–74. doi: 10.1126/science.831256

Honda, Y., Tani, H., Masuda, A., Kobayashi, T., Nishino, T., Kimura, H., et al. (1985). Effect of prior O_2 breathing on ventilatory response to sustained isocapnic hypoxia in adult humans. *J. Appl. Physiol.* 81, 1627–1632. doi: 10.1152/jappl.1996.81.4.1627

Huan, T., Forsberg, E. M., Rinehart, D., Johnson, C. H., Ivanisevic, J., Benton, H. P., et al. (2017). Systems biology guided by XCMS online metabolomics. *Nat. Methods* 14, 461–462. doi: 10.1038/nmeth.4260

Jahan, E., Barua, T., and Salma, U. (2014). An overview on heart rate monitoring and pulse oximeter system. *Int. J. Latest Res. Sci. Technol.* 3, 148–152.

Jia, D., Bai, P., Wan, N., Liu, J., Zhu, Q., He, Y., et al. (2020). Niacin attenuates pulmonary hypertension through H-PGDS in macrophages. *Circ. Res.* 127, 1323–1336. doi: 10.1161/CIRCRESAHA.120.316784

Julian, C. G. (1985). Epigenomics and human adaptation to high altitude. *J. Appl. Physiol.* 123, 1362–1370. doi: 10.1152/japplphysiol.00351.2017

Kanwisher, J. (1957). Oxygen in Antarctic air. *Tellus* 9, 137–138.

Katz, I. R. (1982). Is there a hypoxic affective syndrome? *Psychosomatics* 23, 846–853. doi: 10.1016/S0033-3182(82)73084-1

Kelly, R. S., Dahlin, A., McGeachie, M. J., Qiu, W., Sordillo, J., Wan, E. S., et al. (2017). Asthma metabolomics and the potential for integrative omics in research and the clinic. *Chest* 151, 262–277. doi: 10.1016/j.chest.2016.10.008

Lam, F., Subhi, R., Houdek, J., Schroder, K., Battu, A., and Graham, H. (2020). The prevalence of hypoxemia among pediatric and adult patients presenting to healthcare facilities in low- and middle-income countries: protocol for a systematic review and meta-analysis. *Syst. Rev.* 9:67. doi: 10.1186/s13643-020-01326-5

Lenis, Y. Y., Elmetwally, M. A., Maldonado-Estrada, J. G., and Bazer, F. W. (2017). Physiological importance of polyamines. *Zygote* 25, 244–255. doi: 10.1017/S0967199417000120

Liao, W. T., Liu, B., Chen, J., Cui, J. H., Gao, Y. X., Liu, F. Y., et al. (2016). Metabolite modulation in human plasma in the early phase of acclimatization to hypobaric hypoxia. *Sci. Rep.* 6:22589. doi: 10.1038/srep22589

Lynes, M. D., Shamsi, F., Sustarsic, E. G., Leiria, L. O., Wang, C. H., Su, S. C., et al. (2018). Cold-activated lipid dynamics in adipose tissue highlights a role for cardiolipin in thermogenic metabolism. *Cell Rep.* 24, 781–790. doi: 10.1016/j.celrep.2018.06.073

Maa, E. H. (2010). Hypobaric hypoxic cerebral insults: the neurological consequences of going higher. *NeuroRehabilitation* 26, 73–84. doi: 10.3233/NRE-2010-0537

Margolis, L. M., Karl, J. P., Wilson, M. A., Coleman, J. L., Ferrando, A. A., Young, A. J., et al. (2021). Metabolomic profiles are reflective of hypoxia-induced insulin resistance during exercise in healthy young adult males. *Am. J. Physiol. Regul. Integr. Comp. Physiol.* 321, R1–R11. doi: 10.1152/ajpregu.00076.2021

Moore, L. G. (1985). Measuring high-altitude adaptation. *J. Appl. Physiol.* 123, 1371–1385. doi: 10.1152/japplphysiol.00321.2017

Murray, A. J., Montgomery, H. E., Feelisch, M., Grocott, M. P. W., and Martin, D. S. (2018). Metabolic adjustment to high-altitude hypoxia: from genetic signals to physiological implications. *Biochem. Soc. Trans.* 46, 599–607. doi: 10.1042/BST20170502

Murthi, P., Wallace, E. M., and Walker, D. W. (2017). Altered placental tryptophan metabolic pathway in human fetal growth restriction. *Placenta* 52, 62–70. doi: 10.1016/j.placenta.2017.02.013

Noordam, R., Ramkisoensing, A., Loh, N. Y., Neville, M. J., Rosendaal, F. R., Willems van Dijk, K., et al. (2019). Associations of outdoor temperature, bright sunlight, and cardiometabolic traits in two European population-based cohorts. *J. Clin. Endocrinol. Metab.* 104, 2903–2910. doi: 10.1210/jc.2018-02532

Ottolenghi, S., Zulueta, A., and Caretti, A. (2020). Iron and sphingolipids as common players of (mal)adaptation to hypoxia in pulmonary diseases. *Int. J. Mol. Sci.* 21:307. doi: 10.3390/ijms21010307

Pasiakos, S. M., Berryman, C. E., Carrigan, C. T., Young, A. J., and Carbone, J. W. (2017). Muscle protein turnover and the molecular regulation of muscle mass during hypoxia. *Med. Sci. Sports Exerc.* 49, 1340–1350. doi: 10.1249/MSS.0000000000001228

Pezzatti, J., Gonzalez-Ruiz, V., Codesido, S., Gagnebin, Y., Joshi, A., Guillarme, D., et al. (2019). A scoring approach for multi-platform acquisition in metabolomics. *J. Chromatogr. A* 1592, 47–54. doi: 10.1016/j.chroma.2019.01.023

Pichler Hefti, J., Sonntag, D., Hefti, U., Risch, L., Schoch, O. D., Turk, A. J., et al. (2013). Oxidative stress in hypobaric hypoxia and influence on vessel-tone modifying mediators. *High Alt. Med. Biol.* 14, 273–279. doi: 10.1089/ham.2012.1110

Porcelli, S., Marzorati, M., Healey, B., Terraneo, L., Vezzoli, A., Bella, S. D., et al. (2017). Lack of acclimatization to chronic hypoxia in humans in the Antarctica. *Sci. Rep.* 7:18090. doi: 10.1038/s41598-017-18212-1

Rathor, R., Suryakumar, G., and Singh, S. N. (2021). Diet and redox state in maintaining skeletal muscle health and performance at high altitude. *Free Radic. Biol. Med.* 174, 305–320. doi: 10.1016/j.freeradbiomed.2021.07.024

Samaja, M., Mariani, C., Prestini, A., and Cerretelli, P. (1997). Acid-base balance and O_2 transport at high altitude. *Acta Physiol. Scand.* 159, 249–256. doi: 10.1046/j.1365-201X.1997.574342000.x

Schneider, J. C., Blazy, I., Dechaux, M., Rabier, D., Mason, N. P., and Richalet, J. P. (2001). Response of nitric oxide pathway to L-arginine infusion at the altitude of 4,350 m. *Eur. Respir. J.* 18, 286–292. doi: 10.1183/09031936.01.00073401

Sim, S., Choi, Y., and Park, H. S. (2021). Potential metabolic biomarkers in adult asthmatics. *Meta* 11:430. doi: 10.3390/metabo11070430

Simon-Manso, Y., Lowenthal, M. S., Kilpatrick, L. E., Sampson, M. L., Telu, K. H., Rudnick, P. A., et al. (2013). Metabolite profiling of a NIST standard reference material for human plasma (SRM 1950): GC-MS, LC-MS, NMR, and clinical laboratory analyses, libraries, and web-based resources. *Anal. Chem.* 85, 11725–11731. doi: 10.1021/ac402503m

Storz, J. F. (2021). High-altitude adaptation: mechanistic insights from integrated genomics and physiology. *Mol. Biol. Evol.* 38, 2677–2691. doi: 10.1093/molbev/msab064

Sztormowska-Achranowicz, K., Jankowski, Z., and Kocic, I. (2020). Protective effect of nicotinamide and L-arginine against monocrotaline-induced pulmonary hypertension in rats: gender dependence. *Pharmacol. Rep.* 72, 1334–1346. doi: 10.1007/s43440-020-00125-y

Tsugawa, H., Cajka, T., Kind, T., Ma, Y., Higgins, B., Ikeda, K., et al. (2015). MS-DIAL: data-independent MS/MS deconvolution for comprehensive metabolome analysis. *Nat. Methods* 12, 523–526. doi: 10.1038/nmeth.3393

Vaccari, A., Brotman, S., Cimino, J., and Timiras, P. S. (1978). Adaptive changes induced by high altitude in the development of brain monoamine enzymes. *Neurochem. Res.* 3, 295–311. doi: 10.1007/BF00965576

Venemans-Jellema, A., Schreijer, A. J., Le Cessie, S., Emmerich, J., Rosendaal, F. R., and Cannegieter, S. C. (2014). No effect of isolated long-term supine immobilization or profound prolonged hypoxia on blood coagulation. *J. Thromb. Haemost.* 12, 902–909. doi: 10.1111/jth.12564

Viswan, A., Singh, C., Rai, R. K., Azim, A., Sinha, N., and Baronia, A. K. (2017). Metabolomics based predictive biomarker model of ARDS: a systemic measure of clinical hypoxemia. *PLoS One* 12:e0187545. doi: 10.1371/journal.pone.0187545

Want, E. J., Masson, P., Michopoulos, F., Wilson, I. D., Theodoridis, G., Plumb, R. S., et al. (2013). Global metabolic profiling of animal and human tissues via UPLC-MS. *Nat. Protoc.* 8, 17–32. doi: 10.1038/nprot.2012.135

Wawrzyniak, R., Kosnowska, A., Macioszek, S., Bartoszewski, R., and Jan, M. M. (2018). New plasma preparation approach to enrich metabolome coverage in untargeted metabolomics: plasma protein bound hydrophobic metabolite release with proteinase K. *Sci. Rep.* 8, 1–10. doi: 10.1038/s41598-018-27983-0

Xu, Y., Liu, Y., Liu, J., and Qian, G. (2014). Meta-analysis of clinical efficacy of sildenafil, a phosphodiesterase type-5 inhibitor on high altitude hypoxia and its complications. *High Alt. Med. Biol.* 15, 46–51. doi: 10.1089/ham.2013.1110

14

Cardiorespiratory Coordination in Hypercapnic Test Before and After High-Altitude Expedition

Valentina V. Gultyaeva, Dmitriy Y. Uryumtsev, Margarita I. Zinchenko, Vladimir N. Melnikov, Natalia V. Balioz and Sergey G. Krivoschekov*

Laboratory of Functional Reserves of Human Organism, Scientific Research Institute of Neurosciences and Medicine, Novosibirsk, Russia

***Correspondence:**
Valentina V. Gultyaeva
gultyaevavv@physiol.ru

Coordination of cardiovascular and respiratory systems enables a wide range of human adaptation and depends upon the functional state of an individual organism. Hypoxia is known to elicit changes in oxygen and carbon dioxide sensitivity, while training alters cardiorespiratory coordination (CRC). The delayed effect of high altitude (HA) acclimatization on CRC in mountaineers remains unknown. The objective of this study was to compare CRC in acute hypercapnia in mountaineers before and after a HA expedition. Nine trained male mountaineers were investigated at sea level before (Pre-HA) and after a 20-day sojourn at altitudes of 4,000–7,000 m (Post-HA) in three states (Baseline, Hypercapnic Rebreathing, and Recovery). A principal component (PC) analysis was performed to evaluate the CRC. The number of mountaineers with one PC increased Post-HA (nine out of nine), compared to Pre-HA (five out of nine) [Chi-square (df = 1) = 5.14, $P = 0.023$]; the percentage of total variance explained by PC1 increased [Pre-HA median 65.6 (Q1 64.9/Q3 74.9), Post-HA 75.6 (73.3/77.9), $P = 0.028$]. Post-HA, the loadings of the expired fraction of O2, CO2, and ventilation onto PC1 did not change, and the loading of heart rate increased [Pre-HA 0.64 (0.45/0.68) and Post-HA 0.76 (0.65/0.82), $P = 0.038$]. During the Recovery, the percentage of total variance explained by PC1 was higher than during the Baseline. Post-HA, there was a high correlation between the Exercise addiction scores and the eigenvalues of PC1 ($r = 0.9$, $P = 0.001$). Thus, acute hypercapnic exposure reveals the Post-HA increase in cardiorespiratory coordination, which is highly related to the level of exercise addiction.

Keywords: high altitude, mountaineers, cardiorespiratory coordination, hypercapnia, rebreathing, principal component analysis, exercise addiction

INTRODUCTION

Ascent to high altitude (HA) is accompanied by the process of acclimatization to chronic hypoxia. Hypoxia is known to cause changes in the brain regulatory circuits, leading to alterations in blood flow and ventilatory sensitivity not only to oxygen but also to carbon dioxide (Lindsey et al., 2018). Six hours of hypoxic exposure is sufficient to lower the peripheral and central CO_2 threshold (Richard et al., 2014). Moreover, ventilatory and cerebrovascular hypercapnic response patterns show similar plasticity in CO_2 sensitivity following hypoxic acclimatization, suggesting an integrated control mechanism (Smith et al., 2017). Cerebral blood flow influences ventilation by altering central chemoreceptor stimulation *via* central CO_2 washout at high altitudes (Hoiland et al., 2018). There are studies that describe the hematological (He et al., 2013) and hormonal changes (Liu et al., 2017), increased hypoxic tolerance, hypoxic ventilatory response and cerebral oxygenation (Cheung et al., 2014), and elevated sympathetic nervous system activity (Sander, 2016) after return to sea level. However, we are not aware of any studies that concern the delayed effects of HA acclimatization on the integration of cardiovascular and respiratory systems.

In general, the integration of the cardiovascular and respiratory systems can provide a wide range of adaptation of the human organism to varying environmental conditions and depends upon the individual functional state. The research approaches of modern physiology demonstrate the transition from the study of the organs and systems functioning to their interaction and integration, which help to improve prediction, particularly in sports physiology (Balagué et al., 2020). Cardiorespiratory coordination (CRC), based on the co-variation among cardiorespiratory variables is a new sensitive approach to studying intersystem integration. A principal component analysis of time series of cardiovascular and respiratory variables registered during cardiorespiratory exercise testing has been used for cardiorespiratory coordination determining to reveal training-specific physiological adaptations (Balagué et al., 2016; Garcia-Retortillo et al., 2019a) and manipulation-specific physiological state (Garcia-Retortillo et al., 2017, 2019b).

We have previously demonstrated that in swimming and skiing correlations between the responses of the cardiovascular and respiratory systems to acute hypoxic and hypercapnic tests are training-specific (Divert et al., 2015, 2017). Later we revealed that cardiorespiratory coherence changes in response to hypoxic exposure depend upon fitness status (Uryumtsev et al., 2020). The study of cardiorespiratory interactions is in its initial stage, and the influencing CRC factors are to be investigated. We suppose that acute hypercapnic exposure may reveal the peculiarities of coordination in the cardiorespiratory system due to the stimulation of central chemoreceptors in mountaineers several weeks after the return from HA.

In addition, we suggested that exercise addiction, which has been found in extreme sports (Heirene et al., 2016), could be correlated with cardiorespiratory coordination. Rock climbing athletes appear to experience withdrawal symptoms when they are abstinent from their sport comparable to individuals with substance and behavioral addictions (Heirene et al., 2016). Mountaineers ascent HA despite all the risks associated with this process. We assumed that the period between HA expeditions could be considered similar to the period of exercise deprivation in athletes with exercise addiction. Krivoschekov and Lushnikov (2017) described increased levels of anxiety and sympathetic nervous system activity assessed by Baevsky's Stress Index (Baevsky and Chernikova, 2017) in athletes addicted to exercises during exercise deprivation (withdrawal states). Jerath et al. (2016) suggested that alteration in cardiorespiratory synchronization is the mechanism that underlies the symptoms of anxiety. Therefore, we expected that the higher the addiction score is, the worse the cardiorespiratory coordination would be during the period between HA expeditions.

Thus, the purpose of this study was threefold: (1) to compare the CRC in the hypercapnic test before and after the high-altitude expedition; (2) to compare the CRC before (at baseline) and right after the acute hypercapnia (during the recovery stage); and (3) to evaluate the correlation between the level of exercise addiction and CRC.

MATERIALS AND METHODS

Subjects

The study included nine experienced healthy non-smoking male mountaineers aged 25–42 years. All subjects provided written informed consent prior to participation. The study protocol was approved by the Ethics Committee of the Scientific Research Institute of Neurosciences and Medicine (Novosibirsk) and performed in accordance with the Declaration of Helsinki.

Procedure

The mountaineers were examined twice in June and September at an altitude of 164 m above sea level (Novosibirsk). The first round of investigations took place prior to ascending to a HA (Pre-HA). Then the subjects sojourned for 20 days in the mountains, living under the camp conditions at the altitude of 4,100 m with short-term ascents to the altitude of 6,500–7,000 m (Khan-Tengri, Tien Shan). The second investigation, similar to the first one, was performed on average 2 weeks (range 8–28 days) after descending the HA (Post-HA).

The mountaineers began the first visit by signing informed consent, measuring anthropometric characteristics, filling out the Exercise Addiction Inventory, and measuring office blood pressure. After a 30-minute rest including adaptation to breathing through a mask, we began recording gas exchange, ventilation, heart rate, and blood oxygen saturation. Physiological testing was performed in a sitting position through a facemask. All investigations were performed in the morning 2 h after a light breakfast by the same research assistant at an air temperature of 25°C in three functional states: breathing the ambient air (Baseline, 7 min of steady-state ventilation), hyperoxic hypercapnic rebreathing from a 5-L bag (Rebreathing, 3 min) and breathing the ambient air again (Recovery, 7 min). The entire measurement procedure hence took about 17 min. The Read modified rebreathing procedure was used to create hypercapnia (Read, 1967). An initial concentration of 5% CO_2 and 40% O_2 was created in the bag. To avoid the increased activity of peripheral chemoreceptors, the hyperoxic O_2 concentration in the bag was maintained. The hyperoxic mixture was prepared using a NewLife (AirSep, United States) oxygen concentrator. The technique is described in detail elsewhere (Divert et al., 2015).

Data Recording

A spiroergometric system Oxycon Pro (Erich Jaeger, Germany) was used for recording the following respiratory parameters: minute ventilation (VE), inspired and expired fraction of O_2 (FiO_2 and FeO_2), inspired and expired fraction of CO_2 ($FiCO_2$

and $FeCO_2$), and end-tidal O_2 and CO_2 partial pressure ($P_{ET}O_2$ and $P_{ET}CO_2$). Heart rate (HR) and blood oxygen saturation (SpO_2) data were recorded by Pulse Oximeter BCI 3304 Autocorr (Smiths Medical, United States) and then automatically transferred to the Oxycon Pro. Office blood pressure was obtained by use of a sphygmomanometer (OMRON, Japan). We measured skeletal muscle mass by a multi-frequency tetrapolar bioelectrical impedance analysis device (InBody 370, Korea).

We used the Exercise Addiction Inventory (EAI) (Terry et al., 2004) to identify subjects at-risk from exercise addiction. The EAI consists of six statements based on a modified version of the components of behavioral addiction. Each statement has a five-point response option from "Strongly disagree" (1) to "Strongly agree" (5). The six statements that make up the inventory are: "Exercise is the most important thing in my life," "Conflicts have arisen between me and my family and/or my partner about the amount of exercise I do," "I use exercise as a way of changing my mood," "Over time I have increased the amount of exercise I do in a day," "If I have to miss an exercise session I feel moody and irritable," and "If I cut down the amount of exercise I do, and then start again, I always end up exercising as often as I did before." The EAI cut-off score for individuals considered at-risk of exercise addiction is 24.

Data Analysis

Data analysis was carried out using the STATISTICA10 software package (StatSoft). To evaluate the effect of hypercapnia on the separate cardiorespiratory variables we averaged the data that we received during the last 2 min of the baseline and recovery periods, taking into account the low-frequency fluctuations of the cardiorespiratory variables with a period of about 2 min (Grishin et al., 2019). To describe a hypercapnic ventilatory response, we calculated CO_2 sensitivity during rebreathing as the slope in the regression line of VE vs. $P_{ET}CO_2$ above the ventilatory threshold $P_{ET}CO_2$.

To study cardiorespiratory coordination, we used principal component (PC) analysis, which reflects the degree of coincidence of temporal patterns of physiological responses, that is, how much their increase and decrease are statistically synchronized. The total variance allows us to represent the time patterns of selected cardiorespiratory variables with fewer coordinating variables or PCs. The PC is extracted in descending order of importance. The number of PC reflects the dimension of the system, so a decrease in the number of PCs indicates greater coordination and vice versa. The PC number changes when the system undergoes reconfiguration. PC analysis was performed for each mountaineer on the time series of the following selected cardiorespiratory Pre- and Post-HA variables: VE, FeO_2, $FeCO_2$, and HR. Other recorded variables were excluded from the analysis due to their mathematical relationship with the above variables.

The number of PCs was determined by the Kaiser criterion, which considers a significant PC with eigenvalues $\geq$ 1.00. In the tables, we give the eigenvalues as a percentage of the total variance. The greater this percentage is, the greater the coordination of the variables projected onto PC appears. To analyze the effect of HA, the PC eigenvalues pre- and post-HA were compared over the entire 17-minute measurement. To find out the effect of hypercapnia on CRC, the PC eigenvalues for the time series of two states (Baseline and Recovery) were compared. A Wilcoxon Matched Pairs Test was performed to assess statistically significant differences in the cardiorespiratory variables, eigenvalues and PC loads Pre- vs. Post-HA and between the Baseline and Recovery states. The frequencies of occurrence were compared by the chi-square criterion. To test the suitability of the selected cardiorespiratory data for structure detection, Bartlett's test of sphericity and the Kaiser-Meyer-Olkin Measure of sampling adequacy was used. The relationship between the level of exercise addiction and the eigenvalues of PC1 was evaluated by the Pearson correlation coefficient. To evaluate whether the Post-HA results were influenced by the delay following the high-altitude exposure, we calculated the Pearson correlation coefficient between the days of delay and the variables characterizing the CRC. Statistical significance was considered at a P-value < 0.05.

RESULTS

Anthropometric Characteristics

The anthropometric descriptive characteristics of the subjects expressed as medians (Q1/Q3) are as follows: height 176 (171/180) cm, body weight 70 (65.7/83.1) kg, body mass index 23.8 (21.7/25.7) kg/m^2, and muscle weight 34.6 (31.9/38.8) kg. The Exercise Addiction score was 18.0 (17/19) with a range 15–21.

Effect of HA and Rebreathing on the Cardiorespiratory Parameters

Post-HA baseline blood pressure and recovery heart rate decreased significantly as compared to pre-HA (**Table 1**). There were no differences between studied respiratory variables as well as rebreathing data pre- and Post-HA. When comparing the variables at the recovery and the baseline stage, only one significant difference was found pre-HA. Recovery $FeCO_2$ was lower than that at baseline, but the difference was less than 4%. Post-HA parameters at recovery and baseline were not different.

Principal Component Analysis

Bartlett's test of sphericity (p < 0.01) and the Kaiser-Meyer-Olkin Measure of sampling adequacy (min 0.53, max 0.74) showed the suitability of the selected cardiorespiratory data for structure detection. The PC analysis of the entire Pre-HA measurement revealed five mountaineers with one PC and four mountaineers with two PCs. Post-HA, the number of mountaineers with one PC significantly increased to nine [Chi-square (df = 1) = 5.14, p = 0.023]. There were no participants with two PCs Post-HA. Since we used the Kaiser criterion to determine the number of PCs in the model, the following PC (PC2, etc.) had eigenvalues < 1, i.e., they explained less variance than the original variables. Since one PC includes coordinated variables, one can conclude that the coordination of cardio-respiratory variables in the hypercapnic test increases Post-HA.

TABLE 1 | Cardiorespiratory parameters and rebreathing test data pre- and post- high altitude.

Parameter	State	Pre-HA			Post-HA			P (Pre-post-HA)
		Me	(Q1/Q3)	*P* (1–2)	Me	(Q1/Q3)	*P* (1–2)	
VE (L min^{-1})	1 Baseline	10.5	(10.0/12.7)	NS	9.4	(9.1/10.0)	NS	NS
	2 Recovery	11.8	(7.6/12.8)		9.7	(8.6/10.7)		NS
FeO_2(%)	1 Baseline	17.1	(16.6/17.2)	NS	17.0	(16.5/17.2)	NS	NS
	2 Recovery	17.0	(16.8/17.4)		17.1	(16.7/17.3)		NS
$FeCO_2$ (%)	1 Baseline	3.83	(3.41/4.23)	0.028	3.69	(3.52/3.75)	NS	NS
	2 Recovery	3.69	(3.16/4.08)		3.62	(3.36/3.82)		NS
HR (beats min^{-1})	1 Baseline	69.2	(60.7/71.8)	NS	61.2	(56.4/62.3)	NS	NS
	2 Recovery	68.9	(62.0/74.4)		61.1	(55.3/63.5)		0.021
SBP	Baseline	128	(120/130)	–	117	(107/123)		0.042
DBP	Baseline	76	(66/86)	–	71	(60/76)		0.018
Hypercapnic ventilatory response								
$P_{ET}CO_2$ threshold (kPa)	Rebreathing	6.1	(6.0/6.2)	–	6.1	(5.8/6.1)	–	NS
Sensitivity (L min^{-1} kPa^{-1})	Rebreathing	16.2	(13.2/18.6)	–	21.8	(17.9/23.5)	–	NS

VE, ventilation; HR, heart rate; HA, High altitude; Sensitivity, hypercapnic ventilatory sensitivity; NS, non-significant; P, Wilcoxon Matched Pairs Test.

TABLE 2 | Percentage of total variance explained by PC1 and PC2 pre- and post-high altitude.

	State	Pre HA			Post HA			P (Pre-Post HA)
		Me	(Q1/Q3)	*P* (1–2)	Me	(Q1/Q3)	P (1–2)	
PC1	Entire measurement	65.6	(64.9/74.9)	–	75.6	(73.3/77.9)	–	0.028
	1 Baseline	51.8	(49.0/54.3)	0.021	49.2	(47.1/53.7)	0.015	NS
	2 Recovery	67.0	(59.2/69.2)		62.2	(60.2/65.5)		NS
	Rebreathing	77.4	(75.8/86.2)	–	78.9	(72.7/88.2)	–	NS
PC2	Entire measurement	24.5	(20.6/26.3)	–	17.6	(13.8/19.3)	–	0.008
	1 Baseline	30.7	(25.8/33.2)	NS	32.3	(28.8/33.0)	NS	NS
	2 Recovery	23.8	(22.1/26.2)		24.6	(21.4/26.7)		NS
	Rebreathing	19.3	(11.7/22.6)	–	20.4	(10.0/26.0)	–	NS

PC, principal component; HA, High altitude; NS, non-significant; P, Wilcoxon Matched Pairs Test.

Post-HA, the percentage of total variance explained by PC1 significantly increased (**Table 2**). This also confirms an increase in cardiorespiratory coordination.

The loadings of VE, FeO_2, and $FeCO_2$ onto PC1 did not change Post-HA, and the heart rate loading significantly increased Post-HA (**Table 3**). This indicates that the coordination of respiratory variables with heart rate increased. Pre-HA, VE, FeO_2, and $FeCO_2$ formed PC1, whereas HR was involved in forming PC2 in four mountaineers with two PCs. Post-HA, in all nine mountaineers, all the selected variables (VE, FeO_2, $FeCO_2$, and HR) formed PC1.

TABLE 3 | Projection of the cardiorespiratory variables onto PC1 pre- and post-HA (entire measurement).

	Pre-HA		Post-HA		
	Me	(Q1/Q3)	Me	(Q1/Q3)	P
VE	0.85	(0.84/0.89)	0.87	(0.84/0.90)	NS
FeO_2	0.95	(0.93/0.95)	0.94	(0.94/0.97)	NS
$FeCO_2$	0.91	(0.88/0.96)	0.91	(0.88/0.93)	NS
HR	0.64	(0.45/0.68)	0.76	(0.65/0.82)	0.038

VE, ventilation; HR, heart rate; HA, High altitude; NS, non-significant; P, Wilcoxon Matched Pairs Test.

The entire measurement segmentation by the states Baseline, Rebreathing, and Recovery revealed the maximal percentage of total variance explained by PC1 during Rebreathing (**Table 2**). During the Recovery stage, this percentage was significantly higher than that during the Baseline state. We did not find any significant differences in these percentages before and after the HA expedition.

Relation of Exercise Addiction and Percentage of Total Variance Explained by PC1

Pre-HA, the Pearson correlation coefficients (r) between the exercise addiction score and the percentage of total variance explained by PC1 was 0.67 (p = 0.049), Post-HA r = 0.90 (p = 0.001) (**Figure 1**). The slopes in the regression equations both pre-HA and Post-HA were about 3. The exercise addiction score as well as the percentage of total variance explained by PC1 Pre- and Post-HA did not correlate with age (r = 0.31, 0.32,

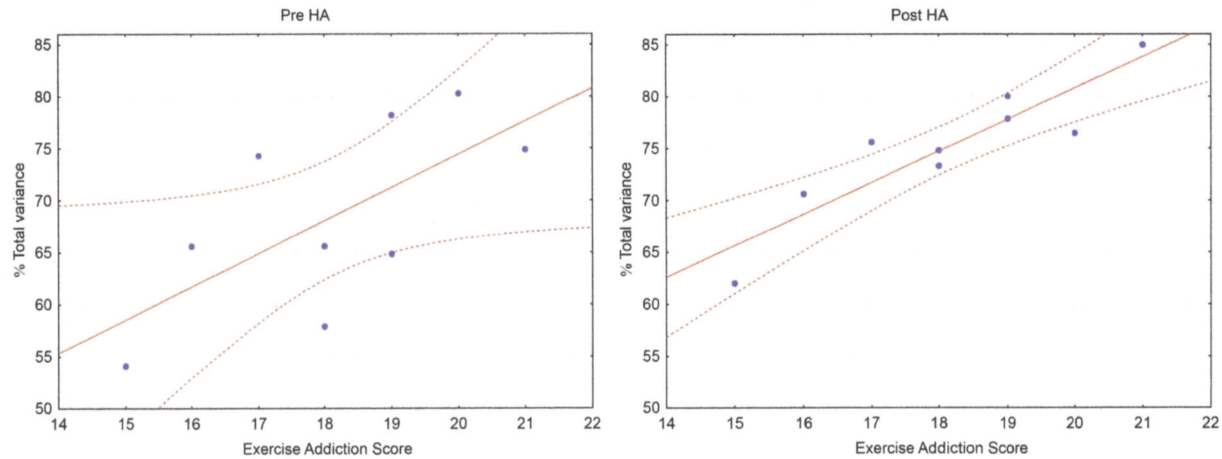

FIGURE 1 | Scatterplot: Percentage of total variance explained by PC1 (% Total variance) vs. Exercise Addiction Score (EAS). Pre-HA: Correlation: $r = 0.67$ ($p = 0.049$), % Total variance = 10.79 + 3.18 • EAS. Post-HA: $r = 0.90$ ($p = 0.001$), % Total variance = 20.03 + 3.04 • EAS. Dashed lines depict 95% confidence interval.

0.31, respectively; NS), weight ($r = -0.23, 0.01, -0.33$; NS), BMI ($r = -0.20, -0.22, -0.25$; NS), and muscle mass ($r = -0.11, -0.02, -0.26$; NS).

Correlation Between the Delay Following the HA Expedition and the Variables Characterizing the CRC Changes

There was a negative correlation between Post- and Pre-HA difference in the percentage of total variance explained by PC1 (Δ% Total variance) on the one hand and the delay following the high-altitude exposure during Rebreathing on the other hand ($r = -0.86$; $p = 0.003$; regression: Δ% Total variance = 16.9–1.3 * Days Post-HA). The regression line crosses the zero level (i.e., CRC return to the Pre-HA value) on the 13th day. We did not find any significant correlation between Δ% Total variance and the delay following the HA exposure during Baseline ($r = -0.02$; NS), Recovery ($r = 0.51$; NS) and Entire measurement ($r = -0.01$; NS). There were no significant correlations between the loadings of VE, HR, FeO_2, $FeCO_2$ onto PC1 and the delay after HA expedition ($r = 0.37, 0.10, 0.16, 0.30$, respectively; NS).

DISCUSSION

Coordination among subsystems is a hallmark of physiologic state and function (Ivanov et al., 2016). Gas exchange, which is the outcome of a more or less coordinated work of the cardiovascular and respiratory systems, is regulated with the participation of the central and peripheral chemoreceptors that respond to the changes in the blood O_2 and CO_2 concentration as well as the pH in the intercellular fluid. The peculiarities of the cardiorespiratory coordination largely determine the individual reserves and physical ability (Balagué et al., 2016; Garcia-Retortillo et al., 2019a). They are of particular importance for mountaineers. Mountaineering is associated with hypoxic high-altitude sojourn, cold, and intense physical activity. The present study was aimed at studying the delayed effect of high-altitude exposure on the peculiarities of cardiorespiratory coordination revealed during central chemoreceptors stimulation. To the best of our knowledge, the results of this pilot study show for the first time an increase of cardiorespiratory coordination revealed by hypercapnic exposure in mountaineers several weeks after the high-altitude expedition. The second result concerns the increase in CRC during the recovery period after acute hypercapnia, which indicates a coordinating effect of acute hypercapnia. The third result demonstrates a high correlation between the exercise addiction scores and the CRC values after the high-altitude expedition.

The value of the ventilation threshold to CO_2 in our study coincides with the value of the central chemoreflex recruitment threshold for ventilation in healthy young men of 46 mmHg (Keir et al., 2019). Previously, researchers considered the features of the influence of hypercapnia on ventilation, using the concepts of threshold, response, reactivity, and sensitivity (slope). This approach has shown some specific ventilatory responses to hypercapnia and hypoxia possibly because of adaptation to frequent high-altitude climbing (Puthon et al., 2016) or training-specific physiological adaptation (Divert et al., 2017), genetic factors (Goldberg et al., 2017), and even the presence of patent foramen ovale (Davis et al., 2019). We have not found any differences in the considered respiratory parameters at rest, as well as ventilatory thresholds and CO_2 sensitivities before and after the high-altitude expedition. Probably, the delayed effect of altitude acclimatization on the studied respiratory parameters varies greatly between individuals. At the same time, heart rate and blood pressure significantly reduced after the expedition. According to He (He et al., 2013) the entire process of deacclimatization may take $\geq$ 100 days.

We revealed the remaining effect of acclimatization on cardiorespiratory coordination several weeks after return from high altitude. Using the principal component analysis, we were able to analyze the cardiorespiratory coordination over the entire measurement, including the transition periods between the baseline, rebreathing, and recovery states. This approach allows obtaining additional information about the CRC, even with the respect to non-stationary states. Various indices obtained as a result of the PC analysis for the entire 17-minute measurement showed the CRC increase Post-HA: the increase in the number of mountaineers with one PC (all the subjects), the increase in the percentage of variance explained by PC1 (eigenvalues), and an increase in the heart rate loading onto PC1. This is consistent with the results obtained by the same method, which has shown the higher sensitivity and responsiveness of cardiorespiratory coordination to exercise effects compared to isolated cardiorespiratory outcomes (Balagué et al., 2016; Garcia-Retortillo et al., 2017, 2019a). The last studies were performed during physical exercise testing. Increasing metabolic demand can be the coordinating factor for cardiorespiratory variables during exercise. In mountaineers Post-HA, changes in cardiorespiratory coordination are presumably associated with the plasticity of medullar regulatory circuits in response to long-term hypoxic stimulation of chemoreceptors (Lindsey et al., 2018).

The negative correlation between the Post- and Pre-HA difference in the percentage of total variance explained by PC1 and days Post-HA during Rebreathing indicates that the Post-HA rebreathing CRC was influenced by the delay following the high-altitude exposure. Meanwhile, we did not find any relationship between Post- and Pre-HA difference in CRC and days Post-HA during Baseline, Recovery, and Entire measurement. Thus, on the one hand, the large variability in the Post-HA exposure re-evaluation delay is a limitation of the study, but on the other hand, this allowed us to estimate the duration of the effects of HA acclimatization on the CRC after returning to the sea level.

The second result concerns an increase in CRC during the recovery period after acute hypercapnia, indicating an acute coordinating effect of hypercapnia. It has long been known that ventilation begins to increase linearly when the concentration of CO_2 increases above the ventilatory threshold (Read, 1967; Duffin, 1990). This fact is used in the rebreathing test. However, we found for the first time that in the period immediately after the rebreathing, the percentage of the total variance, explaining PC1, also increases compared to the baseline level. In addition to ventilation and $FeCO_2$, FeO_2, and heart rate are included in the PC in our study. It should be mentioned that in our CRC study, we do not concern another type of cardiorespiratory coupling, respiratory sinus arrhythmia (RSA). However, hypercapnia is known to increase the amplitude of RSA (Tzeng et al., 2007; Brown et al., 2014), which also indicates an increase in cardiorespiratory coupling.

The third result relates the cardiorespiratory coordination to the exercise addiction score. When we included the EAI in our methods, we expected to identify subjects at-risk of exercise addiction similar to those found in extreme sports (Heirene et al., 2016). We assumed that the higher the addiction score is, the worse the cardiorespiratory coordination would be during the period between HA expeditions. However, the results obtained turned out to be the opposite. There was a high positive correlation between CRC and EAI scores. Moreover, none of the investigated climbers has reached the cut-off score of 24 points to be at-risk of exercise addiction. All examined subjects had a medium EAI score. Therefore, it is not possible to talk about withdrawal states. In our study, the level of exercise addiction as well as CRC did not correlate with age, weight, BMI, and muscle mass. An increase in the exercise addiction score indicates a greater commitment to a training lifestyle. We could assume that the EAI score is a psychological correlate of the fitness level in mountaineers. Therefore, the obtained high positive correlation between exercise addiction scores and CRC could be explained by the interdependence of these indices on the level of fitness. This is confirmed by the fact that it is after the high-altitude expedition that there is a high correlation. The concept of fitness for mountaineers includes the adaptation of the chemoreflex regulation circuit, as well as physical ability. However, this assumption requires further verification.

The practical relevance of the results obtained is that the cardiorespiratory coordination could serve as an additional marker of specific physiological adaptations to different hypoxic states, including high-altitude hypoxia in mountaineers and the pathological state accompanied by hypoxia.

Limitations

The main limitation of the study is the lack of blood pressure time series, which could significantly improve the PC model. Another limitation is the lack of blood and biochemical analyses, including changes in pH, and indices of autonomic nervous system regulation, which could provide a more detailed integration of dynamics across different systems. Large variability in the Post-HA exposure re-evaluation delay could be a limitation of the study, but this allowed us to estimate the duration of the effects of HA acclimatization on the CRC after returning to the sea level. Moreover, this study investigates nine subjects only, which may limit the statistical power of the study.

Further Considerations

In the future, we consider it appropriate to investigate the effect of autonomic nervous regulation on cardiorespiratory coordination.

Conclusion

Acute hypercapnic exposure reveals the Post-HA increase in cardiorespiratory coordination, which is highly related to the level of exercise addiction. Acute hypercapnia provides a coordinating effect on the cardiorespiratory system. The CRC after the acute hypercapnia during the recovery stage is significantly higher than at baseline. These facts require further investigation.

ETHICS STATEMENT

The studies involving human participants were reviewed and approved by Ethics Committee of the Scientific Research Institute of Neurosciences and Medicine (Novosibirsk). The patients/participants provided their written informed consent to participate in this study.

AUTHOR CONTRIBUTIONS

SK: conceptualized the research question, study design, and supervised the entire project. DU: performed the data analysis. VG and MZ: drafted the manuscript. VM and NB: collected data. All authors interpreted the results and critically reviewed and significantly contributed to the manuscript and approved the final version.

ACKNOWLEDGMENTS

We would like to thank Helen Wiebe and Nina Poleeva for their support in the translation of the manuscript, Taissia Chinina-Kelly for her support in the translation of the abstract, and Tamara Komlyagina and Victor Divert for their helpful assistance with data collection.

REFERENCES

Baevsky, R. M., and Chernikova, A. G. (2017). Heart rate variability analysis: physiological foundations and main methods. *Cardiometry* 10, 66–67. doi: 10.12710/cardiometry.2017.10.6676

Balagué, N., González, J., Javierre, C., Hristovski, R., Aragonés, D., Álamo, J., et al. (2016). Cardiorespiratory coordination after training and detraining. A principal component analysis approach. *Front. Physiol.* 7:35. doi: 10.3389/fphys.2016.00035

Balagué, N., Hristovski, R., Almarcha, M., Garcia-Retortillo, S., and Ivanov, P. C. (2020). Network physiology of exercise: vision and perspectives. *Front. Physiol.* 11:611550. doi: 10.3389/fphys.2020.611550

Brown, S. J., Barnes, M. J., and Mündel, T. (2014). Effects of hypoxia and hypercapnia on human HRV and respiratory sinus arrhythmia. *Acta Physiol. Hung.* 101, 263–272. doi: 10.1556/APhysiol.101.2014.3.1

Cheung, S. S., Mutanen, N. E., Karinen, H. M., Koponen, A. S., Kyröläinen, H., Tikkanen, H. O., et al. (2014). Ventilatory chemosensitivity, cerebral and muscle oxygenation, and total hemoglobin mass before and after a 72-day mt. Everest expedition. *High. Alt. Med. Biol.* 15, 331–340. doi: 10.1089/ham.2013.1153

Davis, J. T., Boulet, L. M., Hardin, A. M., Chang, A. J., Lovering, A. T., and Foster, G. E. (2019). Ventilatory responses to acute hypoxia and hypercapnia in humans with a patent foramen ovale. *J. Appl. Physiol.* 126, 730–738. doi: 10.1152/japplphysiol.00741.2018

Divert, V. E., Komlyagina, T. G., Krasnikova, N. V., Martynov, A. B., Timofeev, S. I., and Krivoschekov, S. G. (2017). Cardiorespiratory responses of swimmers to hypoxia and hypercapnia. *Novosibirsk State Pedagog. Univer. Bul.* 7, 207–224. doi: 10.15293/2226-3365.1705.14

Divert, V. E., Krivoshchekov, S. G., and Vodyanitsky, S. N. (2015). Individual-typological assessment of cardiorespiratory responses to hypoxia and hypercapnia in young healthy men. *Hum. Physiol.* 41, 166–174. doi: 10.3389/fphys.2019.0004510.1134/S036211971502005X

Duffin, J. (1990). The chemoreflex control of breathing and its measurement. *Can. J. Anaesth.* 37, 933–942. doi: 10.1007/BF03006641

Garcia-Retortillo, S., Javierre, C., Hristovski, R., Ventura, J. L., and Balagué, N. (2017). Cardiorespiratory coordination in repeated maximal exercise. *Front. Physiol.* 8:387. doi: 10.3389/fphys.2017.00387

Garcia-Retortillo, S., Javierre, C., Hristovski, R., Ventura, J. L., and Balagué, N. (2019a). Cardiorespiratory coordination reveals training-specific physiological adaptations. *Eur. J. Appl. Physiol.* 119, 1701–1709. doi: 10.1007/s00421-019-04160-3

Garcia-Retortillo, S., Javierre, C., Hristovski, R., Ventura, J. L., and Balagué, N. (2019b). Principal component analysis as a novel approach for cardiorespiratory exercise testing evaluation. *Physiol. Meas.* 40:084002. doi: 10.1088/1361-6579/ab2ca0

Goldberg, S., Ollila, H. M., Lin, L., Sharifi, H., Rico, T., Andlauer, O., et al. (2017). Analysis of hypoxic and hypercapnic ventilatory response in healthy volunteers. *PLoS One* 12:e0168930. doi: 10.1371/journal.pone.0168930

Grishin, V. G., Grishin, O. V., Gultyaeva, V. V., Ziinchenko, M. I., and Uryumtsev, D. Y. (2019). Very-low-frequency oscillations of oxygen transport in resting humans. *Russ. J. Physiol.* 105, 1154–1162. doi: 10.1134/S0869813919090061

He, B., Wang, J., Qian, G., Hu, M., Qu, X., Wei, Z., et al. (2013). Analysis of high-altitude de-acclimatization syndrome after exposure to high altitudes: a cluster-randomized controlled trial. *PLoS One* 8:e62072. doi: 10.1371/journal.pone.0062072

Heirene, R. M., Shearer, D., Roderique-Davies, G., and Mellalieu, S. D. (2016). Addiction in extreme sports: an exploration of withdrawal states in rock climbers. *J. Behav. Addict.* 5, 332–341. doi: 10.1556/2006.5.2016.039

Hoiland, R. L., Howe, C. A., Coombs, G. B., and Ainslie, P. N. (2018). Ventilatory and cerebrovascular regulation and integration at high-altitude. *Clin. Auton. Res.* 28, 423–435. doi: 10.1007/s10286-018-0522-2

Ivanov, P. C., Liu, K. K. L., and Bartsch, R. P. (2016). Focus on the emerging new fields of network physiology and network medicine. *New J. Phys.* 18:100201. doi: 10.1088/1367-2630/18/10/100201

Jerath, R., Cearley, S. M., and Jensen, M. (2016). Widespread membrane potential changes and cardiorespiratory synchronization involved in anxiety and sleep-wake transitions. *J. Biol. Regul. Homeost. Agents* 30, 935–944.

Keir, D. A., Duffin, J., Millar, P. J., and Floras, J. S. (2019). Simultaneous assessment of central and peripheral chemoreflex regulation of muscle sympathetic nerve activity and ventilation in healthy young men. *J. Physiol.* 597, 3281–3296. doi: 10.1113/JP277691

Krivoschekov, S. G., and Lushnikov, O. N. (2017). The functional state of athletes addicted to exercises during exercise deprivation. *Hum. Physiol.* 43, 678–685. doi: 10.1134/S0362119717040077

Lindsey, B. G., Nuding, S. C., Segers, L. S., and Morris, K. F. (2018). Carotid bodies and the integrated cardiorespiratory response to hypoxia. *Physiology* 33, 281–297. doi: 10.1152/physiol.00014.2018

Liu, C., Chen, J., Liu, B., Liao, W. T., Liu, J., Xu, G., et al. (2017). Activated corticosterone synthetic pathway is involved in poor responses to re-oxygenation after prolonged hypoxia. *Int. J. Clin. Exp. Pathol.* 10, 8414–8423.

Puthon, L., Bouzat, P., Rupp, T., Robach, P., Favre-Juvin, A., and Verges, S. (2016). Physiological characteristics of elite high-altitude climbers. *Scand. J. Med. Sci. Sports* 26, 1052–1059. doi: 10.1111/sms.12547

Read, D. J. (1967). A clinical method for assessing the ventilatory response to carbon dioxide. *Australas. Ann. Med.* 16, 20–32. doi: 10.1111/imj.1967.16.1.20

Richard, N. A., Sahota, I. S., Widmer, N., Ferguson, S., Sheel, A. W., and Koehle, M. S. (2014). Acute mountain sickness, chemosensitivity, and cardiorespiratory responses in humans exposed to hypobaric and normobaric hypoxia. *J. Appl. Physiol.* 116, 945–952. doi: 10.1152/japplphysiol.00319.2013

Sander, M. (2016). Does the sympathetic nervous system adapt to chronic altitude exposure? *Adv. Exp. Med. Biol.* 903, 375–393. doi: 10.1007/978-1-4899-7678-9_25

Smith, Z. M., Krizay, E., Sá, R. C., Li, E. T., Scadeng, M., Powell, F. L. Jr., et al. (2017). Evidence from high-altitude acclimatization for an integrated cerebrovascular and ventilatory hypercapnic response but different responses to hypoxia. *J. Appl. Physiol.* 123, 1477–1486. doi: 10.1152/japplphysiol.00341.2017

Terry, A., Szabo, A., and Griffiths, M. D. (2004). The exercise addiction inventory: a new brief screening tool. *Addict. Res. Theory* 12, 489–499. doi: 10.1080/16066350310001637363

Tzeng, Y. C., Larsen, P. D., and Galletly, D. C. (2007). Effects of hypercapnia and hypoxia on respiratory sinus arrhythmia in conscious humans during spontaneous respiration. *Am. J. Physiol. Heart Circ. Physiol.* 292, H2397–H2407. doi: 10.1152/ajpheart.00817.2006

Uryumtsev, D. Y., Gultyaeva, V. V., Zinchenko, M. I., Baranov, V. I., Melnikov, V. N., Balioz, N. V., et al. (2020). Effect of acute hypoxia on cardiorespiratory coherence in male runners. *Front. Physiol.* 11:630. doi: 10.3389/fphys.2020.00630

15

Arginine: Glycine Amidinotransferase is Essential for Creatine Supply in Mice during Chronic Hypoxia

Juliane Hannemann[1,2], Kathrin Cordts[1†], Anika Seniuk[3,4], Chi-un Choe[5], Lena Schmidt-Hutten[1], Jorge Duque Escobar[3,6‡], Florian Weinberger[7], Rainer Böger[1,2,3] and Edzard Schwedhelm[1,3]*

[1]Institute of Clinical Pharmacology and Toxicology, University Medical Center Hamburg-Eppendorf, Hamburg, Germany, [2]Institute DECIPHER, German-Chilean Institute for Research on Pulmonary Hypoxia and Its Health Sequelae, Hamburg, Germany, [3]German Centre for Cardiovascular Research (DZHK), Partner Site Hamburg/Kiel/Lübeck, Hamburg, Germany, [4]Institute of Cellular and Integrative Physiology, University Medical Center Hamburg, Hamburg, Germany, [5]Department of Neurology, University Medical Center Hamburg-Eppendorf, Hamburg, Germany, [6]Department of Cardiology, University Heart and Vascular Center, Hamburg, Germany, [7]Insitute of Experimental Pharmacology and Toxicology, University Medical Center Hamburg-Eppendorf, Hamburg, Germany

***Correspondence:**
Edzard Schwedhelm
schwedhelm@uke.de

†Present address:
Kathrin Cordts,
Institute of Forensic Medicine,
University Medical Center Schleswig-Holstein, Kiel, Germany

Objective: Chronic hypoxia induces pulmonary and cardiovascular pathologies, including pulmonary hypertension (PH). L-arginine:glycine amidinotransferase (AGAT) is essential for homoarginine (hArg) and guanidinoacetate synthesis, the latter being converted to creatine by guanidinoacetate methyltransferase. Low hArg concentrations are associated with cardiovascular morbidity and predict mortality in patients with PH. We therefore aimed to investigate the survival and cardiac outcome of AGAT knockout (*Agat*$^{-/-}$) mice under hypoxia and a possible rescue of the phenotype.

Methods: *Agat*$^{-/-}$ mice and wild-type (WT) littermates were subjected to normoxia or normobaric hypoxia (10% oxygen) for 4 weeks. A subgroup of *Agat*$^{-/-}$ mice was supplemented with 1% creatine from weaning. Survival, hematocrit, blood lactate and glucose, heart weight-to-tibia length (HW/TL) ratio, hArg plasma concentration, and *Agat* and *Gamt* expression in lung, liver, and kidneys were evaluated.

Results: After 6 h of hypoxia, blood lactate was lower in *Agat*$^{-/-}$-mice as compared to normoxia ($p < 0.001$). *Agat*$^{-/-}$ mice died within 2 days of hypoxia, whereas *Agat*$^{-/-}$ mice supplemented with creatine and WT mice survived until the end of the study. In WT mice, hematocrit (74 ± 4 vs. 55 ± 2%, mean ± SD, $p < 0.001$) and HW/TL (9.9 ± 1.3 vs. 7.3 ± 0.7 mg/mm, $p < 0.01$) were higher in hypoxia, while hArg plasma concentration (0.25 ± 0.06 vs. 0.38 ± 0.12 μmol/L, $p < 0.01$) was lower. *Agat* and *Gamt* expressions were differentially downregulated by hypoxia in lung, liver, and kidneys.

Conclusion: *Agat* and *Gamt* are downregulated in hypoxia. *Agat*$^{-/-}$ mice are nonviable in hypoxia. Creatine rescues the lethal phenotype, but it does not reduce right ventricular hypertrophy of *Agat*$^{-/-}$ mice in hypoxia.

Keywords: creatine, homoarginine, hypoxia, L-arginine:glycine amidinotransferase, pulmonary hypertension

INTRODUCTION

In patients with newly diagnosed, treatment-naïve pulmonary hypertension (PH), low homoarginine (hArg) plasma concentration was identified as an independent predictor of morbidity and mortality (Atzler et al., 2016). PH is a rare disease with a poor prognosis; it is based on an increase in vascular resistance, which leads to elevated blood pressure in the pulmonary circulation. The increased afterload leads to an increased stress on the right ventricle, causing right ventricular hypertrophy. Eventually, heart failure evolves, which is a major cause of death in PH patients (Giordano, 2005).

The detailed pathophysiological mechanisms leading to idiopathic pulmonary hypertension are not yet fully understood. Pulmonary vasoconstriction is one of the compensatory mechanisms that help to maintain sufficient oxygen supply in focal pulmonary hypoxia; however, excessive and global pulmonary vasoconstriction in global hypoxia may lead to pulmonary hypertension and fatal outcome (Hannemann et al., 2020b). Increased vasoconstriction of the pulmonary vessels is assumed to play an important role, due to an increased release of vasoconstrictor prostaglandins and endothelin-1, and a reduced release of the vasodilator nitric oxide (NO; Lourenco et al., 2012; Giannakoulas et al., 2014). Accumulation of endogenous inhibitors of NO synthesis contributed to this dysregulation, and we and others have shown that chronic hypoxia induces pulmonary and cardiovascular phenotypes that are similar to PH (Hannemann et al., 2020a; Smith et al., 2020); therefore, chronic hypoxia was used as an experimental model in this study.

hArg is a non-proteinogenic amino acid that is synthesized by L-arginine:glycine amidinotransferase (AGAT, Kayacelebi et al., 2015). The same enzyme catalyzes the formation of guanidinoacetic acid, which is further metabolized to creatine by guanidinoacetate methyltransferase (GAMT, Kan et al., 2004). Accordingly, *Agat*-deficient mice (*Agat*$^{-/-}$ mice) are characterized by low circulating hArg and creatine concentrations (Choe et al., 2013a; Nabuurs et al., 2013). hArg is a weak substrate of NO synthase (NOS) and an inhibitor of arginase (Hrabák et al., 1994; Moali et al., 1998). Phosphorylated creatine, on the other hand, plays a key role in energy metabolism and acts as a rapidly available energy buffer due to its capacity to recycle adenosine triphosphate (ATP, Lygate et al., 2013; Stockebrand et al., 2018).

Our group has previously shown that *Agat*$^{-/-}$ mice develop significantly larger stroke areas in a temporary middle cerebral artery occlusion model as compared to WT littermates. Stroke size was significantly reduced to WT size in *Agat*$^{-/-}$ mice supplemented with hArg, but only slightly in creatine-supplemented animals (Choe et al., 2013a). Likewise, Faller and co-workers have shown that impaired cardiac contractile function in *Agat*$^{-/-}$ mice is rescued by hArg, but not creatine (Faller et al., 2018). By contrast, Laasmaa et al. showed that impaired calcium handling by isolated cardiomyocytes from *Agat*$^{-/-}$ mice is normalized by creatine supplementation when creatine is supplemented from weaning (Laasmaa et al., 2021). Taken together, these data suggest that hArg and creatine play differential roles in mediating the pathophysiological phenotypes of *Agat*$^{-/-}$ mice, which are not yet fully understood.

Chronic hypoxia is a condition that is associated with a global dysbalance of energy metabolism. We therefore hypothesized that *Agat*$^{-/-}$ mice may be specifically vulnerable in chronic hypoxia and that creatine or hArg supplementation may help to maintain a healthy phenotype.

MATERIALS AND METHODS

Animals and Study Design

Agat$^{-/-}$ mice used in the present study were described previously and have a life expectancy similar to WT littermates (Choe et al., 2013a,b; Nabuurs et al., 2013). Female mice were kept at 20 to 24°C and a 12:12 light–dark cycle with free access to chow and water. Agat$^{-/-}$ mice and WT littermates aged 3–4 months were placed in normobaric hypoxia (10% O_2) or normoxia (21% O_2) for 4 weeks (8–9 animals per group, **Supplementary Figure 1**). A separate group of *Agat*$^{-/-}$ mice was supplemented with 1% creatine from weaning in standard chow (Ssniff, Soest, Germany) and placed in normoxia or hypoxia, respectively, together with WT littermates in hypoxia (8–9 animals per group). For each group separately, mice from the same litter were kept in one cage. Throughout the study period, all animals were monitored daily for survival and chow was changed from dry to moistened starting 4 to 7 days prior to hypoxia for *Agat*$^{-/-}$ mice. For the first hours of hypoxia, mice were housed on external heating mates. After 6 h of hypoxia, a blood sample was collected by puncture; surviving animals were killed in anesthesia after 4 weeks of hypoxia or normoxia. Blood and tissues were collected and processed for analysis as previously described (Hannemann et al., 2020a). This study was approved by the Animal Care and Use Committee of the Freie und Hansestadt Hamburg (Approval no. 40/16). The use of animals was consistent with the Guide for the Care and Use of Laboratory Animals published by the US National Institutes of Health (NIH publication No. 85-23, revised 1996).

Analysis of Hematocrit, Glucose, Lactate, Cardiac Troponin I, Hypertrophy, and Echocardiography

Hematocrit, glucose, and lactate were determined after puncture of the *Vena facialis* and subsequent blood analysis with an ABL 90 FLEX (Radiometer, Krefeld, Germany) after 6 h of hypoxia and after 4 weeks of hypoxia or normoxia. Cardiac troponin I (cTnI) was determined by ARCHITECT STAT high-sensitive cTnI immunoassay (i2000SR, Abbott Diagnostics, IL, United States) in serum samples diluted 1:5 with 0.9% NaCl. The epitope of the antigen showed 96% similarity between mice and human. Body weight and wet weights of the right ventricle (RV) and left ventricle (LV), septum, and the tibia length were determined. The Fulton index was calculated by dividing the RV to the sum of LV and septum. Cardiac echography was performed using the Vevo 3100 System

(VisualSonics, Toronto, Canada) using standardized procedures (Zacchigna et al., 2021). Mice were anaesthetized with isoflurane (1–2%) and taped to a warming platform in a supine position. B-mode images were obtained using a MX400 transducer. Images were obtained in a parasternal short- and long-axis view, and dimensions of the left ventricle were measured in a short-axis view in diastole and systole. Fractional area shortening (FAS) was calculated as:

$$\mathrm{FAS}\,(\%) = (\mathrm{LVIDd} - \mathrm{LVIDs}) / \mathrm{LVIDd} \times 100$$

Quantification of Homoarginine Plasma Concentration

hArg plasma concentrations were determined from EDTA plasma obtained from cardiac puncture; blood samples were centrifuged at 3,000 × *g* for 3 min at 4°C and stored at −80°C until analysis. hArg concentration was determined by liquid chromatography–tandem mass spectrometry (LC–MS/MS) as previously described (Atzler et al., 2011). Briefly, 25 μl of plasma was diluted with 100 μl of stable isotope-labeled hArg dissolved in methanol. After protein precipitation, hArg was converted to its butyl ester derivative and analyzed by LC–MS/MS (Varian 1200, Agilent Technologies, Santa Clara, CA, United States). Quantification was performed by calculation of peak area ratios and calibration with known concentrations of hArg in dialyzed EDTA plasma (Atzler et al., 2011).

Analysis of *Agat* and *Gamt* mRNA Expression

RNA preparation, reverse transcription, and quantitative real-time PCR (qRT-PCR) were performed as previously described (Hannemann et al., 2020a). Briefly, total RNA was isolated from snap-frozen, homogenized lung, liver, and renal tissues using Trizol (Thermo Fisher Scientific, Waltham, MA, United States). Genomic DNA was removed by an on-column clean-up procedure using PureLink™ RNA Mini Kit in combination with PureLink™ DNase (both Thermo Fisher). RNA was reverse transcribed with SuperScript™ IV VILO™ (Thermo Fisher). qRT-PCR was performed with gene-specific, FAM-labeled Taqman™ assays for Agat (Mm00491882_m1) and Gamt (Mm00487473_m1) and a VIC-labeled control assay (Tbp, Mm01277042_m1) for normalization (all Thermo Fisher). For all experiment, technical triplicates were analyzed. Relative gene expression was calculated using the ΔΔCt method (Schmittgen and Livak, 2008).

Analysis of *Agat* Protein Expression

Preparation of tissue lysates was performed as previously described (Hannemann et al., 2020a). Samples were prepared for SDS-PAGE (kidney, 30 μg total protein; liver, 50 μg total protein per lane) by boiling in beta-mercaptoethanol containing sample buffer; samples were subjected to 10% SDS-PAGE. Subsequently, proteins were transferred onto a 0.2 μm nitrocellulose membrane (GE Healthcare, Munich, Germany). Membranes were incubated with the primary antibody (anti-AGAT, 1:300 in liver, 1:500 in kidney; 12801, Proteintech Chicago, Illinois, United States; anti-β-tubulin: 1:500, Abcam ab6046, Cambridge, United Kingdom) for 1 h at room temperature. Incubation with the secondary antibody (1:10,000; A0545, Merck, Darmstadt, Germany) was done for 1 h at room temperature. Protein was detected using enhanced chemiluminescence detection according to the manufacturer's protocol (GE Healthcare, Munich, Germany).

Statistical Analyses

Data are expressed as mean ± standard deviation (SD). A two-sided independent Student's *t*-test was used to compare two groups. One-way ANOVA with Bonferroni *post-hoc* test was used to compare more than two groups. Chi-square test was used to compare dichotomized variables; Kaplan–Meier curves were generated for survival analysis. $p < 0.05$ was considered statistically significant in all analyses. Statistical analyses were performed by GraphPad Prism 6.0 (La Jolla, CA, United States).

RESULTS

Acute Effects of Hypoxia in *Agat*$^{-/-}$ Mice vs. WT Littermates

We analyzed the acute effects of hypoxia after 6 h of exposure to 10% oxygen. By comparison with normoxia, there was a significant reduction of blood lactate concentration in *Agat*$^{-/-}$ mice (7.5 ± 1.8 vs. 2.6 ± 0.3 mmol/L; $p < 0.001$), while no significant reduction was observed in WT littermates (**Figure 1A**). No significant difference was observed in hematocrit or glucose after 6 h of hypoxia in *Agat*$^{-/-}$ or WT animals (**Figures 1B,C**).

All *Agat*$^{-/-}$ mice died within 48 h of hypoxia, whereas all WT littermates survived until the end of the study after 4 weeks of hypoxia ($p < 0.001$ Chi-square test; **Figure 2A**). The lethal phenotype in hypoxia was completely reversed in *Agat*$^{-/-}$ mice supplemented with creatine (**Figure 2A**). *Agat*$^{-/-}$ mice showed a trend of cTnI increase as compared with WT littermates and *Agat*$^{-/-}$-mice supplemented with creatine in hypoxia (**Figure 2B**).

Effects of Chronic Hypoxia on *Agat* and *Gamt* Expression and hArg Plasma Concentration in WT Mice

Agat mRNA was highly expressed in kidneys and to a lower extent in liver, heart, and lungs, while Gamt showed highest gene expression in liver and low gene expression levels in kidneys, heart, and lungs (**Figure 3**). As compared to normoxia, chronic hypoxia caused a significant reduction of *Agat* mRNA expression in kidneys ($p = 0.001$) and lungs ($p = 0.005$), but not in heart and liver (**Figure 3A**). Likewise, *Gamt* gene expression in liver was lower in chronic hypoxia ($p = 0.001$), but remained unchanged in kidneys, heart, and lungs (**Figure 3B**). In line with the gene expression results, AGAT protein is downregulated in the hypoxic kidney. In the liver, where *Agat* expression is rather low, no effect of hypoxia was

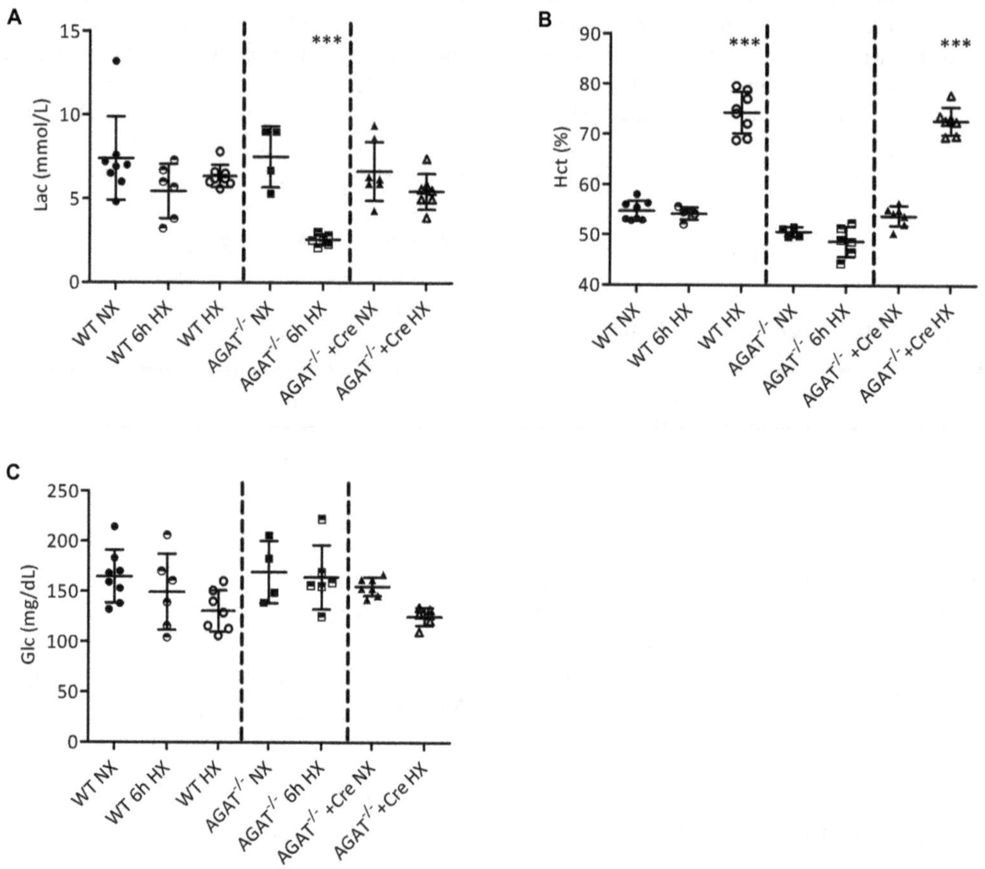

FIGURE 1 | Blood analyses of *Agat*$^{-/-}$ mice and wild-type (WT) littermates. **(A–C)** Mean values ± SD from blood gas analyses under normoxia (NX), after 6 h of hypoxia (6 h HX) and after 4 weeks of hypoxia (HX) in unsupplemented and *Agat*$^{-/-}$ mice supplemented with 1% creatine from weaning (Cre). **(A)** Lactate (Lac). **(B)** Hematocrit (Hct %). **(C)** Glucose (Glc). *Agat*, arginine:glycine amidinotransferase; Cre, supplemented with 1% creatine. ***$p < 0.001$ vs. NX (ANOVA with Bonferroni *post-hoc* test).

obvious (**Figure 3C**). Plasma hArg concentrations were significantly lower in hypoxia as compared to normoxia (0.25 ± 0.06 vs. 0.38 ± 0.12 μmol/L, $p < 0.01$).

Effects of Creatine Supplementation in *Agat*$^{-/-}$ Mice

At the beginning of the intervention, *Agat*$^{-/-}$ mice had a lower mean body weight than their WT littermates (13.3 ± 1.3 vs. 19.0 ± 1.7 g, respectively, $p < 0.001$). Agat$^{-/-}$ mice supplemented with creatine from weaning had a body weight similar to WT littermates (18.0 ± 1.4 g, p = n.s. vs. WT).

After 4 weeks of hypoxia, hematocrit was significantly elevated in *Agat*$^{-/-}$ mice supplemented with creatine (73 ± 3% vs. 54 ± 2%, $p < 0.001$) and their unsupplemented WT littermates (74 ± 4% vs. 55 ± 2%, $p < 0.001$; **Figure 1B**) as compared with normoxic littermates. No significant differences in blood lactate and glucose concentrations were observed between mice of both groups exposed to either normoxia or hypoxia (**Figures 1A,C**).

Heart weight-to-tibia length (HW/TL) ratio was significantly elevated in WT mice exposed to chronic hypoxia; however, it was not significantly different between normoxia and hypoxia in *Agat*$^{-/-}$ mice supplemented with creatine (**Figure 4A**). Of note, there was a significant increase in Fulton index in both, *Agat*$^{-/-}$ mice supplemented with creatine (0.43 ± 0.04 vs. 0.27 ± 0.05, $p < 0.001$) and unsupplemented WT mice after 4 weeks of hypoxia (0.43 ± 0.06 vs. 0.29 ± 0.04, $p < 0.001$; **Figure 4B**) as compared with normoxic littermates. Hypoxia did not change tibia length or the sum of LV and septum (**Supplementary Figure 2**).

Echocardiography revealed higher FAS and ejection fraction in *Agat*$^{-/-}$ mice as compared with WT littermates and *Agat*$^{-/-}$ mice supplemented with creatine (**Figures 5A,B**). Hypoxia did not change FAS and ejection fraction in WT mice or AGAT$^{-/-}$ mice supplemented with creatine.

DISCUSSION

The main findings of our study are threefold: (1) Chronic hypoxia downregulates *Agat* expression and reduces hArg plasma concentrations. (2) *Agat*-deficient mice are not viable in hypoxia. (3) Supplementation with creatine rescues the lethal phenotype and cardiac hypertrophy.

The enzyme AGAT catalyzes the formation of guanidinoacetate from L-glycine and L-arginine; guanidinoacetate is subsequently methylated to creatine by GAMT activity (Kan et al., 2004; Barsunova et al., 2020). AGAT is involved not only in creatine synthesis but also in the formation of hArg from L-arginine and L-lysine (Kayacelebi et al., 2015). Relative mRNA expression of *Agat* and *Gamt* was highest in kidney and liver, respectively (**Figure 3**). Under hypoxia, *Agat* and *Gamt* were found downregulated in kidney and liver, respectively. Downregulation of *Agat* mRNA was paralleled by decreased AGAT protein detected in the kidney. Moreover, we found impaired hArg in the circulation of hypoxic WT mice. We thus conclude that renal AGAT is essential for hArg synthesis and whole body supply *via* the circulation.

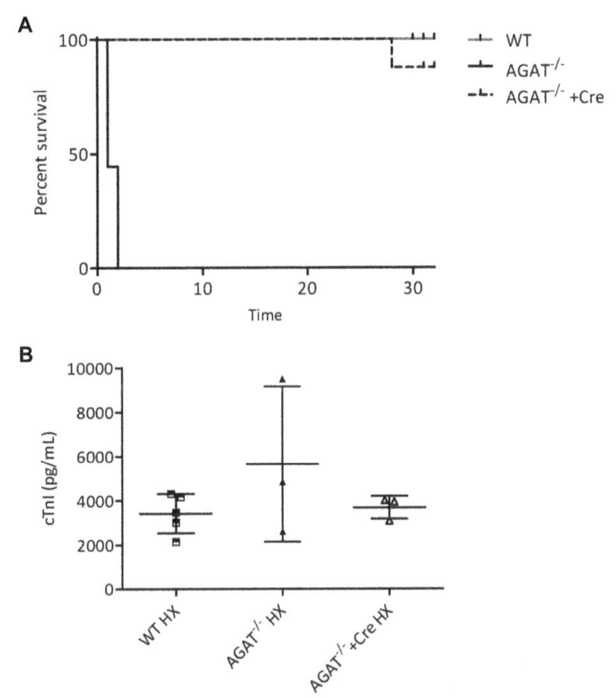

FIGURE 2 | Kaplan–Meier survival analysis and cardiac troponin I (cTnI). **(A,B)** Outcome of *Agat*$^{-/-}$ mice with and w/o creatine (Cre) supplementation and WT littermates in hypoxia (HX). **(A)** Kaplan–Meier survival analysis of *Agat*$^{-/-}$ mice (n = 9), WT littermates (WT, n = 17) and *Agat*$^{-/-}$ mice supplemented with 1% creatine from weaning (*Agat*$^{-/-}$+Cre, n = 8). All mice were kept in hypoxia and followed for up to 32 days. **(B)** cTnI in *Agat*$^{-/-}$ mice (n = 3, 1–2 days of HX), WT littermates (WT, n = 5, 4 weeks of HX) and *Agat*$^{-/-}$ mice supplemented with 1% creatine from weaning (*Agat*$^{-/-}$+Cre, n = 3, 4 weeks of HX) *Agat*, arginine:glycine amidinotransferase; Cre, supplemented with 1% creatine.

hArg is a non-essential amino acid that differs from arginine by an additional methylene group in the carboxylic acid chain (Bell, 1962). Both L-arginine and hArg serve as substrates for NOS, with a 5- to 15-fold higher catalytic efficiency for L-arginine (Moali et al., 1998). Furthermore, hArg has been shown to be a weak inhibitor of the L-arginine-degrading enzyme arginase (Hrabák et al., 1994). In various clinical studies, low hArg concentrations have been associated with an increased risk of cardiovascular disease and mortality, as recently reviewed by our group (Atzler et al., 2015). Moreover, hArg plasma concentrations in treatment-naive PH patients are low and indicate a risk for mortality (Atzler et al., 2016). In line with these observations in PH patients, chronic hypoxia decreased hArg plasma concentration as well as *Agat* mRNA expression in mice. While this decrease in AGAT expression and function might be maladaptive, the absence of AGAT under hypoxia was deleterious. *Agat*$^{-/-}$ mice were not viable in hypoxia for more than 2 days. This phenotype was reversed by supplementation with 1% creatine from weaning and enabled *Agat*$^{-/-}$ mice to survive under hypoxic conditions for the complete study period of 4 weeks.

In neuronal and in muscle cells, creatine is phosphorylated to phosphocreatine by creatine kinase, thus serving as a quickly available energy buffer (Lygate et al., 2013; Nabuurs et al., 2013). Adenosine monophosphate-activated protein kinase (AMPK) is a key enzyme regulating energy metabolism; it downregulates energy-consuming metabolic processes in the presence of ATP deficiency. AMPK has been shown to be involved in hypoxic pulmonary vasoconstriction (Evans et al., 2015). In the event of a lack of energy in the cells, AMPK upregulates

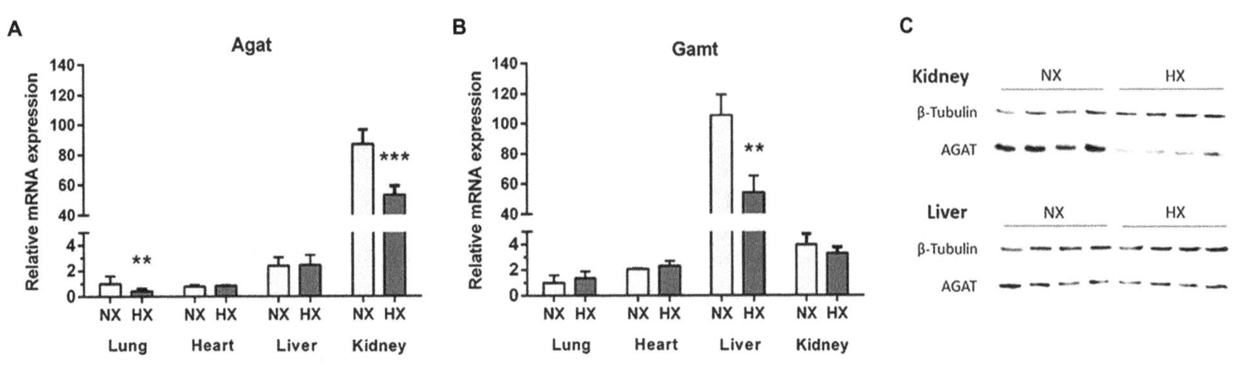

FIGURE 3 | *Agat* and *Gamt* mRNA expression in lungs, liver, heart, and kidneys, and L-arginine:glycine amidinotransferase (AGAT) protein expression in liver and kidneys. mRNA expression of *Agat* **(A)** and *Gamt* **(B)** in normoxia (NX) and hypoxia (HX) as determined by quantitative real-time PCR normalized to Tbp as housekeeping gene. **(C)** Western Blot of AGAT in liver and kidneys as compared to β-tubulin as loading control. $^{**}p < 0.01$ and $^{***}p < 0.001$ vs. NX (ANOVA with Bonferroni *post-hoc* test).

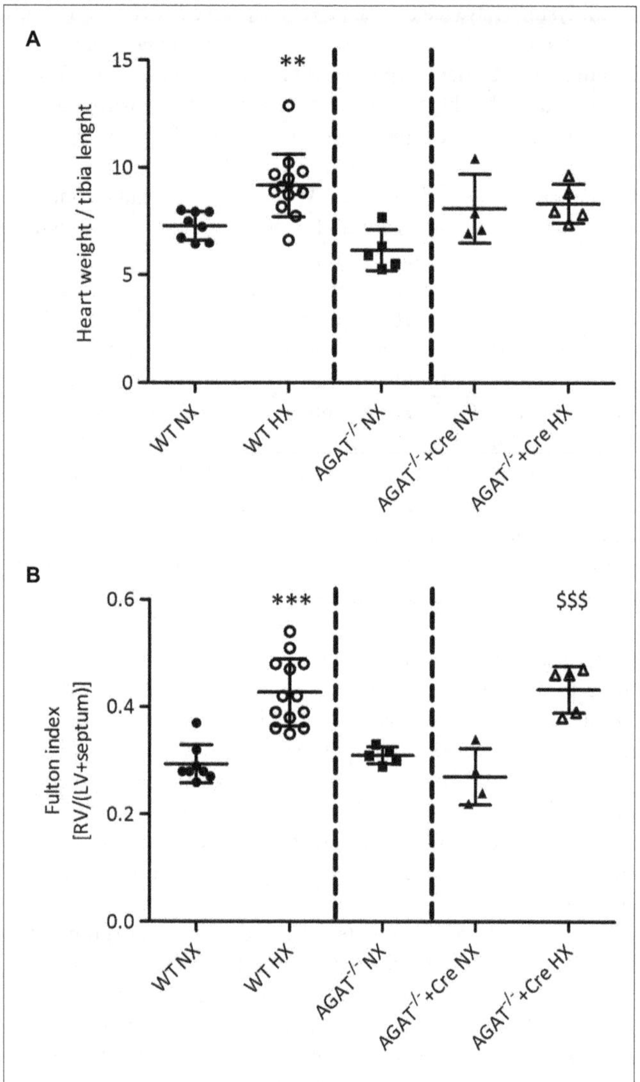

FIGURE 4 | Phenotypes of cardiac hypertrophy of *Agat*$^{-/-}$ mice and WT littermates. **(A,B)** Mean values ± SD from hearts from *Agat*$^{-/-}$ mice supplemented with 1% creatine and WT littermates (WT) under normoxia (NX) and after 4 weeks of hypoxia (HX). **(A)** Heart weight to tibia length. **(B)** Fulton index {right ventricle (RV) weight/[left ventricle (LV) + septum weight]}. *Agat*, arginine:glycine amidinotransferase; Cre, supplemented with 1% creatine. $^{**}p < 0.01$ vs. WT NX, $^{***}p < 0.001$ vs. WT NX, $^{\$\$\$}p < 0.001$ vs. *Agat*$^{-/-}$+Cre NX (ANOVA with Bonferroni *post-hoc* test).

voltage-dependent potassium channels (Kv5.1), which contributes to cellular repolarization in pulmonary artery smooth muscle cells (Firth et al., 2011). In line with this, we previously observed chronic activation of AMPK in skeletal muscle of AGAT-deficient mice (Choe et al., 2013b). Even though we do not show AMPK activation in tissues of *Agat*$^{-/-}$ mice in hypoxia in the current study, we observed a dramatic decrease of blood lactate in *Agat*$^{-/-}$ mice as early as 6 h after the initiation of hypoxia. The heart can utilize glucose, lactate, fatty acids, and creatine for maintaining energy supply (Neubauer, 2007; Branovets et al., 2021). The decrease of blood lactate may thus indicate an increased anaerobic energy demand triggered by hypoxia, which cannot be buffered by cellular stores of creatine/phosphocreatine in the heart of *Agat*$^{-/-}$ mice as previously shown in hypoxic muscle tissue of these mice (Nabuurs et al., 2013).

Four weeks of hypoxia caused a significant increase of hematocrit as well as cardiac and – more specifically – right ventricular hypertrophy, as assessed by the HW/TL ratio for global cardiac hypertrophy and by the Fulton index for right ventricular hypertrophy. Clearly, the same extent of right ventricular hypertrophy was also found in *Agat*$^{-/-}$ mice supplemented with creatine, suggesting that right ventricular hypertrophy is not prevented by creatine but hArg supplementation might have an impact. Global cardiac hypertrophy seemed less pronounced in *Agat*$^{-/-}$ mice supplemented with creatine than in unsupplemented WT mice; however, this finding may have been influenced by the slightly reduced total body growth of the *Agat*$^{-/-}$ mice supplemented with creatine.

Our study has several limitations. Firstly, *Agat*$^{-/-}$ mice were supplemented with creatine from weaning; therefore, we cannot extend our findings to a possible effect of creatine supplementation if initiated after the induction of hypoxia. Secondly, animal welfare prevented us from studying the effects of hArg supplementation on the phenotype of *Agat*$^{-/-}$ mice. Supplementation of WT animals with hArg in hypoxia might be an alternative strategy; however, this was beyond the focus of our study. Although hArg has been implicated with heart failure and cardiomyocyte contractility (Faller et al., 2018), we have no definite proof if the PH-like phenotype, i.e., increase in Fulton index, may be caused, at least in part, by lack of hArg.

CONCLUSION

We show here that creatine rescues lethality of *Agat*$^{-/-}$ mice in hypoxia, showing a pathophysiological significance of creatine-related metabolic pathways. Creatine may therefore be a potentially valuable supplement in individuals having impaired AGAT activity, e.g., caused by genetic missense polymorphisms in the *Agat* gene, during conditions of impaired oxygen availability, e.g., at high altitude. However, creatine supplementation did not affect the PH-like phenotype in hypoxia, suggesting that mechanisms other than creatine-related ones may be involved in its pathogenesis. Further studies in animals and humans are needed to investigate the potentially differential roles of creatine and hArg in PH.

ETHICS STATEMENT

The animal study was reviewed and approved by the Animal Care and Use Committee of the Freie und Hansestadt Hamburg (Approval no. 40/16), BGV, Billestrasse 80, 20539 Hamburg,

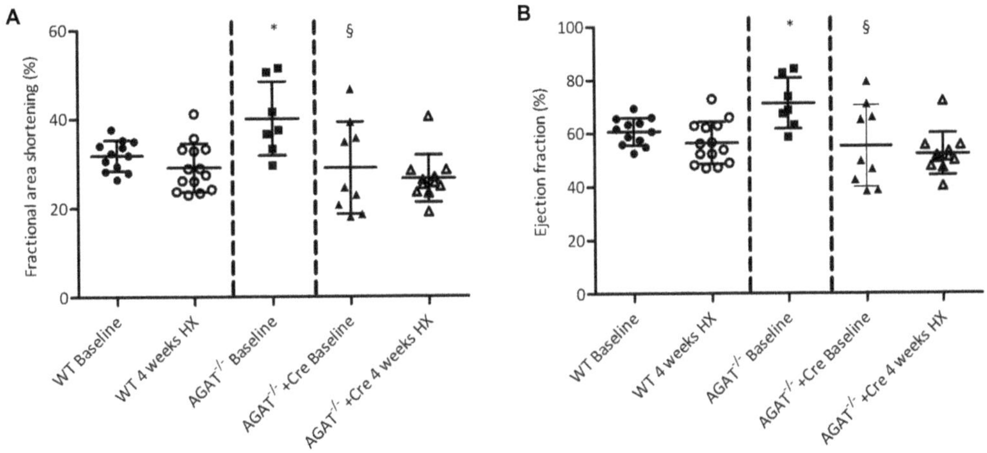

FIGURE 5 | Echocardiography of *Agat*$^{-/-}$ mice and WT littermates. **(A,B)** B-mode images were obtained in a parasternal short- and long-axis view, and dimensions of the left ventricle were measured in a short-axis view in diastole and systole from *Agat*$^{-/-}$ mice supplemented with 1% creatine and WT littermates (WT) at baseline and after 4 weeks of hypoxia (HX). Mean values ± SD are presented. **(A)** Fractional area shortening. **(B)** Ejection fraction. *Agat*, arginine:glycine amidinotransferase; Cre, supplemented with 1% creatine. $^*p < 0.05$ vs. WT baseline, $^§p < 0.05$ vs. *Agat*$^{-/-}$ baseline (ANOVA with Bonferroni *post-hoc* test).

Germany. Written informed consent was obtained from the owners for the participation of their animals in this study.

AUTHOR CONTRIBUTIONS

JH, KC, RB, and ES contributed to the conception and design of the study. KC organized the database. JH, KC, FW, and ES performed the statistical analysis. JH and ES wrote the first draft of the manuscript. KC, AS, JDE, and FW wrote the sections of the manuscript. All authors contributed to manuscript revision, read, and approved the submitted version.

(BMBF grant 01DN17046, DECIPHER, to JH and RB, DZHK grant 81Z1710102 to ES), an Else Kröner Exzellenzstipendiu by the Else Kröner-Fresenius-Stiftung (to C-UC) and the Werner Otto Foundation, Hamburg, Germany (02/96, to JH). JDE was supported by the German Center for Cardiovascular Research (DZHK e.V.) under grant number 81Z0710102.

ACKNOWLEDGMENTS

We thank Mariola Kastner, Fiona Franke, and Birgit Geertz for excellent technical assistance.

REFERENCES

Atzler, D., Cracowski, J. L., Cordts, K., Böger, R. H., Humbert, M., and Schwedhelm, E. (2016). Homoarginine predicts mortality in treatment-naive patients with pulmonary arterial hypertension. *Int. J. Cardiol.* 217, 12–15. doi: 10.1016/j.ijcard.2016.04.161

Atzler, D., Mieth, M., Maas, R., Böger, R. H., and Schwedhelm, E. (2011). Stable isotope dilution assay for liquid chromatography-tandem mass spectrometric determination of L-homoarginine in human plasma. *J. Chromatogr. B Analyt. Technol. Biomed. Life Sci.* 879, 2294–2298. doi: 10.1016/j.jchromb.2011.06.016

Atzler, D., Schwedhelm, E., and Choe, C. U. (2015). L-homoarginine and cardiovascular disease. *Curr. Opin. Clin. Nutr. Metab. Care* 18, 83–88. doi: 10.1097/MCO.0000000000000123

Barsunova, K., Vendelin, M., and Birkedal, R. (2020). Marker enzyme activities in hindleg from creatine-deficient AGAT and GAMT KO mice - differences between models, muscles, and sexes. *Sci. Rep.* 10:7956. doi: 10.1038/s41598-020-64740-8

Bell, E. A. (1962). α,γ-Diaminobutyric acid in seeds of twelve species of Lathyrus and identification of a new natural amino-acid, L-homoarginine, in seeds of other species toxic to man and domestic animals. *Nature* 193, 1078–1079. doi: 10.1038/1931078b0

Branovets, J., Karro, N., Barsunova, K., Laasmaa, M., Lygate, C. A., Vendelin, M., et al. (2021). Cardiac expression and location of hexokinase changes in a mouse model of pure creatine deficiency. *Am. J. Physiol. Heart Circ. Physiol.* 320, H613–H629. doi: 10.1152/ajpheart.00188.2020

Choe, C. U., Atzler, D., Wild, P. S., Carter, A. M., Böger, R. H., Ojeda, F., et al. (2013a). Homoarginine levels are regulated by L-arginine:glycine amidinotransferase and affect stroke outcome: results from human and murine studies. *Circulation* 128, 1451–1461. doi: 10.1161/CIRCULATIONAHA.112.000580

Choe, C. U., Nabuurs, C., Stockebrand, M. C., Neu, A., Nunes, P., Morellini, F., et al. (2013b). L-arginine:glycine amidinotransferase deficiency protects from metabolic syndrome. *Hum. Mol. Genet.* 22, 110–123. doi: 10.1093/hmg/dds407

Evans, A. M., Lewis, S. A., Ogunbayo, O. A., and Moral-Sanz, J. (2015). Modulation of the LKB1-AMPK signalling pathway underpins hypoxic pulmonary vasoconstriction and pulmonary hypertension. *Adv. Exp. Med. Biol.* 860, 89–99. doi: 10.1007/978-3-319-18440-1_11

Faller, K. M. E., Atzler, D., McAndrew, D. J., Zervou, S., Whittington, H. J., Simon, J. N., et al. (2018). Impaired cardiac contractile function in arginine:glycine amidinotransferase knockout mice devoid of creatine is rescued by homoarginine but not creatine. *Cardiovasc. Res.* 114, 417–430. doi: 10.1093/cvr/cvx242

Firth, A. L., Remillard, C. V., Platoshyn, O., Fantozzi, I., Ko, E. A., and Yuan, J. X. (2011). Functional ion channels in human pulmonary artery smooth muscle cells: Voltage-dependent cation channels. *Pulm. Circ.* 1, 48–71. doi: 10.4103/2045-8932.78103

Giannakoulas, G., Mouratoglou, S. A., Gatzoulis, M. A., and Karvounis, H. (2014). Blood biomarkers and their potential role in pulmonary arterial hypertension associated with congenital heart disease. A systematic review. *Int. J. Cardiol.* 174, 618–623. doi: 10.1016/j.ijcard.2014.04.156

Giordano, F. (2005). Oxygen, oxidative stress, hypoxia, and heart failure. *J. Clin. Invest.* 115, 500–508. doi: 10.1172/JCI200524408

Hannemann, J., Glatzel, A., Hillig, J., Zummack, J., Schumacher, U., Lüneburg, N., et al. (2020a). Upregulation of DDAH2 limits pulmonary hypertension and right ventricular hypertrophy during chronic hypoxia in Ddah1 knockout mice. *Front. Physiol.* 11:597559. doi: 10.3389/fphys.2020.597559

Hannemann, J., Zummack, J., Hillig, J., and Böger, R. (2020b). Metabolism of asymmetric dimethylarginine in hypoxia: from bench to bedside. *Pulm. Circ.* 10:2045894020918846. doi: 10.1177/2045894020918846

Hrabák, A., Bajor, T., and Temesi, A. (1994). Comparison of substrate and inhibitor specificity of arginase and nitric oxide (NO) synthase for arginine analogues and related compounds in murine and rat macrophages. *Biochem. Biophys. Res. Commun.* 198, 206–212. doi: 10.1006/bbrc.1994.1029

Kan, H. E., Renema, W. K. J., Isbrandt, D., and Heerschap, A. (2004). Phosphorylated guanidinoacetate partly compensates for the lack of phosphocreatine in skeletal muscle of mice lacking guanidinoacetate methyltransferase. *J. Physiol.* 560, 219–229. doi: 10.1113/jphysiol.2004.067926

Kayacelebi, A. A., Langen, J., Weigt-Usinger, K., Chobanyan-Jürgens, K., Mariotti, F., Schneider, J. Y., et al. (2015). Biosynthesis of homoarginine (hArg) and asymmetric dimethylarginine (ADMA) from acutely and chronically administered free L-arginine in humans. *Amino Acids* 47, 1893–1908. doi: 10.1007/s00726-015-2012-3

Laasmaa, M., Branovets, J., Barsunova, K., Karro, N., Lygate, C. A., Birkedal, R., et al. (2021). Altered calcium handling in cardiomyocytes from arginine-glycine amidinotransferase-knockout mice is rescued by creatine. *Am. J. Physiol. Heart Circ. Physiol.* 320, H805–H825. doi: 10.1152/ajpheart.00300.2020

Lourenco, A. P., Fontoura, D., Henriques-Coelho, T., and Leite-Moreira, A. F. (2012). Current pathophysiological concepts and management of pulmonary hypertension. *Int. J. Cardiol.* 155, 350–361. doi: 10.1016/j.ijcard.2011.05.066

Lygate, C. A., Aksentijevic, D., Dawson, D., Hove, M. T., Phillips, D., Bono, J. D., et al. (2013). Living without creatine unchanged exercise capacity and response to chronic myocardial infarction in creatine-deficient mice. *Circ. Res.* 112, 945–955. doi: 10.1161/CIRCRESAHA.112.300725

Moali, C., Boucher, J. L., Sari, M. A., Stuehr, D. J., and Mansuy, D. (1998). Substrate specificity of NO synthases: detailed comparison of L-arginine, homo-L-arginine, their N omega-hydroxy derivatives, and N omega-hydroxynor-L-arginine. *Biochemistry* 37, 10453–10460. doi: 10.1021/bi980742t

Nabuurs, C. I., Choe, C. U., Veltien, A., Kan, H. E., van Loon, L. J., Rodenburg, R. J., et al. (2013). Disturbed energy metabolism and muscular dystrophy caused by pure creatine deficiency are reversible by creatine intake. *J. Physiol.* 591, 571–592. doi: 10.1113/jphysiol.2012.241760

Neubauer, S. (2007). The failing heart–an engine out of fuel. *N. Engl. J. Med.* 356, 1140–1151. doi: 10.1056/NEJMra063052

Schmittgen, T. D., and Livak, K. J. (2008). Analyzing real-time PCR data by the comparative C(T) method. *Nat. Protoc.* 3, 1101–1108. doi: 10.1038/nprot.2008.73

Smith, K. A., Waypa, G. B., Dudley, V. J., Budinger, G. R. S., Abdala-Valencia, H., Bartom, E., et al. (2020). Role of hypoxia-inducible factors in regulating right ventricular function and remodeling during chronic hypoxia-induced pulmonary hypertension. *Am. J. Respir. Cell Mol. Biol.* 63, 652–664. doi: 10.1165/rcmb.2020-0023OC

Stockebrand, M., Sasani, A., Das, D., Hornig, S., Hermans-Borgmeyer, I., Lake, H. A., et al. (2018). A mouse model of creatine transporter deficiency reveals impaired motor function and muscle energy metabolism. *Front. Physiol.* 9:773. doi: 10.3389/fphys.2018.00773

Zacchigna, S., Paldino, A., Falcão-Pires, I., Daskalopoulos, E. P., Dal Ferro, M., Vodret, S., et al. (2021). Towards standardization of echocardiography for the evaluation of left ventricular function in adult rodents: a position paper of the ESC Working Group on Myocardial Function. *Cardiovasc. Res.* 117, 43–59. doi: 10.1093/cvr/cvaa110

16

The Association Between Notching of the Right Ventricular Outflow Tract Flow Velocity Doppler Envelope and Impaired Right Ventricular Function After Acute High-Altitude Exposure

Fangzhengyuan Yuan[1,2†], Chuan Liu[1,2†], Shiyong Yu[1,2], Shizhu Bian[1,2], Jie Yang[1,2], Xiaohan Ding[3], Jihang Zhang[1], Hu Tan[1,2], Jingbin Ke[1,2], Yuanqi Yang[1,2], Chunyan He[1,2], Chen Zhang[1,2], Rongsheng Rao[4], Zhaojun Liu[4], Jun Yang[4] and Lan Huang[1,2]*

[1] Institute of Cardiovascular Diseases of PLA, The Second Affiliated Hospital, Third Military Medical University (Army Medical University), Chongqing, China, [2] Department of Cardiology, The Second Affiliated Hospital, Third Military Medical University (Army Medical University), Chongqing, China, [3] Department of Geriatric Cardiology, Chinese PLA General Hospital, Beijing, China, [4] Department of Medical Ultrasonics, The Second Affiliated Hospital, Third Military Medical University (Army Medical University), Chongqing, China

***Correspondence:**
Lan Huang
huanglan260@126.com

[†] These authors have contributed equally to this work

Introduction: Pulmonary artery pressure (PAP) is increased and right ventricular (RV) function is well preserved in healthy subjects upon exposure to high altitude (HA). An increase in PAP may trigger notching of the right ventricular outflow tract Doppler flow velocity envelope (RVOT notch), which is associated with impaired RV function in patients with pulmonary hypertension. However, whether HA exposure can induce RVOT notch formation and the subsequent impact on cardiac function in healthy subjects remains unclear.

Methods: A total of 99 subjects (69 males and 30 females) with a median age of 25 years were enrolled in this study; they traveled from 500 to 4100 m by bus over a 2-day period. All subjects underwent a comprehensive physiological and echocardiographic examination 1 day before ascension at low altitude and 15 $\pm$ 3 h after arrival at HA. The RVOT notch was determined by the presence of a notched shape in the RVOT Doppler flow velocity envelope. The systolic PAP (SPAP) was calculated as Bernoulli equation SPAP = 4 $\times$ (maximum tricuspid regurgitation velocity)^2+5 and mean PAP (mPAP) = 0.61 $\times$ SPAP+2. Cardiac output was calculated as stroke volume $\times$ heart rate. Pulmonary capillary wedge pressure (PCWP) was calculated as 1.9+1.24 $\times$ mitral E/e'. Pulmonary vascular resistance (PVR) was calculated as (mPAP-PCWP)/CO.

Results: After HA exposure, 20 (20.2%) subjects had an RVOT notch [notch (+)], and 79 (79.8%) subjects did not have an RVOT notch [notch (−)]. In the multivariate logistic regression analysis, the SPAP, right ventricular global longitude strain (RV GLS), and tricuspid E/A were independently associated with the RVOT notch. The SPAP, mPAP, PVR, standard deviations of the times to peak systolic strain in the four mid-basal RV segments (RVSD4), peak velocity of the isovolumic contraction period (ICV), and the peak systolic velocity (s') at the mitral/tricuspid annulus were increased in all subjects.

Conversely, the pulse oxygen saturation (SpO_2), RV GLS, and tricuspid annulus plane systolic excursion (TAPSE)/SPAP were decreased. However, the increases of SPAP, mPAP, PVR, and RVSD4 and the decreases of SpO_2, RV GLS, and TAPSE/SPAP were more pronounced in the notch (+) group than in the notch (−) group. Additionally, increased tricuspid ICV and mitral/tricuspid s' were found only in the notch (−) group.

Conclusion: HA exposure-induced RVOT notch formation is associated with impaired RV function, including no increase in the tricuspid ICV or s', reduction of RV deformation, deterioration in RV-pulmonary artery coupling, and RV intraventricular synchrony.

Keywords: high altitude, right ventricular function, right ventricular outflow tract, speckle tracking echocardiography, tissue Doppler imaging

INTRODUCTION

Travelers typically flock to high-altitude (HA) areas. However, hypobaric hypoxia at HA stresses the cardiopulmonary system (Parati et al., 2018). Due to HA-induced hypoxic pulmonary vasoconstriction (HPV), the pulmonary artery pressure (PAP) increases (Naeije, 2019), filling of the left ventricle and right ventricle decreases, and the left ventricular (LV)/right ventricular (RV) diastolic function is altered (Maufrais et al., 2017). In contrast, the LV/RV contractile function remains well-preserved (Osculati et al., 2016; Maufrais et al., 2019; Williams et al., 2019; Sareban et al., 2020). According to previous studies, mild pulmonary hypertension (PH) could decrease RV function, and the RV dysfunction progresses regardless of the treatment of lowering pulmonary vascular resistance (PVR) (van de Veerdonk et al., 2011; Huston et al., 2019).

Notching of the right ventricular outflow tract flow velocity Doppler envelope (RVOT notch) has been widely reported in patients with PH. The RVOT notch is caused by the reflected wave propagating to the pulmonary valve prior to the closure of the valve during a systole. The RVOT notch forms in the context of increased PAP and PVR, decreased pulmonary vascular compliance, and the presence of a reflecting site close enough to the pulmonary valve to allow for the velocity of the reflecting wave (Arkles et al., 2011; Ghimire et al., 2016).

The formation of the RVOT notch was mainly attributed to high PAP (Lopez-Candales and Edelman, 2012). As for patients with PH, it has been reported that the presence of an RVOT notch is associated with deteriorated RV function, such as reduced tricuspid annulus plane systolic excursion (TAPSE), RV fractional area change (FAC), peak systolic velocity of the tricuspid annulus (tricuspid s'), and the ratio of stroke volume index to RV end-diastolic area (Arkles et al., 2011; Lopez-Candales and Edelman, 2012). Even though PAP also increased in healthy subjects upon acute HA exposure, the amount of increase only ranged from mild to moderate. It is unclear whether this moderate increase of PAP induced by HPV led to RVOT notch formation. Additionally, since the RV function in healthy subjects upon acute HA exposure was reported to be well preserved; whether the presence of the RVOT notch in healthy subjects upon acute HA exposure is associated with deteriorated RV function is also unclear. Thus, the mechanism of RVOT notch formation and the relationship between RVOT notch and RV function at HA are worthy to investigate.

In a previous study, we had preliminarily reported that compared to the RVOT notch negative population, the correlation between PAP and intraventricular RV dyssynchrony was much greater in people with an RVOT notch. In this study, we tended to formally characterize the RVOT notch and comprehensively unravel the association between HA-induced RVOT notch and cardiac function.

MATERIALS AND METHODS

Participants and Study Design

This study was approved by the Clinical Research Ethics Board of Army Medical University (Identification Code 201907501) and was registered at www.chictr.org.cn (ChiCTR-TRC-No.1900025728). In June 2019, we conducted this prospective cohort study on the Qinhai–Tibet Plateau. Han Chinese people who were born and permanently lived at a low altitude ($\leq$500 m) were invited to participate in this study. A total of 111 participants were recruited at low altitudes (Chengdu, China, 500 m) to ascend to HA (Litang, China, 4100 m). Of all 111 subjects, five subjects withdrew from the study prior to ascending, and two subjects returned to low altitude because of severe HA illness. Ultimately, 104 subjects successfully ascended to 4100 m (Litang, China) by bus over a 2-day period. Due to the lack of suitable echocardiographic images in five subjects, the final analysis included 99 subjects. These subjects were healthy adults without HA exposure history in the past 6 months and had no recent medication use. Exclusion criteria included the presence of cardiopulmonary disease, cerebrovascular disease, liver disease, kidney disease, or malignant tumors. All physiological and transthoracic echocardiography examinations were performed 1 day prior to ascension at low altitude and 15 $\pm$ 3 h after arrived at HA. This study was conducted in accordance with the Declaration of Helsinki, and all subjects provided written informed consent.

Assessment of Physiological Parameters

Pulse oxygen saturation (SpO_2) was recorded using a pulse oximeter (ONYX OR9500, Nonin, Plymouth, MN,

United States). Blood pressure was measured with the subject in a sitting position using an electronic sphygmomanometer (Omron HEM-6200, Japan) after a 10-minute rest period. Heart rate (HR) data were recorded using the synchronous electrocardiogram during echocardiography. We measured height and weight with a height and weight scale (RGZ-120, I WISH, China) 1 day before ascension at a low altitude. The body mass index (BMI) was calculated as weight/(height)^2.

Transthoracic Echocardiography

Echocardiographic examinations were performed by two experienced sonographers equipped with a 2.5 MHz adult transducer using a CX50 ultrasound system (Philips Ultrasound System, Andover, MA, United States) with the subject in the left lateral decubitus position. The dynamic echocardiographic images, which consisted of three consecutive cardiac cycles, were stored digitally for offline analysis using QLAB 10.5 (Philips Healthcare, Andover, MA, United States) in a blinded fashion. All examinations and measurements were performed according to the recommendations of the American Society of Echocardiography (Rudski et al., 2010; Mitchell et al., 2019), and the value of each echocardiographic parameter was averaged from measurements of three consecutive cardiac cycles.

LV end-diastolic volume, LV end-systolic volume, RV basal transverse diameter (RVD base), and RVD mid were measured. RV end-diastolic and end-systolic areas were determined using the apical four-chamber view by manually tracing the RV endocardium. TAPSE was recorded as the peak excursion of the lateral tricuspid annulus, which was measured with M-mode echocardiography. The maximum tricuspid regurgitation velocity (TRV) was evaluated using continuous-wave Doppler. The LV and RV inflow were measured using the apical four-chamber view of pulsed-wave Doppler. The maximum early (E) and late (A) diastolic velocities were recorded. A pulse tissue Doppler was used to assess the velocities of the mitral and tricuspid annuli on the lateral and septal aspects in early diastole and systole. The peak early diastolic velocity of the annulus (e'), peak systolic velocity of the annulus (s'), and peak velocity of the isovolumic contraction period (ICV) were recorded as the average of the lateral and septal values. Stroke volume (SV), left ventricular ejection fraction (LVEF), and cardiac output (CO) were calculated using LV volume data and HR (Lang et al., 2015). RV FAC was calculated as follows: FAC = (end-diastolic area - end-systolic area)/end-diastolic area × 100. Systolic pulmonary artery pressure (SPAP) was calculated with the following modified Bernoulli equation: $SPAP = 4 \times (TRV)^2 + 5$ (Yock and Popp, 1984). The mean PAP (mPAP) was calculated as follows: $mPAP = 0.61 \times SPAP + 2$ (Bossone et al., 2013). Pulmonary capillary wedge pressure (PCWP) was calculated using the following equation: $PCWP = 1.9 + 1.24 \times$ mitral E/e' (Bossone et al., 2013). PVR was derived according to the equation PVR = (mPAP-PCWP)/CO (Bossone et al., 2013).

To investigate the RVOT blood flow, the pulse Doppler sample volume probe was placed 0.5–1 cm proximally to the pulmonic valve in the parasternal short-axis view. The RVOT acceleration time (AT_{RVOT}) and RVOT ejection time (ET_{RVOT}) were measured. The shapes of the RVOT Doppler flow velocity envelope were categorized as notch (+) (in the presence of a notching pattern) and notch (−) (when no notching pattern was present), as previously described (Arkles et al., 2011). The specific notch relevant parameter mid-systolic flow deceleration time (mid-systolic DT) was measured (Takahama et al., 2017).

2D-STE Analysis

Standard 2D grayscale images (frame rate > 60 fps) in the apical two-, three-, and four-chamber views were used for the LV and RV speckle tracking analyses. Apical, basal, and mid-level parasternal short-axis views of three consecutive beats were also recorded. Using QLAB software v10.5, the operator manually adjusted the region of interest to include all segments of the ventricular myocardium. These were then traced by an algorithm, which automatically calculated the peak strain of each segment on different images.

The LV global longitudinal strain (GLS) was defined as the mean of 17 segments that was calculated on the apical two-, three- and four-chamber images. The LV global circumferential strain (GCS) was defined as the average peak strain in each segment of the basal, mid-, and apical levels using parasternal short-axis images. The RV GLS was defined as the mean of six segments on the RV-focused four-chamber image.

To analyze LV/RV dyssynchrony, the time from the onset of the QRS complexes to the peak strain of each segment on ECG was calculated and correlated to the R-R interval according to Bazett's formula: corrected interval = measured time to peak strain/(RR interval)$^{1/2}$. The standard deviation (SD) of the correlated interval for the 12 mid-basal LV segments was termed the TS-12SD (Zoroufian et al., 2014), whereas the SD for the four mid-basal RV segments was termed the RV-SD4 (Badagliacca et al., 2015).

Reproducibility

To determine the intraobserver variability, data from 10 subjects at a low altitude and 10 subjects at a HA were randomly selected and evaluated twice by the same observer with a 1-month interval between evaluations. Interobserver variability was determined by comparing the evaluations conducted by two separate observers blinded to each other. The intra- and interobserver variabilities for the echocardiographic variables are presented in **Supplementary Table S1**.

Statistical Analysis

All statistical analyses were performed using SPSS software (Version 22.0, IBM Corp., Armonk, NY, United States). Continuous variables are presented as mean ± standard error of mean if normally distributed or as median and interquartile range if not normally distributed, according to the Kolmogorov-Smirnov test. The paired t-test or Wilcoxon test was used to analyze the differences between paired variables at low altitude and HA, whereas the unpaired variables in the notch (−) and notch (+) groups at low altitude or HA and the unpaired variables in notch (+) subjects with mid-systolic DT < 120 ms and with mid-systolic DT > 120 ms were compared using the independent sample t-test or Mann-Whitney U test. Univariate logistic regression analysis was used to identify the relevant variables associated with RVOT notch. The variables with P-value < 0.05 were included in the multivariate logistic regression analysis. Category variables are presented as a number (percentage) and compared using the chi-square test. Statistical significance was set at $P < 0.05$.

RESULTS

Subject Characteristics

The 99 subjects consisted of 69 men and 30 women with a median age of 25 years and an average BMI of 22.2 kg/m^2. No subject was found to have an RVOT notch at low altitude. Upon HA exposure, an RVOT notch was identified in 20 subjects (20.2%) (**Figure 1**). There were no significant differences in age, sex, or BMI between the notch (+) and notch (−) groups. Following HA exposure, subjects in all groups had increased systolic blood pressure, diastolic blood pressure, and HR. Both groups also had decreased SpO_2 following HA exposure, with the notch (+) group experiencing a lower SpO_2 level than the notch (−) group ($P = 0.039$) (**Table 1** and **Figure 2**).

LV Function

After HA exposure, SV and LV GLS decreased, GCS did not change, and the LVEF, CO, mitral ICV, and TS-12SD increased in all subjects. The mitral s' in the notch (−) group increased upon HA exposure, but the mitral s' in the notch (+) group did not change. Following HA exposure, the mitral E, mitral E/A, and mitral E/e' decreased in all subjects. However, the mitral A increased in all subjects following HA exposure, with a higher value in the notch (+) group than in the notch (−) group. The mitral E/A at HA in the notch (+) group was lower than that in the notch (−) group (**Table 2**).

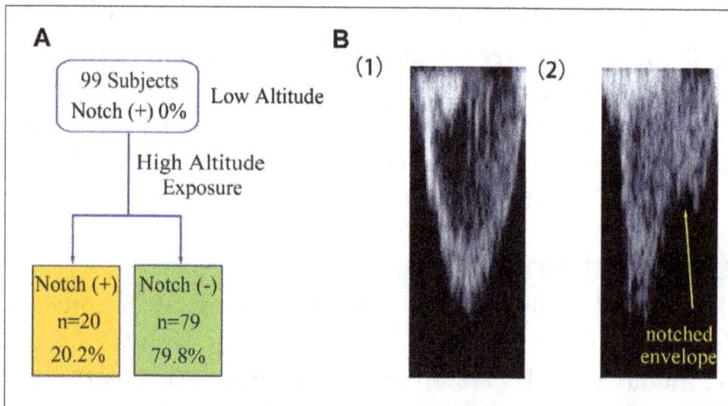

FIGURE 1 | Occurrence of RVOT notch in healthy subjects at low altitude and upon acute HA exposure. **(A)** The occurrence of RVOT notch in healthy subjects was 0% at low altitude. Following HA exposure, the occurrence of RVOT notch in healthy subjects was 20.2%. **(B)** Morphology of the RVOT Doppler flow velocity envelope with or without RVOT notch. **(1)** RVOT Doppler flow velocity envelope in healthy subjects at low altitude was parabolic in shape. **(2)** Healthy subjects upon HA exposure with notched RVOT Doppler flow velocity envelope.

Pulmonary Hemodynamics and RV Function

Upon HA exposure, TRV, SPAP, mPAP, and PVR increased in all subjects; however, this increase was greater in notch (+) subjects. The AT_{RVOT}, ET_{RVOT}, AT_{RVOT}/ET_{RVOT}, and PCWP decreased in all subjects, except for ET_{RVOT} in notch (+) subjects. The RVD base did not change in all subjects. The RVD mid increased in all subjects, which was majorly observed in the notch (+) group. The RV FAC, TAPSE, and RV GLS decreased in both groups, and the change in RV GLS was greater in the notch (+) group. The tricuspid s' and tricuspid ICV increased after HA exposure in the notch (−) group (**Figure 3**). Additionally, the RV GLS decreased in both groups upon HA exposure and was lower in the notch (+) group than in the notch (−) group (**Figure 4**). The two-dimensional strain of the middle segment in the right ventricular free wall (2DS RVFW mid) and 2DS RVFW base in the notch (+) group at HA were lower than those in the notch (−) group. The TAPSE/SPAP decreased in all subjects after HA exposure, with a greater decrease in the notch (+) group (**Figure 2**). The RVSD4 increased in all subjects upon HA exposure, and it was more pronounced in the notch (+) group (**Figure 4**). After HA exposure, the tricuspid A in the notch (+) group was higher than that in the notch (−) group, and the tricuspid E/A in the notch (+) group was lower than that in the notch (−) group (**Table 3**). Categorizing notch (+) subjects into two groups according to mid-systolic DT (Takahama et al., 2017), we determined the RVD base and RVD mid were larger in mid-systolic DT < 120 ms group than those in mid-systolic DT > 120 ms group (**Supplementary Table S2**).

Determinants of RVOT Notch

In multivariate logistic regression analysis, SPAP (OR, 1.14; 95% CI, 1.05 to 1.23; $P = 0.001$), RV GLS (OR, 0.74; 95% CI, 0.60 to 0.93; $P = 0.011$), and tricuspid E/A (OR, 0.13; 95% CI, 0.03 to 0.68; $P = 0.016$) were found to be independently associated with RVOT notch (**Supplementary Table S3**).

DISCUSSION

Following rapid elevation gain, an RVOT notch was found in 20 (20.2%) healthy subjects. SpO_2, RV deformation, the level of RV-PA coupling, and RV intraventricular synchrony were decreased in all subjects, while the RV afterload, biventricular s', and ICV were increased in all subjects. However, the increase in the RV afterload and the decrease in SpO_2, RV deformation, RV-PA coupling, and RV intraventricular synchrony were more pronounced in subjects with an RVOT notch. Moreover, the mitral s', tricuspid s', and tricuspid ICV in subjects with an RVOT notch did not increase upon HA exposure. These results suggest that HA exposure induced the RVOT notch formation, which may be related to impaired RV function.

Association of RVOT Notch, PAP, and SpO_2 Upon HA Exposure

In previous studies, the RVOT notch was mainly observed in patients with chronic PH, especially in those with pulmonary

TABLE 1 | Physiologic parameters in the subjects with or without RVOT notch at low altitude and high altitude.

Baseline variables	Total (n = 99)			Notch (–) (n = 79)			Notch (+) (n = 20)		
	Low altitude	High altitude	P-value	Low altitude	High altitude	P-value	Low altitude	High altitude	P-value
Age, years	25.0 (21.3, 29.0)	–		25.0 (21.5, 28.5)	–		26.0 (21.0, 33.0)	–	
Male, n (%)	69 (69.7)	–		57 (72.2)	–		12 (60.0)	–	
BMI, kg/m^2	22.2 ± 0.2	–		22.2 ± 0.3	–		22.4 ± 0.6	–	
HR, beats/min	63.0 (57.0, 72.5)	81.0 (73.5, 93.0)	**< 0.001**	62.0 (56.5, 72.5)	80.0 (72.5, 92.5)	**< 0.001**	66.0 (63.0, 75.8)	88.0 (79.3, 94.0)	**< 0.001**
SpO_2, %	97.0 (96.0, 98.0)	88.0 (85.0, 90.0)	**< 0.001**	97.0 (96.0, 98.0)	88.0 (85.0, 90.0)	**< 0.001**	97.5 (97.0, 99.0)	86.0 (82.5, 88.0)*	**< 0.001**
SBP, mmHg	117.0 (108.0, 126.0)	121.0 (111.0, 132.0)	**0.004**	117.0 (109.0, 126.0)	120.0 (111.0, 128.0)	**0.033**	122.0 (107.3, 134.3)	131.0 (113.0, 134.8)	**0.048**
DBP, mmHg	73.0 (66.0, 82.5)	81.0 (72.5, 90.5)	**< 0.001**	73.0 (64.5, 81.5)	79.0 (72.5, 89.5)	**< 0.001**	77.5 (67.5, 83.0)	85.0 (72.0, 96.0)	**0.032**

*BMI, body mass index; HR, heart rate; SpO_2, pulse oxygen saturation; SBP, systolic blood pressure; DBP, diastolic blood pressure. Data are presented as mean ± standard error of the mean or median (25th to 75th quartile). *P < 0.05 compared with notch (–) at HA. The bolded values mean p value < 0.05.*

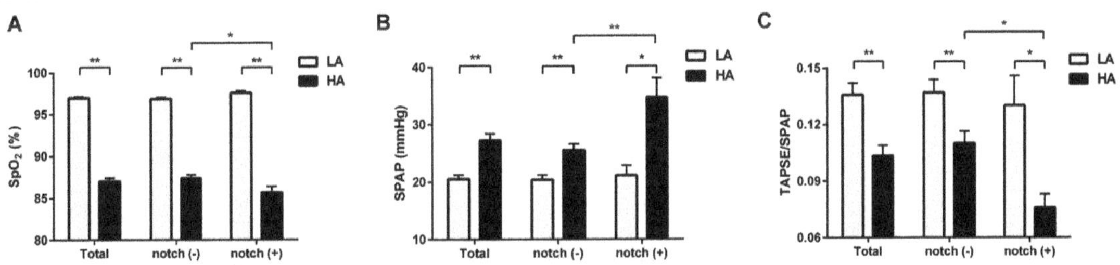

FIGURE 2 | Differences in SpO_2, SPAP, and TAPSE/SPAP between notch (–) and notch (+) groups at low altitude and HA. Different levels of **(A)** SpO_2, **(B)** SPAP, and **(C)** TAPSE/SPAP in total subjects, notch (–) subjects and notch (+) subjects upon HA exposure are shown. Differences between notch (–) subjects and notch (+) subjects in **(A)** SpO_2, **(B)** SPAP, and **(C)** TAPSE/SPAP were compared at low altitude and HA. Values are presented as mean and standard error of mean. *P < 0.05, **P < 0.01. Abbreviations as in **Tables 1, 3**.

vascular disease (Arkles et al., 2011; Takahama et al., 2017). Patients with low arterial compliance, high arterial resistance, and/or a pulmonary embolism proximal to the pulmonary valve may have a pulmonary vascular reflected wave on Doppler, which is seen as a notched Doppler flow velocity contour in the RVOT if the reflected wave rapidly propagates to the pulmonary valve prior to its closure (Torbicki et al., 1999; Arkles et al., 2011). In this study, we found that RVOT notch formation in subjects upon HA exposure is associated with higher SPAP, which is in accordance with the previous finding in PH patients (Lopez-Candales and Edelman, 2012). Upon HA exposure, alveolar hypoxia-induced HPV and inhomogeneous pulmonary vasoconstriction facilitated the ventilation–perfusion matching in the regional lung (Sommer et al., 2008). According to previous studies, SpO_2 decreases and SPAP increases with rising altitude (Penaloza and Arias-Stella, 2007). Furthermore, in patients receiving bosentan for PH, SpO_2 levels significantly increase with an increase in altitude (Modesti et al., 2006; Mellor et al., 2014). Thus, patients with lower SpO_2 are more likely to experience HPV of greater magnitude as an attempt to maintain the ventilation–perfusion balance, which leads to higher SPAP and PVR. Although the presence of an RVOT notch in patients with PH indicates a high SPAP (Kubba et al., 2016), the uneven HPV at HA might induce a reflection site proximal to the pulmonary valve, which leads to the formation of an RVOT notch.

LV Function

Similar to previous studies, our results indicated that LV filling is decreased and LV contractile function is preserved in subjects upon HA exposure (Maufrais et al., 2017, 2019). Although the LV filling is decreased, the HR is increased. The maintained LV function might due to the increase of sympathetic activation. According to a previous study, LV function is not related to RVOT notch formation due to the absence of an RVOT notch in left-heart-disease-associated PH (Kushwaha et al., 2016). However, hypoxia may affect LV function in notch (+) subjects with a lower SpO_2. Thus, the increase of mitral s' in the notch (+) group was blunted in this study. At HA, no difference in TS-12SD was found between the two groups in this study, indicating that upon HA exposure, the SpO_2 has little effect on LV dyssynchrony.

Impact of RVOT Notch on RV Function Evaluated by Conventional Echocardiography

In our study, we found that the presence of an RVOT notch indicates impaired RV function in healthy subjects upon HA

TABLE 2 | Left ventricular parameters in subjects with or without RVOT notch at low altitude and high altitude.

Variables	Total (*n* = 99)			Notch (–) (*n* = 79)			Notch (+) (*n* = 20)		
	Low altitude	High altitude	*P*-value	Low altitude	High altitude	*P*-value	Low altitude	High altitude	*P*-value
Conventional Doppler echocardiography									
SV, ml	65.0 (57.2, 71.45)	57.5 (51., 66.35)	**<0.001**	66.1 (57.2, 73.1)	58.5 (53.6, 66.5)	**<0.001**	64.1 (56.9, 68.3)	55.7 (48.6, 66.4)	0.156
LVEF, %	59.2 (56.4, 61.5)	59.2 (55.8, 61.6)	0.841	58.5 (56.4, 61.5)	59.0 (56.2, 62.0)	0.784	60.0 (57.5, 62.3)	59.3 (54.8, 61.6)	0.458
CO, L/min	4.2 (3.5, 4.9)	4.6 (4.1, 5.5)	**<0.001**	4.2 (3.5, 5.0)	4.6 (4.1, 5.4)	**<0.001**	4.3 (3.5, 4.6)	4.7 (4.4, 6.1)	**0.008**
Mitral E, cm/s	93.4 (81.0, 110.4)	81.6 (71.9, 97.4)	**<0.001**	93.4 (82.1, 111.0)	83.0 (72.6, 98.1)	**<0.001**	92.7 (74.8, 107.6)	78.3 (64.9, 93.8)	**0.001**
Mitral A, cm/s	51.7 (44.4, 63.5)	59.4 (50.8, 68.4)	**<0.001**	50.9 (44.3, 63.0)	57.2 (49.1, 67.0)	**<0.001**	52.7 (48.8, 66.1)	64.5 (58.4, 73.7)*	**0.007**
Mitral E/A ratio	1.7 (1.5, 2.1)	1.4 (1.2, 1.6)	**<0.001**	1.7 (1.6, 2.1)	1.5 (1.2, 1.7)	**<0.001**	1.6 (1.2, 2.2)	1.3 (1.1, 1.5)*	**<0.001**
Pulse tissue Doppler imaging									
Mitral s', cm/s	10.5 (9.6, 11.6)	11.6 (10.3, 12.7)	**<0.001**	10.5 (9.6, 11.7)	11.6 (10.3, 13.1)	**<0.001**	10.6 (9.4, 11.5)	10.9 (9.6, 12.4)	0.297
Mitral e', cm/s	15.1 (13.6, 16.3)	14.5 (13.4, 16.1)	0.663	15.1 (13.7, 16.2)	14.9 (13.4, 16.9)	0.346	14.1 (10.8, 16.7)	14.1 (13.4, 15.3)*	0.701
Mitral E/e' ratio	6.4 (5.7, 7.2)	5.6 (4.9, 6.4)	**<0.001**	6.4 (5.6, 7.3)	5.5 (4.7, 6.4)	**<0.001**	6.6 (5.9, 7.1)	5.7 (5.3, 6.5)	**0.006**
Mitral ICV, cm/s	8.6 ± 0.2	9.6 ± 0.2	**<0.001**	8.7 ± 0.2	9.5 ± 0.2	**0.005**	8.5 ± 0.5	10.0 ± 0.6	**0.035**
Speckle tracking imaging									
LV GLS, %	−20.9 (−19.9, −21.7)	−19.1 (−17.8, −20.6)	**<0.001**	−20.8 (−19.9, −21.6)	−19.2 (−18.1, −20.6)	**<0.001**	−21.3 (−20.4, −22.3)	−18.7 (−17.3, −20.3)	**0.001**
LV GCS, %	−24.8 (−23.6, −26.7)	−24.6 (−23.3, −25.9)	0.118	−24.8 (−23.8, −26.9)	−24.6 (−23.6, −26.0)	0.106	−24.8 (−21.4, −26.7)	−23.6 (−22.6, −25.8)	0.520
TS-12SD, ms	19.7 ± 0.9	25.7 ± 1.0	**<0.001**	20.1 ± 1.0	25.7 ± 1.2	**<0.001**	18.3 ± 1.9	25.5 ± 2.2	**0.015**

*SV, stroke volume; LVEF, left ventricular ejection fraction; CO, cardiac output; E, early diastolic transmitral or transtricuspid flow velocity; A, late diastolic transmitral or transtricuspid flow velocity; s', mitral or tricuspid annulus systolic velocity; e', mitral or tricuspid annulus early diastolic velocity; ICV, peak velocity of isovolumic contraction period at mitral or tricuspid annulus; LV, left ventricular; GLS, global longitude strain; GCS, global circumferential strain; TS-12SD, the standard deviation of time to peak systolic strain in 12 LV segments; Data are presented as mean ± standard error of the mean or median (25th to 75th quartile). *P < 0.05 compared with notch (–) at HA. The bolded values mean p value < 0.05.*

exposure, which is consistent with previous studies that reported advanced RV dysfunction in PH patients with RVOT notch (Arkles et al., 2011; Lopez-Candales and Edelman, 2012). Previous reports of the changes in RV FAC and TAPSE vary from a decrease (Kurdziel et al., 2017; Netzer et al., 2017), to no change (Maufrais et al., 2017, 2019), and to an increase upon HA exposure (Sareban et al., 2020). These inconsistent results may be due to different exposure times and ascending altitudes, or states of dehydration, all of which have been associated with RV adaptation upon HA exposure. In the present study, we found that the TAPSE and RV FAC decreased upon HA exposure. Although RV contractility may increase in response to the acutely increased RV afterload to maintain the pump function and RV-PA coupling (Naeije et al., 2014), the appropriately increased RV contractility upon HA exposure that is mirrored by load-dependent RV FAC and TAPSE may be under detected due to hypovolemia-induced RV FAC and TAPSE reduction via the Frank-Starling mechanism in patients with moderately increased PAP (Rudski et al., 2010; Najafian et al., 2015; Stembridge et al., 2016; Zhao et al., 2019).

TAPSE/SPAP is noninvasively measured for the evaluation of RV-PA coupling and correlates well with the gold standard multi-beat end-systolic/arterial elastance ratio in patients with PH (Tello et al., 2019; Richter et al., 2020). In this study, the decrease of TAPSE/SPAP in all subjects indicates that the level of RV-PA coupling was decreased in healthy subjects upon HA exposure. The more significant decrease of TAPSE/SPAP in the notch (+) group was attributed to the higher SPAP. The comparable TAPSE between notch (−) and notch (+) groups suggests that the RV contractility in the notch (+) group is maladaptive to the higher RV afterload upon HA exposure. TAPSE/SPAP has been reported to be positively correlated with VO_2 peak and workload during cardiopulmonary exercise testing (Martens et al., 2018; Tello et al., 2018). Thus, although TAPSE/SPAP was maintained within a normal range, lower TAPSE/SPAP in the notch (+) subjects upon HA exposure may indicate lower work capacity.

Impact of RVOT Notch on RV Function Evaluated by TDI

Upon HA exposure, the load-independent tricuspid s' and ICV increased in the context of increased PAP (Abali et al., 2005; Rudski et al., 2010; Negishi et al., 2017), which indicates an increased RV inotropic function in response to the elevated RV afterload (Vonk Noordegraaf et al., 2017). This enhancement of myocardial contractility may be attributed to homeometric autoregulation or sympathetic activation (Rex et al., 2007, 2008). The association of RV contractility with sympathetic activation

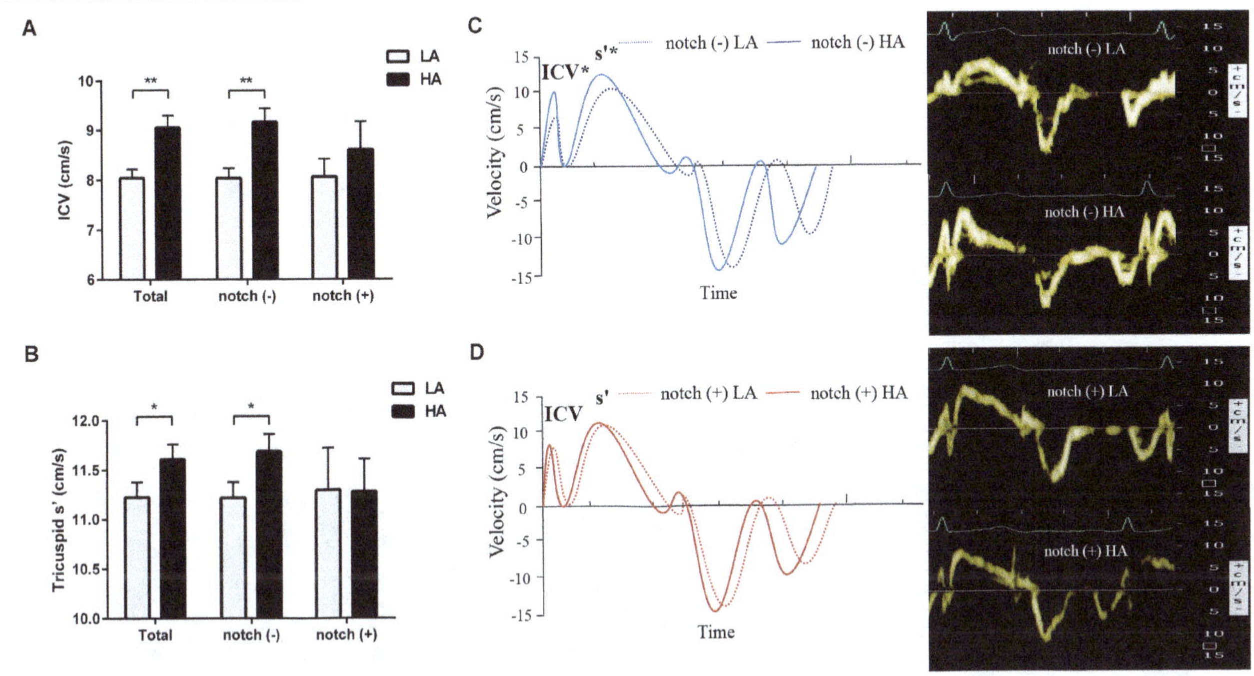

FIGURE 3 | Tricuspid pulse Doppler velocity analysis in subjects with and without RVOT notch. Different changes in tricuspid ICV **(A)** and s' **(B)** in notch (–) subjects and notch (+) subjects upon HA exposure. **(C)** and **(D)** Left panel: pulse tissue Doppler velocity curves of the tricuspid annulus in notch (–) and notch (+) subjects at low altitude and HA. Right panel: examples of the pulse TDI at tricuspid annulus in a subject without RVOT notch **(C)** and a subject with RVOT notch **(D)**. TDI, tissue Doppler imaging; *$P < 0.05$, **$P < 0.01$. Other abbreviations as in **Table 3**.

upon HA exposure is supported by a previous report, which suggests that the tricuspid s' is correlated with HR (Sareban et al., 2020). However, in the notch (+) group, the tricuspid s' and ICV did not increase to match the increased RV afterload, leading to a blunted RV contractile response upon HA exposure. This may be due to the fact that the positive inotropic effect of homeometric autoregulation or sympathetic activation was overwhelmed by the negative inotropic effect of hypoxia in notch (+) subjects with lower SpO_2 (Silverman et al., 1997).

Impact of RVOT Notch on RV Function Evaluated by 2D-STE

Although the conventional RV function parameters RV FAC and TAPSE were comparable in both groups at HA in this study, the 2D-STE RV function parameter RV GLS was lower in the notch (+) group, especially in the base and mid segments of RVFW. This may be due to the fact that the RV GLS is a more sensitive and accurate assessment for detecting subclinical RV dysfunction than TAPSE and RV FAC (Giusca et al., 2010; Li et al., 2018; Tamulenaite et al., 2018). Even in mild PH, when FAC does not change, the RV GLS begins to decrease (Li et al., 2013). Moreover, the correlation of RV GLS with the gold standard cardiac magnetic resonance-derived RV ejection fraction (RVEF) is better than the correlation of RV FAC and TAPSE with RVEF (Tong et al., 2018; Kavurt et al., 2019); a lower RV GLS may indicate a lower RVEF in notch (+) subjects. These findings are consistent with those of a previous study which reported that the presence of an RVOT notch was related to a reduced RV SV index in patients with PH (Arkles et al., 2011). Intraventricular RV dyssynchrony is an early sign of RV contractile dysfunction. In our previous study, we had found that notch (+) cases in RV dyssynchrony (−) subjects and RV dyssynchrony (+) subjects were comparable. However, in this study, we found that the RVOT notch was associated with higher RVSD4, which is the indicator of RVD. This inconsistency may be attributed to the different ascending modes, exposure times, and ratio of males and females. In the present 2-day period HA exposure study, the subjects with an RVOT notch are more prone to suffer intraventricular RV mechanical dyssynchrony (RVSD4 > 18.7 ms) compared with subjects without an RVOT notch (Badagliacca et al., 2015; Yang et al., 2020). In this study, higher RV dyssynchrony was accompanied by a lower RV GLS. A similar observation was reported in patients after hemodialysis (Unlu et al., 2019).

Impact of Mid-Systolic DT on Cardiac Function

Previous studies reported that PH patients with mid-systolic DT < 120 ms had worse clinical outcomes compared with those subjects with mid-systolic DT > 120 ms (Takahama et al., 2017). In this study, the RVD base and RVD mid in mid-systolic DT < 120 ms group were larger than those in mid-systolic DT > 120 ms group. RV dilation is a sign of RV maladaptation in response to high PAP; however, the outcomes of subjects

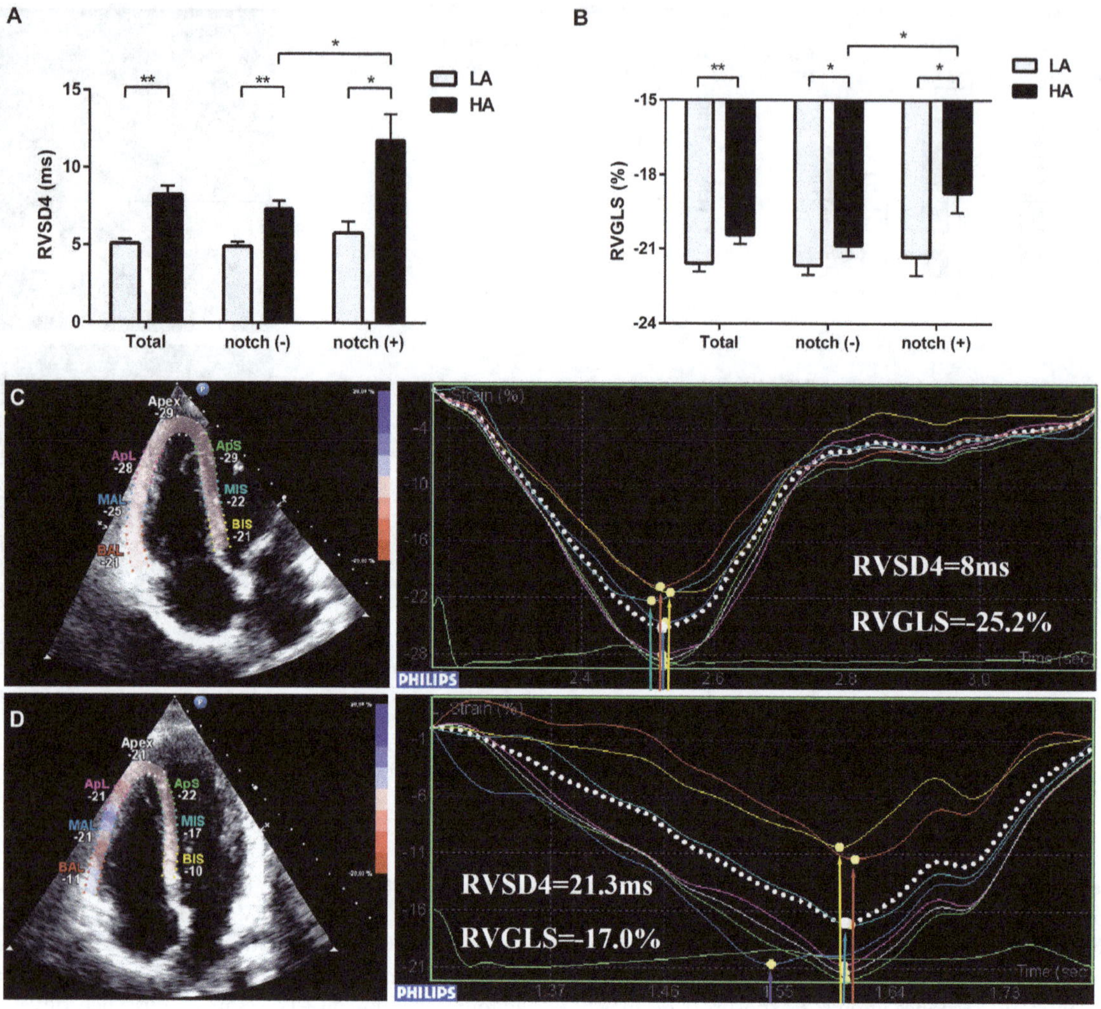

FIGURE 4 | Evaluation of RV GLS and dyssynchrony in subjects with and without RVOT notch from low altitude to HA. Different levels of **(A)** RVSD4 and **(B)** RV GLS in total subjects, notch (−) subjects, and notch (+) subjects upon HA exposure are shown. **(C)** and **(D)** Examples illustrating the 2D-STE measurements of RV GLS and RV dyssynchrony in a subject without RVOT notch **(C)** and a subject with RVOT notch **(D)** at HA. $^{*}P < 0.05$, $^{**}P < 0.01$. Abbreviations as in **Table 3**.

with mid-systolic DT < 120 ms upon HA exposure still need long-term follow-up studies to investigate.

Several limitations in this study should be noted. For ethical reasons, cardiac catheterization, the gold standard for the measurement of cardiac hemodynamics, was not performed in this study. As 30 females (30.3% of total subjects) were included in this study and the menstrual cycle in female participants may affect heart physiology, menstrual cycle information should be collected, and its association with RVOT notch needs to be investigated. Acute mountain sickness was reported to be associated with reduced LV function, whereas, as this study mainly focused on the association of RVOT notch with RV function, acute mountain sickness cases were not excluded. As the subjects in this study returned to low altitude within two months, the long-term association of an RVOT notch with RV function was not studied. It is not clear whether the subjects with RVOT notch are more likely to develop HA heart disease. Furthermore, the cardiopulmonary exercise test to investigate RV contractile reserves in subjects with an RVOT notch should be performed in future studies as the RV function in these subjects is maladapted to HA exposure. It would be valuable to see whether the RVOT notch would reverse to normal after notch (+) subjects returned to sea level and whether a lower exercise capacity could be observed in the notch (+) subjects at sea level via cardiopulmonary exercise test.

CONCLUSION

Our study revealed that HA exposure-induced RVOT notch formation may be attributed to high PAP and low SpO_2. The presence of an RVOT notch upon HA exposure was associated with impaired RV function as the tricuspid ICV and s' did not increase, the RV deformation reduced, the RV-PA coupling deteriorated, and RV intraventricular dyssynchrony was observed. Therefore, an RVOT notch may be a potential

TABLE 3 | Pulmonary circulation and right ventricular parameters in subjects with or without RVOT notch at low altitude and high altitude.

Variables	Total (n = 99)			Notch (-) (n = 79)			Notch (+) (n = 20)		
	Low altitude	High altitude	P-value	Low altitude	High altitude	P-value	Low altitude	High altitude	P-value
Pulmonary hemodynamics									
TR, n (%)	63 (63.6)	91 (91.9)	**< 0.001**	53 (67.1)	74 (93.7)	**< 0.001**	10 (50.0)	17 (85.0)	**0.018**
TRV, cm/s	196 (174, 220)	231 (202, 261)	**< 0.001**	195 (173, 220)	229 (194, 257)	**< 0.001**	209 (181, 226)	243 (222, 312)**	**0.020**
SPAP, mmHg	20.5 ± 0.7	27.2 ± 1.1	**< 0.001**	20.4 ± 0.8	25.5 ± 1.1	**< 0.001**	21.2 ± 1.7	34.8 ± 3.3**	**0.020**
mPAP, mmHg	14.4 (12.5, 16.9)	18.1 (15.0, 21.7)	**< 0.001**	14.3 (12.3, 16.9)	17.8 (14.2, 21.2)	**< 0.001**	15.7 (13.0, 17.6)	19.5 (17.0, 28.8)**	**0.020**
PVR, WU	1.2 (0.8, 1.8)	1.9 (1.3, 2.9)	**< 0.001**	1.2 (0.8, 1.7)	1.9 (1.3, 2.4)	**< 0.001**	1.3 (0.6, 1.8)	3.1 (1.4, 4.3)*	**0.037**
AT_{RVOT}, ms	146.5 (135.1, 161.3)	116.0 (96.6, 134.4)	**< 0.001**	146.6 (135.1, 162.6)	118.1 (96.6, 134.1)	**< 0.001**	141.3 (131.8, 157.6)	112.9 (96.7, 137.6)	**0.002**
ET_{RVOT}, ms	372.2 ± 35.96	360.0 ± 35.51	**0.001**	374.3 ± 33.8	361.7 ± 36.7	**0.002**	364.1 ± 43.5	353.4 ± 30.5	0.311
AT_{RVOT}/ET_{RVOT}	0.40 (0.35, 0.43)	0.32 (0.27, 0.38)	**< 0.001**	0.40 (0.35, 0.43)	0.32 (0.26, 0.37)	**< 0.001**	0.39 (0.36, 0.43)	0.33 (0.27, 0.40)	**0.002**
PCWP, mmHg	9.9 (8.9, 10.9)	8.9 (8.0, 9.8)	**< 0.001**	9.8 (8.9, 11.0)	8.7 (7.7, 9.8)	**< 0.001**	10.0 (9.2, 10.7)	9.0 (8.5, 10.0)	**0.006**
Conventional Doppler echocardiography									
RVD base, cm	3.5 ± 0.05	3.4 ± 0.06	0.378	3.6 ± 0.06	3.4 ± 0.07	0.055	3.3 ± 0.11##	3.5 ± 0.09	0.079
RVD mid, cm	3.2 ± 0.08	3.4 ± 0.08	**0.017**	3.2 ± 0.09	3.4 ± 0.09	0.119	3.0 ± 0.18	3.5 ± 0.14	**0.031**
RV EDA, cm^2	20.2 (17.7, 23.0)	20.0 (17.3, 22.8)	0.380	20.4 (17.7, 24.2)	20.0 (17.7, 22.9)	0.129	19.3 (17.4, 21.1)	19.7 (17.1, 22.3)	0.458
RV ESA, cm^2	10.9 (9.0, 12.5)	11.4 (9.8, 13.0)	0.065	11.2 (9.1, 12.9)	11.4 (9.8, 13.1)	0.273	9.8 (8.5, 11.8)	11.2 (9.6, 12.8)	0.065
RV FAC, %	46.6 ± 0.6	43.2 ± 0.5	**< 0.001**	46.5 ± 0.6	43.5 ± 0.5	**< 0.001**	47.1 ± 1.5	42.2 ± 1.1	**0.021**
TAPSE, mm	25.9 ± 0.4	23.8 ± 0.4	**< 0.001**	25.7 ± 0.4	24.1 ± 0.4	**0.003**	26.6 ± 0.9	22.9 ± 0.9	**0.002**
TAPSE/SPAP	1.2 (1.1, 1.5)	0.9 (0.7, 1.2)	**< 0.001**	1.2 (1.1, 1.5)	0.9 (0.8, 1.3)	**< 0.001**	1.1 (1.1, 1.4)	0.8 (0.5, 1.0)*	**0.023**
Tricuspid E, cm/s	66.6 ± 1.2	60.9 ± 1.5	**< 0.001**	67.0 ± 1.3	61.6 ± 1.6	**0.004**	65.1 ± 2.8	58.4 ± 3.7	**0.017**
Tricuspid A, cm/s	36.3 (30.5, 42.8)	42.1 (33.0, 52.5)	**< 0.001**	36.5 (30.6, 42.4)	39.7 (31.8, 48.5)	**< 0.001**	32.7 (29.3, 49.0)	51.5 (42.7, 57.7)*	**0.006**
Tricuspid E/A ratio	1.5 (1.8, 2.2)	1.5 (1.2, 1.7)	**< 0.001**	1.5 (1.8, 2.2)	1.5 (1.3, 1.7)	**< 0.001**	1.7 (1.4, 2.4)	1.2 (1.0, 1.6)**	**0.001**
Pulse tissue Doppler imaging									
Tricuspid s', cm/s	11.2 ± 0.2	11.6 ± 0.2	**0.020**	11.2 ± 0.2	11.7 ± 0.2	**0.017**	11.3 ± 0.4	11.3 ± 0.3	0.662
Tricuspid e', cm/s	14.3 ± 0.2	14.1 ± 0.3	0.211	14.5 ± 0.2	14.3 ± 0.3	0.403	13.7 ± 0.6	13.2 ± 0.7	0.229
Tricuspid E/e' ratio	4.7 (4.1, 5.2)	4.5 (3.8, 4.9)	**0.046**	4.7 (4.1, 5.2)	4.4 (3.7, 4.9)	0.082	4.7 (4.3, 5.1)	4.6 (3.9, 5.0)	0.270
Tricuspid ICV, cm/s	7.9 (7.3, 8.8)	8.8 (7.3, 10.7)	**< 0.001**	7.9 (7.1, 8.7)	9.2 (7.3, 10.8)	**< 0.001**	7.8 (7.4, 9.1)	8.4 (6.7, 40.6)	0.341
Speckle tracking imaging									
RV GLS, %	−21.7 (−19.8, −23.9)	−20.1 (−17.7, −22.9)	**0.003**	−21.7 (−20.0, −24.2)	−20.5 (−18.6, −22.9)	**0.035**	−22.2 (−19.3, −23.3)	−18.4 (−16.0, −22.4)*	**0.015**
2DS RVFW apex, %	−23.6 ± 0.4	−21.9 ± 0.5	**0.005**	−23.5 ± 0.5	−22.3 ± 0.5	0.079	−23.9 ± 0.7	−20.3 ± 1.0	**0.004**
2DS RVFW mid, %	−23.3 ± 0.4	−22.2 ± 0.5	0.063	−23.5 ± 0.5	−22.8 ± 0.6	0.183	−22.6 ± 0.9	−20.0 ± 1.1*	0.057
2DS RVFW base, %	−18.0 (−15.0, −21.0)	−17.0 (−14.0, −20.0)	0.274	−18.0 (−15.0, −20.0)	−18.0 (−15.0, −20.0)	0.684	−18.0 (−14.3, −21.8)	−14.0 (−13.0, −19.0)*	0.093
RVSD4, ms	4.2 (3.1, 7.0)	6.6 (4.4, 11.6)	**< 0.001**	4.2 (3.1, 6.9)	6.4 (4.3, 9.8)	**< 0.001**	4.1 (3.4, 7.7)	12.1 (5.1, 18.0)*	**0.005**

TR, tricuspid regurgitation; TRV, tricuspid regurgitation velocity; SPAP, systolic pulmonary artery pressure; mPAP, mean pulmonary artery pressure; PVR, pulmonary vascular resistance; AT_{RVOT}, acceleration time of RVOT; ET_{RVOT}, ejection time of RVOT; PCWP, pulmonary capillary wedge pressure; RV, right ventricular; EDA, end-diastolic area; ESA, end-systolic area; FAC, fraction area change; TAPSE, tricuspid annulus plane systolic excursion; RVD, right ventricular transverse diameter; 2DS RVFW, two-dimensional strain of right ventricular free wall. RVSD4, standard deviation of the time to peak systolic strain in the 4 mid-basal RV segments; Other abbreviation as in ***Table 2****. Data are presented as mean ± standard error of the mean or median (25th to 75th quartile). ##$P < 0.01$ compared with notch (−) at low altitude, *$P < 0.05$, **$P < 0.01$ compared with notch (−) at HA. The bolded values mean p value < 0.05.*

echocardiographic sign representing impaired RV function at HA. However, whether the impaired RV function in subjects with RVOT notch upon HA exposure persists or is transient still needs further investigation.

ETHICS STATEMENT

The studies involving human participants were reviewed and approved by the Clinical Research Ethics Board of Army Medical University. The patients/participants provided their written informed consent to participate in this study.

AUTHOR CONTRIBUTIONS

LH, FY, and CL contributed to the conception or design of the work. FY, CL, JK, YY, CH, CZ, RR, ZL, and JuY conducted the experiments. FY and CL performed the statistical analyses and drafted the manuscript. SY, SB, JiY, XD, JZ, and HT interpreted the results of the statistical analyses. LH critically revised the manuscript. All authors approved of the final version of the manuscript and agreed to be accountable for all aspects of the work.

ACKNOWLEDGMENTS

We thank all participants in this study for their contributions to medical science.

REFERENCES

Abali, G., Tokgozoglu, L., Ozcebe, O. I., Aytemir, K., and Nazli, N. (2005). Which Doppler parameters are load independent? a study in normal volunteers after blood donation. *J. Am. Soc. Echocardiogr.* 18, 1260–1265. doi: 10.1016/j.echo.2005.06.012

Arkles, J. S., Opotowsky, A. R., Ojeda, J., Rogers, F., Liu, T., Prassana, V., et al. (2011). Shape of the right ventricular doppler envelope predicts hemodynamics and right heart function in pulmonary hypertension. *Am. J. Respir. Crit. Care Med.* 183, 268–276. doi: 10.1164/rccm.201004-0601oc

Badagliacca, R., Reali, M., Poscia, R., Pezzuto, B., Papa, S., Mezzapesa, M., et al. (2015). Right intraventricular dyssynchrony in idiopathic, heritable, and anorexigen-induced pulmonary arterial hypertension: clinical impact and reversibility. *JACC Cardiovasc. Imaging* 8, 642–652. doi: 10.1016/j.jcmg.2015.02.009

Bossone, E., D'andrea, A., D'alto, M., Citro, R., Argiento, P., Ferrara, F., et al. (2013). Echocardiography in pulmonary arterial hypertension: from diagnosis to prognosis. *J. Am. Soc. Echocardiogr.* 26, 1–14. doi: 10.1016/j.echo.2012.10.009

Ghimire, A., Andersen, M. J., Burrowes, L. M., Bouwmeester, J. C., Grant, A. D., Belenkie, I., et al. (2016). The reservoir-wave approach to characterize pulmonary vascular-right ventricular interactions in humans. *J. Appl. Physiol.* 121, 1348–1353. doi: 10.1152/japplphysiol.00697.2016

Giusca, S., Dambrauskaite, V., Scheurwegs, C., D'hooge, J., Claus, P., Herbots, L., et al. (2010). Deformation imaging describes right ventricular function better than longitudinal displacement of the tricuspid ring. *Heart* 96, 281–288. doi: 10.1136/hrt.2009.171728

Huston, J. H., Maron, B. A., French, J., Huang, S., Thayer, T., Farber-Eger, E. H., et al. (2019). Association of mild echocardiographic pulmonary hypertension with mortality and right ventricular function. *JAMA Cardiol.* 4, 1112–1121. doi: 10.1001/jamacardio.2019.3345

Kavurt, A. V., Paç, F. A., Koca, S., Mutlu Mıhçıoðlu, A., and Yiðit, H. (2019). The evaluation of right ventricular systolic function in patients with repaired tetralogy of fallot by conventional echocardiographic methods and speckle tracking echocardiography: compared with the gold standard cardiac mangenetic resonance. *Echocardiography* 36, 2251–2258. doi: 10.1111/echo.14532

Kubba, S., Davila, C. D., and Forfia, P. R. (2016). Methods for evaluating right ventricular function and ventricular-arterial coupling. *Prog. Cardiovasc. Dis.* 59, 42–51. doi: 10.1016/j.pcad.2016.06.001

Kurdziel, M., Wasilewski, J., Gierszewska, K., Kazik, A., Pytel, G., Waclawski, J., et al. (2017). Echocardiographic assessment of right ventricle dimensions and function after exposure to extreme altitude: is an expedition to 8000 m hazardous for right ventricular function? *High Alt. Med. Biol.* 18, 330–337. doi: 10.1089/ham.2017.0019

Kushwaha, S. P., Zhao, Q. H., Liu, Q. Q., Wu, W. H., Wang, L., Yuan, P., et al. (2016). Shape of the pulmonary artery doppler-flow profile predicts the hemodynamics of pulmonary hypertension caused by left-sided heart disease. *Clin. Cardiol.* 39, 150–156. doi: 10.1002/clc.22493

Lang, R. M., Badano, L. P., Mor-Avi, V., Afilalo, J., Armstrong, A., Ernande, L., et al. (2015). Recommendations for cardiac chamber quantification by echocardiography in adults: an update from the American society of echocardiography and the European association of cardiovascular imaging. *Eur. Heart J. Cardiovasc. Imaging* 16, 233–270. doi: 10.1093/ehjci/jev014

Li, A. L., Zhai, Z. G., Zhai, Y. N., Xie, W. M., Wan, J., and Tao, X. C. (2018). The value of speckle-tracking echocardiography in identifying right heart dysfunction in patients with chronic thromboembolic pulmonary hypertension. *Int. J. Cardiovasc. Imaging* 34, 1895–1904. doi: 10.1007/s10554-018-1423-0

Li, Y., Xie, M., Wang, X., Lu, Q., and Fu, M. (2013). Right ventricular regional and global systolic function is diminished in patients with pulmonary arterial hypertension: a two-dimensional ultrasound speckle tracking echocardiography study. *Int. J. Cardiovasc. Imaging* 29, 545–551. doi: 10.1007/s10554-012-0114-5

Lopez-Candales, A., and Edelman, K. (2012). Shape of the right ventricular outflow doppler envelope and severity of pulmonary hypertension. *Eur. Heart J. Cardiovasc. Imaging* 13, 309–316. doi: 10.1093/ejechocard/jer235

Martens, P., Verbrugge, F. H., Bertrand, P. B., Verhaert, D., Vandervoort, P., Dupont, M., et al. (2018). Effect of cardiac resynchronization therapy on exercise-induced pulmonary hypertension and right ventricular-arterial coupling. *Circ. Cardiovasc. Imaging* 11:e007813.

Maufrais, C., Rupp, T., Bouzat, P., Doucende, G., Verges, S., Nottin, S., et al. (2017). Heart mechanics at high altitude: 6 days on the top of Europe. *Eur. Heart J. Cardiovasc. Imaging* 18, 1369–1377. doi: 10.1093/ehjci/jew286

Maufrais, C., Rupp, T., Bouzat, P., Esteve, F., Nottin, S., Walther, G., et al. (2019). Medex 2015: the key role of cardiac mechanics to maintain biventricular function at high altitude. *Exp. Physiol.* 104, 667–676. doi: 10.1113/ep087350

Mellor, A., Boos, C., Holdsworth, D., Begley, J., Hall, D., Lumley, A., et al. (2014). Cardiac biomarkers at high altitude. *High Alt. Med. Biol.* 15, 452–458. doi: 10.1089/ham.2014.1035

Mitchell, C., Rahko, P. S., Blauwet, L. A., Canaday, B., Finstuen, J. A., Foster, M. C., et al. (2019). Guidelines for performing a comprehensive transthoracic echocardiographic examination in adults: recommendations from the american society of echocardiography. *J. Am. Soc. Echocardiogr.* 32, 1–64. doi: 10.1016/j.echo.2018.06.004

Modesti, P. A., Vanni, S., Morabito, M., Modesti, A., Marchetta, M., Gamberi, T., et al. (2006). Role of endothelin-1 in exposure to high altitude: acute mountain sickness and endothelin-1 (ACME-1) study. *Circulation* 114, 1410–1416. doi: 10.1161/circulationaha.105.605527

Naeije, R. (2019). Pulmonary hypertension at high altitude. *Eur. Respir. J.* 53:1900985.

Naeije, R., Brimioulle, S., and Dewachter, L. (2014). Biomechanics of the right ventricle in health and disease (2013 grover conference series). *Pulm. Circ.* 4, 395–406. doi: 10.1086/677354

Najafian, J., Taheri, S., Mahaki, B., Molavi, S., Alami, S., Khalesi, S., et al. (2015). Comparing right ventricular function and pulmonary artery pressure before and shortly after hemodialysis in patients with end-stage renal disease. *Adv. Biomed. Res.* 4:197.

Negishi, K., Borowski, A. G., Popoviæ, Z. B., Greenberg, N. L., Martin, D. S., Bungo, M. W., et al. (2017). Effect of gravitational gradients on cardiac filling and performance. *J. Am. Soc. Echocardiogr.* 30, 1180–1188. doi: 10.1016/j.echo.2017.08.005

Netzer, N. C., Strohl, K. P., Hogel, J., Gatterer, H., and Schilz, R. (2017). Right ventricle dimensions and function in response to acute hypoxia in healthy human subjects. *Acta Physiol.* 219, 478–485. doi: 10.1111/apha.12740

Osculati, G., Revera, M., Branzi, G., Faini, A., Malfatto, G., Bilo, G., et al. (2016). Effects of hypobaric hypoxia exposure at high altitude on left ventricular twist in healthy subjects: data from HIGHCARE study on mount everest. *Eur. Heart J. Cardiovasc. Imaging* 17, 635–643. doi: 10.1093/ehjci/jev166

Parati, G., Agostoni, P., Basnyat, B., Bilo, G., Brugger, H., Coca, A., et al. (2018). Clinical recommendations for high altitude exposure of individuals with pre-existing cardiovascular conditions: a joint statement by the european society of cardiology, the council on hypertension of the european society of cardiology, the european society of hypertension, the international society of mountain medicine, the italian society of hypertension and the italian society of mountain medicine. *Eur. Heart J.* 39, 1546–1554.

Penaloza, D., and Arias-Stella, J. (2007). The heart and pulmonary circulation at high altitudes: healthy highlanders and chronic mountain sickness. *Circulation* 115, 1132–1146. doi: 10.1161/circulationaha.106.624544

Rex, S., Missant, C., Segers, P., and Wouters, P. F. (2007). Thoracic epidural anesthesia impairs the hemodynamic response to acute pulmonary hypertension by deteriorating right ventricular–pulmonary arterial coupling. *Crit. Care Med.* 35, 222–229. doi: 10.1097/01.ccm.0000250357.35250.a2

Rex, S., Missant, C., Segers, P., Rossaint, R., and Wouters, P. F. (2008). Epoprostenol treatment of acute pulmonary hypertension is associated with a paradoxical decrease in right ventricular contractility. *Intensive Care Med.* 34, 179–189. doi: 10.1007/s00134-007-0831-8

Richter, M. J., Peters, D., Ghofrani, H. A., Naeije, R., Roller, F., Sommer, N., et al. (2020). Evaluation and prognostic relevance of right ventricular-arterial coupling in pulmonary hypertension. *Am. J. Respir. Crit. Care Med.* 201, 116–119. doi: 10.1164/rccm.201906-1195le

Rudski, L. G., Lai, W. W., Afilalo, J., Hua, L., Handschumacher, M. D., Chandrasekaran, K., et al. (2010). Guidelines for the echocardiographic assessment of the right heart in adults: a report from the American society of echocardiography endorsed by the european association of echocardiography, a registered branch of the european society of cardiology, and the canadian society of echocardiography. *J. Am. Soc. Echocardiogr.* 23, 685–713. doi: 10.1016/j.echo.2010.05.010

Sareban, M., Perz, T., Macholz, F., Reich, B., Schmidt, P., Fried, S., et al. (2020). Preserved right ventricular function but increased right atrial contractile demand in altitude-induced pulmonary hypertension. *Int. J. Cardiovasc. Imaging* 36, 1069–1076. doi: 10.1007/s10554-020-01803-x

Silverman, H. S., Wei, S., Haigney, M. C., Ocampo, C. J., and Stern, M. D. (1997). Myocyte adaptation to chronic hypoxia and development of tolerance to subsequent acute severe hypoxia. *Circ. Res.* 80, 699–707. doi: 10.1161/01.res.80.5.699

Sommer, N., Dietrich, A., Schermuly, R. T., Ghofrani, H. A., Gudermann, T., Schulz, R., et al. (2008). Regulation of hypoxic pulmonary vasoconstriction: basic mechanisms. *Eur. Respir. J.* 32, 1639–1651.

Stembridge, M., Ainslie, P. N., and Shave, R. (2016). Mechanisms underlying reductions in stroke volume at rest and during exercise at high altitude. *Eur. J. Sport Sci.* 16, 577–584. doi: 10.1080/17461391.2015.1071876

Takahama, H., Mccully, R. B., Frantz, R. P., and Kane, G. C. (2017). Unraveling the RV ejection doppler envelope: insight into pulmonary artery hemodynamics and disease severity. *JACC Cardiovasc. Imaging* 10, 1268–1277. doi: 10.1016/j.jcmg.2016.12.021

Tamulenaite, E., Zvirblyte, R., Ereminiene, R., Ziginskiene, E., and Ereminiene, E. (2018). Changes of left and right ventricle mechanics and function in patients with end-stage renal disease undergoing haemodialysis. *Medicina* 54:87. doi: 10.3390/medicina54050087

Tello, K., Axmann, J., Ghofrani, H. A., Naeije, R., Narcin, N., Rieth, A., et al. (2018). Relevance of the TAPSE/PASP ratio in pulmonary arterial hypertension. *Int. J. Cardiol.* 266, 229–235. doi: 10.1016/j.ijcard.2018.01.053

Tello, K., Wan, J., Dalmer, A., Vanderpool, R., Ghofrani, H. A., Naeije, R., et al. (2019). Validation of the tricuspid annular plane systolic excursion/systolic pulmonary artery pressure ratio for the assessment of right ventricular-arterial coupling in severe pulmonary hypertension. *Circ. Cardiovasc. Imaging* 12:e009047.

Tong, X., Poon, J., Li, A., Kit, C., Yamada, A., Shiino, K., et al. (2018). Validation of cardiac magnetic resonance tissue tracking in the rapid assessment of RV function: a comparative study to echocardiography. *Clin. Radiol.* 73, 324 e329–324 e318. .

Torbicki, A., Kurzyna, M., Ciurzynski, M., Pruszczyk, P., Pacho, R., Kuch-Wocial, A., et al. (1999). Proximal pulmonary emboli modify right ventricular ejection pattern. *Eur. Respir. J.* 13, 616–621. doi: 10.1183/09031936.99.13361699

Unlu, S., Pagourelias, E., Sezenoz, B., Sahinarslan, A., Uludag, O. M., Gokalp, G., et al. (2019). Higher ultrafiltration rate is associated with right ventricular mechanical dispersion. *Anatol. J. Cardiol.* 21, 206–213.

van de Veerdonk, M. C., Kind, T., Marcus, J. T., Mauritz, G. J., Heymans, M. W., Bogaard, H. J., et al. (2011). Progressive right ventricular dysfunction in patients with pulmonary arterial hypertension responding to therapy. *J. Am. Coll. Cardiol.* 58, 2511–2519. doi: 10.1016/j.jacc.2011.06.068

Vonk Noordegraaf, A., Westerhof, B. E., and Westerhof, N. (2017). The relationship between the right ventricle and its load in pulmonary hypertension. *J. Am. Coll. Cardiol.* 69, 236–243. doi: 10.1016/j.jacc.2016.10.047

Williams, A. M., Ainslie, P. N., Anholm, J. D., Gasho, C., Subedi, P., and Stembridge, M. (2019). Left ventricular twist is augmented in hypoxia by beta1-adrenergic-dependent and beta1-adrenergic-independent factors, without evidence of endocardial dysfunction. *Circ. Cardiovasc. Imaging* 12:e008455.

Yang, Y., Liu, C., Tian, J., Ding, X., Yu, S., Bian, S., et al. (2020). Preliminary study of right ventricular dyssynchrony under high-altitude exposure: determinants and impacts. *Front. Physiol.* 11:703.

Yock, P. G., and Popp, R. L. (1984). Noninvasive estimation of right ventricular systolic pressure by doppler ultrasound in patients with tricuspid regurgitation. *Circulation* 70, 657–662. doi: 10.1161/01.cir.70.4.657

Zhao, H., Kang, Y., Pickle, J., Wang, J., and Han, Y. (2019). Tricuspid annular plane systolic excursion is dependent on right ventricular volume in addition to function. *Echocardiography* 36, 1459–1466. doi: 10.1111/echo.14439

Zoroufian, A., Razmi, T., Taghavi-Shavazi, M., Lotfi-Tokaldany, M., and Jalali, A. (2014). Evaluation of subclinical left ventricular dysfunction in diabetic patients: longitudinal strain velocities and left ventricular dyssynchrony by two-dimensional speckle tracking echocardiography study. *Echocardiography* 31, 456–463. doi: 10.1111/echo.12389

17

Comparison Between Pressure Swing Adsorption and Liquid Oxygen Enrichment Techniques in the Atacama Large Millimeter/Submillimeter Array Facility at the Chajnantor Plateau (5,050 m)

*Ivan Lopez[1], Reinaldo Aravena[1], Daniel Soza[1], Alicia Morales[1], Silvia Riquelme[2], Rodrigo Calderon-Jofré[3] and Fernando A. Moraga[3]**

[1] Atacama Large Millimeter/Submillimeter Array, San Pedro de Atacama, Chile, [2] Departamento de Medicina, Facultad de Ciencias de la Salud, Universidad de Tarapacá, Arica, Chile, [3] Laboratorio de Fisiología, Hipoxia y Función Vascular, Departamento de Ciencias Biomédicas, Facultad de Medicina, Universidad Católica del Norte, Coquimbo, Chile

Correspondence:
Fernando A. Moraga
fmoraga@ucn.cl

The Chilean workforce has over 200,000 people that are intermittently exposed to altitudes over 4,000 m. In 2012, the Ministry of Health provided a technical guide for high-altitude workers that included a series of actions to mitigate the effects of hypoxia. Previous studies have shown the positive effect of oxygen enrichment at high altitudes. The Atacama Large Millimeter/submillimeter Array (ALMA) radiotelescope operates at 5,050 m [Array Operations Site (AOS)] and is the only place in the world where pressure swing adsorption (PSA) and liquid oxygen technologies have been installed at a large scale. These technologies reduce the equivalent altitude by increasing oxygen availability. This study aims to perform a retrospective comparison between the use of both technologies during operation in ALMA at 5,050 m. In each condition, variables such as oxygen (O_2), temperature, and humidity were continuously recorded in each AOS rooms, and cardiorespiratory variables were registered. In addition, we compared portable O_2 by using continuous or demand flow during outdoor activities at very high altitudes. The outcomes showed no differences between production procedures (PSA or liquid oxygen) in regulating oxygen availability at AOS facilities. As a result, big-scale installations have difficulties reaching the appropriate O_2 concentration due to leaks in high mobility areas. In addition, the PSA plant requires adequacy and maintenance to operate at a very high altitude. A continuous flow of 2–3 l/min of portable O_2 is recommended at 5,050 m.

Keywords: pressure swing adsorption (PSA), liquid oxygen, oxygen generation, operation at 5050 m, heart rate, oxygen saturation (SpO_2), portable oxygen, chronic intermittent hypobaric hypoxia

INTRODUCTION

High altitude is a geographical condition where barometric pressure and inspired partial pressure of oxygen (PiO_2) are reduced with altitude. Today, about 140 million people live or work at altitudes above 2,500 m (Moore, 2001). According to the periodicity of exposure, hypoxia can be acute (observed in tourists, climbers, and hikers), chronic (people who live permanently at high altitudes, between 3,000 and 4,500 m), and intermittent (people who alternate exposure between hypoxia and normoxia) (Gassmann et al., 2021). However, the term "intermittent hypoxia" refers to a wide spectrum of contexts: episodic intermittent hypoxia (EIH), in obstructive sleep apnea-hypopnea syndrome (OSAHS); intervallic intermittent hypoxia (IIH), during intercontinental commercial flight crews; and the chronic intermittent hypobaric hypoxia (CIHH), in people who work under a shift system at high altitude and rest at sea level (Viscor et al., 2018).

The CIHH model of exposure is common in the mining industry in the Andes and the Central Asian regions but is also observed in astronomical observatories and border control personnel (including military, police, and customs) in many high-elevation countries (Moraga et al., 2014, 2018). In Chile, over 200,000 people ascend to high altitudes for work (Consejo de Competencias Mineras, 2017, available at http://www.ccm.cl/ReporteCCM_13-11_FINAL). Nowadays, we know that this exposure model is associated with acute mountain sickness, sleep disorders, polycythemia, pulmonary hypertension, and an acute increase in arterial pressure (Ministry of Health Chile, 2014, available at https://www.minsal.cl/sites/default/files/guia_hipobaria_altitud.pdf). These symptoms are present each time workers arrive at their high altitude worksite and do not disappear over time (Richalet et al., 2002; Moraga et al., 2014, 2018). To meet the requirements of the work unions of mining companies and studies about the safety of work at high altitudes, the Chilean Ministry of Health recognized altitude exposure as a health risk and by Decree 28 of 2013 defined chronic intermittent hypoxia exposure when workers are exposed to altitudes over 3,000 m for business reasons for more than 6 months, with a minimum stay of 30% of the time in rotating work shifts at high altitude and rest at low altitude (Ministry of Health Chile, 2013, available at http://bcn.cl/1vgrd). Considering this, in 2014, the Ministry of Health provided a technical guide for high altitude workers that includes a series of recommendations to reduce malaise or risk during exposure to altitudes over 3,000 m and considers altitudes over 5,500 m as extreme altitudes. In regard to environmental oxygenation, the oxygen equivalent must be below 3,000 m with permanent control of temperature, relative humidity, and room ventilation (Ministry of Health Chile, 2014, available at https://www.minsal.cl/sites/default/files/guia_hipobaria_altitud.pdf).

One way to avoid the consequences of high-altitude hypoxemia is to reduce the equivalent altitude (altitude that provides the same PiO_2 when ambient air with an oxygen concentration of 21% is inhaled) (West, 2002). The first physiological response is increased pulmonary ventilation, which can be reduced by increasing the room PiO_2 with an artificial increase in oxygen supply (Cudaback, 1984). West (2016) explored the possibility of oxygen supplementation at high altitudes to reduce the malaise associated with high altitude exposure, i.e., miners camps, observatories, hotels, trains, schools, and hospitals. He defined that each increase of oxygen concentration by 1% resulted in a reduction equivalent to 300 m (West, 1995, 2002; Luks et al., 1998). In an oxygen-enriched ambient air room, the oxygen is a comburent and significantly increases the risk of ignition and fire. However, the fire hazard in ambient air decreases at higher altitudes than sea level since the decrease in oxygen partial pressure reduces the number of oxygen molecules available for combustion (West, 1995, 2015). Thus, despite oxygen enrichment of the atmosphere at high altitudes, the PiO_2 is still far below that of air at sea level.

Nowadays, it is possible to recognize two different procedures to reduce the equivalent altitude by oxygen enrichment in the air ambient of a workplace at high altitudes (i.e., room dormitories, office): First, an oxygen concentrator, a device that increases oxygen concentration to 90–95%, through a separation process that employs a technology called pressure swing adsorption (PSA). In this system, a non-flammable ceramic material (zeolite) adsorbs N_2 more readily than O_2, increasing oxygen concentration in the delivered gas mixture (West, 1995). In a series of studies, oxygen concentrators were considered as low-cost systems in installation and maintenance and only required electrical power (West, 1995, 2002; Luks et al., 1998). Second, the use of liquid oxygen, which requires the installation of bigger tanks with liquid oxygen obtained from a cryogenic plant. In both the cases (oxygen concentrators or liquid oxygen), it is required to install pipelines, valves, sensors, and control systems to maintain O_2, CO_2, temperature, and humidity (West, 1995, 2002; Moraga et al., 2014, 2018).

The Atacama Large Millimeter/submillimeter Array (ALMA) is a radiotelescope operating at 5,050 m in the Chajnantor Plateau. The ALMA operation is carried out by near of 400 workers and has two locations: the first is the base camp or Operations Support Facility (OSF), located 16 km from the town of San Pedro de Atacama and situated at 2,900 m, providing all the personnel facilities (residential, food services, and leisure facilities) and the second is the Array Operations Site (AOS), located 30 km from the OSF at an altitude of 5,050 m. The ALMA is the only place in the world where both the technologies (PSA and liquid oxygen) have been installed at a large scale to reduce equivalent altitude by increasing oxygen availability at very high altitudes. In this way, the aim of this study is a retrospective comparison between the use of both technologies for oxygen supplementation during the operation of the ALMA laborers at 5,050 m.

SUBJECTS, MATERIALS, AND METHODS

All the evaluated workers lived at a low altitude (<1,000 m) and worked at the ALMA (2,900 and 5,050 m), with a shift pattern of 8 days of work at high altitude followed by 6 days of rest at sea level. All the subjects worked as operators and maintenance crew with CIHH exposure experience for more than 4 years and were free of cardiovascular, pulmonary, hematological, renal, or hepatic diseases. This study complied with the Helsinki guidelines and was previously approved by the Ethics Committee of the Facultad de Medicina of Universidad Catoìlica del Norte and the ALMA Safety Department.

Oxygen Enrichment Inside the AOS Building Areas at 5,050 m

In 2008, the ALMA installed an onsite oxygen generator machine capable of producing oxygen by using PSA technology to satisfy oxygenation requirements in all the AOS rooms at 5,050 m, obtaining an oxygen concentration of 28%, equivalent to an altitude of 2,900 m. The installed oxygen system has two external tanks (2,498 L × 2). The maximum oxygen pressure is 75 psi with a delivery of 850 l/min with 90–95% oxygen purity and 45 psi outlet pressure. The oxygen concentration in the ambient air was controlled by a wide range oxygen sensor (0–50%, accuracy ± 0.05%, Area Safety Monitor, model 221, Advanced Micro Instruments, Costa Mesa, CA, United States) and maintained by a precise servo control system that increased oxygen concentration to 28 ± 0.5%. All the ambient variables (O_2, temperature, and humidity) were recorded continuously in the available AOS rooms (corridor, hall, office, and correlator; **Figure 1**). All the variables recorded, such as O_2, temperature, and humidity, were compiled monthly for at least 1 year for each AOS room. After installing and operating the PSA, we performed cardiorespiratory evaluations in 9 of 13 acclimatized AOS workers of 30.5 ± 6.4 years. A nurse or paramedic measured variables such as heart rate (HR) (bpm) and pulse oxygen saturation (SpO_2) (%) using a multiparameter monitor (model BM3, Bionet, Tustin, CA, United States). However, in 2011, the ALMA shut down the oxygen administration procedure in the building areas at 5,050 m due to problems in the operation of the PSA plant.

In 2015, one liquid oxygen tank was installed with a maximal net volume of 14.75 m^3, enabling a 70 normalized m^3/h (or Nm^3/h) flow rate (installation and liquid oxygen supply was performed by Indura). The ambient oxygen concentration, temperature, and humidity were controlled and maintained, as previously described. Additionally, we evaluated cardiorespiratory parameters routinely at the arrival of 40 workers to AOS rooms and values represent the mean of 1 year of operation. In this case, the evaluation of variables such as HR (bpm) and SpO_2 (%) was measured by a nurse or paramedic using a multiparameter monitor (model BM3, Bionet, Tustin, CA, United States).

Use of Portable Oxygen in Outdoor Operations at 5,050 m

We evaluated efficiency during a period of workers' activity (changing an antenna). We defined the oxygen flow requirements using two different pieces of equipment: first is a piece of equipment that supplies oxygen by continuous flow (range

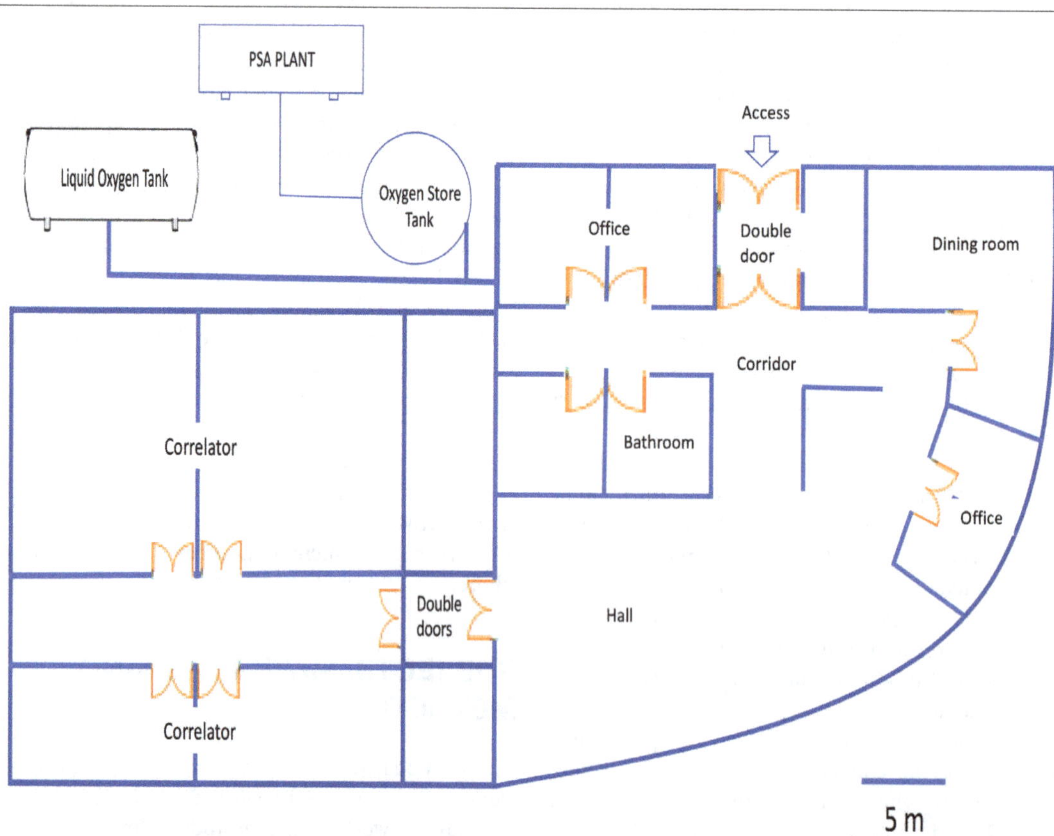

FIGURE 1 | The scheme represents a diagram of oxygen enrichment inside Array Operations Site (AOS) facilities at 5,050 m.

flow of 0.5–15 l/min, model 108 MF 870, Corpus™ INDURA, Santiago, Chile) and the second the CHAD® Evolution™ Motion Auto-Adjusting Oxygen Conserver (probably model OM-900M; Drive DeVilbiss Healthcare, Somerset, PA, United States), both gaseous medicinal oxygen, compressed in the high-pressure cylinder, were administrated *via* a nasal cannula. We performed dose-response curves of oxygen saturation vs. flow breathing between 0 and 6 l/min in six antenna maintenance personnel. We continuously recorded the subjects while changing an antenna with a pulse oximeter (Wristox 3100, Nonin, MN, United States). All the recordings were analyzed by nVision software (Nonin, MN, United States).

Statistical Analysis

All the results were expressed as mean ± SD. Variables compiled of AOS rooms O_2, temperature, and humidity of PSA or liquid oxygen were analyzed using the paired *t*-test. Cardiorespiratory variables SpO_2 and HR recorded in AOS rooms or taken outdoors were analyzed using the paired *t*-test. All the differences were considered statistically significant when $p < 0.05$. Data analyses were performed using the GraphPad Prism version 5.03 (GraphPad Software Incorporation, San Diego, CA, United States).

TABLE 1 | Conditioning and ambient oxygen (O_2) enrichment in the Array Operations Site (AOS) building areas.

	O_2 enrichment in rooms (%)	
	PSA	**Liquid oxygen**
Areas in AOS		
Corridor	26.5 ± 1.0	25.5 ± 1.5
Hall	26.5 ± 1.4	26.3 ± 1.3
Dining room	-	26.5 ± 1.2
Office	26.6 ± 1.3	27.5 ± 0.8
Correlator	27.8 ± 0.5	28.0 ± 0.5
All AOS	26.8 ± 1.1	26.8 ± 1.1
Temperature (°C)	17.5 ± 1.5	18.5 ± 1.2
Relative Humidity (%)	33.2 ± 7.5	29.1 ± 3.1

Mean ± SD.

TABLE 2 | Comparison of cardiorespiratory variables in O_2-enriched AOS rooms.

	Arrive at 5050 m	
	(Outside AOS)	**(Inside AOS + O_2)**
PSA		
Oxygen saturation (%)	83.1 ± 2.3	92.8 ± 1.2*
Heart rate (bpm)	102 ± 13	93.1 ± 10.6
Liquid oxygen		
Oxygen saturation (%)	82.6 ± 2.8	89.5 ± 1.4*
Heart rate (bpm)	110.0 ± 9.2	78.6 ± 8.6*

*Mean ± SD, *p < 0.05 outside vs. inside.*

RESULTS

Oxygen Enrichment Inside Array Operations Site Facilities at 5,050 m

A similar oxygenation pattern was observed in both the procedures to increase oxygen concentration (PSA or liquid oxygen) inside AOS rooms. **Table 1** shows ambient measurements of O_2, relative humidity, and temperature at all the AOS sites without an observed difference. O_2 variations in the corridor, hall room, and office were not significantly different between the PSA and liquid oxygen system 26.5 ± 1.2 and 26.1 ± 1.3%, respectively. Furthermore, when evaluating cardiorespiratory responses such as oxygen saturation and HR in all the subjects during ascents to AOS, subjects presented increased arterial oxygenation and reduction in the HR in both the conditions (PSA and liquid oxygen) (**Table 2**).

Use of Portable Oxygen in Outdoor Operations

The use of individual oxygen supplementation showed that efficient oxygenation, equivalent to 2,900 m, was obtained using a continuous flow (3 l/min) rather than the demand flow that obtained equivalent values at 5 l/min (**Figure 2**).

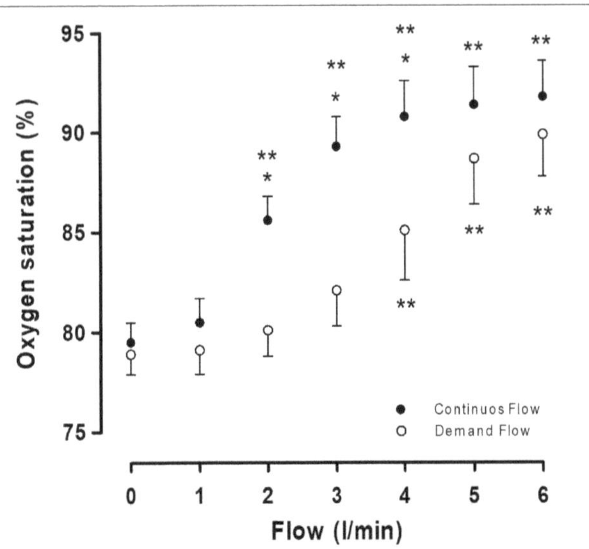

FIGURE 2 | Oxygen saturation dose-response curve vs. inhalatory flow (l/min). Closed circle represents the use of a continuous flow and open circle represents the use of a demand flow. Each circle represents a mean ± SD. *$p < 0.05$ continuous vs. demand and **$p < 0.05$ vs. 0 flow.

DISCUSSION

Oxygen Enrichment Within Array Operations Site Facilities at 5,050 m

Our results demonstrate that both the oxygen production procedures (PSA or liquid oxygen) effectively increase the fraction of inspired oxygen (FiO_2) at very high altitudes, protecting the health of the workers as noted by the increase in oxygen saturation and reduced HR.

The use of an oxygen concentrator (PSA plant) vs. liquid oxygen for oxygen enrichment produced similar oxygenation patterns at AOS facilities at 5,050 m. These patterns were characterized by a variation in the oxygen concentration within AOS facilities. Even though these facilities have double door access, these oxygen variations could be explained by the movement of personnel, resulting in the doors being constantly opened and closed and promoting a fall in FiO_2 to 26.5%. In contrast, offices and correlators have access through doors that are usually maintained shut. In this pilot study, we used a comfortable and mobile module in the AOS facilities at 5,050 m where liquid oxygen was administered to the room air to increase oxygen concentration to 28 ± 0.5%. This oxygen concentration represents an equivalent altitude of 2,900 m (for more detail, see Moraga et al., 2018), with higher precision and maintenance of the oxygen concentration, potentially explained by a reduced module size where the leakage is lower. However, when we measured cardiorespiratory response before or after access to oxygenated AOS facilities, a similar increase in oxygen saturation was observed in both the oxygenation procedures. In contrast, we only observed a reduced HR in workers within AOS facilities with liquid oxygen, similar to previous reports (Moraga et al., 2018).

The PSA plant oxygen concentrator was shut down, even though a series of studies emphasize that oxygen concentrators are low cost in installation and maintenance and only require electrical power support (West, 1995, 2002; Luks et al., 1998). It was also proposed that the molecular sieve will last indefinitely (West, 1995, 2015), as long as it does not become contaminated with water and oil vapors (Litch and Bishop, 2000). However, after installation in 2008, a series of operational troubles were reported such as not reaching the required oxygenation. Inspection of the PSA plant following shutdown reported a series of malfunctions, starting with oil contamination along the air preparation route. This fact was unacceptable due to the risk of rapid self-ignition and possible explosions with fatal consequences for the ALMA operating staff. In addition, zeolite beds, O_2 storage tanks, and pipelines needed to be exchanged due to the oil and water contamination mentioned in the same report. This experience was corroborated in an article that mentioned regular maintenance is required such as cleaning cabinet filters, changing bacterial and particulate filters, and zeolite columns after 15,000–20,000 h of use, depending on local conditions (Litch and Bishop, 2000). The same authors indicated that output oxygen concentration at high altitudes decreases by approximately 10% for each 2,000 m gain in elevation (Litch and Bishop, 2000). Therefore, we expect a decrease in oxygen concentration by 25% at 5,050 m. This suggests that the PSA plant at very high altitude its efficiency decreases. Then, how is it possible that this technology is not helpful at very high altitudes? In our opinion, the studies that supported this technology did not consider the loss in equipment efficiency at very high altitudes, as mentioned by Litch and Bishop (2000). In this sense, we believe that installing the PSA plant at high and very high altitudes requires that the efficiency of this technology is validated in real ambient conditions such as very low pressure, dust, and air dry and consider periodic maintenance.

Previous studies developed in real conditions at 4,200 m used liquid oxygen to enhance sleep quality (Moraga et al., 2014). In the Collahuasi mine, the same solution was taken at a large scale with 60 oxygen-enriched dormitory rooms using liquid oxygen at 3,800 m (West, 2004). However, we recognize the major weakness of this procedure for oxygen-enrichment areas given by the complications associated with refilling liquid oxygen tanks due to road accessibility and weather conditions. However, programming delivery, having backup tanks, and providing supplemental oxygen equipment could cover any delays.

Use of Portable Oxygen in Outdoor Operations

Our results show that oxygen administration was more efficient when using a continuous flow than a demand flow. This was proven by arterial oxygen saturation, where values of 2–3 l/min for continuous flow reached saturation values over 85%, but 5 l/min was necessary with the demand flow. A similar pattern was observed in a study showing that the administration of low-flow oxygen (1 or 3 l/min) *via* a face mask enhances physical performance in unacclimatized subjects following rapid ascent to the ALMA in the Chajnantor plateau (Silva-Urra et al., 2011). However, previous studies reported oxygen saturation values lower than expected at 5,050 m (Moraga et al., 2018), suggesting that a flow of 1 or 3 l/min was insufficient. An explanation based on the results reported by Silva-Urra et al. (2011) is that the study was performed in acutely exposed subjects to 5,050 m. In contrast, our results were obtained in acclimatized personal evaluated in AOS. The outcomes of this study are that all the subjects that ascend (visitors and operators) to AOS and outdoor activities and drivers of light or heavy trucks must use oxygen with a continuous O_2 flow of 2.0–3.0 l/min to maintain an O_2 saturation of 85–91%, supporting that the demand flow is not recommended at very high altitude.

CONCLUSION

No differences were observed between both the oxygen production procedures (PSA or liquid oxygen) in regular operations. Big-scale installations have difficulties reaching the oxygen concentration due to leaks in areas of high mobility. However, the PSA plant requires adequacy and maintenance to operate at a very high altitude. At 5,050 m, portable oxygen should operate with a continuous flow of 2–3 l/min. In addition, new equipment for individual oxygen supplementation at 5,050 m must be evaluated, considering ergonomics and autonomy during exposure/operation.

ETHICS STATEMENT

The studies involving human participants were reviewed and approved by Ethics Committee of the Facultad de Medicina of Universidad Católica del Norte. The patients/participants provided their written informed consent to participate in this study.

AUTHOR CONTRIBUTIONS

IL and FM were the guarantors and conceived and designed the study. RA, SR, and AM supervised the overall study. RC-J and DS contributed to sample and data collections. RC-J performed the statistical analysis. All authors drafted the report, interpreted the results, critically revised the manuscript, and approved the final manuscript.

ACKNOWLEDGMENTS

We are grateful to all the volunteers from the ALMA who participated in this study, the nurses and paramedics who participated in all the evaluations performed at the OSF and AOS rooms, and the facility support by the safety manager, ALMA.

REFERENCES

Consejo de Competencias Mineras (2017). *Fuerza Laboral de la Gran Mineriìa Chilena 2017-2026*. Available online at: http://www.ccm.cl/ReporteCCM_13-11_FINAL

Cudaback, D. M. (1984). Four-km altitude effects on performance and health. *Publ. Astronom. Soc. Pacif.* 96, 463–477.

Gassmann, M., Cowburn, A., Gum, H., Li, J., Rodriguez, M., Babicheva, A., et al. (2021). Hypoxia-induced pulmonary hypertension - utilizing experiments of nature. *Br. J. Pharmacol.* 178, 121–131. doi: 10.1111/bph.15144

Litch, J. A., and Bishop, R. A. (2000). Oxygen concentrators for delivery of supplemental oxygen in remote high-altitude areas. *Wilderness Environ. Med.* 11, 189–191.

Luks, A. M., van Melick, H., Batarse, R. R., Powell, F. L., Grant, I., and West, J. B. (1998). Room oxygen enrichment improves sleep and subsequent day-time performance at high altitude. *Respir. Physiol.* 113, 247–258. doi: 10.1016/s0034-5687(98)00068-1

Ministry of Health Chile (2013). Decreto 28 Modifica Decreto N° 594 de 1999. Reglamento Sobre Condiciones Sanitarias y Ambientales Básicas en los Lugares de Trabajo. Available online at: http://www.leychile.cl/N?i=1045465&f=2013-11-08&p=

Ministry of Health Chile (2014). *Guía Técnica Sobre Exposición Ocupacional a Hipobaria Intermitente Crónica por Gran altitud*. Available online at: https://www.minsal.cl/sites/default/files/guia_hipobaria_altitud.pdf

Moore, L. G. (2001). Human genetic adaptation to high altitude. *High Alt. Med. Biol.* 2, 257–279.

Moraga, F. A., Jiménez, D., Richalet, J. P., Vargas, M., and Osorio, J. (2014). Periodic breathing and oxygen supplementation in Chilean miners at high altitude (4200m). *Respir. Physiol. Neurobiol.* 203, 109–115. doi: 10.1016/j.resp.2014.09.001

Moraga, F. A., López, I., Morales, A., Soza, D., and Noack, J. (2018). The effect of oxygen enrichment on cardiorespiratory and neuropsychological responses in workers with chronic intermittent exposure to high altitude (ALMA, 5,050 m). *Front. Physiol.* 9:187. doi: 10.3389/fphys.2018.00187

Richalet, J. P., Vargas Donoso, M., Jiménez, D., Antezana, A. M., Hudson, C., Cortès, G., et al. (2002). Chilean miners commuting from sea level to 4500 m: a prospective study. *High Alt. Med. Biol.* 3, 159–166. doi: 10.1089/15270290260131894

Silva-Urra, J. A., Urizar, C., Basualto-Alarcón, C., Torrella, J. R., Pagés, T., Behn, C., et al. (2011). Effects of oxygen supplementation on acute mountain sickness symptoms and functional capacity during a 2-kilometer walk test on Chajnantor plateau (5050 meters. Northern Chile). *Wilderness Environ. Med.* 22, 250–256. doi: 10.1016/j.wem.2011.05.004

Viscor, G., Torrella, J. R., Corral, L., Ricart, A., Javierre, C., Pages, T., et al. (2018). Physiological and biological response to short-term intermittent hypobaric hypoxia exposure: from sport and mountain medicine to new biomedical application. *Front. Physiol.* 9:814. doi: 10.3389/fphys.2018.00814

West, J. B. (1995). Oxygen enrichment of room air to relieve the hypoxia of high altitude. *Respir. Physiol.* 99, 225–232. doi: 10.1016/0034-5687(94)00094-g

West, J. B. (2002). Commuting to high altitude: value of oxygen enrichment of room air. *High Alt. Med. Biol.* 3, 223–235. doi: 10.1089/15270290260131948

West, J. B. (2004). Working at high altitude: medical problems, misconceptions, and solutions. *Observatory* 124, 1–14.

West, J. B. (2015). A strategy for oxygen conditioning at high altitude: comparison with air conditioning. *J. Appl. Physiol.* 119, 719–723. doi: 10.1152/japplphysiol.00421.2015

West, J. B. (2016). Oxygen conditioning: a new technique for improving living and working at high altitude. *Physiology* 31, 216–222. doi: 10.1152/physiol.00057.2015

18

Enhanced Placental Mitochondrial Respiration in Tibetan Women at High Altitude

Huifang Liu[1,2,3]*, Noryung Tenzing*[1,2,3]*, Martha Tissot van Patot*[4]*, Muge Qile*[1,2]*, Ri-li Ge*[1,2] *and Tana Wuren*[1,2*]

[1] *Research Center for High Altitude Medicine, Qinghai University, Xining, China,* [2] *Key Laboratory for Application of High-Altitude Medicine, Qinghai University, Xining, China,* [3] *Affiliated Hospital of Qinghai University, Xining, China,* [4] *Retired, Fort Collins, CO, United States*

Correspondence:
Tana Wuren
tanna.mgl@gmail.com

Living at high altitudes is extremely challenging as it entails exposure to hypoxia, low temperatures, and high levels of UV radiation. However, the Tibetan population has adapted to such conditions on both a physiological and genetic level over 30,000–40,000 years. It has long been speculated that fetal growth restriction is caused by abnormal placental development. We previously demonstrated that placentas from high-altitude Tibetans were protected from oxidative stress induced by labor compared to those of European descent. However, little is known about how placental mitochondria change during high-altitude adaptation. In this study, we aimed to uncover the mechanism of such adaptation by studying the respiratory function of the placental mitochondria of high-altitude Tibetans, lower-altitude Tibetans, and lower-altitude Chinese Han. We discovered that mitochondrial respiration was greater in high-altitude than in lower-altitude Tibetans in terms of OXPHOS via complexes I and I+II, ETS_{max} capacity, and non-phosphorylating respiration, whereas non-ETS respiration, LEAK/ETS, and OXPHOS via complex IV did not differ. Respiration in lower-altitude Tibetans and Han was similar for all tested respiratory states. Placentas from high-altitude Tibetan women were protected from acute ischemic/hypoxic insult induced by labor, and increased mitochondrial respiration may represent an acute response that induces mitochondrial adaptations.

Keywords: Tibetan, mitochondria respiration, placenta, hypoxia, high altitude adaptation

INTRODUCTION

The oxygen content of the atmosphere is 21% regardless of altitude, while the barometric pressure decreases as the altitude increases. In medical research, high altitude is defined as ≥2,500 m above sea level (Julian and Moore, 2019). The main challenges at high altitudes are hypoxia, low temperatures, and high levels of UV radiation (Peacock, 1998; Butaric and Klocke, 2018; Song et al., 2020). The Tibetan population is considered both physiologically and genetically adapted to such hypoxic conditions since they have lived and successfully reproduced at high altitudes for 30,000–40,000 years (Zhang et al., 2018; Bhandari and Cavalleri, 2019). Tibetans are protected from polycythemia, pulmonary hypertension, low birth weight, and other hypoxia-related diseases that normally result from prolonged exposure to such inhospitable environments (Yang et al., 2017; Jeong et al., 2018; Bhandari and Cavalleri, 2019; Song et al., 2020). Most research has focused on

Tibetans living permanently at high altitudes, and there have been few studies of Tibetans living at relatively low altitudes. Therefore, we decided to devote a study to the differences between lower- and high-altitude Tibetans, as well as between lower-altitude Tibetans and other ethnic groups, such as Chinese Han, living at the same altitude.

At high altitudes, an insufficient maternal supply of O_2 and nutrients leads to fetal growth restriction (Bailey et al., 2019; Lorca et al., 2019, 2020; Lane et al., 2020a,b). Fetal growth restriction is a condition in which the fetus fails to reach its full growth potential, related to the increased risk of development of metabolic syndrome in childhood and multiple diseases in adulthood; therefore, it has received increasing attention (de Rooij et al., 2007; Veenendaal et al., 2013; Sayama et al., 2020). The placenta plays an essential role in fetal growth (Shaw et al., 2018; Sferruzzi-Perri et al., 2019). It has long been speculated that fetal growth restriction is initially caused by abnormal placental development and functional deficiency (Tong and Giussani, 2019; Sangkhae et al., 2020; Turner et al., 2020). Most Tibetans experience unrestricted fetal growth at high altitudes and our previous study indicated that placentas of Tibetans living at high altitudes are protected from labor-induced oxidative stress compared to those of other high-altitude residents (Tana et al., 2021). Placental mitochondria are critical to the healthy development of the fetus; however, little is known about mitochondrial respiration in populations adapted to high altitudes. Impaired placental mitochondrial function can have a detrimental effect on fetal development (Tissot van Patot et al., 2010). Therefore, etiologic studies of hypoxia-related pregnancy diseases, such as pre-eclampsia and intrauterine growth restriction, should include focus on the mitochondria.

The aim of this study was to investigate mitochondrial respiration in Tibetan women permanently residing at high altitudes and compare it with those permanently residing at lower altitudes. We hypothesized that Tibetan placenta possesses enhanced mitochondria respiration capacity to remedy the increased energy demand of labor and oxidative stress during the labor in the oxygen deprived environment. This was done in the attempt to further our understanding of the mechanism of adaptation to high altitudes and the risk factors that change the growth trajectory of the fetus. Ultimately, we strived to identify opportunities to improve the health of children and reduce the risk of many adult diseases related to fetal growth restriction.

MATERIALS AND METHODS

Materials and Sample Collection

All chemical substrates were purchased from Sigma Aldrich, Australia. This study was approved by the Qinghai University Affiliated Hospital Ethics Committee. In total, 21 human full-term (37–40 weeks) placentas were collected after laboring vaginal delivery, with the written consent of donors after receiving an explanation from local doctors in their native language. Placental tissues from high-altitude Tibetan women ($n = 9$) were collected at Yushu Bayi Hospital (3780 m); those from lower-altitude Tibetan ($n = 7$) and Han ($n = 5$) woman were collected at the Guide County Hospital (2200 m) and Qinghai University Affiliated Hospital (2261 m). The general characteristics of the pregnancies are provided in **Table 1**. All neonates had Apgar scores between 7 and 9.

Each placenta was weighed immediately after delivery and divided into six sections for random sampling. Samples from the fetal side of the placenta were biopsied within 15 min, placed on ice and in PBS, and delivered to the laboratory.

High-Resolution Respirometry

In order to most accurately assess the metabolic characteristics of mitochondrial activity in placentas delivered at high altitude, we installed a respirometer in a laboratory at the delivery site. The respirometer was carefully recalibrated for optimal accuracy in the low-O_2 environment.

The samples were washed in ice-cold PBS to remove blood. The plasma membranes were permeabilized for 40 min on ice and mixed with 50 μg/mL saponin in 1 mL biopsy preservation solution containing CaK_2EGTA (2.77 mM), K_2EGTA (7.23 mM), Na_2ATP (5.77 mM), $MgCl_2{\cdot}6H_2O$ (6.56 mM), taurine (20 mM), sodium phosphocreatine (15 mM), imidazole (20 mM), dithiothreitol (0.5 mM), and MES (50 mM) at pH 7.1. The samples were washed twice for 10 min on ice in mitochondria respiration medium (MiR05) containing 0.5 mM EGTA, 3 mM $MgCl_2{\cdot}6H_2O$, 60 mM K-lactobionate, 20 mM taurine, 10 mM KH_2PO_4, 20 mM HEPES, 110 mM sucrose, and 1 g/L BSA (fatty acid free) at pH 7.1, after which the tissue was used for respirometry.

To measure mitochondrial respiration, 5–10 mg wet-weight tissue was added to the chamber of an Oxygraph-2k respirometer (Oroboros Instruments, Austria) containing MiR05 at 37°C, and a substrate-uncoupler-inhibitor titration protocol was used, as illustrated in **Figure 1** (from a high-altitude Tibetan sample) (**Supplementary Figure 1A** for low altitude Tibetan and **Supplementary Figure 1B** for low altitude Han).

Glutamate (10 mM), malate (5 mM), and pyruvate (5 mM) were added to stimulate non-phosphorylating (LEAK) respiration mediated by complex I (CI). Subsequently, ADP (5 mM) was added to activate the phosphorylation of ADP to ATP through CI. Cytochrome c (10 μM) was added to confirm the integrity of the outer mitochondrial membrane; Succinate (10 mM) was added to stimulate oxidative phosphorylation (OXPHOS) through complex II (CII). Carbonyl cyanide m-chloro phenyl hydrazine (stepwise titration of 1 mM) was used to uncouple OXPHOS and investigate the capacity of the electron transfer system (ETS). CI was inhibited using rotenone (1 mM), to separately determine the succinate-linked ETS capacity. Complex III was inhibited using antimycin A (2.5 μM) to determine the residual O_2 consumption. Finally, 1-*N*,1-*N*,2-*N*,2-*N*-tetramethylbenzene-1,2-diamine; dihydrochloride (0.5 mM) and ascorbate (2 mM) were added to measure OXPHOS through complex IV (CIV).

Thus, the main outcome measures were LEAK respiration and OXPHOS capacity through CI, CII, ETS maximum capacity, and CIV. The respiratory control ratio (RCR) was calculated as OXPHOS capacity with CI substrates and saturating ADP as a fraction of LEAK respiration with CI substrates.

TABLE 1 | Maternal and infant characteristics.

	Tibetan		Chinese Han	*P*-values	
	3780 m	2200 m	2200 m	Altitude	Nationality
Maternal characteristics					
n	9	7	5		
Age (years)	28.2 ± 2.4	26.6 ± 1.8	28.6 ± 2.1	NS	NS
Parity	3.3 ± 0.7	1.7 ± 0.3	1.8 ± 0.4	NS	NS
Height (cm)	161 ± 2	167 ± 1	165 ± 2	<0.05	NS
Non-pregnant weight (kg)	55 ± 3	54 ± 2	61 ± 4	NS	NS
Non-pregnant body mass index (kg m^{-2})	34 ± 2	33 ± 1	37 ± 3	NS	NS
Weight gain with pregnancy (kg)	13 ± 1	13 ± 2	14 ± 2	NS	NS
Systolic BP (mmHg)	111 ± 2	108 ± 2	103 ± 5	NS	NS
Diastolic BP (mmHg)	72 ± 2	66 ± 2	66 ± 3	NS	NS
Infant characteristics					
Birth weight (g)	3318 ± 125	3253 ± 150	3423 ± 186	NS	NS
Birth/Placental weight ratio	5.5 ± 0.2	5.6 ± 0.3	5.7 ± 0.4	NS	NS
Apgar score	8.778 ± 0.443	8.857 ± 0.35	8.8 ± 0.4	NS	NS

All values are either numbers or means ± standard errors of the mean. BP, blood pressure.

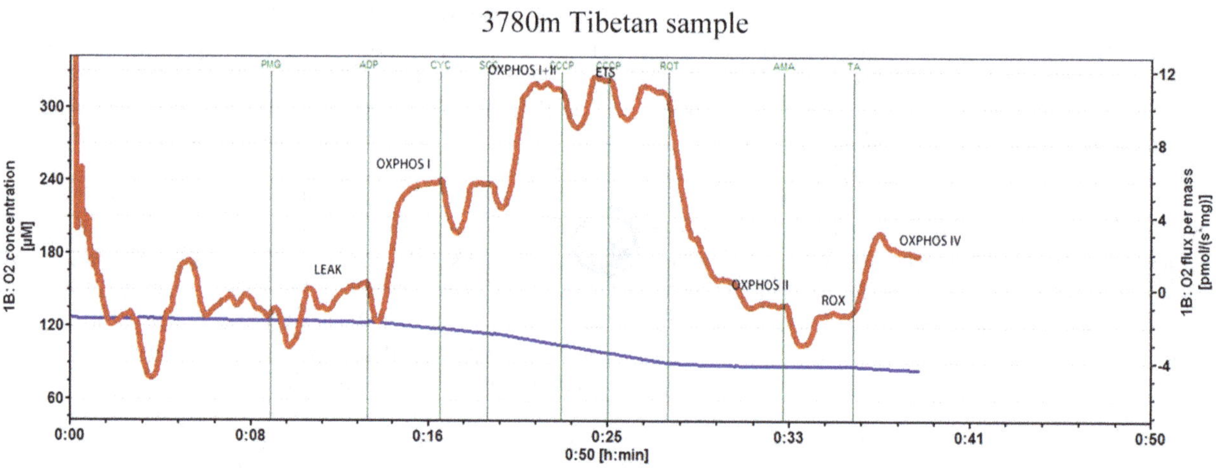

FIGURE 1 | Substrate-uncoupler-inhibitor titration (SUIT) protocol. Representative oxygraph traces of oxygen flux relative to tissue mass. The vertical lines show the introduction of various substrates or inhibitors. LEAK refers to non-phosphorylating respiration; OXPHOS CI, CII, and CIV represent oxidative phosphorylation through mitochondrial complexes I, II, and IV, respectively; ETS_{max} represents electron transfer system maximum capacity; ROX represents non-ETS respiration; PMG represents pyruvate, glutamate, and malate; CYC represents cytochrome c; ROT represents rotenone; SCC represents succinate; CCCP represents the uncoupler, 2-[(3-chlorophenyl)hydrazinylidene]propanedinitrile (CCCP); AMA represents antimycin A; TA represents 1-*N*,1-*N*,2-*N*,2-*N*-tetramethylbenzene-1,2-diamine;dihy drochloride and ascorbate.

Statistical Analysis

GraphPad Prism version 8 (GraphPad Software, San Diego, California, USA)[1] was used for statistical analyses. Values are expressed as means ± standard errors of the mean. Data were analyzed using the D'Agostino-Pearson omnibus normality test, and Student's *t*-tests were used to evaluate the differences between two groups at a time. Statistical significance was defined as $p < 0.05$.

[1] www.graphpad.com.

RESULTS

Respiration of Placental Mitochondria at Different Altitudes

As illustrated in **Figure 2A**, the mitochondrial respiration capacity in the high-altitude Tibetan group was greater than that in the lower-altitude Tibetan group in terms of OXPHOS with substrates for CI and CI+II, as well as for ETS maximum capacity and LEAK. Non-ETS respiration and OXPHOS with substrates for CIV, however, remained stable across different altitude Tibetan groups. As displayed

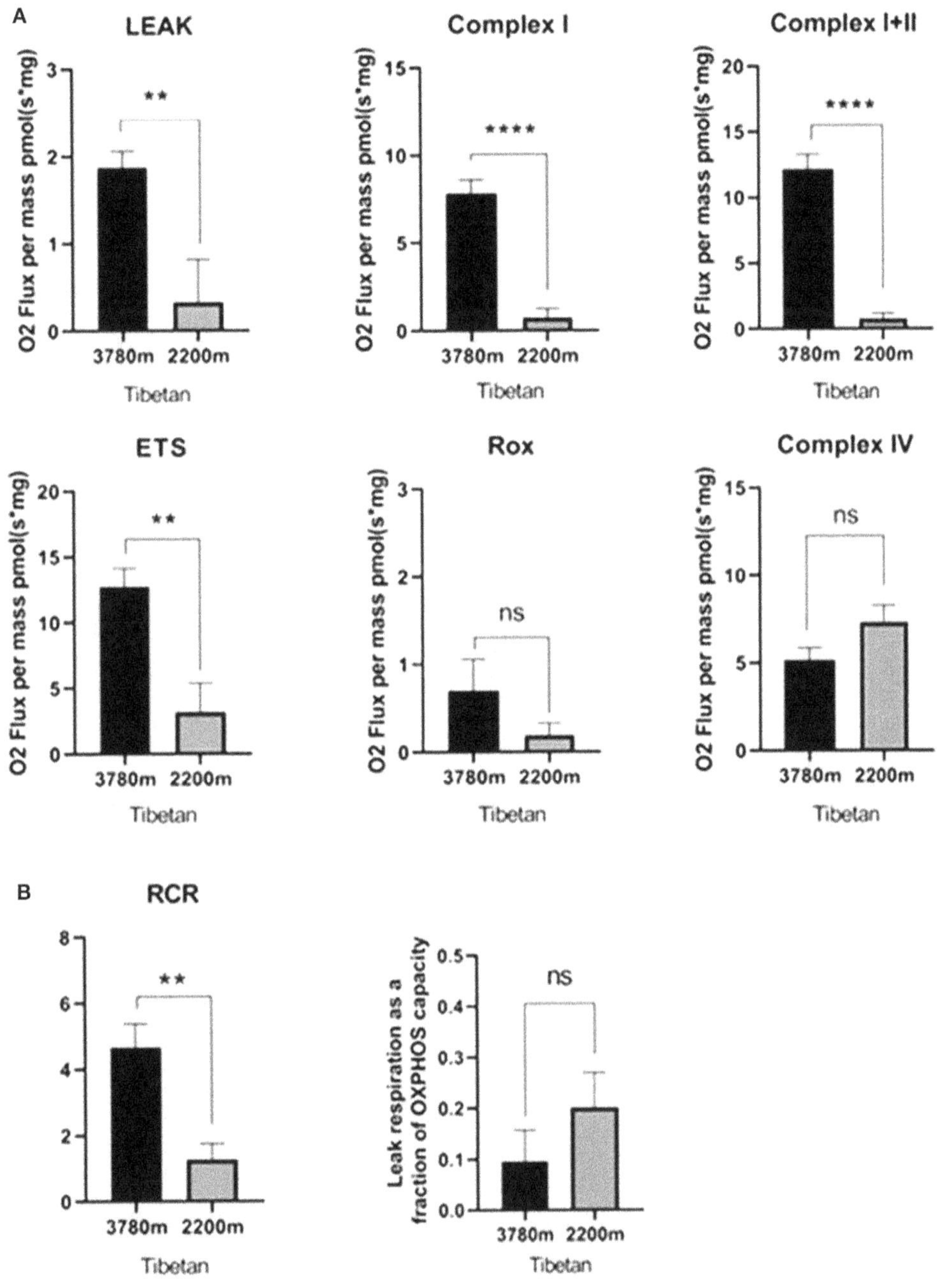

FIGURE 2 | Respiration in high- vs. lower-altitude Tibetan groups. **(A)** Oxidative phosphorylation (OXPHOS) through mitochondrial complex I, complex I+II, non-phosphorylating (LEAK) respiration, and electron transfer system (ETS) maximum capacity respiration were statistically significantly increased in high-altitude Tibetan group compared to lower-altitude Tibetan group. Non-ETS respiration (ROX) and OXPHOS through mitochondrial complex IV did not change with altitude. **(B)** The respiratory control ration (RCR) was statistically significantly increased in the high-altitude Tibetan group compared to the lower-altitude Tibetan group. But the LEAK/ETS was not significant change. ns: $p \geq 0.05$; $^{**}p < 0.01$; $^{****}p < 0.0001$. Statistical significance was determined via Student's *t*-test. Columns represent means and error bars present standard errors of the mean.

in **Figure 2B**, the RCR in the high-altitude Tibetan group was higher than that in the lower-altitude Tibetan group, LEAK/ETS was not change, which suggests stronger coupling of mitochondrial respiration and ATP synthesis in the high-altitude Tibetan group.

Respiration of Placental Mitochondria in Different Nationality

Respiration in the lower-altitude Tibetan and Han groups was similar for all measured respiratory states (**Figure 3**). The respiratory function of mitochondria in Tibetan and Han women

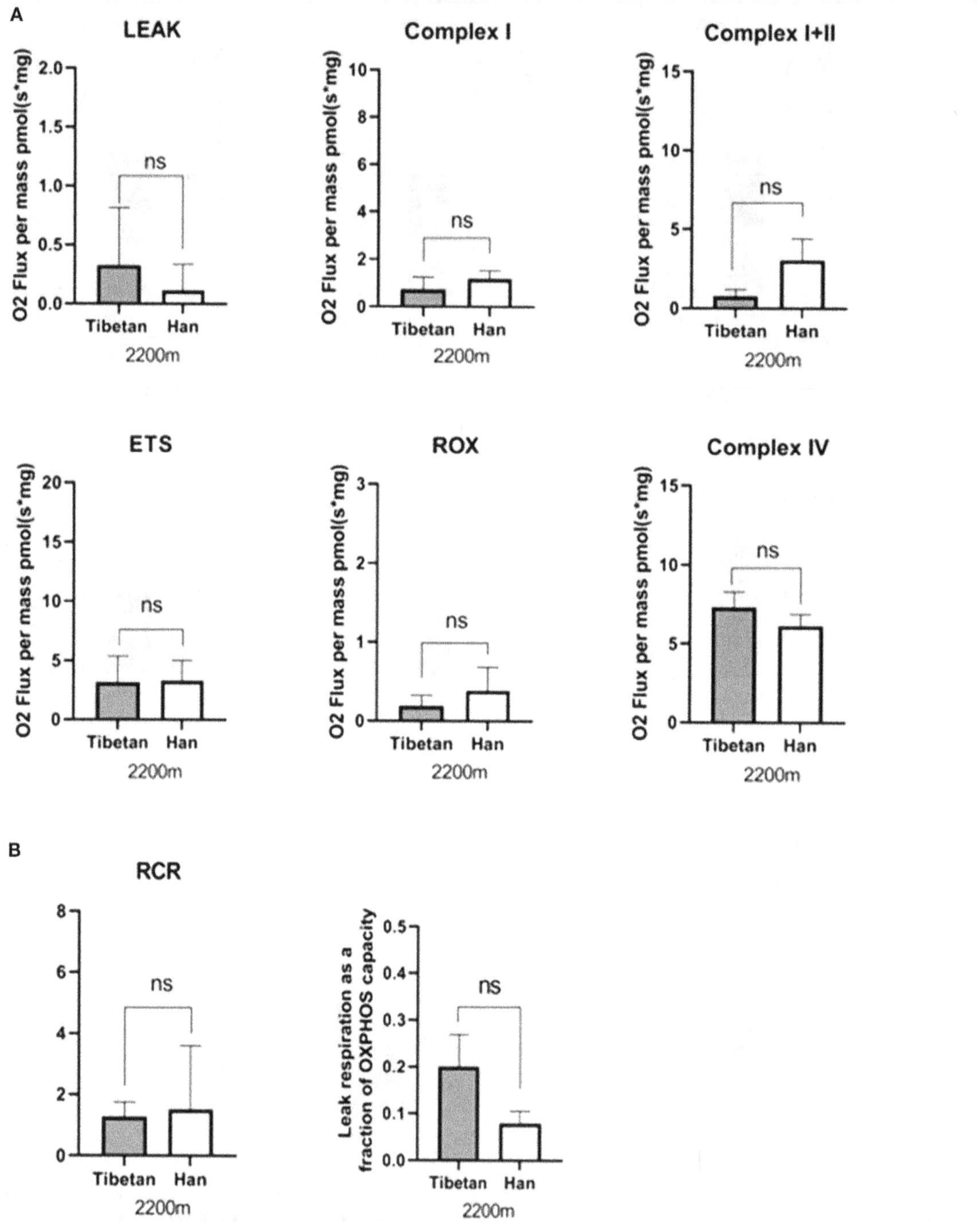

FIGURE 3 | Respiration in lower-altitude Tibetan vs. Han groups. **(A)** Oxidative phosphorylation (OXPHOS) with substrates for mitochondrial complexes I (CI), C I+II, and CIV; non-phosphorylating respiration (LEAK); ETS maximum capacity respiration; and non-ETS respiration (ROX) were not statistically significantly different between the lower-altitude Tibetan and Han groups. ns: $p \geq 0.05$. **(B)** The respiratory control ration (RCR) and LEAK/ETS was not statistically significantly different between the lower-altitude Tibetan and Han groups.

at the same altitude and mode of delivery was similar. We observed a low RCR in lower-altitude Tibetan (RCR: 1.4) and Han (RCR: 1.5) mitochondria using substrates for CI, suggesting that these mitochondria have impaired respiratory efficiency.

DISCUSSION

Our study provides evidence that significant differences in human placental mitochondrial respiration exist between Tibetan women living at high and those at lower altitudes. Specifically, through the utilization of mitochondrial complexes.

The energy metabolism of cardiac and skeletal muscles is altered at high altitudes. Hypoxic rats (13% O_2, 2 weeks) exhibited a loss of fatty acid oxidation capacity, complex I-supported respiration, and ATP levels in the left ventricle, and experienced increased oxidative stress (Ashmore et al., 2014). Further investigations have been carried out on the metabolic response of human skeletal muscle at high altitudes. At moderately high altitudes, respiratory capacity of fatty acid oxidation decreased without changes in mitochondrial volume density (Murray, 2016). In high altitude residents, pregnant women had increased O_2 demand and blood O_2 saturation compared to pregnant women at sea level. However, the decrease in arterial blood oxygen content during high-altitude pregnancies may lead to physiologic anemia due to the expansion of circulating plasma volume in the second trimester, which is also related to an insufficient increase in cardiac output. Interestingly, it was observed that women who lived on the Tibetan plateau for less than three generations had less hemoglobin and arterial blood O_2 content during pregnancy, compared with those who live in a multi generations there (McAuliffe et al., 2001). Tibetan women at high altitudes also have a greater uterine artery blood flow than women at low altitude, providing more O_2 and nutrients to the fetus (Moore, 1990). There is evidence to suggest that they may also have an increased mitochondrial activity and a larger RCR to use O_2 more efficiently, ensuring sufficient growth of the fetus and a higher birth weight (Moore, 1990).

Our results suggest that mitochondrial respiration was higher in all tested states, except for non-ETS and CIV-mediated respiration, in the high- compared to the lower-altitude Tibetan group. The RCR was also greater in the high- as compared with the lower-altitude Tibetan group, suggesting improved coupling to ATP production and/or less oxidative damage. A decrease in the RCR often coincides with elevated oxidative stress. These findings are consistent with those of Bustamante et al. (2014). The respiratory function of mitochondria at lower altitudes was less than that in high-altitude Tibetans. This may be related to the oxidative stress experienced by mitochondria in response to labor-induced placental ischemia and reperfusion. However, previous studies have indicated a decrease in placental ATP (Bloxam and Bobinski, 1984) and an increase in placental oxidative stress markers during vaginal delivery (Diamant et al., 1980; Cindrova-Davies et al., 2007). The placental mitochondria of high-altitude Tibetans appear to make more efficient use of O_2 than do those of lower-altitude Tibetans when there is oxygen shortage at higher altitude, which may be the outcome of adaptation to high altitudes. Mitochondria in the skeletal muscles have been demonstrated to adapt to strength and endurance training (Zoll et al., 2002; Pesta et al., 2011). Changes in placental mitochondria have been reported for several disease states (Mandò et al., 2014; Mele et al., 2014; Holland et al., 2017), many of which are thought to include hypoxia/reperfusion injury (Holland et al., 2017). Our data indicate that mitochondrial respiration is less robust in Tibetans residing at an altitude of 2,200 m as compared with those living at 3780 m. Sufficient O_2 supply, a high partial pressure of arterial O_2, and sufficient uterine artery blood flow maintain the physiological needs of the fetus without increasing the activity of mitochondria. Additionally, our previous study suggested that placentas from Tibetan women living at high altitudes were better protected from labor-induced oxidative stress than were high-altitude residents of European descent (Tana et al., 2021). The reproductive success of Tibetans is therefore likely to be, at least in part, due to cardiac-related traits and placental adaptation, via increased mitochondrial respiration (Burton et al., 2016; Jeong et al., 2018).

Our data suggests that the result might be of genetic selection. We intend to examine the correlation between gene variants, fetal birth weight and placental function. Limited by the interrelatedness of the geographical location, environment surroundings and one's ethnic cultural background, very few Han women are known to live at high altitude during their pregnancy so that collecting appropriate placental specimens and data of the high plateau Han women became extremely difficult for us. Meanwhile our study is also restricted by the fact that as majority of Tibetan women are permanent residents at an altitude above 2000 m, the chance of them living at sea level was rare, therefore recruiting sea level Tibetan pregnant women for our research had been impossible for years. That being said, our study still provides strong evidence that the adaptation of mitochondrial respiration in high altitude Tibetans is likely to contribute to reproductive success at plateau.

ETHICS STATEMENT

The studies involving human participants were reviewed and approved by Qinghai University Affiliated Hospital Ethics Committee. The patients/participants provided their written informed consent to participate in this study.

AUTHOR CONTRIBUTIONS

TW designed the experiments. HL, NT, and MQ performed the experiments and HL and TW analyzed the data. HL, NT, MP, TW, and R-lG wrote, read, edited, and approved the final version of manuscript. All authors contributed to the article and approved the submitted version.

ACKNOWLEDGMENTS

We thank all study participants and the great support of all staff in the obstetrics departments of Yushu Bayi Hospital, Guide County Hospital, and Qinghai University Affiliated Hospital without whom this study could not have been performed.

REFERENCES

Ashmore, T., Fernandez, B. O., Branco-Price, C., West, J. A., Cowburn, A. S., HeaHeHeather, L. C., et al. (2014). Dietary nitrate increases arginine availability and protects mitochondrial complex I and energetics in the hypoxic rat heart. *J. Physiol.* 592, 4715–4731. doi: 10.1113/jphysiol.2014.275263

Bailey, B. A., Donnelly, M., Bol, K., Moore, L. G., and Julian, C. G. (2019). High altitude continues to reduce birth weights in Colorado. *Matern. Child Health J.* 23, 1573–1580. doi: 10.1007/s10995-019-02788-3

Bhandari, S., and Cavalleri, G. L. (2019). Population history and altitude-related adaptation in the Sherpa. *Front. Physiol.* 10:1116. doi: 10.3389/fphys.2019.01116

Bloxam, D. L., and Bobinski, P. M. (1984). Energy metabolism and glycolysis in the human placenta during ischaemia and in normal labour. *Placenta* 5, 381–394. doi: 10.1016/S0143-4004(84)80018-1

Burton, G. J., Fowden, A. L., and Thornburg, K. L. (2016). Placental origins of chronic disease. *Physiol. Rev.* 96, 1509–1565. doi: 10.1152/physrev.00029.2015

Bustamante, J., Ramírez-Vélez, R., Czerniczyniec, A., Cicerchia, D., Aguilar de Plata, A. C., and Lores-Arnaiz, S. (2014). Oxygen metabolism in human placenta mitochondria. *J. Bioenerg. Biomembr.* 46, 459–469. doi: 10.1007/s10863-014-9572-x

Butaric, L. N., and Klocke, R. P. (2018). Nasal variation in relation to high-altitude adaptations among Tibetans and Andeans. *Am. J. Hum. Biol.* 30:e23104. doi: 10.1002/ajhb.23104

Cindrova-Davies, T., Yung, H.-W., Johns, J., Spasic-Boskovic, O., Korolchuk, S., Jauniaux, E., et al. (2007). Oxidative stress, gene expression, and protein changes induced in the human placenta during labor. *Am. J. Pathol.* 171, 1168–1179. doi: 10.2353/ajpath.2007.070528

de Rooij, S. R., Painter, R. C., Holleman, F., Bossuyt, P. M. M., and Roseboom, T. J. (2007). The metabolic syndrome in adults prenatally exposed to the Dutch famine. *Am. J. Clin. Nutr.* 86, 1219–1224. doi: 10.1093/ajcn/86.4.1219

Diamant, S., Kissilevitz, R., and Diamant, Y. (1980). Lipid peroxidation system in human placental tissue: general properties and the influence of gestational age. *Biol. Reprod.* 23, 776–781. doi: 10.1095/biolreprod23.4.776

Holland, O., Dekker Nitert, M., Gallo, L. A., Vejzovic, M., Fisher, J. J., and Perkins, A. V. (2017). Review: placental mitochondrial function and structure in gestational disorders. *Placenta* 54, 2–9. doi: 10.1016/j.placenta.2016.12.012

Jeong, C., Witonsky, D. B., Basnyat, B., Neupane, M., Beall, C. M., Childs, G., et al. (2018). Detecting past and ongoing natural selection among ethnically Tibetan women at high altitude in Nepal. *PLoS Genet.* 14:e1007650. doi: 10.1371/journal.pgen.1007650

Julian, C. G., and Moore, L. G. (2019). Human genetic adaptation to high altitude: evidence from the Andes. *Genes* 10:150. doi: 10.3390/genes10020150

Lane, S. L., Doyle, A. S., Bales, E. S., Lorca, R. A., Julian, C. G., and Moore, L. G. (2020a). Increased uterine artery blood flow in hypoxic murine pregnancy is not sufficient to prevent fetal growth restriction. *Biol. Reprod.* 102, 660–670. doi: 10.1093/biolre/ioz208

Lane, S. L., Houck, J. A., Doyle, A. S., Bales, E. S., Lorca, R. A., Julian, C. G., et al. (2020b). AMP-activated protein kinase activator AICAR attenuates hypoxia-induced murine fetal growth restriction in part by improving uterine artery blood flow. *J. Physiol.* 598, 4093–4105. doi: 10.1113/JP279341

Lorca, R. A., Lane, S. L., Bales, E. S., Nsier, H., Yi, H., Donnelly, M. A., et al. (2019). High altitude reduces NO-dependent myometrial artery vasodilator response during pregnancy. *Hypertension* 73, 1319–1326. doi: 10.1161/HYPERTENSIONAHA.119.12641

Lorca, R. A., Matarazzo, C. J., Bales, E. S., Houck, J. A., Orlicky, D. J., Euser, A. G., et al. (2020). AMPK activation in pregnant human myometrial arteries from high-altitude and intrauterine growth-restricted pregnancies. *Am. J. Physiol. Heart Circ. Physiol.* 319, H203–H212. doi: 10.1152/ajpheart.00644.2019

Mandò, C., De Palma, C., Stampalija, T., Anelli, G. M., Figus, M., Novielli, C., et al. (2014). Placental mitochondrial content and function in intrauterine growth restriction and preeclampsia. *Am. J. Physiol. Endocrinol. Metab.* 306, E404–E413. doi: 10.1152/ajpendo.00426.2013

McAuliffe, F., Kametas, N., Krampl, E., Ernsting, J., and Nicolaides, K. (2001). Blood gases in pregnancy at sea level and at high altitude. *BJOG* 108, 980–985. doi: 10.1111/j.1471-0528.2001.00225.x

Mele, J., Muralimanoharan, S., Maloyan, A., and Myatt, L. (2014). Impaired mitochondrial function in human placenta with increased maternal adiposity. *Am. J. Physiol. Endocrinol. Metab.* 307, E419–E425. doi: 10.1152/ajpendo.00025.2014

Moore, L. G. (1990). Maternal O_2 transport and fetal growth in Colorado, Peru, and Tibet high-altitude residents. *Am. J. Hum. Biol.* 2, 627–637. doi: 10.1002/ajhb.1310020606

Murray, A. J. (2016). Energy metabolism and the high-altitude environment. *Exp. Physiol.* 101, 23–27. doi: 10.1113/EP085317

Peacock, A. J. (1998). Oxygen at high altitude. *BMJ* 317:1063. doi: 10.1136/bmj.317.7165.1063

Pesta, D., Hoppel, F., Macek, C., Messner, H., Faulhaber, M., Kobel, C., et al. (2011). Similar qualitative and quantitative changes of mitochondrial respiration following strength and endurance training in normoxia and hypoxia in sedentary humans. *Am. J. Physiol. Regul. Integr. Comp. Physiol.* 301, R1078–R1087. doi: 10.1152/ajpregu.00285.2011

Sangkhae, V., Fisher, A. L., Wong, S., Koenig, M. D., Tussing-Humphreys, L., Chu, A., et al. (2020). Effects of maternal iron status on placental and fetal iron homeostasis. *J. Clin. Invest.* 130, 625–640. doi: 10.1172/JCI127341

Sayama, S., Song, A., Brown, B. C., Couturier, J., Cai, X., Xu, P., et al. (2020). Maternal erythrocyte ENT1-mediated AMPK activation counteracts placental hypoxia and supports fetal growth. *JCI Insight* 5:e130205. doi: 10.1172/jci.insight.130205

Sferruzzi-Perri, A. N., Higgins, J. S., Vaughan, O. R., Murray, A. J., and Fowden, A. L. (2019). Placental mitochondria adapt developmentally and in response to hypoxia to support fetal growth. *Proc. Natl. Acad. Sci. U.S.A.* 116, 1621–1626. doi: 10.1073/pnas.1816056116

Shaw, S., Ghosh, D., Kumar, U., Panjwani, U., and Kumar, B. (2018). Impact of high altitude on key determinants of female reproductive health: a review. *Int. J. Biometeorol.* 62, 2045–2055. doi: 10.1007/s00484-018-1609-0

Song, D., Navalsky, B. E., Guan, W., Ingersoll, C., Wang, T., Loro, E., et al. (2020). Tibetan PHD2, an allele with loss-of-function properties. *Proc. Natl. Acad. Sci. U.S.A.* 117, 12230–12238. doi: 10.1073/pnas.1920546117

Tana, W., Noryung, T., Burton, G. J., Tissot van Patot, M., and Ri-Li, G. (2021). Protective effects from the ischemic/hypoxic stress induced by labor in the high-altitude Tibetan placenta. *Reprod. Sci.* 28, 659–664. doi: 10.1007/s43032-020-00443-9

Tissot van Patot, M. C., Murray, A. J., Beckey, V., Cindrova-Davies, T., Johns, J., Zwerdlinger, L., et al. (2010). Human placental metabolic adaptation to chronic hypoxia, high altitude: hypoxic preconditioning. *Am. J. Physiol. Regul. Integr. Comp. Physiol.* 298, R166–R172. doi: 10.1152/ajpregu.00383.2009

Tong, W., and Giussani, D. A. (2019). Preeclampsia link to gestational hypoxia. *J. Dev. Orig. Health Dis.* 10, 322–333. doi: 10.1017/S204017441900014X

Turner, J. M., Mitchell, M. D., and Kumar, S. S. (2020). The physiology of intrapartum fetal compromise at term. *Am. J. Obstet. Gynecol.* 222, 17–26. doi: 10.1016/j.ajog.2019.07.032

Veenendaal, M. V. E., Painter, R. C., de Rooij, S. R., Bossuyt, P. M., van der Post, J. A. M., Gluckman, P. D., et al. (2013). Transgenerational effects of prenatal exposure to the 1944-45 Dutch famine. *BJOG* 120, 548–553. doi: 10.1111/1471-0528.12136

Yang, J., Jin, Z.-B., Chen, J., Huang, X.-F., Li, X.-M., Liang, Y.-B., et al. (2017). Genetic signatures of high-altitude adaptation in Tibetans. *Proc. Natl. Acad. Sci. U.S.A.* 114, 4189–4194. doi: 10.1073/pnas.1617042114

Zhang, X. L., Ha, B. B., Wang, S. J., Chen, Z. J., Ge, J. Y., Long, H., et al. (2018). The earliest human occupation of the high-altitude Tibetan Plateau 40 thousand to 30 thousand years ago. *Science* 362, 1049–1051. doi: 10.1126/science.aat8824

Zoll, J., Sanchez, H., N'Guessan, B., Ribera, F., Lampert, E., Bigard, X., et al. (2002). Physical activity changes the regulation of mitochondrial respiration in human skeletal muscle. *J. Physiol.* 543, 191–200. doi: 10.1113/jphysiol.2002.019661

19

Metabotropic Glutamate Receptors 1 Regulates Rat Carotid Body Response to Acute Hypoxia *via* Presynaptic Mechanism

*Chaohong Li[1], Baosheng Zhao[2], Chenlu Zhao[1], Lu Huang[1] and Yuzhen Liu[1]**

[1] Henan Key Laboratory of Neural Regeneration and Repairment, Life Science Research Center, The First Affiliated Hospital of Xinxiang Medical University, Weihui, China, [2] Department of Thoracic Surgery, The First Affiliated Hospital of Xinxiang Medical University, Weihui, China

***Correspondence:**
Yuzhen Liu
yuzhenliu@xxmu.edu.cn

Background: The carotid body (CB) plays a critical role in oxygen sensing; however, the role of glutamatergic signaling in the CB response to hypoxia remains uncertain. We previously found that functional multiple glutamate transporters and inotropic glutamate receptors (iGluRs) are expressed in the CB. The aim of this present research is to investigate the expression of group I metabotropic glutamate receptors (mGluRs) (mGluR1 and 5) in the CB and its physiological function in rat CB response to acute hypoxia.

Methods: RT-PCR and immunostaining were conducted to examine the mRNA and protein expression of group I mGluRs in the human and rat CB. Immunofluorescence staining was performed to examine the cellular localization of mGluR1 in the rat CB. *In vitro* carotid sinus nerve (CSN) discharge recording was performed to detect the physiological function of mGluR1 in CB response to acute hypoxia.

Results: We found that (1) mRNAs of mGluR1 and 5 were both expressed in the human and rat CB. (2) mGluR1 protein rather than mGluR5 protein was present in rat CB. (3) mGluR1 was distributed in type I cells of rat CB. (4) Activation of mGluR1 inhibited the hypoxia-induced enhancement of CSN activity (CSNA), as well as prolonged the latency time of CB response to hypoxia. (5) The inhibitory effect of mGluR1 activation on rat CB response to hypoxia could be blocked by $GABA_B$ receptor antagonist.

Conclusion: Our findings reveal that mGluR1 in CB plays a presynaptic feedback inhibition on rat CB response to hypoxia.

Keywords: carotid body, hypoxia, glutamate, group I metabotropic glutamate receptors, DHPG

Abbreviations: ACh, acetylcholine; AMPARs, alpha-amino-3-hydroxy-5-methyl-4-isoxazole propionic acid receptors; CB, carotid body; CIH, cyclic intermittent hypoxia; CSN, carotid sinus nerve; CSNA, carotid sinus nerve activity; DHPG, (S)-3,5-dihydroxyphenylglycine; EAAT, excitatory amino acid transporter; GFAP, glial fibrillary acidic protein; iGluRs, ionotropic glutamate receptors; JNJ, JNJ16258685, (3,4-dihydro-2H-pyrano[2,3-b]quinolin-7-yl)-(cis-4-methoxycyclohexyl)-methanone; KARs, kainite receptors; GRM, mGluRs, metabotropic glutamate receptors; NC, negative control; NMDARs, *N*-methyl-D-aspartate receptors; nAChR, nicotinic ACh receptors; VGluT, vesicular glutamate transporter; PBS, phosphate-buffered saline; RT, reverse transcription; SD, Sprague-Dawley; TH, tyrosine hydroxylase; TASK-1, TWIK-related acid-sensitive potassium channel 1.

INTRODUCTION

Oxygen sensing mediated by central and peripheral chemoreceptors is essential for survival of multicellular organisms. Carotid body (CB), a highly vascular tissue, is mainly a peripheral chemoreceptor located in the adventitia of the bifurcation of the common carotid artery. CB is usually organized in glomeruli clusters, which are composed of four to eight neuron-like glomus cells (type I cells) and one to two glia-like sustentacular cells (type II cells) (Ortega-Sáenz and López-Barneo, 2020). Type I glomus cells are tyrosine hydroxylase (TH)-positive O_2 sensing cells, and their cytoplasm is rich in abundant synaptic vesicles that contain neurotransmitters and neuromodulators. Type II sustentacular cells that encase clusters of type I cells are glial fibrillary acidic protein (GFAP) positive cells and can be transformed into type I glomus cells under certain conditions (Platero-Luengo et al., 2014).

Evidence supports that the type I glomus cells, as presynaptic neuroendocrine cells, establish synapses with afferent sensory fibers of carotid sinus nerve (CSN) (as postsynaptic nerve endings) (Ortega-Sáenz and López-Barneo, 2020). There is general acceptance that transduction of the hypoxic stimulus in the CB involves closure of O_2-sensitive K^+ channels, which leads to membrane depolarization of type I cells. This process induces Ca^{2+}-dependent release of neurotransmitters from type I cells; subsequently, the neurotransmitters act on specific postsynaptic receptors on CSN afferent fibers (Chang et al., 2015). It is established that these neurotransmitters [such as ATP, GABA, and acetylcholine (ACh)] in type I cells regulate CB oxygen sensing not only by acting on the corresponding ionotropic receptors of chemosensory nerve endings (Zhang et al., 2000, 2009; Rong et al., 2003; Varas et al., 2003; Alcayaga et al., 2007; Sacramento et al., 2019) but also by acting on non-ionotropic receptors of chemosensory nerve endings (such as ATP and ACh) (Alcayaga et al., 2000; Shirahata et al., 2004) or non-ionotropic receptors of type I cells themselves (such as GABA and ATP) (Fearon et al., 2003; Tse et al., 2012). Studies show that neurotransmitters acting on non-ionotropic receptors of type I cells provide feedback mechanisms to regulate the CB hypoxia response. Xu et al. (2005) found that ATP exert strong negative feedback regulation on CB hypoxia response by restricting the increase in $[Ca^{2+}]$i during hypoxia or acting on P2Y receptors on type I cells to close the background ion channels. GABA was also demonstrated to play a negative feedback role by acting on $GABA_B$ receptors located on type I cells to inhibit the hypoxia-induced release of ATP and ACh (Fearon et al., 2003). Although evidence supports numerous mechanisms by which hypoxia-triggered depolarization of type I cells leads to excitation of the CSN, the glutamatergic neurotransmitter system its expression in CB as well as its effect on the hypoxia-triggered excitation of the CSN has not been systematically explored.

In the central nervous system, glutamate is the major neurotransmitter. In the process of glutamatergic synaptic transmission, once an action potential depolarizes the presynaptic membrane, glutamate accumulated in presynaptic transmitter vesicles by the vesicular glutamate transporters (VGluTs) is released into the synaptic cleft by exocytosis and then acts on the corresponding postsynaptic receptors to transmit neuronal signaling. Excitatory amino acid transporters (EAATs) on adjacent glial cells scavenge glutamate from the synaptic cleft to terminate glutamate's functions (Zhou and Danbolt, 2014; Reiner and Levitz, 2018). Glutamate receptors are divided into two families: ionotropic glutamate receptors (iGluRs) and metabotropic glutamate receptors (mGluRs) (Reiner and Levitz, 2018). Playing an important role in synaptic transmission/plasticity, iGluRs are ligand-gated ion channels, which once activated leads to a rapid ion flux, and are further divided into three main subfamilies: alpha-amino-3-hydroxy-5-methyl-4-isoxazole propionic acid receptors (AMPARs), *N*-methyl-D-aspartate receptors (NMDARs), and kainate receptors (KARs) (Traynelis et al., 2010; Reiner and Levitz, 2018). mGluRs belong to the G protein-coupled receptor family and are divided into group I mGluRs (GluR1/5), group II mGluRs (mGluR2/3) and group III mGluRs (mGluR4, mGluR6–8) (Niswender and Conn, 2010; Reiner and Levitz, 2018). mGluRs activate the G protein-coupled signal cascades leading to changes in synaptic function/excitability by inhibiting the presynaptic transmitter release (Sladeczek et al., 1993; Gereau and Conn, 1995) or by regulating the postsynaptic response (Sheng et al., 2017; Jin et al., 2018).

It is established that glutamatergic signaling functions not only in the central nervous system but also in the peripheral nervous system (Tremolizzo et al., 2012; Chen and Kukley, 2020). Multiple VGluTs, EAATs (Li et al., 2020), and iGluRs (Liu et al., 2009, 2018) have been demonstrated to exist in the rat CB. We found that exposure of rats to cyclic intermittent hypoxia (CIH) alters the expression of some of these molecules. iGluRs in the CB are functional because blockading with the NMDAR antagonist MK801 reduces endothelin-induced CSN activity (CSNA) (Liu et al., 2018). These data suggested that iGluR-mediated glutamatergic signaling might occur in the CB, but the information regarding the mGluRs expression in the CB and its physiological function in the CB reponse to hypoxia is unknown.

We previously demonstrated that group I mGluRs exist in human and rat adrenal glands and that mGluR1 is involved in hypoxia-induced upregulation of TH in cultured rat adrenal medulla (Fan et al., 2020). Both adrenal medulla and CB originate from the neural crest and function as peripheral chemoreceptors in acute oxygen sensing (Gao et al., 2019). Taken together, these observations led us to speculate that group I mGluRs might be present in the CB and are involved in the carotid chemoreflex. In this study, we examined the expression of group I mGluRs in the human and rat CB and its cellular localization in the rat CB by RT-PCR and immunostaining. Moreover, we investigated the physiological function of mGluR1 in rat CB response to acute hypoxia.

MATERIALS AND METHODS

Human Carotid Body

Human surgical specimens were obtained from The First Affiliated Hospital of Xinxiang Medical University with consent from patients (grant approval number: 2016008). Human

CB specimen was obtained from a patient with left CB paraganglioma, and human cerebral cortex tissue was obtained from a patient with craniocerebral trauma. The protocol related to human subjects was conducted in accordance with the declaration of Helsinki and approved by the Human Ethics Committee of The First Affiliated Hospital of Xinxiang Medical University.

Animals and Rat Carotid Body Harvest

Adult male Sprague-Dawley (SD) rats were ordered from Beijing Vital River Laboratory Animal Technology Co., Ltd. (Beijing, China). The age of the rats was 8 weeks, and the body weight was 240–250 g at entry into the protocol. Rats were housed under room temperature and standard humidity (50 ± 5%) with a 12-h day/night cycle with laboratory chow and water *ad libitum*. All procedures performed in this study were in accordance with national animal research regulations, and all animal experimental protocols were approved by the Institutional Animal Ethics Committee at The First Affiliated Hospital of Xinxiang Medical University.

After the SD rat was anesthetized by inhalation of 2% isoflurane (RWD Life Science, Shenzhen, China), the rat was decapitated and the bilateral carotid bifurcations were rapidly removed and placed into 95% O_2–5% CO_2 saturated ice-cold phosphate-buffered saline (PBS). The CBs were dissected (within 4 min) and immediately soaked in RNAlater (Qiagen, Valencia, CA, United States), then stored at −80°C until analyzed.

RNA Extraction and Reverse Transcription-PCR

Total RNA was extracted from human CB specimens and rat CBs (total 16 CBs pooled from 8 rats) using TRIzol reagent (Thermo Fisher Scientific, Waltham, MA, United States) according to the manufacturer's protocol. After removal of gDNA, 500 ng of total RNA was reversely transcribed into cDNA by using QuantiTect Reverse Transcription Kit (Qiagen, Valencia, CA, United States), in accordance with the manufacturer's protocol. The RNA without reverse transcriptase was used in reverse transcription (RT) reaction to obtain a negative cDNA control. The mRNA expression level was detected by semi-quantitative PCR in a Veriti® 96-well Thermal Cycler (Applied Biosystems, Foster City, CA, United States) using HotStarTaq® Master Mix Kit (Qiagen, Valencia, CA, United States). Two microliters of cDNA samples was mixed with 10 μl of HotStarTaq Master Mix and 1 μl of gene-specific primer pairs in a final reaction volume of 20 μl to amplify the target gene. The PCR reactive conditions included an initial step at 95°C for 10 min, followed by 40 cycles at 94°C for 50 s, proper annealing temperature for 50 s, extension at 72°C for 1 min, and then ending at 72°C for 10 min. An equal volume of the negative cDNA control was used in the PCR reaction as negative PCR control. The PCR product was loaded into 1.2% agarose gel. A total of three technical replicates were conducted for each target gene. All primers were exon spanning and designed using Primer-BLAST.[1] Details of all primers are listed in **Tables 1, 2**.

Immuno-Staining

After the rats were fixed with 4% neutral buffered formalin by cardiac perfusion, the carotid bifurcations containing the CB were removed and embedded in paraffin. The paraffin-embedded carotid bifurcations were cut by Shandon™ Finesse™ 325 Microtomes (Thermo Fisher Scientific, Waltham, MA, United States) to prepare CB sections (3 μm).

For immunohistochemistry staining, after being deparaffinized, hydrated, and antigen retrieved, the CB sections were blocked with 10% goat serum at room temperature for 1 h, then incubated at 4°C overnight with the following primary antibodies: rabbit anti-mGluR1 (1:300, Abcam, Cambridge, United Kingdom, Cat No. ab82211) and anti-mGluR5 (1:100, Abcam, Cambridge, United Kingdom, Cat No. ab76316). After being washed three times in PBS, sections were incubated with GTVision™ III Detection System Mouse & Rabbit Kit (HRP/DAB) (GeneTech, Shanghai, China), according to the manufacturer's instruction, to yield a brown crystalline antigen–antibody complex product. The paraffin-embedded rat brain sections were incubated with primary antibodies as the positive control. The negative staining control was prepared by replacing the primary antibody to PBS containing 5% normal goat serum. The staining was examined through the Nikon H600L microscope and photographed with Nikon digital camera DS-Fi1c (Nikon, Tokyo, Japan).

For double immunofluorescence staining, after blocking with 10% goat serum, the CB sections were exposed to a mixture of two primary antibodies as follows: rabbit anti-mGluR1 (1:100, CST, Danvers, MA, United States, Cat No. 12551) with mouse anti-TH (1:2,000, Sigma, St. Louis, MO, United States, Cat No. T2928); rabbit anti-mGluR1 (1:100, CST, Danvers, MA, United States, Cat No. 12551) with mouse anti-GFAP (1:200, CST, Danvers, MA, United States, Cat No. 3670). After washing with PBS, the sections were incubated with a mixture of second antibody of Alexa Fluor 488 goat anti-rabbit IgG (1:400, CST, Danvers, MA, United States, Cat No. 4412) with Alexa Fluor 555 goat anti-mouse IgG (1:400, CST, Danvers, MA, United States, Cat No. 4409). The negative staining control was prepared by omitting the primary antibody. The staining was examined and photographed with the Nikon C2 confocal microscope (Nikon, Tokyo, Japan).

In vitro Carotid Sinus Nerve Discharge Recording

The CB response to hypoxia was recorded by *in vitro* CSN discharge recording similar to the method described in a previous report (Rong et al., 2003). Briefly, SD rat was anesthetized by inhalation of 2% isoflurane, and then decapitated. The bilateral carotid bifurcations containing the CB were then rapidly removed and placed into 95% O_2–5% CO_2 saturated ice-cold Kreb's solution (in mM: NaCl 113, KCl 5.9, NaH_2PO_4 1.2, $MgSO_4$ 1.2, $NaHCO_3$ 25, glucose 11.5, $CaCl_2$ 2, and pH 7.4). The sinus nerve attached to the CB was dissected

[1] https://www.ncbi.nlm.nih.gov/

TABLE 1 | Sequence of human primers used in RT-PCR experiment.

Gene	Accession No.	Primer sequence	PCR Cycle no.	Annealing Tm (°C)
GRM1	**NM_001278065.2**	F: 5′-CAGCCGATTCGCTTTAGCC-3′ R: 5′-GGGATCGCGGTACTGAAGTTG-3′	40	57
GRM5	**NM_000842.5**	F: 5′-TCCAGAATTTGCTCCAGCTT-3′ R: 5′-CTTCCATCCCACTTTCTCCA-3′	40	60
GAPDH	**NM_002046.7**	F: 5′-GCAGGGGGGAGCCAAAAGGGT-3′ R: 5′-TGGGTGGCAGTGATGGCATGG-3′	40	53

GRM, glutamate metabotropic receptor; Tm, temperature; F, forward primer; R, reverse primer.

TABLE 2 | Sequence of rat primers used in RT-PCR experiment.

Gene	Accession No.	Primer sequence	PCR Cycle no.	Annealing Tm (°C)
GRM1	**NM_001114330.1**	F: 5′-CCAGTGATGTTCTCCATACC-3′ R: 5′-CACTCTGGGTAGACTTGAGTG-3′	40	50
GRM5	**NM_017012.1**	F: 5′-CCCCAAACTCTCCAGTCT-3′ R: 5′-ATTTTTCACCTCGGGTTC-3′	40	49
β-actin	**NM_031144.3**	F: 5′-GGGAAATCGTGCGTGACATT-3′ R: 5′-CGGATGTCAACGTCACACTT-3′	40	55

GRM, glutamate metabotropic receptor; Tm, temperature; F, forward primer; R, reverse primer.

under a microscope, and the bifurcation was placed into a recording chamber (3 ml) perfused with 95% O_2–5% CO_2 saturated warm Kreb's solution (15 ml/min) with the chamber temperature being kept at 33°C. The CSN discharge was recorded using a suction electrode (Warner Instruments, Hamden, CT, United States). The signaling was amplified (1,000×) and filtered (100–1,000 Hz) by a DP-311 differential amplifier (Warner Instruments, Hamden, CT, United States), then collected by PowerLab 8/35 (AD Instruments, Bella Vista, NSW, Australia) and analyzed and integrated by LabChart 8 software (AD Instruments, Bella Vista, NSW, Australia). To detect the CB response to hypoxia, the CB was exposed to 5% O_2–5% CO_2–90% N_2 saturated Kreb's solution for a period of 90 s at an interval of 15 min. Hypoxia-induced CSNA was normalized by integrated CSNA under hypoxia divided by the integrated baseline CSNA under 95% O_2–5% CO_2 condition. Group I receptor agonist (S)-3,5-dihydroxyphenylglycine (DHPG, 40 μM) (Sigma, St. Louis, MO, United States), mGluR1 antagonist (3,4-dihydro-2H-pyrano[2,3-b]quinolin-7-yl)-(cis-4-methoxycyclohexyl)-methanone (JNJ16259685, 20 μM) (Santa Cruz Biotechnology, Dallas, TX, United States), and DHPG (40 μM) combined with JNJ or DHPG combined with $GABA_B$ receptor antagonist CGP52432 (10 μM) (Selleck Chemicals, Houston, TX, United States) were applied by switching the basal perfusate to 95% O_2–5% CO_2 saturated Kreb's solution containing the compound for 10 min before switching to 5% O_2–5% CO_2–90% N_2 saturated Kreb's solution containing the compound.

Statistical Analysis

The Shapiro–Wilk normality tests of all data could be conducted with the SPSS statistical software. All data were normally distributed, and the normality test results were shown in the online supplementary tables. The data were presented as mean ± SEM. Statistical evaluation was conducted by one-way ANOVA with repeated measures. $p < 0.05$ was considered significant.

RESULTS

mRNA Expression of Group I Metabotropic Glutamate Receptors in Human and Rat Carotid Body

Reverse transcription-PCR was performed to detect the mRNA expression of group I mGluRs (*GRM1* and *GRM5*) in human and rat CB. As shown in **Figure 1**, PCR-amplified transcripts corresponding to the predicted sizes of *GRM1* and *GRM5* were detected in human (**Figure 1A**) and rat CB (**Figure 1B**) as well as brain cerebral cortex, which was used as positive control. These results indicate that both human and rat CB express all group I mGluR mRNAs.

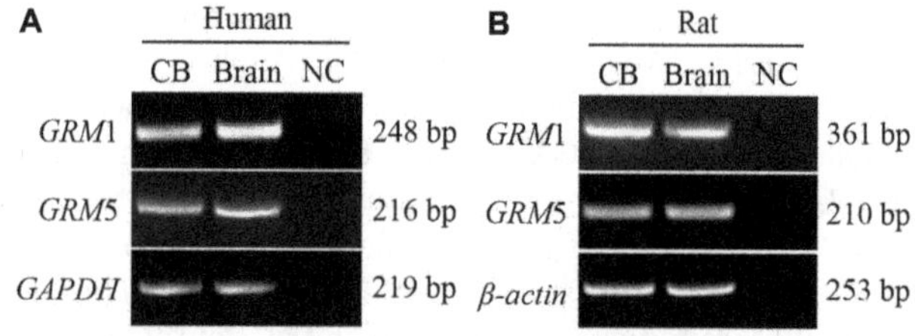

FIGURE 1 | mRNA expression of group I mGluRs in human and rat CB. **(A,B)** Representative agarose gel images show the RT-PCR results of group I mGluR mRNA expression in human and rat CB. CB, left lanes in **(A,B)**. RNA extracted from the human brain cerebral cortex was used as positive control (brain, middle lanes in **A,B**). An equal volume of the negative cDNA control was used in the PCR as PCR negative control (NC; right lanes in **A,B**). GRM, glutamate metabotropic receptor.

Protein Expression of Group I Metabotropic Glutamate Receptors in Rat Carotid Body

To detect the protein expression of group I mGluRs (mGluR1 and mGluR5) in rat CB, immunohistochemistry was performed. Representative photomicrographs in **Figures 2A1,A2** showed that mGluR1-positive immunoreaction was ubiquitously detected in the clustering glomeruli of rat CB. However, mGluR5-specific immunostaining was not observed in rat CB (**Figures 2B1,B2**). The representative negative controls (NCs) in the absence of the anti-mGluR1 or mGluR5 antibody did not yield specific staining in rat CB (**Figures 2C1,C2**). Rat brain sections with intense immunoreactive mGluR1 (**Figure 2D**) or mGluR5 (**Figure 2E**) were used as positive controls. These results indicate that mGluR1 protein rather than mGluR5 protein is present in rat CB.

Cellular Localization of Metabotropic Glutamate Receptors 1 in Rat Carotid Body

The CB is composed of type I glomus cells and type II sustentacular cells. To further ascertain the localization of mGluR1 in rat CB, double immunofluorescence was performed. TH was used as the type I glomus cell marker and GFAP was used as the type II cell marker. As shown in **Figure 3**, the mGluR1 immunoreactive signal was diffusely present in the cytoplasm of round-shaped cells which are clustered in rat CB and co-localized with TH-positive immunoreactivity (**Figures 3A–C**), but not detected with GFAP-positive signals (**Figures 3D–F**), thus indicating that mGluR1 distributes in type I cells rather in type II cells in rat CB.

Activation of Group I Metabotropic Glutamate Receptors Attenuates Carotid Body Response to Hypoxia

As a chemoreceptor, the CB senses the reduction of arterial PO_2 during hypoxia, resulting in afferent activation of the CSN, which is also known as the CB response to hypoxia. To investigate the effect of mGluR1 on the CB response to hypoxia, CSN discharge was recorded from CB-sinus nerve preparations *ex vivo*. A representative trace of CSNA is shown in **Figure 4A**. Similar to a previous study (Rong et al., 2003), the baseline CSNA under 95% O_2 was increased sharply after exposure to 5% O_2 hypoxia. The time from exposure to hypoxia to the onset of CSNA increase is referred to as latency time (*t*; **Figure 4C**) of CB response to hypoxia. After application of selective group I mGluR agonist DHPG into basal perfusate (95% O_2–5% CO_2 saturated Kreb's solution) for 10 min, DHPG (40 μM) significantly inhibited the CSNA under hypoxia conditions (normalized integrated CSNA before treatment with DHPG vs. normalized integrated CSNA while treatment with DHPG: 248.80 ± 26.17 vs. 175.03 ± 19.23%; $n = 9$, $p < 0.005$) (**Figures 4A,B**). The latency time of CB response to hypoxia was 47.78 ± 2.52 s before treatment with DHPG, 83.89 ± 1.82 s during treatment with DHPG, and 45.56 ± 2.36 s after treatment with DHPG (**Figures 4C,D**; $n = 9$, $p < 0.01$). These results indicate that group I mGluR activation inhibits CSNA under hypoxia and increases the latency time of CB response to hypoxia; that is, activation of group I mGluRs attenuates the CB response to hypoxia.

Activation of Metabotropic Glutamate Receptors 1 Attenuates Carotid Body Response to Hypoxia

To assess the role of mGluR1 in DHPG-attenuated CB response to hypoxia, we first investigated the effects of mGluR1 antagonist

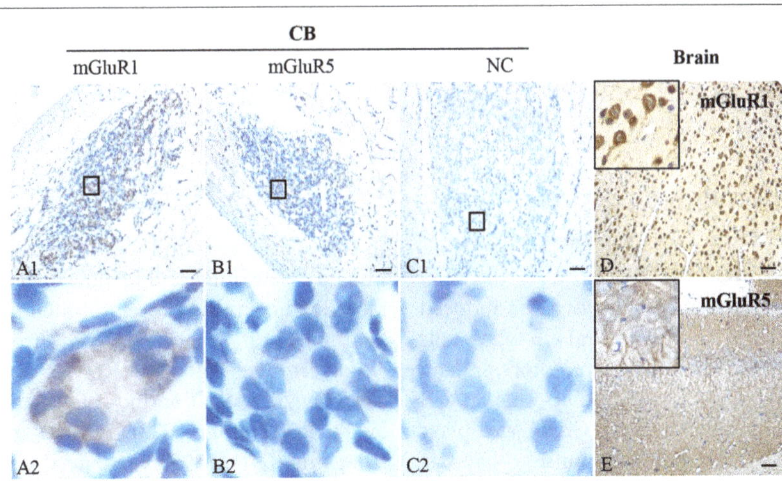

FIGURE 2 | Immunohistochemical staining of mGluR1 and mGluR5 in rat CB. Representative images of rat CB and brain sections were immunostained with mGluR1 and mGluR5. Panels **(C1,C2)** are negative staining controls obtained by omitting the primary antibody. mGluR1 **(D)** or mGluR5 **(E)** staining of rat brain sections were used as positive controls. Panels **(A2–C2)** are higher-magnification images of framed areas in **(A1–C1)**, respectively. The brown staining represents the mGluR1 or mGluR5, while the blue staining represents hematoxylin-stained cell nuclei. mGluR, glutamate metabotropic receptor; NC, negative control. Scale bar, 50 μm for all images.

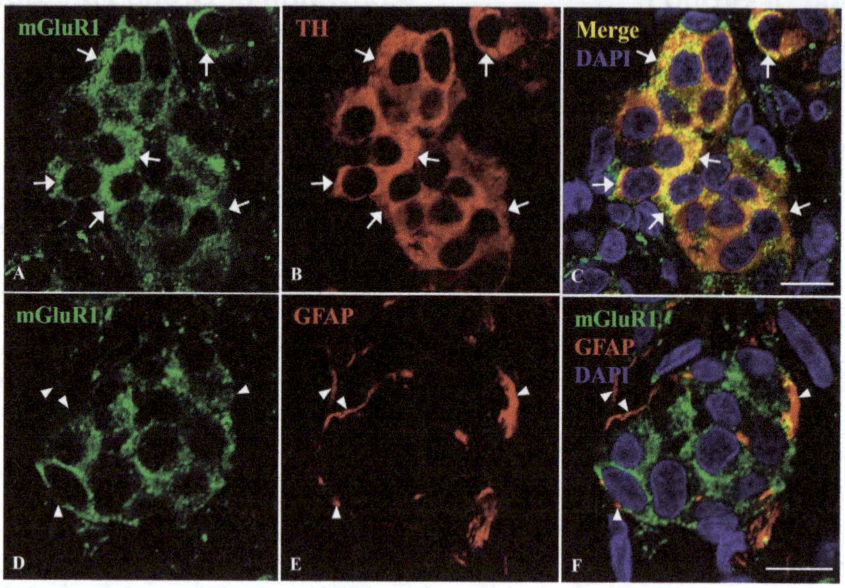

FIGURE 3 | Distribution of mGluR1 in rat CB. Panels **(A–C)** are double immunofluorescence staining of mGluR1 (green) with TH (red) in rat CB. Panels **(D–F)** are double immunofluorescence staining of mGluR1 (green) and GFAP (red) in rat CB. Some TH-immunoreactive type I cells are immunoreactive for mGluR1 (arrows), whereas the GFAP-immunoreactive type II cells are not immunoreactive for mGluR1 (arrowheads). TH, tyrosine hydroxylase, the CB type I cells marker; GFAP, glial fibrillary acidic protein, the CB type II cells marker; mGluR, glutamate metabotropic receptor. Scale bar, 10 μm for all images.

JNJ16259685 (JNJ) on CB response to hypoxia by applying JNJ (20 μM) in basal perfusate for 10 min before exposing it to hypoxia. We found that JNJ enhanced the CSNA under hypoxia conditions, as indicated by an increase in normalized integrated CSNA from 186.72 ± 13.72 to 232.77 ± 17.61% ($n = 7, p < 0.005$) (**Figures 5A,B**). The inhibitory effect of DHPG on CSNA under hypoxia conditions was also blocked by pre-perfusion with JNJ for 5 min, as the normalized integrated CSNA increased from 144.60 ± 8.05 (treatment with DHPG only) to 200.87 ± 15.77% (treatment with DHPG and JNJ) ($n = 4, p < 0.05$) (**Figures 5C,D**). These results indicate that DHPG attenuates CB response to hypoxia by activating mGluR1; that is, mGluR1 in CB may act as an inhibitory feedback regulator to modulate CB chemoreflex.

Inhibitory Effect of (S)-3,5-Dihydroxyphenylglycine on Carotid Body Response to Hypoxia Involves the $GABA_B$ Receptor

Previous studies found that GABA inhibits hypoxia-induced postsynaptic sensory responses in coculture of rat CB type I cells with petrosal neurons by acting on $GABA_A$ receptors (Zhang et al., 2009). We also found that GABA inhibits the rat CB hypoxia response *in vitro* (unpublished data). GABA also plays an autoreceptor feedback inhibition in CB response to hypoxia *via* acting on the $GABA_B$ receptor in CB type I cells (Fearon et al., 2003), and the cross talk has been demonstrated between the $GABA_B$ receptor and other receptors (such as $GABA_A$ receptor, mGluR1, and NMDA receptor) (Xu et al., 2014). Therefore, we speculate that the $GABA_B$ receptor may be involved in the DHPG-induced inhibitory effect on CB response to hypoxia by activating mGluR1. To determine whether activated mGluR1 exerts its inhibitory effect on CB response to hypoxia through $GABA_B$ receptor, we applied the $GABA_B$ receptor antagonist CGP52432 (10 μM) for 5 min before DHPG treatment. As shown in **Figure 6**, compared with normalized integrated CSNA during treatment with DHPG (148.96 ± 21.28%), the normalized integrated CSNA was increased to 208.00 ± 36.18% ($n = 5$, $p < 0.05$) after pre-perfusion with CGP52432. That is, CGP52432 could prevent the inhibitory effect of DHPG on CB response to hypoxia. This result indicates that the $GABA_B$ receptor in CB may be involved in the mGluR1-induced feedback inhibition in CB response to hypoxia.

DISCUSSION

In this study, we found for the first time that mRNAs of group I mGluRs (mGluR1 and mGluR5) were expressed in human and rat CB, whereas the protein of mGluR1 instead of mGluR5 was detected in rat CB and scattered throughout the CB. Moreover, we determined that mGluR1 was distributed in type I glomus cells. Our investigation indicates that group I mGluR activation by DHPG inhibited CB response to hypoxia, while mGluR1 antagonist JNJ16259685 enhanced CB response to hypoxia and blocked the inhibitory effect of DHPG on CB response to hypoxia. We also found that the inhibitory effect of DHPG on CB response to hypoxia might be related to the $GABA_B$ receptor in CB type I cells, as the inhibitory effect could be blocked by inhibition of the $GABA_B$ receptor. Taken together, these results indicate that, rather than mGluR5, functional mGluR1 exists in

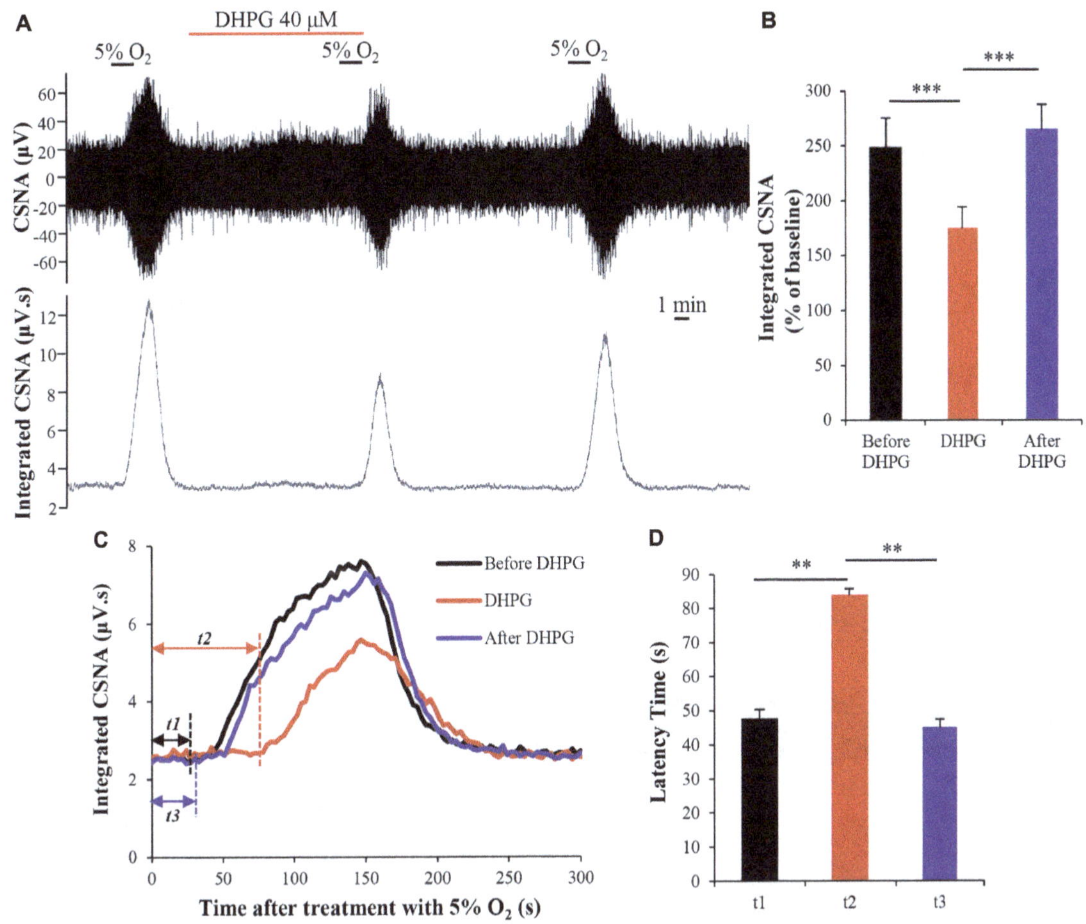

FIGURE 4 | DHPG attenuates CB response to hypoxia. **(A)** Effect of DHPG (40 μM) on the CSNA under hypoxia conditions. Note that DHPG reversibly reduces the CSNA under hypoxia condition. **(B)** DHPG (40 μM) reduces the integrated CSNA during hypoxia. **(C)** Changes in integrated CSNA within 5 min of switching to 5% O_2–5% CO_2–90% N_2 saturated Kreb's solution. *t1*, latency time of CB response to hypoxia before treatment with DHPG (40 μM); *t2*, latency time of CB response to hypoxia while treatment with DHPG; *t3*, latency time of CB response to hypoxia after treatment with DHPG. **(D)** DHPG (40 μM) reversibly increases the latency time of CB response to hypoxia. DHPG, group I mGluRs agonist; CSNA, carotid sinus nerve activity; *t*, time. The data were presented as mean ± SEM. $n = 9$, $^{**}p < 0.01$ and $^{***}p < 0.005$ indicate significant difference (one-way ANOVA with repeated measures).

the CB and may play a role in presynaptic feedback inhibition in rat CB hypoxia sensitivity.

The CB transmits the changes of oxygen levels in arterial blood through chemosensory synapses formed by type I cells (as presynaptic neuroendocrine cells) with CSN afferent fibers (as postsynaptic nerve endings). Hypoxia-induced depolarization of type I cells releases a variety of neurotransmitters, which are the material basis of CB oxygen sensory transmission (Ortega-Sáenz and López-Barneo, 2020), acting on the corresponding receptors of CSN afferent fibers. Studies have confirmed that neurotransmitters in CB type I cells such as ATP, ACh, 5-HT, and GABA regulate CB response to hypoxia by acting on P2X receptors (Zhang et al., 2000; Prasad et al., 2001; Iturriaga et al., 2007), nicotinic ACh receptors (nAChR; Zhang et al., 2000; Varas et al., 2003; Iturriaga et al., 2007), 5-HT_2 receptors (Jacono et al., 2005), and $GABA_A$ receptors (Zhang et al., 2009) on postsynaptic CSN afferent fibers, respectively. Nonetheless, the role of glutamate and its receptors, the most important neurotransmitter in the central nervous system, in CB response to hypoxia is unclear.

Torrealba et al. (1996) report that type I cells in the cat CB had high concentrations of glutamate, but glutamate release from *in vitro* cat CB superfusion with high potassium within 2 min was not observed. The perfusate used in this study was 50 or 70 mM potassium Krebs–Ringer–HEPES (KRH) solution. Accordingly, they speculated that glutamate could not be released as a neurotransmitter from type I cells. Interestingly, when Kim et al. (2004) measured the ACh release from rabbit CB, they found that 30 or 60 mM KCl stimulation for 15 min had no effect on ACh release, but increasing the KCl concentration to 100 mM significantly induced the ACh release from the CB, indicating whether or not a transmitter release from the CB triggered by high potassium *in vitro* might be dependent on potassium concentration and duration time. Hence, it cannot entirely exclude the possibility that the superfusion condition in the study by Torrealba was not optimum to induce glutamate

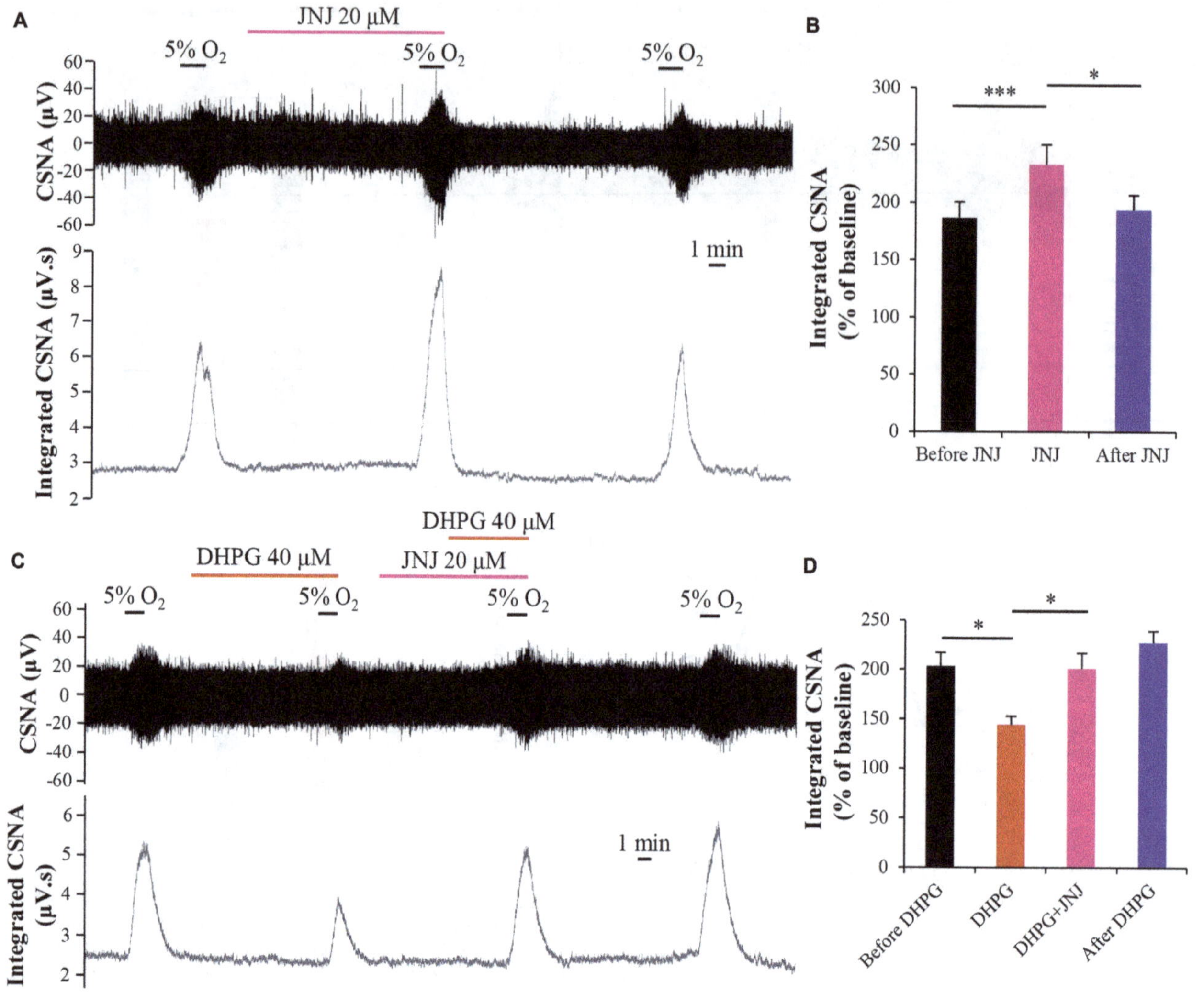

FIGURE 5 | mGluR1 antagonist JNJ blocks the inhibitory effect of DHPG on CB response to hypoxia. **(A)** Effect of JNJ (20 μM) on the CSNA under hypoxia conditions. Note that DHPG reversibly enhances the CSNA under hypoxia conditions. **(B)** JNJ (20 μM) increases the normalized integrated CSNA during hypoxia. $n = 7$. **(C,D)** Pretreatment with JNJ prevents the inhibitory effect of DHPG on CB response to hypoxia. The data were presented as mean ± SEM. $n = 4$. *$p < 0.05$ and ***$p < 0.05$ indicate significant difference (one-way ANOVA with repeated measures). CSNA, carotid sinus nerve activity; JNJ, JNJ16259685, mGluR1 antagonist.

release from the CB stimulated with high-potassium solution *in vitro*. Interestingly, Yokoyama et al. (2014) found that VGluT2 is localized in the carotid sinus afferent nerve terminals. Recently, we have demonstrated multiple subtypes of VGluTs (VGluT3) and EAATs (EAAT2 and 3) being present in the CB (Li et al., 2020). These data suggested that glutamate might be releasing from CB itself or carotid sinus afferent nerve terminals, and then acting as a neurotransmitter. We also found that functional NMDAR1 and AMPAR1 in rat CB might regulate the CB chemoreflex plasticity (Liu et al., 2009, 2018). In this study, we further discovered that mRNAs of group I mGluRs (mGluR1 and 5) were also expressed in human and rat CB (**Figure 1**); this finding is consistent with our previous report; i.e., the adrenal medulla, another oxygen sensor originating similarly with the CB, expresses both mGluR1 and 5 (Fan et al., 2020). Among group I mGluRs, only mGluR1 protein was detected in rat CB by immunostaining (**Figure 2**). Awobuluyi et al. (2003) reported that glutamate inotropic receptor NMDAR1 (NR1) mRNA was present in PC12 cells but not its protein, and the underlying mechanism might be from the 3′ untranslated region of NR1 blocking the translation of NR1 mRNA at initiation in PC12 cells. Therefore, rat CB expressing mGluR5 mRNA but lacking obviously expression of mGluR5 protein implies translational or posttranscriptional modification. Additional work will be necessary to characterize the discrepancy expression between mGluR5 mRNA and protein in rat CB.

As members of the G protein-coupled receptor family, mGluRs are divided into three subtypes, groups I, II, and III, based on its receptor structure and physiological activity (Ohashi et al., 2002). In the central nervous system, the three groups of

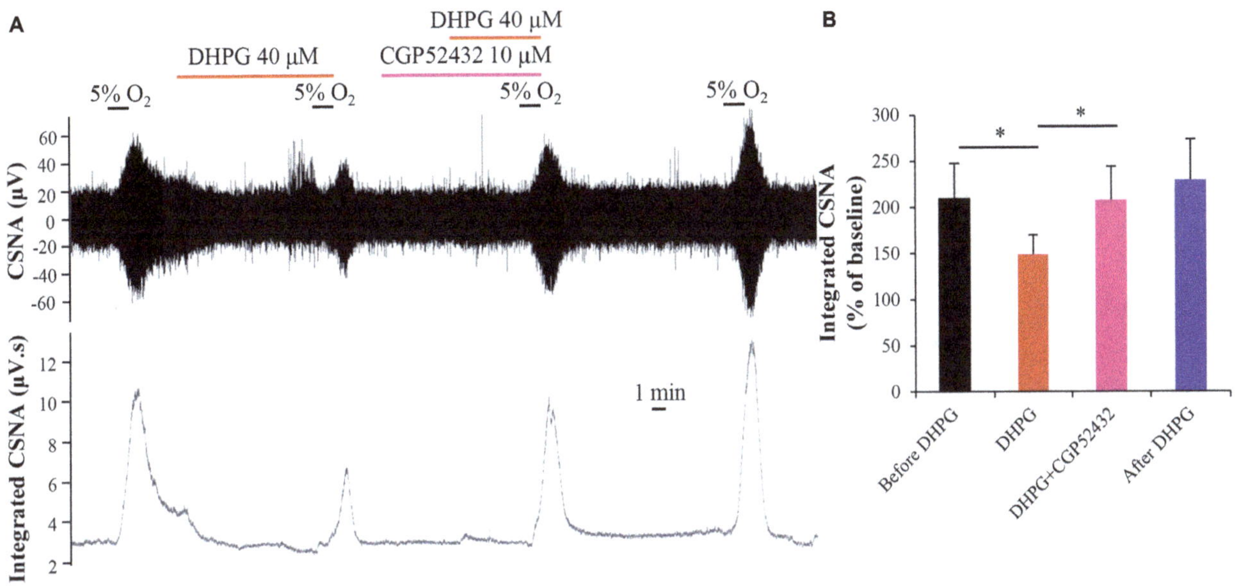

FIGURE 6 | $GABA_B$ receptor antagonist CGP52432 blocks inhibitory effect of DHPG on CB response to hypoxia. **(A)** Representative traces of changes in raw CSNA and integrated CSNA recordings. Note that pretreatment with CGP52432 prevents the inhibitory effect of DHPG on CSNA under hypoxia conditions. **(B)** Statistical analysis of normalized integrated CSNA after difference treatment. The data were presented as mean ± SEM. $n = 5$, $^*p < 0.05$ indicates significant difference (one-way ANOVA with repeated measures). CSNA, carotid sinus nerve activity; CGP52432, $GABA_B$ receptor antagonist; DHPG, group I mGluRs agonist.

mGluRs have different precise synaptic site locations. Generally, group I mGluRs are located primarily on the postsynaptic membrane, and groups II and III mGluRs are primarily on the presynaptic membrane (Shigemoto et al., 1997). However, some studies have shown presynaptic group I mGluRs. Romano et al. (1995) reported that some mGluR5 were located in the presynaptic axon terminal. Wittmann et al. (2001) also found that mGluR1 was localized on presynaptic elements of the excitatory synapses of substantia nigra pars reticulata by immunohistochemistry at the electron microscope level. In this study, mGluR1 immunoreactive signals were co-localized with TH immunoreactives, and moreover, both signals were diffusely present in the cytoplasm of clustered round-shaped cells (**Figure 3**), demonstrating the ubiquitous presence of mGluR1 in type I cells of rat CB. However, we cannot rule out that mGluR1 is also present in TH-positive nerve terminals projected from petrosal ganglion neurons, which has been shown to express TH (Czyzyk-Krzeska et al., 1991; Finley et al., 1992). Additional co-staining of mGluR1 with a specific marker of postsynaptic nerve ending, such as the P2X2 receptor, will help answer this question. Due to type I cells being presynaptic neuroendocrine cells to the afferent nerve terminal of CSN, we thus speculate that mGluR1 in the carotid chemoreflex might regulate the synaptic transmission *via* a presynaptic mechanism.

Group I mGluRs play an important role in synaptic transmission and synaptic plasticity through G protein coupling (Anwyl, 2009; Reiner and Levitz, 2018) or through non-canonical effector pathways (Eng et al., 2016). Previous studies demonstrated that group I mGluRs participated in pathogenic and adaptogenic response to hypoxia in rat brain development (Simonyi et al., 1999; Vetrovoy et al., 2021) and mGluR1/5 was involved in the enhancement of respiratory rhythm during early hypoxia by concomitant activation of L-type Ca(2+) channels in inspiratory brainstem neurons (Mironov and Richter, 2000). Our previous study also found that inhibition of mGluR1 blocked the hypoxia-induced activation of ERK1/2 in rat adrenal medulla (Fan et al., 2020). These data suggested that group I mGluRs are likely to be involved in hypoxic modification of channel activity or regulation of hypoxia response molecules in some conditions. In this study, we observed that superfusion of rat CB *in vitro* with DHPG, an agonist of group I mGluRs, decreased the acute hypoxia-evoked discharge activity of CSN (**Figure 4**), and this effect was blocked by mGluR1 antagonist JNJ16259685 (**Figure 5**), indicating an inhibitory effect of mGluR1 on CB response to acute hypoxia. There is evidence shown that, *via* activation of the G protein-coupled receptor downstream protein kinase C, postsynaptic mGluR1 mediates the potentiation of NMDAR activity in hippocampus glutamatergic synapses (Skeberdis et al., 2001) or the hyper-excitability of layer 5 pyramidal neurons in the rat anterior cingulate cortex (Gao et al., 2016). In contrast, some evidence showed that mGluR1 or 5 inhibits excitatory or inhibitory synaptic transmission in the hippocampus CA1 (Gereau and Conn, 1995; Manzoni and Bockaert, 1995) and the superior colliculus (White et al., 2003) *via* presynaptic mechanism. Studies also found that activation of group I mGluRs by DHPG induces a long-term depression of excitatory synaptic transmission in the hippocampus (Fitzjohn et al., 2001; Faas et al., 2002) or hippocampal interneurons *via* presynaptic P/Q-type Ca^{2+} channels (Le Duigou et al., 2011). Thus, activation of group I mGluRs results in different functions in the central and peripheral nervous systems, which depends

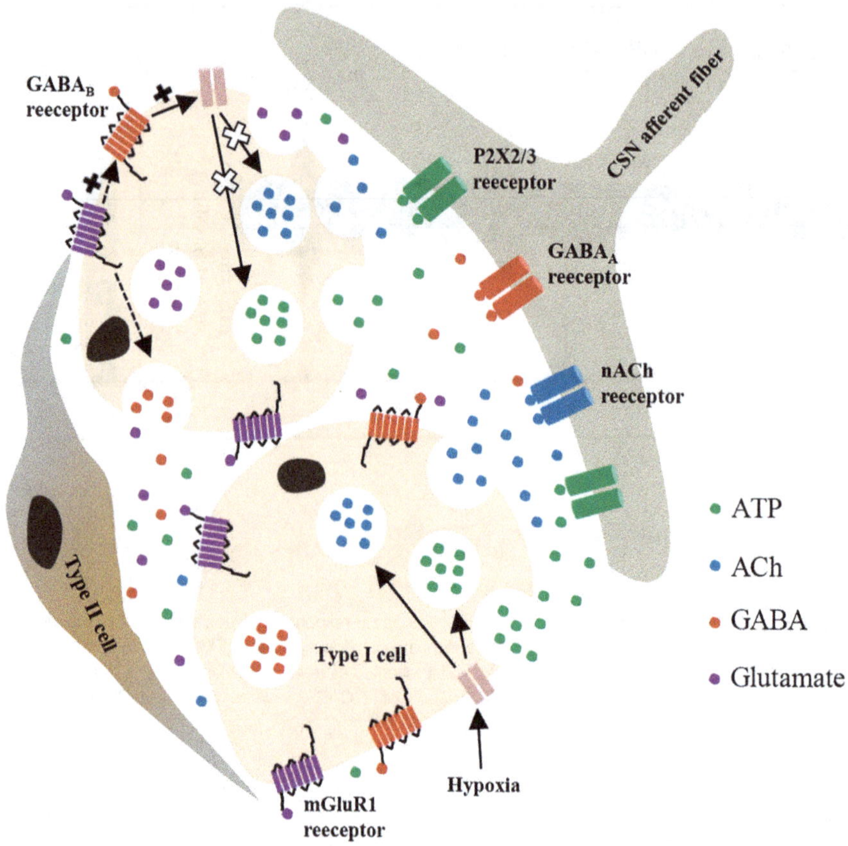

FIGURE 7 | Schematic representation of mGluR1-mediated regulation of neurotransmitter release from rat CB type I cells during hypoxia. Inhibition of TASK-1 in type I cells by hypoxia leads to membrane depolarization and release of various neurotransmitters. Among these neurotransmitters, glutamate and GABA act on presynaptic mGluR1 and $GABA_B$ receptors in themselves or in adjacent type I cells. $GABA_B$ activation further activates TASK-1, thus leading to an increase of potassium outflow, then limiting the degree of depolarization of type I cells in order to inhibit the further release of ATP and ACh induced by hypoxia. Additionally, mGluR1 activation may enhance the activation effect of $GABA_B$ receptor on TASK-1 through synergistic enhancement or modulate the release of GABA. In other words, both mGluR1 and $GABA_B$ receptors on type I cells regulate the CSN afferent signals of CB response to hypoxia through a presynaptic feedback mechanism. P2X2/3, purinergic P2X2/3 receptor; nACh, nicotinic ACh receptor.

on its localization on the synaptic site. Based on these above studies and our results in this study, we speculate that activation of mGluR1 likely reduces hypoxia-induced CB response by regulating the release of other neurotransmitters in presynaptic type I cells or by regulating P/Q-type Ca^{2+} channels in type I cells.

We also found that activation of mGluR1 by DHPG prolonged the latency time of CB response to hypoxia (**Figures 4C,D**). Hypoxia induces Ca^{2+}-dependent release of a variety of excitatory (such as ATP and ACh) (Zhang et al., 2000) and inhibitory (such as GABA and dopamine) (Zhang et al., 2009, 2018) transmitters in rat CB. These transmitters, which released from rat CB, act on postsynaptic P2X2/3 receptors and nAChR to produce excitatory effects or on $GABA_A$ receptors and D2 receptors to produce inhibitory effects on CSNA to regulate the final CSN afferent signal. Jacono et al. (2005) detected the release of neurotransmitters in the perfusion solution after treatment with acute hypoxia by using high-performance liquid chromatography coupled with an electrochemical detection system. They found that hypoxia induced the release of different neurotransmitters from type I cells in a time-dependent manner, i.e., different neurotransmitters released at different times following hypoxia. Therefore, we speculated that DHPG may inhibit the release of some neurotransmitters in CB type I cells under early hypoxia, subsequently leading to the prolonged latency of CB response to hypoxia.

Carotid body has a complex regulatory network. A variety of neurotransmitters or neuromodulators act on the corresponding receptors in type I cells or CSN afferent fibers to produce excitatory or inhibitory effects and ultimately regulate the input of CB type I cells' oxygen-sensitive signals (Aldossary et al., 2020; Ortega-Sáenz and López-Barneo, 2020). Many of these receptors are G protein-coupled receptors located not only in CSN afferent fibers but also in type I cells and type II cells (Guidolin et al., 2018). For example, GABA inhibits hypoxia-induced release of ATP and ACh by acting on presynaptic $GABA_B$ receptor-mediated activation of TWIK-related acid-sensitive potassium channel 1 (TASK-1) (Fearon et al., 2003). Evidence showed that G protein-coupled receptors may interact with each other under various physiological and pathological conditions (Guidolin et al., 2018, 2019). Based on a varietyof G protein-coupled receptors located in CB, the researchers suggested that there may be receptor–receptor interactions in CB (Porzionato et al., 2018). Previous studies found that there is also an interaction between $GABA_B$ and mGluR1, which is not a direct physical interaction between both receptors but rather a synergistic enhancement effect between G protein-coupled receptors (Rives et al., 2009; Xu et al., 2014). In this study, our results showed that pre-blocking $GABA_B$ receptor activity by superfusion with its antagonist CGP52432 at least partially blocked the inhibitory effect of DHPG on acute hypoxia-evoked discharge of CSN (**Figure 6**). This suggests that the inhibitory effect of mGluR1 activation on CB hypoxia response is at least partially related to the $GABA_B$ receptor. Future studies will determine how mGluR1 activates $GABA_B$ directly or indirectly.

Taken together, our results in this study provide a novel candidate molecule that is involved in regulating CB response to hypoxia. We speculate that hypoxia not only stimulates the release of ATP, ACh, and GABA from CB type I cells but also stimulates the release of glutamate, which activates mGluR1 receptors on the surface of type I cells. Subsequently, mGluR1 may enhance the effect of $GABA_B$ receptors by directly interacting with $GABA_B$ receptors or indirectly modulating the release of GABA, and ultimately attenuates hypoxia-evoked enhancement of CSN afferent discharges (**Figure 7**).

Although this study found that $GABA_B$ receptors may be involved in the inhibitory effect of mGluR1 on CB response to hypoxia, we cannot rule out other presynaptic mechanisms involved in this inhibitory effect. Further studies *via* single unit electrophysiological recording, along with primary coculture of type I cells with petrosal ganglion cells, will hopefully clarify the specific mechanism of mGluR1 on CB response to hypoxia. In addition, we cannot rule out that glutamate, like 5-HT (Jacono et al., 2005), participates in CB response to hypoxia as a modulator rather than an initiator. Therefore, further work on detecting glutamate release from CB after hypoxia treatment is necessary.

CONCLUSION

In summary, our study found that the protein of mGluR1, rather than mGluR5, is mainly expressed in the CB and plays a presynaptic feedback inhibition on CB response to hypoxia.

ETHICS STATEMENT

The studies involving human participants were reviewed and approved by the Ethics Committee of The First Affiliated Hospital of Xinxiang Medical University. The patients/participants provided their written informed consent to participate in this study. The animal study was reviewed and approved by the Institutional Animal Ethics Committee at The First Affiliated Hospital of Xinxiang Medical University.

AUTHOR CONTRIBUTIONS

YL designed the study. YL and BZ supervised the study execution. CL, CZ, and LH performed the experiments and analyzed the data. CL and YL wrote the manuscript. CL, BZ, and YL reviewed the manuscript. All authors read and approved the final manuscript.

ACKNOWLEDGMENTS

We thank Weifang Rong (Department of Anatomy and Physiology, Shanghai Jiao Tong University School of Medicine, Shanghai, China) for the technical guidance of *in vitro* carotid sinus nerve recording. We thank Chenfang Qi (Intensive Care Unit, Lowell General Hospital, Lowell, United States) for providing language editorial assistance.

REFERENCES

Alcayaga, J., Cerpa, V., Retamal, M., Arroyo, J., Iturriaga, R., and Zapata, P. (2000). Adenosine triphosphate-induced peripheral nerve discharges generated from the cat petrosal ganglion in vitro. *Neurosci. Lett.* 282, 185–188. doi: 10.1016/s0304-3940(00)00896-x

Alcayaga, C., Varas, R., Valdés, V., Cerpa, V., Arroyo, J., Iturriaga, R., et al. (2007). ATP- and ACh-induced responses in isolated cat petrosal ganglion neurons. *Brain Res.* 1131, 60–67. doi: 10.1016/j.brainres.2006.11.012

Aldossary, H. S., Alzahrani, A. A., Nathanael, D., Alhuthail, E. A., Ray, C. J., Batis, N., et al. (2020). G-protein-coupled receptor (GPCR) signaling in the carotid body: roles in hypoxia and cardiovascular and respiratory disease. *Int. J. Mol. Sci.* 21:6012. doi: 10.3390/ijms21176012

Anwyl, R. (2009). Metabotropic glutamate receptor-dependent long-term potentiation. *Neuropharmacology* 56, 735–740. doi: 10.1016/j.neuropharm.2009.01.002

Awobuluyi, M., Vazhappilly, R., and Sucher, N. J. (2003). Translational activity of N-methyl-D-aspartate receptor subunit NR1 mRNA in PC12 cells. *Neurosignals* 12, 283–291. doi: 10.1159/000075310

Chang, A. J., Ortega, F. E., Riegler, J., Madison, D. V., and Krasnow, M. A. (2015). Oxygen regulation of breathing through an olfactory receptor activated by lactate. *Nature* 527, 240–244. doi: 10.1038/nature15721

Chen, T. J., and Kukley, M. (2020). Glutamate receptors and glutamatergic signalling in the peripheral nerves. *Neural Regen. Res.* 15, 438–447. doi: 10.4103/1673-5374.266047

Czyzyk-Krzeska, M. F., Bayliss, D. A., Lawson, E. E., and Millhorn, D. E. (1991). Expression of messenger RNAs for peptides and tyrosine hydroxylase in primary sensory neurons that innervate arterial baroreceptors and chemoreceptors. *Neurosci. Lett.* 129, 98–102. doi: 10.1016/0304-3940(91)90729-d

Eng, A. G., Kelver, D. A., Hedrick, T. P., and Swanson, G. T. (2016). Transduction of group I mGluR-mediated synaptic plasticity by beta-arrestin2 signalling. *Nat. Commun.* 7:13571. doi: 10.1038/ncomms13571

Faas, G. C., Adwanikar, H., Gereau, R. W. IV, and Saggau, P. (2002). Modulation of presynaptic calcium transients by metabotropic glutamate receptor activation: a differential role in acute depression of synaptic transmission and long-term depression. *J. Neurosci.* 22, 6885–6890. doi: 10.1523/JNEUROSCI.22-16-06885.2002

Fan, Y. N., Li, C., Huang, L., Chen, L., Tang, Z., Han, G., et al. (2020). Characterization of group I metabotropic glutamate receptors in rat and human adrenal glands. *Front. Physiol.* 11:401. doi: 10.3389/fphys.2020.00401

Fearon, I. M., Zhang, M., Vollmer, C., and Nurse, C. A. (2003). GABA mediates autoreceptor feedback inhibition in the rat carotid body via presynaptic GABAB receptors and TASK-1. *J. Physiol.* 553, 83–94. doi: 10.1113/jphysiol.2003.048298

Finley, J. C., Polak, J., and Katz, D. M. (1992). Transmitter diversity in carotid body afferent neurons: dopaminergic and peptidergic phenotypes. *Neuroscience* 51, 973–987. doi: 10.1016/0306-4522(92)90534-9

Fitzjohn, S. M., Palmer, M. J., May, J. E., Neeson, A., Morris, S. A., and Collingridge, G. L. (2001). A characterisation of long-term depression induced by metabotropic glutamate receptor activation in the rat hippocampus in vitro. *J. Physiol.* 537, 421–430. doi: 10.1111/j.1469-7793.2001.00421.x

Gao, L., Ortega-Sáenz, P., and López-Barneo, J. (2019). Acute oxygen sensing-role of metabolic specifications in peripheral chemoreceptor cells. *Respir. Physiol. Neurobiol.* 265, 100–111. doi: 10.1016/j.resp.2018.08.007

Gao, S. H., Wen, H. Z., Shen, L. L., Zhao, Y. D., and Ruan, H. Z. (2016). Activation of mGluR1 contributes to neuronal hyperexcitability in the rat anterior cingulate cortex via inhibition of HCN channels. *Neuropharmacology* 105, 361–377. doi: 10.1016/j.neuropharm.2016.01.036

Gereau, R. W. IV, and Conn, P. J. (1995). Multiple presynaptic metabotropic glutamate receptors modulate excitatory and inhibitory synaptic transmission in hippocampal area CA1. *J. Neurosci.* 15, 6879–6889. doi: 10.1523/JNEUROSCI.15-10-06879.1995

Guidolin, D., Marcoli, M., Tortorella, C., Maura, G., and Agnati, L. F. (2018). G protein-coupled receptor-receptor interactions give integrative dynamics to intercellular communication. *Rev. Neurosci.* 29, 703–726. doi: 10.1515/revneuro-2017-0087

Guidolin, D., Marcoli, M., Tortorella, C., Maura, G., and Agnati, L. F. (2019). Receptor-receptor interactions as a widespread phenomenon: novel targets for drug development? *Front. Endocrinol. (Lausanne)* 10:53. doi: 10.3389/fendo.2019.00053

Iturriaga, R., Varas, R., and Alcayaga, J. (2007). Electrical and pharmacological properties of petrosal ganglion neurons that innervate the carotid body. *Respir. Physiol. Neurobiol.* 157, 130–139. doi: 10.1016/j.resp.2006.12.006

Jacono, F. J., Peng, Y. J., Kumar, G. K., and Prabhakar, N. R. (2005). Modulation of the hypoxic sensory response of the carotid body by 5-hydroxytryptamine: role of the 5-HT2 receptor. *Respir. Physiol. Neurobiol.* 145, 135–142. doi: 10.1016/j.resp.2004.10.002

Jin, L. E., Wang, M., Galvin, V. C., Lightbourne, T. C., Conn, P. J., Arnsten, A. F. T., et al. (2018). mGluR2 versus mGluR3 metabotropic glutamate receptors in primate dorsolateral prefrontal cortex: postsynaptic mGluR3 strengthen working memory networks. *Cereb. Cortex* 28, 974–987. doi: 10.1093/cercor/bhx005

Kim, D. K., Prabhakar, N. R., and Kumar, G. K. (2004). Acetylcholine release from the carotid body by hypoxia: evidence for the involvement of autoinhibitory receptors. *J. Appl. Physiol. (1985)* 96, 376–383. doi: 10.1152/japplphysiol.00726.2003

Le Duigou, C., Holden, T., and Kullmann, D. M. (2011). Short- and long-term depression at glutamatergic synapses on hippocampal interneurons by group I mGluR activation. *Neuropharmacology* 60, 748–756. doi: 10.1016/j.neuropharm.2010.12.015

Li, C., Huang, L., Jia, X., Zhao, B., Chen, L., and Liu, Y. (2020). Functional glutamate transporters are expressed in the carotid chemoreceptor. *Respir. Res.* 21:208. doi: 10.1186/s12931-020-01468-z

Liu, Y., Ji, E. S., Xiang, S., Tamisier, R., Tong, J., Huang, J., et al. (2009). Exposure to cyclic intermittent hypoxia increases expression of functional NMDA receptors in the rat carotid body. *J. Appl. Physiol. (1985)* 106, 259–267. doi: 10.1152/japplphysiol.90626.2008

Liu, Y., Li, C., Jia, X., Huang, L., and Weiss, J. W. (2018). AMPA receptor-dependent glutamatergic signaling is present in the carotid chemoreceptor. *Neuroscience* 382, 59–68. doi: 10.1016/j.neuroscience.2018.04.032

Manzoni, O., and Bockaert, J. (1995). Metabotropic glutamate receptors inhibiting excitatory synapses in the CA1 area of rat hippocampus. *Eur. J. Neurosci.* 7, 2518–2523. doi: 10.1111/j.1460-9568.1995.tb01051.x

Mironov, S. L., and Richter, D. W. (2000). Hypoxic modulation of L-type Ca(2+) channels in inspiratory brainstem neurones: intracellular signalling pathways and metabotropic glutamate receptors. *Brain Res.* 869, 166–177. doi: 10.1016/s0006-8993(00)02396-9

Niswender, C. M., and Conn, P. J. (2010). Metabotropic glutamate receptors: physiology, pharmacology, and disease. *Annu. Rev. Pharmacol. Toxicol.* 50, 295–322. doi: 10.1146/annurev.pharmtox.011008.145533

Ohashi, H., Maruyama, T., Higashi-Matsumoto, H., Nomoto, T., Nishimura, S., and Takeuchi, Y. (2002). A novel binding assay for metabotropic glutamate receptors using [3H] L-quisqualic acid and recombinant receptors. *Z. Naturforsch. C J. Biosci.* 57, 348–355. doi: 10.1515/znc-2002-3-425

Ortega-Sáenz, P., and López-Barneo, J. (2020). Physiology of the carotid body: from molecules to disease. *Annu. Rev. Physiol.* 82, 127–149. doi: 10.1146/annurev-physiol-020518-114427

Platero-Luengo, A., González-Granero, S., Durán, R., Díaz-Castro, B., Piruat, J. I., García-Verdugo, J. M., et al. (2014). An O2-sensitive glomus cell-stem cell synapse induces carotid body growth in chronic hypoxia. *Cell* 156, 291–303. doi: 10.1016/j.cell.2013.12.013

Porzionato, A., Stocco, E., Guidolin, D., Agnati, L., Macchi, V., and De Caro, R. (2018). Receptor–receptor interactions of G protein-coupled receptors in the carotid body: a working hypothesis. *Front. Physiol.* 9:697. doi: 10.3389/fphys.2018.00697

Prasad, M., Fearon, I. M., Zhang, M., Laing, M., Vollmer, C., and Nurse, C. A. (2001). Expression of P2X2 and P2X3 receptor subunits in rat carotid body afferent neurones: role in chemosensory signalling. *J. Physiol.* 537, 667–677. doi: 10.1111/j.1469-7793.2001.00667.x

Reiner, A., and Levitz, J. (2018). Glutamatergic signaling in the central nervous system: ionotropic and metabotropic receptors in concert. *Neuron* 98, 1080–1098. doi: 10.1016/j.neuron.2018.05.018

Rives, M. L., Vol, C., Fukazawa, Y., Tinel, N., Trinquet, E., Ayoub, M. A., et al. (2009). Crosstalk between GABAB and mGlu1a receptors reveals new insight into GPCR signal integration. *EMBO J.* 28, 2195–2208. doi: 10.1038/emboj.2009.177

Romano, C., Sesma, M. A., McDonald, C. T., O'Malley, K., Van den Pol, A. N., and Olney, J. W. (1995). Distribution of metabotropic glutamate receptor mGluR5 immunoreactivity in rat brain. *J. Comp. Neurol.* 355, 455–469. doi: 10.1002/cne.903550310

Rong, W., Gourine, A. V., Cockayne, D. A., Xiang, Z., Ford, A. P., Spyer, K. M., et al. (2003). Pivotal role of nucleotide P2X2 receptor subunit of the ATP-gated ion channel mediating ventilatory responses to hypoxia. *J. Neurosci.* 23, 11315–11321. doi: 10.1523/JNEUROSCI.23-36-11315.2003

Sacramento, J. F., Olea, E., Ribeiro, M. J., Prieto-Lloret, J., Melo, B. F., Gonzalez, C., et al. (2019). Contribution of adenosine and ATP to the carotid body chemosensory activity in ageing. *J. Physiol.* 597, 4991–5008. doi: 10.1113/JP274179

Sheng, N., Yang, J., Silm, K., Edwards, R. H., and Nicoll, R. A. (2017). A slow excitatory postsynaptic current mediated by a novel metabotropic glutamate receptor in CA1 pyramidal neurons. *Neuropharmacology* 115, 4–9. doi: 10.1016/j.neuropharm.2016.08.028

Shigemoto, R., Kinoshita, A., Wada, E., Nomura, S., Ohishi, H., Takada, M., et al. (1997). Differential presynaptic localization of metabotropic glutamate receptor subtypes in the rat hippocampus. *J. Neurosci.* 17, 7503–7522. doi: 10.1523/JNEUROSCI.17-19-07503.1997

Shirahata, M., Hirasawa, S., Okumura, M., Mendoza, J. A., Okumura, A., Balbir, A., et al. (2004). Identification of M1 and M2 muscarinic acetylcholine receptors in the cat carotid body chemosensory system. *Neuroscience* 128, 635–644. doi: 10.1016/j.neuroscience.2004.06.068

Simonyi, A., Zhang, J. P., and Sun, G. Y. (1999). Changes in mRNA levels for group I metabotropic glutamate receptors following in utero hypoxia-ischemia. *Brain Res. Dev. Brain Res.* 112, 31–37. doi: 10.1016/s0165-3806(98)00152-7

Skeberdis, V. A., Lan, J., Opitz, T., Zheng, X., Bennett, M. V., and Zukin, R. S. (2001). mGluR1-mediated potentiation of NMDA receptors involves a rise in intracellular calcium and activation of protein kinase C. *Neuropharmacology* 40, 856–865. doi: 10.1016/s0028-3908(01)00005-3

Sladeczek, F., Momiyama, A., and Takahashi, T. (1993). Presynaptic inhibitory action of a metabotropic glutamate receptor agonist on excitatory transmission in visual cortical neurons. *Proc. Biol. Sci.* 253, 297–303. doi: 10.1098/rspb.1993.0117

Torrealba, F., Bustos, G., and Montero, V. M. (1996). Glutamate in the glomus cells of the cat carotid body: immunocytochemistry and in vitro release. *Neurochem. Int.* 28, 625–631. doi: 10.1016/0197-0186(95)00130-1

Traynelis, S. F., Wollmuth, L. P., McBain, C. J., Menniti, F. S., Vance, K. M., Ogden, K. K., et al. (2010). Glutamate receptor ion channels: structure, regulation, and function. *Pharmacol. Rev.* 62, 405–496. doi: 10.1124/pr.109.002451

Tremolizzo, L., Sala, G., Zoia, C. P., and Ferrarese, C. (2012). Assessing glutamatergic function and dysfunction in peripheral tissues. *Curr. Med. Chem.* 19, 1310–1315. doi: 10.2174/092986712799462702

Tse, A., Yan, L., Lee, A. K., and Tse, F. W. (2012). Autocrine and paracrine actions of ATP in rat carotid body. *Can. J. Physiol. Pharmacol.* 90, 705–711. doi: 10.1139/y2012-054

Varas, R., Alcayaga, J., and Iturriaga, R. (2003). ACh and ATP mediate excitatory transmission in cat carotid identified chemoreceptor units in vitro. *Brain Res.* 988, 154–163. doi: 10.1016/s0006-8993(03)03366-3

Vetrovoy, O., Stratilov, V., Nimiritsky, P., Makarevich, P., and Tyulkova, E. (2021). Prenatal hypoxia induces premature aging accompanied by impaired function of the glutamatergic system in rat hippocampus. *Neurochem. Res.* 46, 550–563. doi: 10.1007/s11064-020-03191-z

White, A. M., Kylänpää, R. A., Christie, L. A., McIntosh, S. J., Irving, A. J., and Platt, B. (2003). Presynaptic group I metabotropic glutamate receptors modulate synaptic transmission in the rat superior colliculus via 4-AP sensitive K(+) channels. *Br. J. Pharmacol.* 140, 1421–1433. doi: 10.1038/sj.bjp.0705570

Wittmann, M., Hubert, G. W., Smith, Y., and Conn, P. J. (2001). Activation of metabotropic glutamate receptor 1 inhibits glutamatergic transmission in the substantia nigra pars reticulata. *Neuroscience* 105, 881–889. doi: 10.1016/s0306-4522(01)00254-8

Xu, C., Zhang, W., Rondard, P., Pin, J. P., and Liu, J. (2014). Complex GABAB receptor complexes: how to generate multiple functionally distinct units from a single receptor. *Front. Pharmacol.* 5:12. doi: 10.3389/fphar.2014.00012

Xu, J., Xu, F., Tse, F. W., and Tse, A. (2005). ATP inhibits the hypoxia response in type I cells of rat carotid bodies. *J. Neurochem.* 92, 1419–1430. doi: 10.1111/j.1471-4159.2004.02978.x

Yokoyama, T., Nakamuta, N., Kusakabe, T., and Yamamoto, Y. (2014). Vesicular glutamate transporter 2-immunoreactive afferent nerve terminals in the carotid body of the rat. *Cell Tissue Res.* 358, 271–275. doi: 10.1007/s00441-014-1921-x

Zhang, M., Clarke, K., Zhong, H., Vollmer, C., and Nurse, C. A. (2009). Postsynaptic action of GABA in modulating sensory transmission in co-cultures of rat carotid body via GABA(A) receptors. *J. Physiol.* 587, 329–344. doi: 10.1113/jphysiol.2008.165035

Zhang, M., Vollmer, C., and Nurse, C. A. (2018). Adenosine and dopamine oppositely modulate a hyperpolarization-activated current I(h) in chemosensory neurons of the rat carotid body in co-culture. *J. Physiol.* 596, 3101–3117. doi: 10.1113/JP274743

Zhang, M., Zhong, H., Vollmer, C., and Nurse, C. A. (2000). Co-release of ATP and ACh mediates hypoxic signalling at rat carotid body chemoreceptors. *J. Physiol.* 525(Pt 1), 143–158. doi: 10.1111/j.1469-7793.2000.t01-1-00143.x

Zhou, Y., and Danbolt, N. C. (2014). Glutamate as a neurotransmitter in the healthy brain. *J. Neural Transm. (Vienna)* 121, 799–817. doi: 10.1007/s00702-014-1180-8

20

Tribbles Homolog 3-Mediated Vascular Insulin Resistance Contributes to Hypoxic Pulmonary Hypertension in Intermittent Hypoxia Rat Model

Fang Fan[1†], Jinxiao He[1†], Hui Su[2†], Haifeng Zhang[3], Hao Wang[1], Qianqian Dong[4], Minghua Zeng[1], Wenjuan Xing[5,6] and Xin Sun[1]**

[1]Department of Pediatrics, Xijing Hospital, Fourth Military Medical University, Xi'an, China, [2]Department of Geratology, Xijing Hospital, Fourth Military Medical University, Xi'an, China, [3]Teaching Experiment Center, Fourth Military Medical University, Xi'an, China, [4]Department of Natural Medicine, School of Pharmacy, Fourth Military Medical University, Xi'an, China, [5]School of Aerospace Medicine, Fourth Military Medical University, Xi'an, China, [6]State Key Laboratory of Space Medicine Fundamentals and Application, China Astronaut Research and Training Center, Beijing, China

***Correspondence:**
Xin Sun
sunxin6@fmmu.edu.cn
Wenjuan Xing
xwjfmmu@126.com

[†]These authors have contributed equally to this work

This study aimed to investigate the role of vascular insulin resistance (VIR) and Tribbles homolog 3 (TRIB3) in the pathogenesis of hypoxia-induced pulmonary hypertension (HPH). Rats were subjected to low air pressure and low oxygen intermittently for 4 weeks to induce HPH. The mean right ventricular pressure (mRVP), mean pulmonary arterial pressure (mPAP), and right ventricular index (RVI) were significantly increased in HPH rats. Pulmonary arteries from HPH rats showed VIR with reduced vasodilating effect of insulin. The protein levels of peroxisome proliferator-activated receptor gamma (PPARγ), phosphoinositide 3-kinase (PI3K), phosphorylations of Akt, and endothelial nitric oxide (NO) synthase (eNOS) were decreased, and TRIB3 and phosphorylated extracellular signal-regulated protein kinases (ERK1/2) were increased in pulmonary arteries of HPH rats. Early treatment of pioglitazone (PIO) partially reversed the development of HPH, improved insulin-induced vasodilation, and alleviated the imbalance of the insulin signaling. The overexpression of TRIB3 in rat pulmonary arterial endothelial cells (PAECs) reduced the levels of PPARγ, PI3K, phosphorylated Akt (p-Akt), and phosphorylated eNOS (p-eNOS) and increased p-ERK1/2 and the synthesis of endothelin-1 (ET-1), which were further intensified under hypoxic conditions. Moreover, TRIB3 knockdown caused significant improvement in Akt and eNOS phosphorylations and, otherwise, a reduction of ERK1/2 activation in PAECs after hypoxia. In conclusion, impaired insulin-induced pulmonary vasodilation and the imbalance of insulin-induced signaling mediated by TRIB3 upregulation in the endothelium contribute to the development of HPH. Early PIO treatment improves vascular insulin sensitivity that may help to limit the progression of hypoxic pulmonary hypertension.

Keywords: hypoxic pulmonary hypertension, proliferator-activated receptor gamma, pulmonary arterial endothelium, vascular insulin resistance, Tribbles homolog 3

INTRODUCTION

Pulmonary hypertension (PH) is a progressive disease featuring vascular remodeling of small pulmonary arteries, elevated pulmonary arterial resistance, and right ventricle hypertrophy (Latus et al., 2015). The mortality and morbidity of PH are remarkable. The etiology of PH is very complicated; it can be idiopathic, heritable, drug/toxin-induced, or associated with HIV infection, congenital heart diseases, lung diseases, and high-altitude habitancy. The development of pulmonary circulation disorders in hypoxia-induced pulmonary hypertension (HPH) is a response unique to the hypoxic environment. This pathological condition triggers the hypoxic vasoconstriction of pulmonary arteries to redistribute the blood flow from hypoxic alveoli to ample alveoli so as to fully oxygenate the blood (Serne et al., 1999; Kekalainen et al., 2000). In the long term, this compensatory strategy can intensify the constriction of pulmonary vessels and eventually cause endothelial dysfunction, remodeling, and stenosis of vessels. Therefore, acute and chronic hypoxia is one of the most effective and reproducible method to induce PH.

Insulin is a key regulator of blood glucose in the body. The condition of insulin resistance is a precursor to developing type 2 diabetes and many cardiovascular disorders. Insulin also has a vasoactive effect on the vascular endothelium in parallel with the metabolic effect on tissues (Munir and Quon, 2013; Xing et al., 2013a,b). It stimulates the production and release of nitric oxide (NO) from the vascular endothelial cells through protein kinase B (also known as Akt) mediated phosphorylation of endothelial NO synthase (eNOS) in a phosphoinositide 3-kinases (PI3K) dependent manner (Yu et al., 2011). Simultaneously, insulin triggers the activation of the mitogen-activated protein kinase (MAPK) pathway to promote the secretion of endothelin-1 (ET-1). The overall response of insulin on the healthy vascular endothelium depends on a balance of the two pathways and presents a vasodilated effect (Muniyappa et al., 2007). Abated vasodilatory effects and augmented vasoconstrictor actions of insulin are referred to as vascular insulin resistance (VIR). The molecular basis of VIR is selectively impaired in insulin-induced PI3K-dependent and intact or even enhanced MAPK-dependent signaling pathways (Muniyappa et al., 2020). The underproduction of NO and the imbalance of NO/ET-1 production are the signposts of endothelial dysfunction. VIR and endothelial dysfunction are vicious cycles in the development of diabetes, cardiovascular disease, and hypertension. However, whether VIR participated in the development of pulmonary circulation disorders and HPH remains largely elusive.

Tribbles homolog 3 (TRIB3) is a pseudokinase of the Tribbles family (Du et al., 2003). It is involved in various cellular functions, including endoplasmic reticulum stress, cell proliferation, and differentiation. TRIB3 is coupled to insulin resistance in oxidative stress, antioxidant stress, inflammation, adiponectin actions, peroxisome proliferator-activated receptor (PPAR) actions, SIRT1 actions, and insulin signal transduction (Koh et al., 2013; Zhang et al., 2016). Overexpression of TRIB3 downregulates insulin-induced Akt phosphorylation, and subsequent downstream insulin signaling and suppression of TRIB3 enhances insulin-stimulated signaling. Several studies demonstrated the key role of TRIB3 in regulating insulin's metabolic function. High-fat diet induced the high TRIB3 expression, which consequently affects insulin-induced glucose uptake and oxidation in muscle and fat tissues in rats (Liu et al., 2012a). TRIB3 proteins are upregulated in diabetic rats and distorted phosphorylation of Akt, and MAPK in diabetic rats is restored by the suppression of TRIB3 (Ti et al., 2011). Hypoxia was reported that induced TRIB3 expression (Wennemers et al., 2011). However, whether TRIB3 is responsible for VIR in HPH is still unknown.

Life style like exercise and intervention such as PPAR gamma (PPARγ) agonist pioglitazone (PIO) have been shown to improve cardiovascular insulin sensitivity and benefit cardiovascular function (Zhang et al., 2008). Most recently, PIO has been reported to reverse pulmonary arterial hypertension, another type of PH, and reverse vascular remodeling *via* fatty acid oxidation (Legchenko et al., 2018), inhibiting transforming growth factor-β (TGFβ1) signaling (Calvier et al., 2019) and 5-HT receptor signaling (Liu et al., 2012b). In addition, systemic insulin resistance (i.e., elevated fasting blood glucose and insulin levels) is associated with the development of pulmonary arterial hypertension (Hansmann et al., 2007) and treatment with PIO abnormal pulmonary artery muscularization. Whether PIO limited VIR in the development of hypoxia-induced pulmonary arterial disorders and HPH is still unknown. This study aimed to investigate the alterations and the mechanisms of the vascular insulin sensitivity of pulmonary arteries in an HPH rat model and the potential role of PIO in HPH.

MATERIALS AND METHODS

Animals

The 6-week male Sprague-Dawley rats (body weight: 200–220 g) were purchased from the Experimental Animal Center of the Fourth Military Medical University (Xi'an, Shaanxi province, China). They were fed with normal diet and water *ad libitum*. The experimental protocol was approved by the ethics committee of the Animal Experimentation of the Fourth Military Medical University and conducted according to the Guidelines of the Animal Experimentation of the Fourth Military Medical University.

Design of the Experiment

The rats were randomly assigned to four groups with seven rats in each group: normal control, HPH, HPH + PIO (E), and HPH + PIO (L). The rats in the last three groups were subjected to low air pressure (50 kPa) and low oxygen (10%) intermittently in an auto-modulating plastic cabin for 8 h and normoxia for 16 h every day, for a total of 4 weeks (Li et al., 2020). Anhydrous calcium chloride and soda lime were used in the plastic box to absorb water and CO_2. PIO pellets were dissolved in physiological saline to form a solution (1.5 mg/ml). Besides, HPH + PIO (E) group rats received early (E) PIO solution [10 mg/(kg d)] once daily for 7 days a week through intragastric administration in the 2nd week of the experiment. HPH + PIO (L) group rats received late (L) treatment of PIO in the same way in the last week of the experiment. HPH group rats were given saline as control. The normal control group was maintained in the same room under normal conditions (at atmospheric pressure and oxygen concentration).

Hemodynamic Measurement and Right Ventricular Hypertrophy

The mean pulmonary arterial pressure (mPAP) and mean right ventricular pressure (mRVP) were measured by jugular vein catheterization and followed the methodology in the previous study (Michelakis et al., 2002).

In addition, the right ventricular index (RVI) was calculated as an indicator of right ventricular hypertrophy. RVI represents the weight of the RV relative to LV + septum.

Morphometric Analysis

The same full section in the mid-portion of the lung parallel to the hilum was taken from all rats and embedded in paraffin. Transverse 10-μm left lung sections were stained using Verhoeff-van Gieson staining and H&E staining. The external diameter (ED), medial wall thickness (MT), medial cross-sectional area (MA), and total arterial cross-sectional area (TAA) of the peripheral pulmonary artery were measured in micrographs. Then, the MT (%) and MA (%) were calculated as follows: MT% = (MT/ED) × 100% and MA% = (MA/TAA) × 100%. The two ratios indicated the level of pathological thickening and remodeling of pulmonary arteries. Further, 7–10 pulmonary arteries were picked from random views of every lung, and the averages of morphometric parameters were used for conducting the statistical analysis.

Isometric Tension Measurement

The pulmonary arteries were isolated from rats and cut into 3-mm rings. Vascular responses to insulin in arteries were studied by exposing pulmonary arterial segments to insulin ($10^{-10} \sim 10^{-6}$ mol/L; Sigma-Aldrich, MO, United States), sodium nitroprusside (SNP) (10^{-10}~10^{-6} mol/L; Sigma-Aldrich, MO, United States), or PE (10^{-10}~10^{-5} mol/L; Sigma-Aldrich, MO, United States). PE (10^{-7} mol/L) was used before testing relaxation to insulin and SNP. The resulting changes in isometric tension were recorded using an RM6240 multichannel physiological recording and processing system (Chengdu Instrument Factory, China).

Primary Culture of Rat Pulmonary Microvascular Endothelial Cells

Rat primary pulmonary microvascular endothelial cells were cultured and maintained as previously described with modifications. The rats were anesthetized by the intraperitoneal injection of 0.3–0.5 ml/100 g chloral hydrate. The thoracic and abdominal regions were sterilized by applying 1% povidone-iodine on the skin. The abdominal cavity was opened, and the abdominal aorta was cut off to drain the blood. Subsequently, the thoracic cavity was opened, and the lungs were immediately removed and rinsed in phosphate-buffered saline (PBS) at pH equal to 7.4 thoroughly. About 1 mm of the fringe of the lung was cut off and cut into pieces of 0.5 × 0.5 × 0.5 mm^3 in fetal bovine serum (FBS). Small pieces of lung tissue were placed evenly at the bottom of the cell culture flask. The flask was placed upside down for incubation at 37°C (210 ml/L O_2) with minimal cell culture medium (M200; Sigma-Aldrich; 15% FBS and 20 g/L LSGS) at the bottom. The flask was reverted back after 4 h. The medium was replaced after 24 h to wash off erythrocytes. Small pieces of lung tissues were removed after 2 days of incubation. Light microscopic images showed the cobblestone morphology of cultured cells typical for endothelial cells. Factor VIII was positive in immunofluorescence staining. The cells were split after >80% confluence at the ratio of 1:2 and used for experiments between passages 2 and 4. A rabbit anti-human factor VIII antibody was purchased from Santa Cruz Biotechnology (TX, United States). Fluorescein isothiocyanate (FITC)-conjugated goat anti-rabbit immunoglobulin G was purchased from Abcam (Cambridge, United Kingdom).

In vitro Experiment Design

Experimental design No. 1: healthy pulmonary arterial endothelial cells (PAECs) at passages 2–4 were plated in a 60-mm cell culture dish (Corning) in 10% FBS M200 medium. After the cells grew to 60% confluence, a fresh medium with 10^{-7} mmol/L insulin was replaced. The dishes were then divided into normoxia and hypoxia groups and placed in a normoxia incubator (37°C, 210 ml/L O_2) and a hypoxia incubator (37°C, 100 ml/L O_2), respectively. The cells and culture media were collected after 6, 24, 48, and 96 h of incubation.

Experimental design No. 2: healthy PAECs at passages 2–4 were plated in a 60-mm cell culture dish (Corning) in 10% FBS M200 medium. For exposure to hypoxia, PAECs were placed in a hypoxia incubator (Thermo Fisher, Boston, MA, United States) filled with a mixture of 10% O2 and 5% CO2 at 37°C. The normoxic control group was filled with a mixture of 21% O2 and 5% CO2 at 37°C. Cells were treated with 10^{-7} mmol/L insulin. The cells were harvested after 48 h of incubation. The proteins were extracted for the immunoblotting test.

Small Interfering RNA Transfection

For gene silencing assay, small interfering RNA (siRNA) for TRIB3 messenger RNA (mRNA) was designed and purchased from GenePharma (ShangHai, China). The target sequence used for TRIB3 siRNA knockdown was 5'-GAAGAAACCGUUGGA GUUTT-3'. PAECs were transfected with TRIB3 siRNA or scramble control by Lipofectamine™ RNAiMAX (Invitrogen) following the manufacturer's instructions. Cells were harvested for western blot analyses 48 h later.

Quantification of NO and ET-1 Expression

The NO concentration in the cell culture media was quantified using a commercial NO assay kit (nitrate reductase method) from Nanjing Jiancheng Bioengineering Institute (Jiangsu Province, China).

Total RNA was isolated from cells using TRIzol reagent according to the manufacturer's protocol (TaKaRa, Japan). Total RNA (0.5 μg) was converted into first-strand complementary DNA in a 20-μl reaction mixture using a One-step Reverse Transcriptase kit (TaKaRa). ET-1 expression was determined by real-time quantitative PCR (forward: 5'-CAAACCGATGTCCTCGTA-3' and reverse: 5'-ACCAAACACATTTCCCTATT-3'). The quantitative expression of the genes was normalized against glyceraldehyde 3-phosphate dehydrogenase (GAPDH; forward: 5'-GATTTGGCCGTATCGGAC-3' and reverse: 5'-GAAGACGCCAGTAGACTC-3'). The reactions were carried out using SYBR Green as a fluorescence dye on a real-time PCR thermal cycler (CFX96 Real-Time PCR cycler; Bio-Rad Laboratories, CA, United States). The $2^{-\Delta\Delta}$CT method was used for relative expression analysis. The experiment was repeated three times.

Western Blot Analysis

To analyze the insulin-induced signaling pathway, mice were given hypodermic injections of 5 mU/g body weight insulin (Novo Nordisk, Plainsboro, NJ, United States) and sacrificed 30 min later to collected vascular tissues. Tissues or cells were lysed with western radio immunoprecipitation assay (RIPA) lysis buffer (Beyotime Institute of Biotechnology, China) supplemented with Complete Mini Protease Inhibitor mixture (Roche Applied Science, Penzberg, Germany) and 1% phosphatase inhibitor mixture (Roche Applied Science). The protein concentration was determined using a bicinchoninic acid (BCA) Protein Quantification Kit (Beyotime Institute of Biotechnology, China). Each lysate containing an equal amount of total protein was loaded and separated using the sodium dodecyl sulfate-polyacrylamide gel electrophoresis method, transferred to polyvinylidene fluoride (Invitrogen, CA, United States) membrane, and probed with specific antibodies. After incubation with horseradish peroxidase-conjugated secondary antibodies (Boster Biological Technology, CA, United States), the blots were visualized with enhanced chemiluminescence detection reagents (Millipore, MA, United States), followed by autoradiography using a Kodak developing system. The intensity of images was quantified using Quantity One 4.0. Western blot analysis was performed using antibodies against Akt (60 kDa, 1:1000), phosphorylated Akt (p-Akt; 60 kDa, 1:1000), extracellular signal-regulated protein kinases 1 and 2 (ERK1/2, 42 and 44 kDa, 1:1000), p-ERK1/2 (42 and 44 kDa, 1:1000), and PI3K (110 kDa, 1:1000) obtained from Cell Signaling Technology (MA, United States); phosphorylated eNOS (p-eNOS; 130 kDa, 1:1000) and eNOS (130 kDa, 1:1000) from BD Biosciences (CA, United States); and TRIB3 (45 kDa, 1:200) and PPARγ (55 kDa, 1:500) from Santa Cruz Biotechnology.

Overexpression of TRIB3 With Lentivirus

Primary PAECs at the second passage were plated into six-well plates. They were infected with the lentivirus harboring *TRIB3* (GeneChem, Shanghai, China) gene according to the manufacturer's protocol. PAECs (80%) were positively infected with lentivirus (green fluorescence) after 3 days of incubation. The cell culture medium was replaced with fresh M200 medium (Gibco, Invitrogen, CA, United States) with 10% FBS (Hyclone, South Logan, UT, United States) and insulin (10^{-7} mmol/L).

Statistical Analysis

All values are presented as means ± SEM of *n* independent experiments. Statistical significance was determined by Student's *t*-test (analysis of two groups) or ANOVA (analysis of four groups), and *post hoc* comparisons, adjusted for multiple comparisons by Bonferroni's correction, were performed if ANOVAs revealed significances. Repetitive measure ANOVA was used in analyzing vascular tension at different points. In all statistical comparisons, probabilities of 0.05 or less were considered to be statistically significant.

RESULTS

Chronic Hypoxia Induced Pulmonary Hypertension and Impaired Insulin-Induced Vasodilation in Pulmonary Arteries

Chronic hypoxia was induced by exposing animals in HPH group to both hypobaric pressure and oxygen-poor air for 4 weeks. The pathological features of pulmonary vascular function and hypertrophy mimic the ones observed in human PH. The main parameters to define PH were tested in all the studied groups. The mPAP, mRVP, and RVI all significantly increased in rats in the HPH group compared with the control group ($p < 0.01$). Vascular remodeling is an important pathological feature of PH, which leads to increased pulmonary vascular resistance. The histological structure and thickness of pulmonary arteries from the control group were normal. Remodeling of the arteries in the HPH group was manifested by a significant alteration in the ratio of MT to ED (MT%) and the ratio of MA to TAA (MA%; **Table 1**). The media thickened, and the arterial lumen was narrowed in the HPH group compared with the control group (**Figures 1D,E**). We also detected RV mRNA levels of brain natriuretic peptide (BNP) and β-myosin heavy chain (β-MHC). Chronic hypoxia caused increased BNP and β-MHC levels (**Figures 1F,G**), indicating right ventricular hypertrophy.

Insulin has a vasodilated effect on arterial rings *in vitro*. VIR is manifested by the reduced vasodilating response to insulin (Wang et al., 2011). Insulin induced a dose-dependent vasodilation in pulmonary arteries from rats of all groups.

TABLE 1 | Comparing MT and MA% between different study groups ($n = 6$, $\bar{x} \pm s$).

Group	MT%	MA%
Control	11.0 ± 1.4	25.6 ± 2.6
HPH	24.7 ± 2.2*	54.0 ± 2.3*
HPH + PIO (E)	13.7 ± 2.1*#	30.5 ± 1.8*#
HPH + PIO (L)	23.0 ± 2.8*	52.9 ± 2.2*

*$p < 0.01$ vs. control group.
#$p < 0.05$ vs. HPH group.
The external diameter (ED), medial wall thickness (MT), medial cross-sectional area (MA), and total arterial cross-sectional area (TAA) of peripheral pulmonary artery were measured. Then, MT and MA% were calculated as follows: MT% = (MT/ED) × 100%; MA% = (MA/TAA) × 100%.

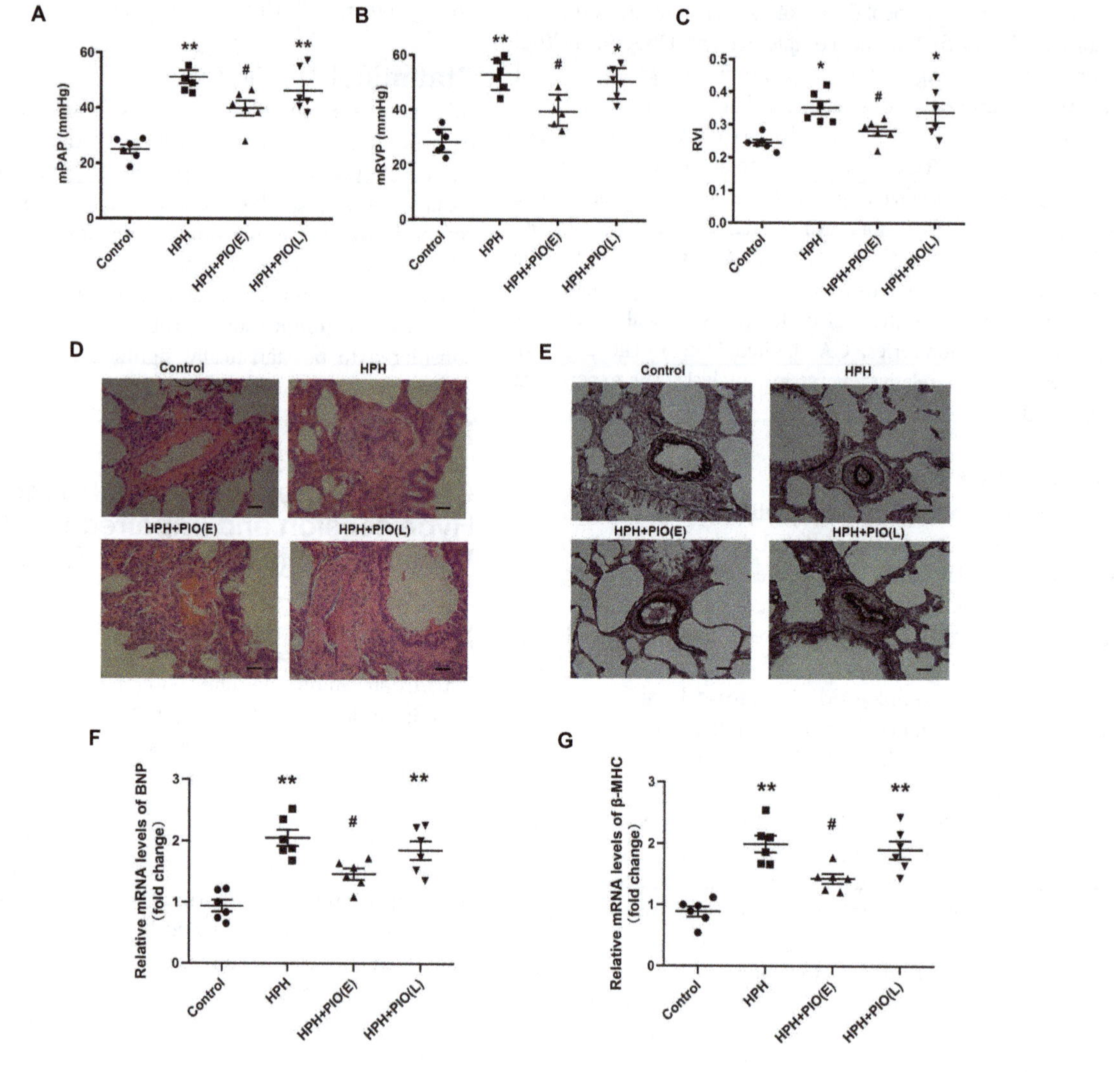

FIGURE 1 | Early treatment with peroxisome proliferator-activated receptor gamma (PPARγ) agonist pioglitazone (PIO) partly reversed the hypoxia-induced pulmonary hypertension (HPH). **(A)** Mean pulmonary artery pressure (mPAP) of different study groups; **(B)** Mean right ventricular pressure (mRVP) of different study groups; **(C)** Right ventricle index (RVI) of different study group. **(D)** Representative microphotographs of pulmonary arteries in rats obtained from four study groups (H&E staining), scale bar = 25 μm; **(E)** Representative microphotographs of pulmonary arteries in rats obtained from four study groups (Verhoeff-van Gieson staining), scale bar = 25 μm. **(F)** and **(G)** messenger RNA (mRNA) levels of brain natriuretic peptide (BNP) and β-myosin heavy chain (β-MHC) in right ventricular of hearts. Data were presented as means ± SEM. $n = 6$–8. $^{*}p < 0.05$, $^{**}p < 0.01$ vs. control group; $^{\#}p < 0.05$ vs. HPH group.

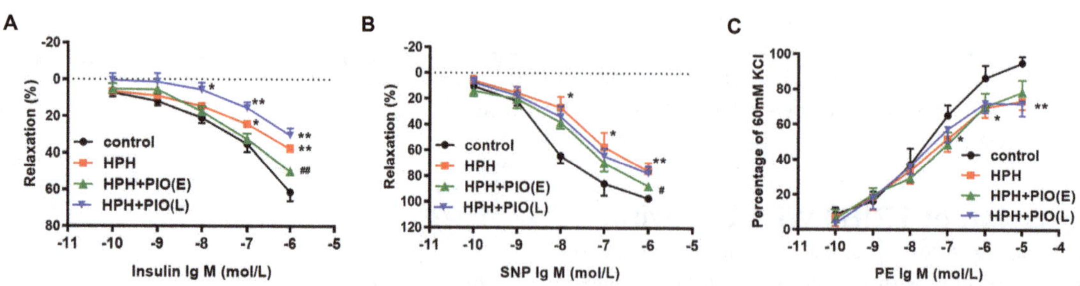

FIGURE 2 | Early treatment of PIO partly reversed the system insulin resistance and the pulmonary arterial insulin resistance. **(A)** Response of the pulmonary artery of each study group to insulin. **(B)** Response of the pulmonary artery of each study group to SNP. **(C)** Response of the pulmonary artery of each study group to PE. Arterial segments of 2–5 from each rat were used. Data were presented as means ± SEM. $n = 6$. $^{*}p < 0.05$, $^{**}p < 0.01$ vs. control group; $^{\#}p < 0.05$, $^{\#\#}p < 0.01$ vs. HPH group.

The insulin-induced relaxation was significantly attenuated in the pulmonary arteries from HPH rats compared with the control group (**Figures 2A–C**), indicating VIR occurred in the pulmonary arteries in HPH rat models.

Early Treatment of PIO Partly Alleviated Vascular Insulin Resistance and Pulmonary Hypertension

Considering PIO is a potent insulin-sensitizing agent, we next treated the HPH rats with PIO. After exposure to chronic hypoxia for 4 weeks, treatment with PIO at early stage of HPH significantly reduced mPAP and RVI (**Figure 1**; $p < 0.05$). However, treatment with PIO at late stage did not improve the HPH as no significant differences were found in these parameters between the HPH + PIO (L) and HPH groups. Consistently, the histopathological alterations were alleviated after early treatment of PIO in the HPH + PIO (E) group. Early treatment with PIO attenuated hypoxia-induced increases in both BNP and β-MHC levels (**Figures 1F,G**). However, PIO treatment in the late stage failed to reverse the

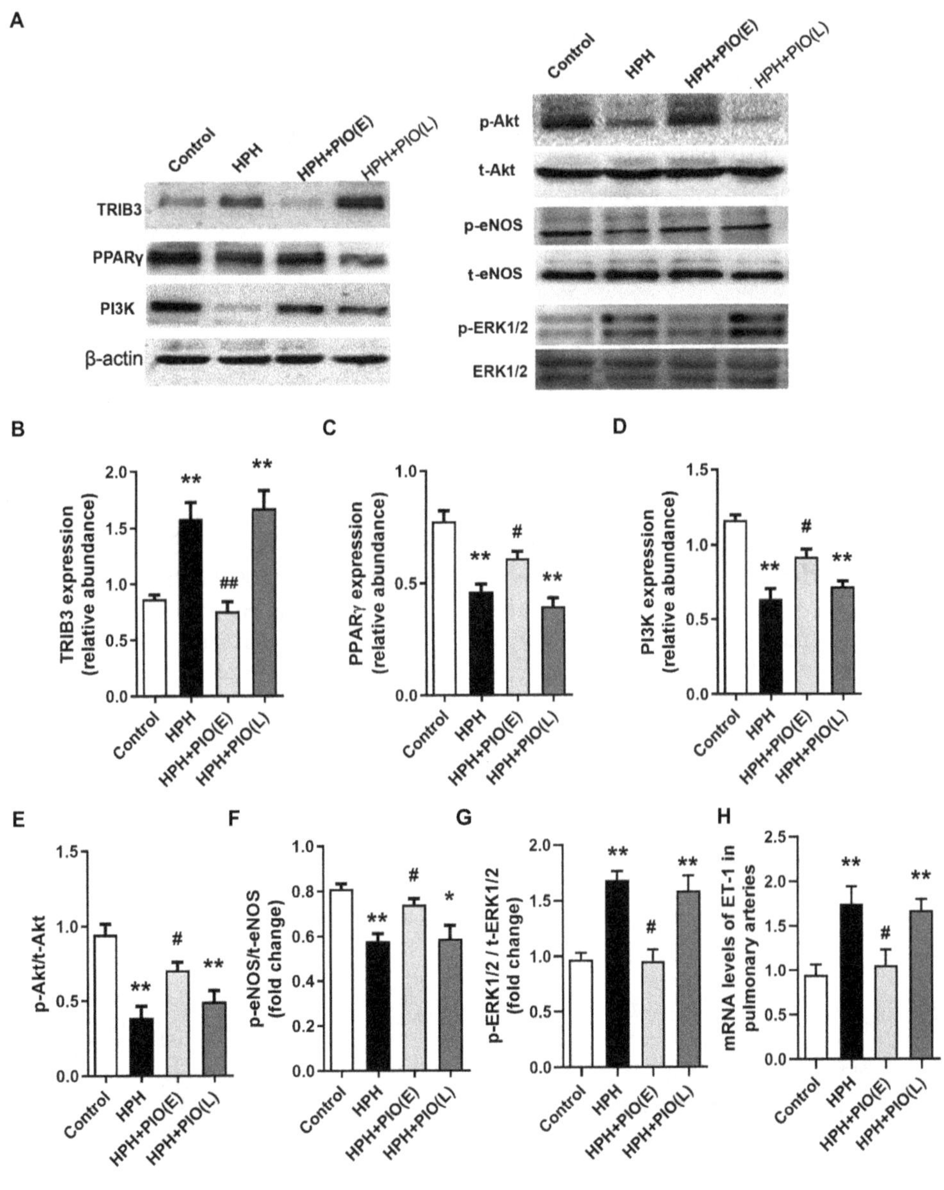

FIGURE 3 | Changes in the protein levels of tribbles homolog 3 (TRIB3), PPARγ, and insulin signaling pathways in the pulmonary arteries of HPH rats. **(A)** Representative western blots showing the expressions of TRIB3, PPARγ, phosphoinositide 3-kinase (PI3K), Akt, and endothelial NO synthase (eNOS), and phosphorylations of Akt and eNOS. **(B)** Western blotting analyzing the protein TRIB3 expression. **(C)** Western blotting analyzing the protein PPARγ expression. **(D)** Western blotting analyzing the protein PI3K expression. **(E)** Western blotting analyzing ratio of phosphorylated Akt (p-Akt) to total Akt. **(F)** Western blotting analyzing ratio of phosphorylated eNOS (p-eNOS) to total eNOS. **(G)** Western blotting analyzing ratio of phosphorylated ERK1/2 (p-ERK1/2) to total ERK1/2. **(H)** mRNA levels of ET-1. Data were presented as means ± SEM. $n = 4$. *$p < 0.05$, **$p < 0.01$ vs. control group; #$p < 0.05$, ##$p < 0.01$ vs. HPH group.

histopathological alterations in the pulmonary arteries of rats in the HPH + PIO (L) group.

We next checked the insulin's effect on pulmonary arterial rings *in vitro*. Early treatment with PIO improved insulin-induced pulmonary arterial relaxation in the HPH rats. While the insulin-induced relaxation of pulmonary arterial rings from rats in the HPH + PIO (L) group was not significantly different from that in the HPH group. In addition, responses to SNP and PE were also impaired in HPH pulmonary arteries. Early treatment with PIO partially improved SNP induced vasodilation but not PE induced vasoconstriction. These data suggested that PIO treatment in the early stage partly alleviate VIR and pulmonary hypertension.

Dysregulation of TRIB3, PPARγ, and Insulin Signaling in the Pulmonary Arteries of Rats With HPH

Tribbles homolog 3 expression significantly increased, while PPARγ expression decreased remarkably in the pulmonary arteries from HPH rat models compared with the control group. Early PIO treatment partly reversed the protein levels of both TRIB3 and PPARγ; however, no effect was noted when PIO was given in the late stage of the HPH. The levels of PI3K, p-Akt, and p-eNOS significantly reduced in the pulmonary arteries of rats with HPH compared with those in the control group. Early PIO treatment reversed the reduction of p-Akt, PI3K, and p-eNOS compared with those in the HPH group; however, late treatment failed to act in the same way (**Figure 3**).

NO Production Decreased and ET-1 Production Increased in Hypoxic Primary Pulmonary Artery Endothelial Cells

In the presence of insulin in the cell culture medium, the NO production by PAECs under the normoxic condition was similar for four time points. After 6 h, hypoxia induced higher NO production than that under the normoxic condition. After 24 h, the concentrations of NO under the hypoxic condition declined dramatically over time and were lower than those under the normoxic condition at each time point (**Figure 4A**). No significant difference in the mRNA levels of ET-1 was observed between different time intervals under the normoxic condition. ET-1 mRNA levels significantly increased under the hypoxic condition than under the normoxic condition with the same time interval; it progressively increased over time under the hypoxic condition (**Figure 4B**).

Dysregulation of Proteins in PAECs in the Insulin Signaling Pathway at Different Time Intervals Under the Normoxic or Hypoxic Condition

Pulmonary arterial endothelial cells were cultured in the medium with 10^{-7} mmol/L of insulin. Among groups with different time intervals under the normoxic condition, the protein levels of TRIB3, PPARγ, PI3K, p-Akt, p-ERK1, and p-eNOS were comparable. In the acute phase of hypoxia (6 or 8 h), the protein level of TRIB3 increased significantly compared with that at the same time interval under the normoxic condition and further increased over time under the hypoxic condition. The protein levels of p-Akt, PI3K, and p-eNOS showed similar trends, which significantly increased after 6 h compared with the same time interval under the normoxic condition, and decreased over time under the hypoxic condition (**Figures 5C–F**). In the acute phase of hypoxia, the protein level of PPARγ was comparable with that under the normoxic condition. It decreased after 24 h under the hypoxic condition compared with the same time point under the normoxic condition, and further decreased over time (**Figure 5B**). The protein level of p-ERK1/2 increased at every time point under the hypoxic condition compared with the normoxic condition; it dramatically increased over time under the hypoxic condition (**Figure 5**).

PPARγ and PI3K/Akt/eNOS in PAECs Were Reduced With TRIB3 Overexpression Under Normoxic and Hypoxic Conditions

Pulmonary arterial endothelial cells were cultured in a medium with 10^{-7} mmol/L of insulin under hypoxic or normoxic condition, with the overexpression of TRIB3 or control vehicle. TRIB3 level was increased and PPARγ levels was decreased in PAECs under hypoxia condition. Hypoxia caused reduced PPARγ and the protein levels of PI3K, p-Akt, and p-eNOS. Importantly, overexpression of TRIB3 further decreased the protein levels of PPARγ, PI3K, p-Akt, and p-eNOS. The p-ERK1/2 levels increased in the TRIB3 + hypoxia, TRIB3 + normoxia, and control + hypoxia groups compared with the control + normoxia group, with the highest level detected in the TRIB3 + hypoxia group (**Figure 6**).

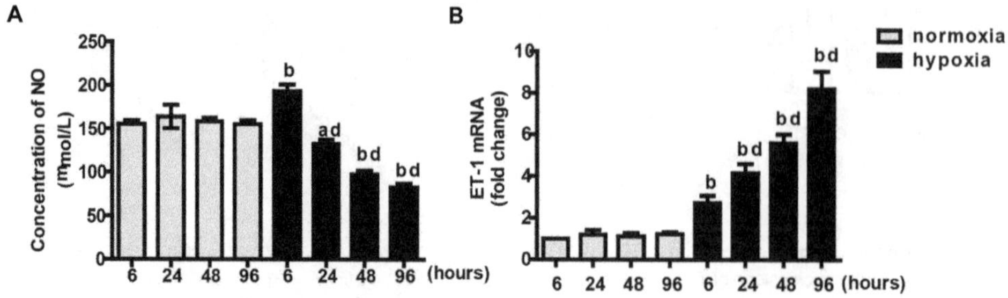

FIGURE 4 | Measurements of NO concentration **(A)** and endothelin-1 (ET-1) mRNA **(B)** at different time intervals under normoxia or hypoxia condition. Values are presented as mean ± SEM, $n = 7$. [a]$p < 0.05$, [b]$p < 0.01$ vs. the same time point under normoxia condition; [d]$p < 0.01$ vs. 6 h under hypoxia condition.

TRIB3 Knockdown Improved Akt and eNOS Phosphorylations and Reduced ERK1/2 Activation in PAECs After Hypoxia

To determine whether TRIB3 is responsible for the impaired insulin signaling, PAECs were cultured in a medium with 10^{-7} mmol/L of insulin under hypoxic condition and measured the activation of insulin signaling with TRIB3 knockdown by siRNA. The results showed that TRIB3 was significantly reduced by siRNA in PAECs. The effect of knockdown of TRIB3 with siTRIB3 or scrambled siRNA on insulin signaling pathway in hypoxia treated PAECs was detected by western blot. p-Akt and p-eNOS were significantly enhanced in the PAECs after knockdown of TRIB3, while activation of ERK1/2 was markedly decreased after siTRIB3 treatment (**Figure 7**).

DISCUSSION

The present study has novel findings that VIR mediated by TRIB3 played an important role in the development of HPH.

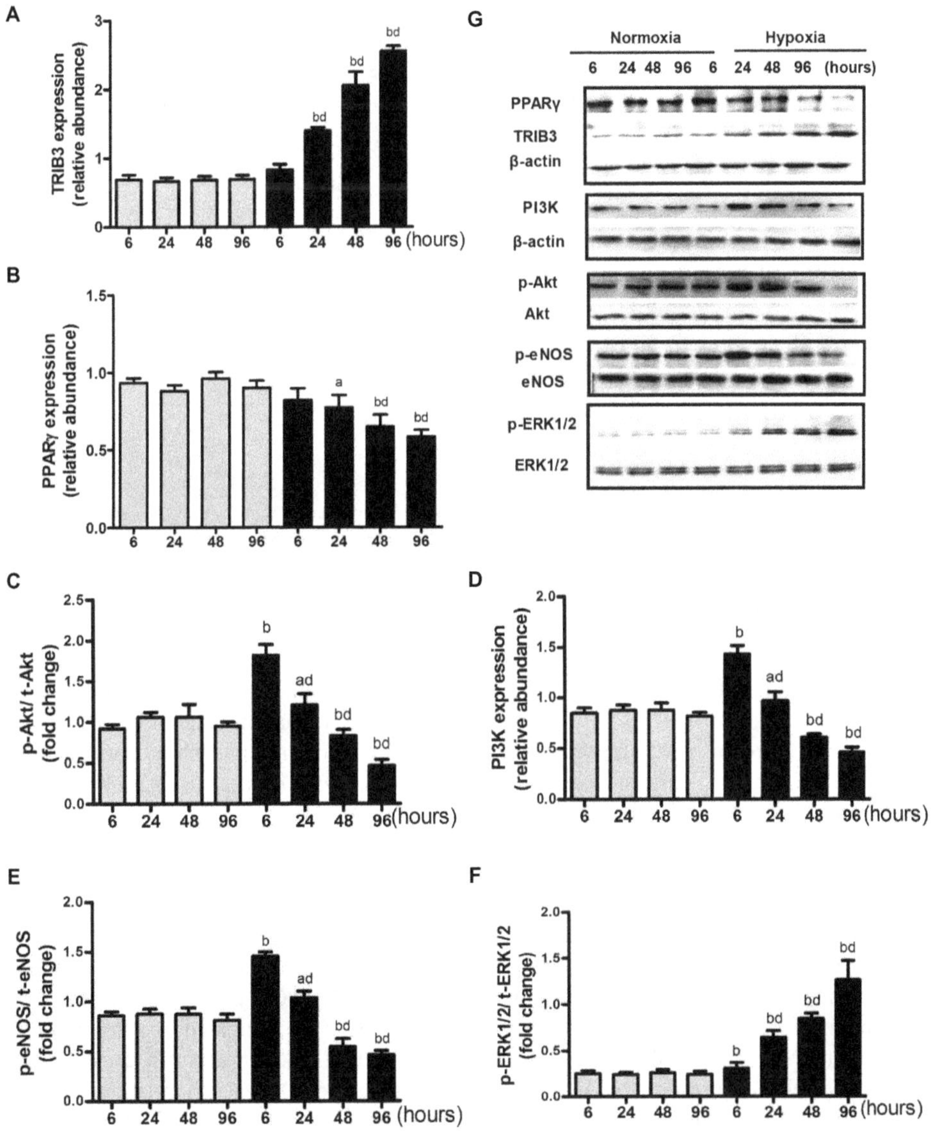

FIGURE 5 | Expression of proteins in insulin signaling pathway under normoxia or hypoxia condition. **(A)** Western blotting analyzing the protein TRIB3 expression. **(B)** Western blotting analyzing the protein PPARγ expression. **(C)** Western blotting analyzing ratio of phosphorylated Akt to total Akt. **(D)** Western blotting analyzing the protein PI3K expression. **(E)** Western blotting analyzing ratio of phosphorylated eNOS to total eNOS. **(F)** Western blotting analyzing ratio of phosphorylated ERK1/2 (p-ERK1/2) to total ERK1/2. **(G)** Representative western blots showing the expressions of TRIB3, PPARγ, PI3K, Akt, eNOS, and ERK1/2, and phosphorylations of Akt, eNOS, and ERK1/2. $^{a}p < 0.05$, $^{b}p < 0.01$ vs. the same time point under normoxia condition; Values are presented as mean ± SEM, $n = 7$. $^{d}p < 0.01$ vs. 6 h under hypoxia condition.

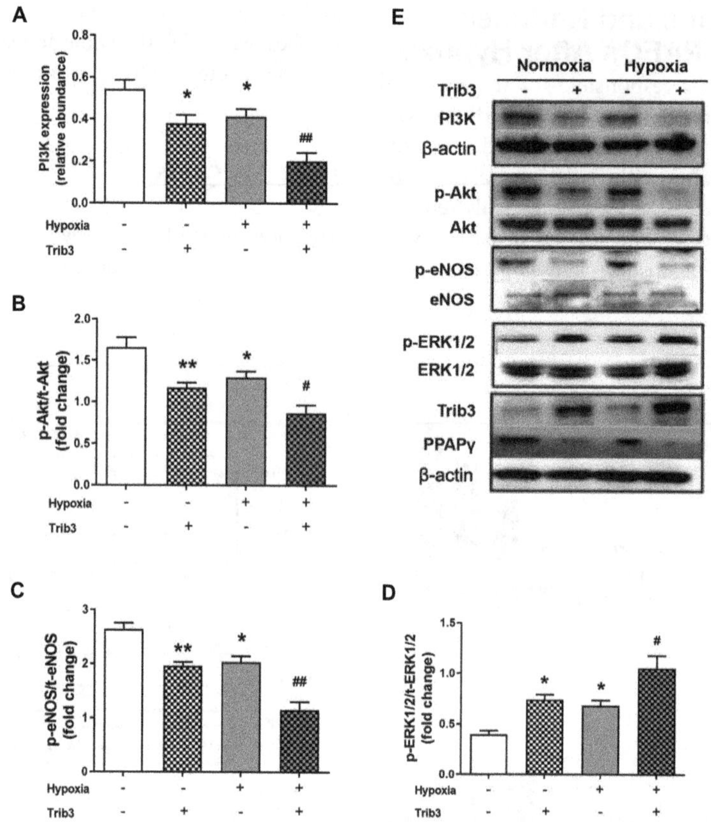

FIGURE 6 | The effect of over-expression of TRIB3 with lentivirus on the protein levels of insulin signaling pathway in PAECs. **(A)** Western blotting analyzing the protein PI3K expression. **(B)** Western blotting analyzing ratio of p-Akt to total Akt. **(C)** Western blotting analyzing ratio of p-eNOS to total eNOS. **(D)** Western blotting analyzing ratio of phosphorylated extracellular signal-regulated protein kinases 1 and 2 (ERK1/2) to total ERK1/2. **(E)** Representative western blots showing the expressions of PI3K, Akt, eNOS, and ERK1/2 and phosphorylations of Akt, eNOS, and ERK1/2. Values are presented as mean ± SEM, $n = 6$. $^{*}p < 0.05$, $^{**}p < 0.01$ vs. normoxia control group; $^{\#}p < 0.05$, $^{\#\#}p < 0.01$ vs. hypoxia control group.

And improvement of the vascular insulin sensitivity at early stage by PIO alleviated HPH.

Insulin's actions on vascular are of great importance as it enhances the compliance of arteries, relaxes arterioles to increase tissue blood flow, and expands perfusion. The present study reveals that VIR is closely associated with the development of HPH. The disturbance of the balance between ET-1 and NO weakened the vasodilating activity and increased the vasoconstrictive activity of the vessels. Disturbance of endothelium may further lead to vessel injury, remodeling, thrombogenesis, and occlusion. We also observed increased systemic blood glucose and insulin levels in HPH rats. Research has shown that hypoxia acutely or chronically influences the control of blood glucose and related hormones. In our study, the increase of glucose is likely due to the intermittent nature of the hypoxia challenge. This is a limitation of the study.

The present study showed an association between hypoxia-induced TRIB3 expression and VIR in pulmonary arteries. TRIB3 levels were increased in pulmonary arteries from HPH rats, accompanied with reduced PPARγ, and imbalance between insulin-induced Akt/eNOS/NO and ERK1/2/ET-1 signaling. Overexpression of TRIB3 in PAECs caused impaired Akt and eNOS activation. These findings were consistent with previous observations that pathological overexpression of TRIB3 blocked insulin-induced Akt phosphorylation, negatively regulated insulin action, and contributed to hyperglycemia and insulin resistance in liver and skeletal muscle (Du et al., 2003; Liu et al., 2010). Therefore, upregulated TRIB3 decreased the level of p-Akt and distorted subsequent signaling pathways. On the other hand, overexpression of TRIB3 in PAECs enhanced insulin-stimulated ERK1/2 phosphorylation. TRIB3 is a known regulator of MAPK–ERK pathway in cancer and cardiomyopathy models (Tang et al., 2008; Izrailit et al., 2013) by directly interacted with ERK or increased posttranslational phosphorylation. Moreover, TRIB3 knockdown caused significant improvement in Akt and eNOS phosphorylations and otherwise a reduction of ERK1/2 activation in PAECs after hypoxia, suggesting that TRIB3 mediates hypoxia-induced VIR and endothelial dysfunction.

Most recent study found that PPARγ activation by PIO prevents pulmonary arterial hypertension, the pathogenesis of which is different from that HPH. The present study for the first time identified PIO treatment at the early stage benefits hypoxia-induced pulmonary arterial dysfunction and HPH, which is at least partially relies on the improvement of vascular

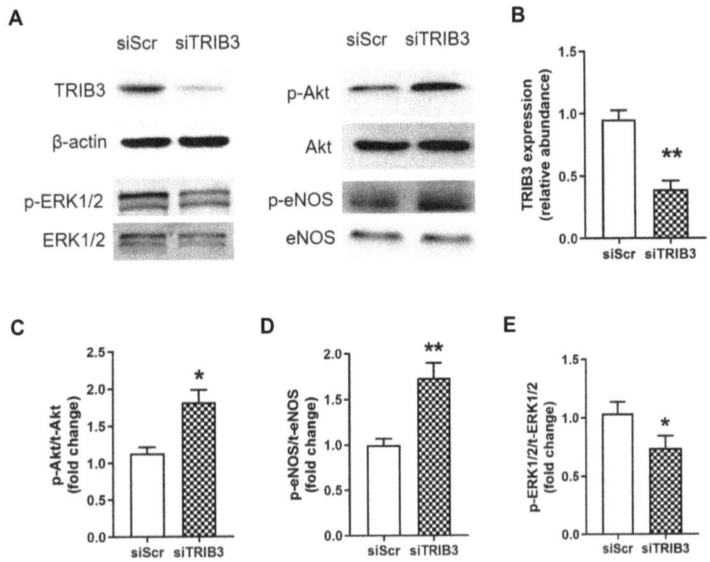

FIGURE 7 | The effect of knockdown of TRIB3 with siTRIB3 or scrambled siRNA on the protein levels of insulin signaling pathway in PAECs after hypoxia. **(A)** Representative western blots showing the expressions of TRIB3, Akt, eNOS, and ERK1/2 and phosphorylations of Akt, eNOS, and ERK1/2. **(B)** Western blotting analyzing the protein TRIB3 expression. **(C)** Western blotting analyzing ratio of p-Akt to total Akt. **(D)** Western blotting analyzing ratio of p-eNOS to total eNOS. **(E)** Western blotting analyzing ratio of phosphorylated ERK1/2 to total ERK1/2. Values are presented as mean ± SEM, $n = 4$. $^{*}p < 0.05$, $^{**}p < 0.01$ vs. siScr control group.

insulin sensitivity and vasodilation. TRIB3 has been identified acting as a potent negative regulator of PPARγ (Takahashi et al., 2008), indicating that the increase of TRIB3 level may be responsible for the limit effects of late PIO treatment.

The present study provided new insights into the development of therapeutics for HPH. Hypoxia-induced TRIB3 upregulation is a potential molecular basis of HPH. TRIB3 suppresses PPARγ and regulates insulin signaling pathway, resulting in the reduction of vascular NO production and raise of ET-1 secretion. Nevertheless, whether other subtypes of PH can benefit from improving insulin sensitivity or TRIB3 reduction need further study. TRIB3 is also a positive regulator of canonical TGF-β signaling to regulate fibroblast activation and tissue fibrosis (Tomcik et al., 2016). PPARγ, which could be regulated by TRIB3, was reported that inhibited TGF-β signaling and acted as a link between pro-proliferative TGF-β and anti-proliferative bone morphogenetic protein 2 (BMP2) signalings in vascular smooth muscle cells and inhibited pulmonary arterial hypertension (Calvier et al., 2017). Additionally, TRIB3 deficiency ameliorates metabolic disturbance inflammation, fibrosis, and myocardial hypertrophy in rats with dilated cardiomyopathy (Ti et al., 2011) indicating the potential benefits of TRIB3 regarding its anti-fibrotic and metabolic modulating effects.

In summary, this study indicated that VIR plays an important role in the development of HPH. The impaired insulin-induced pulmonary vasodilation and the imbalance of insulin-induced signalings are mediated by TRIB3 upregulation in the endothelium of HPH. PIO treatment beginning at the early stage improves vascular insulin sensitivity that may help to limit the progression of hypoxic pulmonary hypertension, which could provide a new perspective in managing patients with HPH, focusing on improving the pulmonary vascular IR in the early stage.

ETHICS STATEMENT

The animal study was reviewed and approved by the ethics committee of the Animal Experimentation of the Fourth Military Medical University.

AUTHOR CONTRIBUTIONS

FF, JH, and HS carried out the studies, collected data, and drafted the manuscript. HW, QD, and MZ collected data and performed the statistical analysis. HZ, WX, and XS designed the study and revised the manuscript. All authors contributed to the article and approved the submitted version.

REFERENCES

Calvier, L., Boucher, P., Herz, J., and Hansmann, G. (2019). LRP1 deficiency in vascular SMC leads to pulmonary arterial hypertension that is reversed by PPARgamma activation. *Circ. Res.* 124, 1778–1785. doi: 10.1161/CIRCRESAHA.119.315088

Calvier, L., Chouvarine, P., Legchenko, E., Hoffmann, N., Geldner, J., Borchert, P., et al. (2017). PPARgamma links BMP2 and TGFbeta1 pathways in vascular smooth muscle cells, regulating cell proliferation and glucose metabolism. *Cell Metab.* 25, 1118.e7–1134.e7. doi: 10.1016/j.cmet.2017.03.011

Du, K., Herzig, S., Kulkarni, R. N., and Montminy, M. (2003). TRB3: a tribbles homolog that inhibits Akt/PKB activation by insulin in liver. *Science* 300, 1574–1577. doi: 10.1126/science.1079817

Hansmann, G., Wagner, R. A., Schellong, S., Perez, V. A., Urashima, T., Wang, L., et al. (2007). Pulmonary arterial hypertension is linked to insulin resistance and reversed by peroxisome proliferator-activated receptor-gamma activation. *Circulation* 115, 1275–1284. doi: 10.1161/CIRCULATIONAHA.106.663120

Izrailit, J., Berman, H. K., Datti, A., Wrana, J. L., and Reedijk, M. (2013). High throughput kinase inhibitor screens reveal TRB3 and MAPK-ERK/TGFbeta pathways as fundamental notch regulators in breast cancer. *Proc. Natl. Acad. Sci. U. S. A.* 110, 1714–1719. doi: 10.1073/pnas.1214014110

Kekalainen, P., Sarlund, H., and Laakso, M. (2000). Long-term association of cardiovascular risk factors with impaired insulin secretion and insulin resistance. *Metabolism* 49, 1247–1254. doi: 10.1053/meta.2000.9514

Koh, H. J., Toyoda, T., Didesch, M. M., Lee, M. Y., Sleeman, M. W., Kulkarni, R. N., et al. (2013). Tribbles 3 mediates endoplasmic reticulum stress-induced insulin resistance in skeletal muscle. *Nat. Commun.* 4:1871. doi: 10.1038/ncomms2851

Latus, H., Delhaas, T., Schranz, D., and Apitz, C. (2015). Treatment of pulmonary arterial hypertension in children. *Nat. Rev. Cardiol.* 12, 244–254. doi: 10.1038/nrcardio.2015.6

Legchenko, E., Chouvarine, P., Borchert, P., Fernandez-Gonzalez, A., Snay, E., Meier, M., et al. (2018). PPARgamma agonist pioglitazone reverses pulmonary hypertension and prevents right heart failure via fatty acid oxidation. *Sci. Transl. Med.* 10:eaao0303. doi: 10.1126/scitranslmed.aao0303

Li, J., Jia, M., Liu, M., Cao, Z., Wang, X., Feng, N., et al. (2020). The effect of activated kappa-opioid receptor (kappa-OR) on the role of calcium sensing receptor (CaSR) in preventing hypoxic pulmonary hypertension development. *Biomed. Pharmacother.* 125:109931. doi: 10.1016/j.biopha.2020.109931

Liu, Y., Tian, X. Y., Mao, G., Fang, X., Fung, M. L., Shyy, J. Y., et al. (2012b). Peroxisome proliferator-activated receptor-gamma ameliorates pulmonary arterial hypertension by inhibiting 5-hydroxytryptamine 2B receptor. *Hypertension* 60, 1471–1478. doi: 10.1161/HYPERTENSIONAHA.112.198887

Liu, J., Wu, X., Franklin, J. L., Messina, J. L., Hill, H. S., Moellering, D. R., et al. (2010). Mammalian Tribbles homolog 3 impairs insulin action in skeletal muscle: role in glucose-induced insulin resistance. *Am. J. Physiol. Endocrinol. Metab.* 298, E565–E576. doi: 10.1152/ajpendo.00467.2009

Liu, J., Zhang, W., Chuang, G. C., Hill, H. S., Tian, L., Fu, Y., et al. (2012a). Role of TRIB3 in regulation of insulin sensitivity and nutrient metabolism during short-term fasting and nutrient excess. *Am. J. Physiol. Endocrinol. Metab.* 303, E908–E916. doi: 10.1152/ajpendo.00663.2011

Michelakis, E. D., Mcmurtry, M. S., Wu, X. C., Dyck, J. R., Moudgil, R., Hopkins, T. A., et al. (2002). Dichloroacetate, a metabolic modulator, prevents and reverses chronic hypoxic pulmonary hypertension in rats: role of increased expression and activity of voltage-gated potassium channels. *Circulation* 105, 244–250. doi: 10.1161/hc0202.101974

Munir, K. M., and Quon, M. J. (2013). Distinct mechanisms for globular adiponectin that integrate vascular and metabolic actions of insulin to help maintain coordinated cardiovascular and glucose homeostasis. *Circ. Res.* 112, 1205–1207. doi: 10.1161/CIRCRESAHA.113.301316

Muniyappa, R., Chen, H., Montagnani, M., Sherman, A., and Quon, M. J. (2020). Endothelial dysfunction due to selective insulin resistance in vascular endothelium: insights from mechanistic modeling. *Am. J. Physiol. Endocrinol. Metab.* 319, E629–E646. doi: 10.1152/ajpendo.00247.2020

Muniyappa, R., Montagnani, M., Koh, K. K., and Quon, M. J. (2007). Cardiovascular actions of insulin. *Endocr. Rev.* 28, 463–491. doi: 10.1210/er.2007-0006

Serne, E. H., Stehouwer, C. D., Ter Maaten, J. C., Ter Wee, P. M., Rauwerda, J. A., Donker, A. J., et al. (1999). Microvascular function relates to insulin sensitivity and blood pressure in normal subjects. *Circulation* 99, 896–902. doi: 10.1161/01.cir.99.7.896

Takahashi, Y., Ohoka, N., Hayashi, H., and Sato, R. (2008). TRB3 suppresses adipocyte differentiation by negatively regulating PPARgamma transcriptional activity. *J. Lipid Res.* 49, 880–892. doi: 10.1194/jlr.M700545-JLR200

Tang, M., Zhong, M., Shang, Y., Lin, H., Deng, J., Jiang, H., et al. (2008). Differential regulation of collagen types I and III expression in cardiac fibroblasts by AGEs through TRB3/MAPK signaling pathway. *Cell. Mol. Life Sci.* 65, 2924–2932. doi: 10.1007/s00018-008-8255-3

Ti, Y., Xie, G. L., Wang, Z. H., Bi, X. L., Ding, W. Y., Wang, J., et al. (2011). TRB3 gene silencing alleviates diabetic cardiomyopathy in a type 2 diabetic rat model. *Diabetes* 60, 2963–2974. doi: 10.2337/db11-0549

Tomcik, M., Palumbo-Zerr, K., Zerr, P., Sumova, B., Avouac, J., Dees, C., et al. (2016). Tribbles homologue 3 stimulates canonical TGF-beta signalling to regulate fibroblast activation and tissue fibrosis. *Ann. Rheum. Dis.* 75, 609–616. doi: 10.1136/annrheumdis-2014-206234

Wang, Y., Cheng, K. K., Lam, K. S., Wu, D., Wang, Y., Huang, Y., et al. (2011). APPL1 counteracts obesity-induced vascular insulin resistance and endothelial dysfunction by modulating the endothelial production of nitric oxide and endothelin-1 in mice. *Diabetes* 60, 3044–3054. doi: 10.2337/db11-0666

Wennemers, M., Bussink, J., Scheijen, B., Nagtegaal, I. D., Van Laarhoven, H. W., Raleigh, J. A., et al. (2011). Tribbles homolog 3 denotes a poor prognosis in breast cancer and is involved in hypoxia response. *Breast Cancer Res.* 13:R82. doi: 10.1186/bcr2934

Xing, W., Li, Y., Zhang, H., Mi, C., Hou, Z., Quon, M. J., et al. (2013a). Improvement of vascular insulin sensitivity by downregulation of GRK2 mediates exercise-induced alleviation of hypertension in spontaneously hypertensive rats. *Am. J. Physiol. Heart Circ. Physiol.* 305, H1111–H1119. doi: 10.1152/ajpheart.00290.2013

Xing, W., Yan, W., Liu, P., Ji, L., Li, Y., Sun, L., et al. (2013b). A novel mechanism for vascular insulin resistance in normotensive young SHRs: hypoadiponectinemia and resultant APPL1 downregulation. *Hypertension* 61, 1028–1035. doi: 10.1161/HYPERTENSIONAHA.111.00728

Yu, Q., Gao, F., and Ma, X. L. (2011). Insulin says NO to cardiovascular disease. *Cardiovasc. Res.* 89, 516–524. doi: 10.1093/cvr/cvq349

Zhang, H., Li, J., Li, R., Zhang, Q., Ma, H., Ji, Q., et al. (2008). Reduced cardiotropic response to insulin in spontaneously hypertensive rats: role of peroxisome proliferator-activated receptor-gamma-initiated signaling. *J. Hypertens.* 26, 560–569. doi: 10.1097/HJH.0b013e3282f343e1

Zhang, W., Wu, M., Kim, T., Jariwala, R. H., Garvey, W. J., Luo, N., et al. (2016). Skeletal muscle TRIB3 mediates glucose toxicity in diabetes and high-fat diet-induced insulin resistance. *Diabetes* 65, 2380–2391. doi: 10.2337/db16-0154

21

Activation of Astrocytes in the Persistence of Post-Hypoxic Respiratory Augmentation

Isato Fukushi[1,2], Kotaro Takeda[2,3], Mieczyslaw Pokorski[4,5], Yosuke Kono[2,6], Masashi Yoshizawa[2,6], Yohei Hasebe[2,6], Akito Nakao[7], Yasuo Mori[7], Hiroshi Onimaru[8] and Yasumasa Okada[2]*

[1]Faculty of Health Sciences, Uekusa Gakuen University, Chiba, Japan, [2]Clinical Research Center, Murayama Medical Center, Musashimurayama, Japan, [3]Faculty of Rehabilitation, School of Healthcare, Fujita Health University, Toyoake, Japan, [4]Institute of Health Sciences, University of Opole, Opole, Poland, [5]Faculty of Health Sciences, The Jan Dlugosz University in Czestochowa, Czestochowa, Poland, [6]Department of Pediatrics, Faculty of Medicine, University of Yamanashi, Yamanashi, Japan, [7]Laboratory of Molecular Biology, Department of Synthetic Chemistry and Biological Chemistry, Graduate School of Engineering, Kyoto University, Kyoto, Japan, [8]Department of Physiology, Showa University School of Medicine, Tokyo, Japan

***Correspondence:**
Isato Fukushi
fukushi@1998.jukuin.keio.ac.jp

Acute hypoxia increases ventilation. After cessation of hypoxia loading, ventilation decreases but remains above the pre-exposure baseline level for a time. However, the mechanism of this post-hypoxic persistent respiratory augmentation (PHRA), which is a short-term potentiation of breathing, has not been elucidated. We aimed to test the hypothesis that astrocytes are involved in PHRA. To this end, we investigated hypoxic ventilatory responses by whole-body plethysmography in unanesthetized adult mice. The animals breathed room air, hypoxic gas mixture (7% O_2, 93% N_2) for 2 min, and again room air for 10 min before and after i.p. administration of low (100 mg/kg) and high (300 mg/kg) doses of arundic acid (AA), an astrocyte inhibitor. AA suppressed PHRA, with the high dose decreasing ventilation below the pre-hypoxic level. Further, we investigated the role of the astrocytic TRPA1 channel, a putative ventilatory hypoxia sensor, in PHRA using astrocyte-specific *Trpa1* knockout (as*Trpa1*$^{-/-}$) and floxed *Trpa1* (*Trpa1*$^{f/f}$) mice. In both *Trpa1*$^{f/f}$ and as*Trpa1*$^{-/-}$ mice, PHRA was noticeable, indicating that the astrocyte TRPA1 channel was not directly involved in PHRA. Taken together, these results indicate that astrocytes mediate the PHRA by mechanisms other than TRPA1 channels that are engaged in hypoxia sensing.

Keywords: astrocyte, hypoxia, post-hypoxic respiratory augmentation, plasticity, short-term potentiation, respiratory control, arundic acid, TRPA1

INTRODUCTION

Acute hypoxia increases ventilation. After brief hypoxic exposure, a switchback to room air is accompanied by a ventilatory fall-off in the recovery phase, but ventilation remains above the pre-hypoxic baseline for a time. Post-hypoxic persistent respiratory augmentation (PHRA) is a form of neural plasticity, which is defined as a change in the neural control system based on the memory-like experience (Mitchell and Johnson, 2003). The poststimulus overshoot in ventilatory activity may even go above the stimulus level as is evident in the acute hypoxic ventilatory response (HVR) to static exercise, with the mechanism ascribed to the interaction with the cardiovascular brain control or rapid release of the volitional hypothalamic control over sustained muscle tension (Pokorski et al., 1990). Neural plasticity is essential for stabilizing respiratory control, but the underlying mechanisms are not yet well known (Eldridge and Millhorn, 1986; Dahan et al., 1995; Eldridge, 1996; Powell et al., 1998).

There are plastic interactions in relay circuits of hypoxic stimulus between peripheral chemoreceptors, among which carotid body chemoreceptors are most engaged in creating the HVR, and brain respiratory control pathways (Pamenter and Powell, 2016). The multipronged complexity of PHRA is highlighted by increased carotid chemoreceptor sensitivity due to the withdrawal of the central efferent activity component running down the sinus nerve to the carotid body (Lahiri et al., 1983). That feature has been unraveled in adaptive plasticity to chronic hypoxia but is plausibly also present in repeat acute hypoxic episodes characteristic of sleep apnea syndrome, the disease that distinctly affects brain function and increases chemoreflex sensitivity (Prabhakar, 2016).

Limited understanding of peripheral and central underliers of respiratory plasticity spurred novel lines of research, one of which is the role of transient receptor potential ankyrin 1 (TRPA1) channel. These channels participate in shaping the acute HVR (Pokorski et al., 2014). However, the channels have never been verified in carotid chemoreceptor cells and their effects on the HVR are mediated by mechanisms other than the carotid body (Pokorski et al., 2014). It has been shown that TRPA1 is localized in the chemosensitive parafacial respiratory group (pFRG/RTN) astrocytes in which hypoxia-induced TRPA1 activation facilitates exocytosis of ATP-containing vesicles (Uchiyama et al., 2020). On the basis of these findings, TRPA1 channels in astrocytes have been proposed as an oxygen sensor for respiratory control (Uchiyama et al., 2020). The proposition is in line with studies that show the role of astrocytes in brain synaptic plasticity (De Pittà et al., 2016; Schiera et al., 2020). Astrocytes are also influential for various aspects of respiratory control, including rhythm generation (Okada et al., 2012; Sheikhbahaei et al., 2018) and hypoxic and hypercapnic ventilatory responses (Gourine et al., 2010; Funk et al., 2015; Pokorski et al., 2016; Beltrán-Castillo et al., 2017; Gourine and Funk, 2017; Funk and Gourine, 2018; Sheikhbahaei et al., 2018; Guyenet et al., 2019). It has been reported that astrocytes can detect hypoxia (Tadmouri et al., 2014; Angelova et al., 2015; Fukushi et al., 2016; Onimaru et al., 2021). Therefore, we aimed to test the hypothesis that astrocytes are involved in PHRA and define the role of astrocytes, notably through TRPA1 channels, in the PHRA phenomenon. We used arundic acid (AA) as a pharmacological tool to inhibit astrocytic function in wild-type mice. We also used astrocyte *Trpa1* knockout mice to investigate the role of astrocytic TRPA1 channels in PHRA. We found that the presence of active astrocytes is indispensable for the expression of PHRA, but their action is mediated by mechanisms other than TRPA1 channels.

MATERIALS AND METHODS

Animal Welfare

All animal experiments were performed with the approval of the Ethics Committee for Animal Experiments of the Murayama Medical Center in Tokyo and complied with the Guidelines for Care and Use of Laboratory Animals released by the National Research Council of the National Academies (8th edition, revised 2011) and with the Guiding Principles for Care and Use of Animals of the Physiological Society of Japan. A total of 34 mice (including the mice in experiments for **Supplementary Figures 1, 2**) were used in the experiments. All efforts were made to minimize the number of animals used.

Experiments With Arundic Acid

We used unanesthetized adult male C57BL/6 mice aged 24.0 ± 3.0 weeks (mean ± SE). It should be the same weeks, weighing 29.6 ± 0.7 g (n = 9). The respiratory flow was measured noninvasively using an "open flow" whole-body plethysmograph (PLY 310, EMMS, Bordon, United Kingdom) consisting of recording (volume of 530 ml) and reference chambers as previously described (Oyamada et al., 2008; Pokorski et al., 2014; Fukushi et al., 2016, 2020). Briefly, the chambers were placed inside a transparent acrylic box (size 20 × 20 × 20 cm). Each mouse was placed in the pre-calibrated recording chamber. The chamber temperature was maintained at 25°C throughout. The air in the recording chamber was suctioned with a constant flow generator (MV-6005VP, E.M.P-Japan, Tokyo, Japan), with a flow rate of 250 ml/min. To calculate the airflow, the pressure difference between the recording and reference chambers was measured with a differential pressure transducer (TPF100, EMMS) connected to an amplifier (AIU060, Information & Display Systems, Bordon, United Kingdom) and was bandpass filtered at 0.1–20 Hz. We calculated tidal volume (V_T; μl/g b.w.) for each breath by integrating the airflow whose changes are proportional to those in the chamber pressure (Lundblad et al., 2002). We counted the number of breaths and obtained respiratory rate (RR; breaths/min). Minute ventilation (V_E; ml/g/min) was calculated as $V_T \times RR$ for each minute. The V_E during hypoxia was calculated as a 2-min average and during the recovery phase as an average of the first 5 min (Recovery 1) and second 5 min (Recovery 2). The O_2 concentration in the chamber was monitored with an O_2 analyzer incorporating a polarographic sensor (Respina IH 26, San-ei, Tokyo, Japan) and was adjusted by controlling the mixing of N_2 and air blown into the acrylic box. The pressure and O_2 concentration data were simultaneously digitized at a 400 Hz sampling rate with an A/D converter (PowerLab4/26) and stored in a PC with LabChart7 software. The signal processing was performed using MATLAB 2020a (MathWorks, Natick, MA).

To evaluate the HVR, mice breathed room air, then a hypoxic gas mixture (7% O_2, 93% N_2 for 2 min), and room air again before and after i.p. administration of AA. The experimental protocol consisted of three repeats of hypoxic challenges. First, dimethyl sulfoxide (DMSO), a vehicle for AA diluted in saline, was injected and the mouse was placed into the chamber to acclimatize in room air for 60 min. Then, after recording normoxic baseline data for 1 min, N_2 gas was blown into the acrylic box. The chamber O_2 concentration rapidly declined to 7%, which was maintained for 2 min and followed by a switchback to room air. The measurement for the recovery continued for 10 min. This protocol was repeated after injections of two doses of AA solubilized in a mixture of DMSO and saline (1:4:5 *v*/*v*) at 30-min intervals. Thus, injections were made in the following sequence (1) vehicle - 0.45 ml/kg DMSO, (2) AA - 100 mg/kg, and (3) AA - 200 mg/kg (cumulative AA dose of 300 mg/kg). Although DMSO alone can affect the brain function when the dose is high, a total dose of DMSO used in the present experiment did not exceed 2.0 g/kg, which is much below the 3.5 g/kg, a dose that starts affecting respiration (Takeda et al., 2016). The total volume of saline used in the experiment was 2.24 ml/kg, which is much below the 10 ml/kg reported to affect respiration in mice (Receno et al., 2018). The dosing of AA was chosen according to previous studies using this agent in *in-vivo* rodents (Higashino et al., 2009; Fukushi et al., 2016, 2020). Any apparent movement and sniffing artifacts interfering with breathing patterns were discarded off-line from the recording traces during the final data elaboration. The mean values of V_E were submitted to a two-factor within-subject analysis of variance (ANOVA), with three pharmacological conditions: DMSO vehicle and the two doses of AA, and four air phases (Baseline room air, Hypoxia, Recovery 1, and Recovery 2). The same statistical tests were performed for RR and V_T as for V_E. A Greenhouse–Geisser adjustment was used to correct for violations of sphericity whenever necessary. Then, to quantitatively evaluate the magnitude of PHRA, we calculated the difference in V_E between the post-hypoxic recovery and pre-hypoxic baseline levels. This difference was divided by the difference in V_E between the hypoxic loading and pre-hypoxic levels to normalize for the degree of hypoxic ventilatory augmentation. The calculation provided the parameter $\Delta V_{ERecovery}/\Delta V_{EHypoxia}$ to compare the PHRA magnitude among three drug conditions (without AA and with low and high doses of AA) in the post-hypoxic Recovery 1 and Recovery 2 phases. Statistical differences were assessed with a paired t-test. Bonferroni correction was performed for the multiple comparisons.

Experiments Using Astrocyte-Specific *Trpa1* Knockout Mice

We examined the role of astrocyte TRPA1 channels in HVR and PHRA using astrocyte-specific *Trpa1* knockout mice (as*Trpa1*$^{-/-}$). To generate the as*Trpa1*$^{-/-}$, two lines of mice were crossed: a transgenic mouse GFAP-Cre (mGFAP-Cre) and a recombinant *Trpa1* floxed (*Trpa1*$^{f/f}$) mouse (Gregorian et al., 2009; Zappia et al., 2017; Uchiyama et al., 2020). We conducted 7% hypoxia loading experiments in as*Trpa1*$^{-/-}$ mice (seven males and five females, aged 21.8 ± 0.4 weeks, weighing 25.8 ± 1.1 g) and *Trpa1*$^{f/f}$ mice (two males and four females, aged 22.7 ± 1.3 weeks, weighing 24.2 ± 0.9 g) according to the same protocol and measurement methods as outlined above for the AA experiments. The mean values of V_E, V_T, and RR were submitted to two-way ANOVA with two TRPA1 conditions (as*Trpa1*$^{-/-}$ and *Trpa1*$^{f/f}$) as between-factor and with four air phases (Baseline room air, Hypoxia, Recovery 1, and Recovery 2) as within-factor. A Greenhouse–Geisser adjustment was used to correct for violations of sphericity. We calculated the $\Delta V_{ERecovery}/\Delta V_{EHypoxia}$ to compare the PHRA magnitude between the two TRPA1 conditions (as*Trpa1*$^{-/-}$ and *Trpa1*$^{f/f}$) in the post-hypoxic Recovery 1 and Recovery 2 phases using the Welch test. The Bonferroni correction was used for multiple comparisons in *post hoc* tests. A $p < 0.05$ defined statistically significant differences. The analysis was performed using SPSS 24.0 (IBM, Armonk, NY).

RESULTS

Effects of Arundic Acid on HVRs

The exemplary recordings of V_E profiles in the two AA conditions vs. the control condition with no AA across the baseline room air, hypoxia, and Recovery 1 and 2 phases are shown in **Figure 1**. There was a significant interaction between pharmacological conditions × ventilatory phases [$F(6, 42) = 8.08$, $p < 0.001$]. On average, AA failed to affect V_E, despite some increases in RR after the higher dose of AA in room air. While V_E increased during hypoxia on the background of AA, there were differences in the post-hypoxia recovery course. In the control condition, V_E decreased from the hypoxic hyperventilation level but remained higher than the pre-hypoxic baseline level in both recovery phases. In the low-dose AA condition, V_E immediately returned to the pre-hypoxic baseline level during Recovery 1 but increased again above it during Recovery 2. In the high-dose AA condition, V_E decreased significantly below the pre-hypoxic baseline level during Recovery 1 and then tended to revert to the baseline level in Recovery 2 failing to reach it. The time courses of V_E, V_T, and RR as outlined in the example shown above are summarized in **Figure 2**. **Figure 3A** shows that the $\Delta V_{ERecovery}/\Delta V_{EHypoxia}$, assessing the PHRA magnitude, was significantly smaller in Recovery 1 between control (no AA) and 100 mg/kg AA ($p < 0.01$) or 300 mg/kg AA ($p < 0.001$), and between 100 and 300 mg/kg AA ($p < 0.05$). The differences between control (no AA) and 300 mg/kg AA and between 100 and 300 mg/kg AA distinctly persisted in Recovery 2 (**Figure 3B**). Thus, blockade of astrocyte activation significantly attenuated PHRA; the effect was greatly potentiated at the higher AA dose.

HVRs in as*Trpa1*$^{-/-}$ Mice

V_E profiles in as*Trpa1*$^{-/-}$ and *Trpa1*$^{f/f}$ mice are shown in **Figures 4A,B**. There was a significant main effect of the ventilatory response phases [$F(3, 48) = 85.011$, $p < 0.001$] but not between the TRPA1 conditions [$F(1, 16) = 1.843$, $p = 0.193$]. In both as*Trpa1*$^{-/-}$ and *Trpa1*$^{f/f}$ mice, V_E increased during hypoxia when compared to the pre-hypoxic baseline level ($p < 0.001$) and then decreased in Recovery 1. However, V_E stayed above the baseline level throughout the recovery phases in both as*Trpa1*$^{-/-}$ and *Trpa1*$^{f/f}$ mice. Both V_T and RR components drove ventilatory changes throughout the hypoxic course in both as*Trpa1*$^{-/-}$ and *Trpa1*$^{f/f}$ mice (**Figures 4C,D**).

Although there was no significant interaction of TRPA1 conditions × ventilatory phases [$F(3, 48) = 2.352$, $p = 0.084$], we performed a between-TRPA1 comparison in each phase.

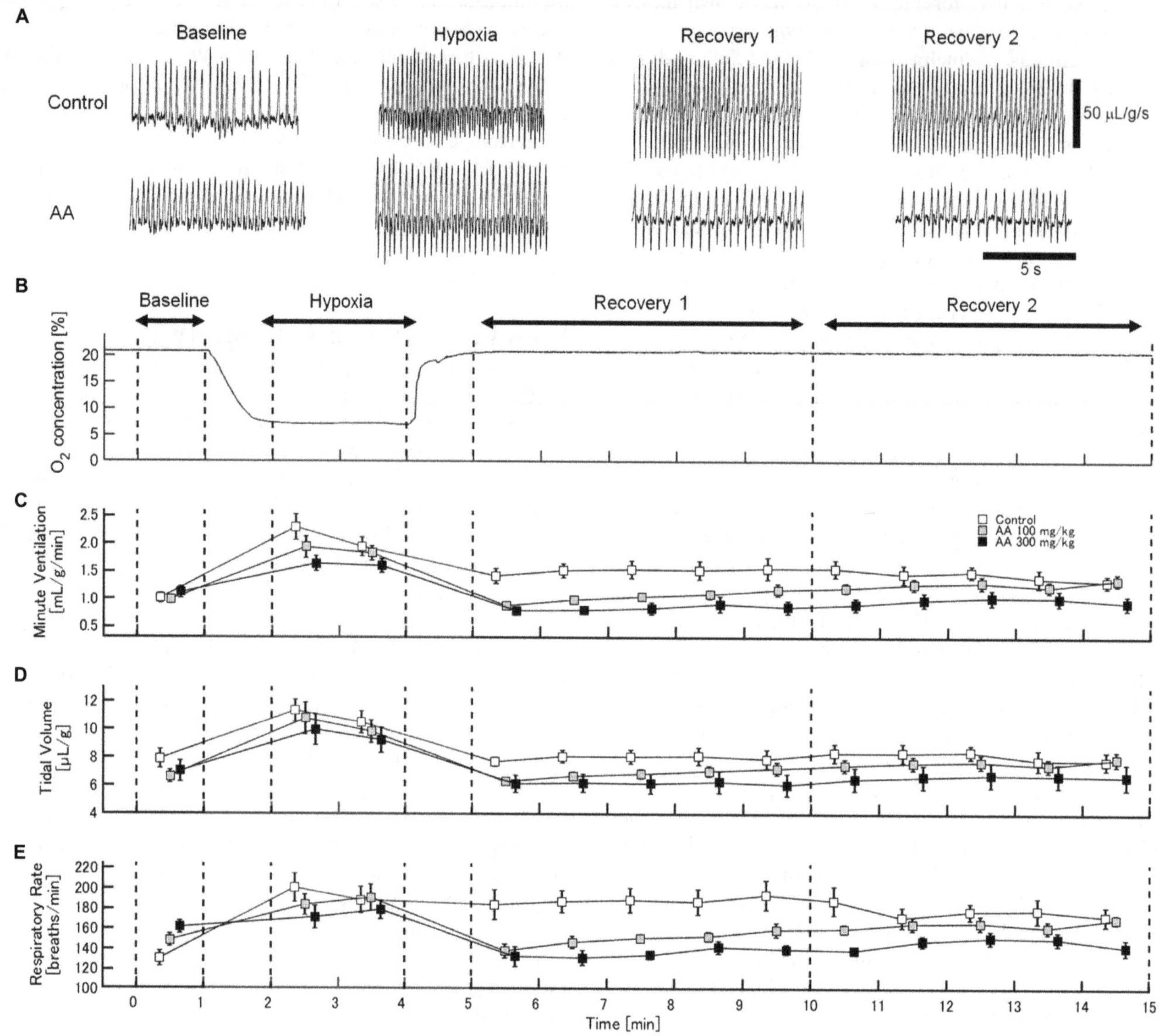

FIGURE 1 | Effects of arundic acid (AA) on hypoxic ventilatory responses (HVRs) in mice by whole-body plethysmography. **(A)** Representative recordings of respiratory flow (inspiration upward) in mice without and with the higher dose of AA in room air (baseline), 7% hypoxia, Recovery 1 (first 5 min), and Recovery 2 (second 5 min). AA did not affect minute ventilation (V_E) at pre-hypoxic baseline but tended to suppress the acute hypoxic hyperventilation. After the lower AA dose, V_E immediately returned to the pre-hypoxic baseline in Recovery 1 but rebounded in Recovery 2. After the higher AA dose, V_E decreased below the pre-hypoxic baseline in Recovery 1 and tended to revert to the baseline level in Recovery 2 failing to reach it. **(B)** Time-profile of chamber oxygen changes. **(C–E)** Time-series data for minute ventilation, tidal volume, and respiratory rate (RR), respectively, in the control (no AA) and low- and high-AA dose conditions.

V_E tended to be smaller in *Trpa1*$^{f/f}$ than as*Trpa1*$^{-/-}$ mice during hypoxia, but the difference was not significant ($p=0.158$). V_E became significantly smaller in as*Trpa1*$^{-/-}$ mice during Recovery 1 ($p=0.034$), but the PHRA phenomenon remained noticeable in both as*Trpa1*$^{-/-}$ and *Trpa1*$^{f/f}$ mice (**Figure 4B**). On average, $\Delta V_{ERecovery}/\Delta V_{EHypoxia}$ percentage values denoting PHRA magnitude were little different between as*Trpa1*$^{-/-}$ and *Trpa1*$^{f/f}$ in post-hypoxic Recovery 1 and 2 phases (**Figures 5A,B**, respectively). Although we did not conduct statistical analysis because the number of *Trpa1*$^{f/f}$ mice was small, there seems to be a gender difference; $\Delta V_{ERecovery1}/\Delta V_{EHypoxia}$ values in male and female *Trpa1*$^{f/f}$, and male and female as*Trpa1*$^{-/-}$ mice were 52, 61, 67, and 16%, respectively. $\Delta V_{ERecovery2}/\Delta V_{EHypoxia}$ values in these mice were 38, 36, 51, and 40%, respectively.

DISCUSSION

This study investigated the role of astrocytes in the PHRA, representing short-term potentiation of respiration. The findings show that astrocytes mediate PHRA. Pharmacological blockade of astrocyte activation by AA inhibited PHRA. The knockout as*Trpa1*$^{-/-}$ mice showed less increase in ventilation in response to hypoxia than *Trpa1*$^{f/f}$ mice. However, the magnitude of PHRA

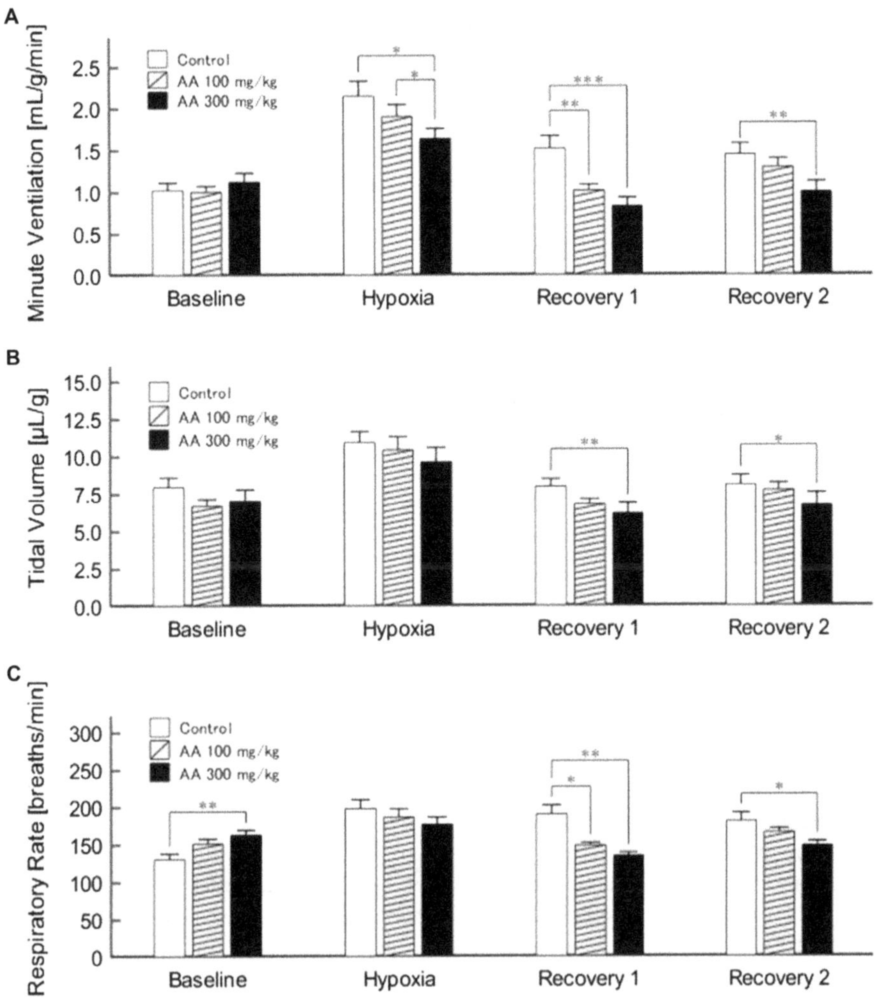

FIGURE 2 | (A) Minute ventilation (V_E) profiles ($n = 9$) in the control (no AA) and low- and high-AA dose conditions across the successive ventilatory phases. V_E differed significantly in the following pairwise comparisons: Control vs. AA 100 and AA 100 vs. AA 300 in hypoxia (both $p < 0.05$); Control vs. AA 100 ($p < 0.01$) and Control vs. AA 300 ($p < 0.001$) in Recovery 1; and Control vs. AA 300 ($p < 0.01$) in Recovery 2. **(B)** The time-course of tidal volume (V_T). There were main effects on V_T of the AA condition ($F_{2,16} = 6.596$, $p < 0.01$) and oxygen concentration ($F_{3,24} = 89.579$, $\varepsilon_{GG} = 0.424$, $p < 0.001$), but no interaction between the two ($F_{6,48} = 1.205$, $\varepsilon_{GG} = 0.522$, $p = 0.329$). V_T differed significantly in the following comparisons: Control vs. AA 300 in Recovery 1 and Control vs. AA 300 in Recovery 2 (both $p < 0.01$). **(C)** Time-course of RR. There was a significant interaction between control (no AA) and two AA conditions × HVR phases ($F_{6,42} = 12.208$, $p < 0.001$). RR differed significantly in the following comparisons: Control vs. AA 300 at baseline ($p < 0.01$); Control vs. AA 100 ($p < 0.05$) and Control vs. AA 300 ($p < 0.01$) in Recovery 1; and Control vs. AA 300 ($p < 0.05$) in Recovery 2. $^{*}p < 0.05$, $^{**}p < 0.01$, and $^{***}p < 0.001$, Bonferroni corrected.

was not attenuated in as*Trpa1*$^{-/-}$ when compared to *Trpa1*$^{f/f}$ mice. Our findings demonstrate the putative role of the astrocyte TRPA1 channels in hypoxia sensing, which confirms the recent findings by Uchiyama et al. (2020). We expanded the role of astrocytes to the mediation of PHRA as well. However, TRPA1 detects mild hypoxia (13%) more closely than severe hypoxia (7%; Takahashi et al., 2011; Pokorski et al., 2014). This suggests that PHRA is more likely to occur under conditions of severe hypoxia. Astrocyte-related action on the short-term PHRA occurs through yet unsettled mechanisms other than TRPA1 channels. The involvement of astrocyte TRPA1 channels has been reported in the hippocampal long-term potentiation in mice (Shigetomi et al., 2013). The contribution of these channels may vary depending on the type of brain plasticity.

In the present study, we used AA, as an inhibitory modulator of astrocyte function. AA inhibits the inflammatory response of astrocytes by reducing GFAP and S100 protein synthesis, increasing the expression of the astroglial glutamate transporter GLAST and releases the glutamate receptor antagonist kynurenic acid from astrocytes (Tateishi et al., 2002; Mori et al., 2004; Asano et al., 2005; Wajima et al., 2013; Yamamura et al., 2013; Yanagisawa et al., 2015). We have previously reported that AA delays the occurrence of seizures and prevents respiratory arrest in severe hypoxia (Fukushi et al., 2020).

The present finding of counteracting the PHRA by AA indicates that astrocytes are influential in shaping respiratory neural plasticity. Hypoxia activates the carotid body, and the information is relayed *via* the carotid sinus nerve to the

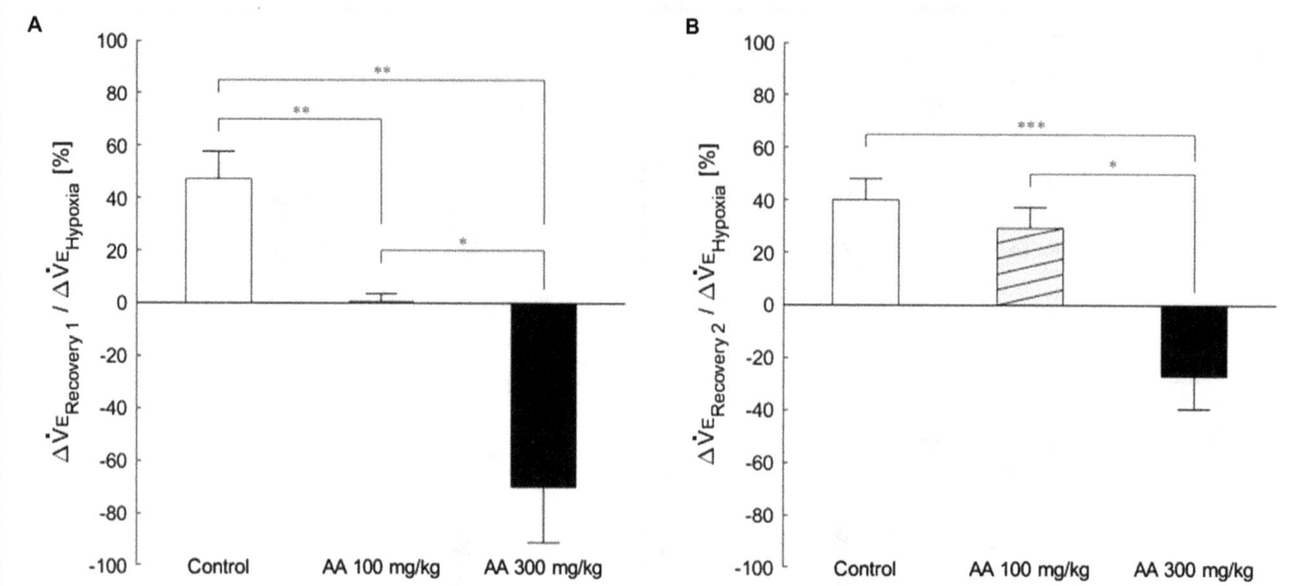

FIGURE 3 | The magnitude of effects of AA on post-hypoxic persistent respiratory augmentation (PHRA) evaluated according to the formula $\Delta V_{ERecovery}/\Delta V_{EHypoxia}$ (see Materials and Methods for details). **(A)** Recovery 1 – PHRA differed between control (no AA) vs. AA 100, control vs. AA 300, and AA 100 vs. AA 300 conditions. **(B)** Recovery 2 – PHRA differed between control (no AA) vs. AA 300. Data are means ± SE. $^{*}p<0.05$, $^{**}p<0.01$, and $^{***}p<0.001$, Bonferroni corrected.

medullary solitary tract nucleus, emanating to other respiratory regions in the brainstem and spinal cord (Guyenet, 2014). Astrocytes around the excited neurons are activated *via* neurotransmitters spilled from neurons. Once activated, they release gliotransmitters that in turn activate respiratory neurons responsible for the sustenance of respiratory potentiation. Of note, the hitherto mechanistic studies on respiratory neural plasticity have been explicitly focused on neurons but not on glial cells. The present study is the first to demonstrate that astrocytes mediate the neural plasticity of respiration.

The short-term potentiation of brain excitability, leading to the continuation of respiratory augmentation after the stimulus cessation, referred to as neural plasticity, has been previously reported (Eldridge, 1973, 1976; Tawadrous and Eldridge, 1974; Eldridge and Gill-Kumar, 1980; Wagner and Eldridge, 1991). The mechanisms of respiratory plasticity are also present in the spinal cord (Feldman et al., 2003; Mitchell and Johnson, 2003; Fuller and Mitchell, 2017). One of the most extensively investigated phenomena in this context is the phrenic long-term facilitation following acute intermittent hypoxia. Regarding the cellular mechanism of facilitation, the Q and S signaling cascades in the phrenic motor nucleus have been proposed, induced by activation of metabotropic receptors coupled to Gq and Gs proteins, respectively, interacting *via* crosstalk inhibition. The serotonin-dependent Q pathway dominates in the phrenic facilitation during mild-to-moderate hypoxia. In contrast, the S pathway is serotonin-independent and dominates during severe hypoxia (Devinney et al., 2013; Fuller and Mitchell, 2017).

Recent studies have revealed an active role of astrocytes in brain plasticity related to other than respiratory functions, with a notable reference to hippocampal memory (Magistretti, 2006; Ota et al., 2013; Croft et al., 2015; Sims et al., 2015; De Pittà et al., 2016). Astrocytes secrete synapse-modulating gliotransmitters such as glutamate, ATP, D-serine, and GABA (Jourdain et al., 2007; Henneberger et al., 2010; Takata et al., 2011; Kang et al., 2013; Shigetomi et al., 2013; Verkhratsky et al., 2016; Zorec et al., 2018; Santello et al., 2019). The regulation of postsynaptic glutamate receptors, particularly α-amino-3-hydroxy-5-methyl-4-isoxazolepropionic acid (AMPA) receptors, is dependent on ATP released from astrocytes. The elevation in astrocytic Ca^{2+}, occurring slowly in the order of seconds, stimulates glutamate release which activates astrocytic metabotropic glutamate receptors (Agulhon et al., 2012; Navarrete et al., 2012). The classical form of neural plasticity also depends on *N*-methyl-D-aspartate (NMDA) receptors and Ca^{2+}-dependent slow release of D-serine from astrocytes (Henneberger et al., 2010). Further, astrocytes express a variety of receptors such as acetylcholine, ATP, GABA, and endocannabinoids (Porter and McCarthy, 1997; Haydon, 2001; Charles et al., 2003).

There are an increasing number of studies referring to the functional role of astrocytes in respiratory control other than respiratory plasticity. Astrocytes in the brainstem are sensitive to hypoxia and involved in HVR (Tadmouri et al., 2014; Angelova et al., 2015; Marina et al., 2015; Fukushi et al., 2016; Pokorski et al., 2016; Rajani et al., 2018; Uchiyama et al., 2020). Astrocytes in the ventral respiratory network, including the pre-Bötzinger complex, release ATP, which increases respiratory activity during hypoxia, putatively counteracting the depressive effects of hypoxia (Gourine et al., 2005; Marina et al., 2016a; Gourine and Funk, 2017; Funk and Gourine, 2018; Rajani et al., 2018). ATP acts *via* $P2Y_1$ receptors in the pre-Bötzinger complex to increase the respiratory burst rate with increases in intracellular Ca^{2+} and glutamate release (Lorier et al., 2007; Huxtable et al., 2010). Astrocytes also are strongly

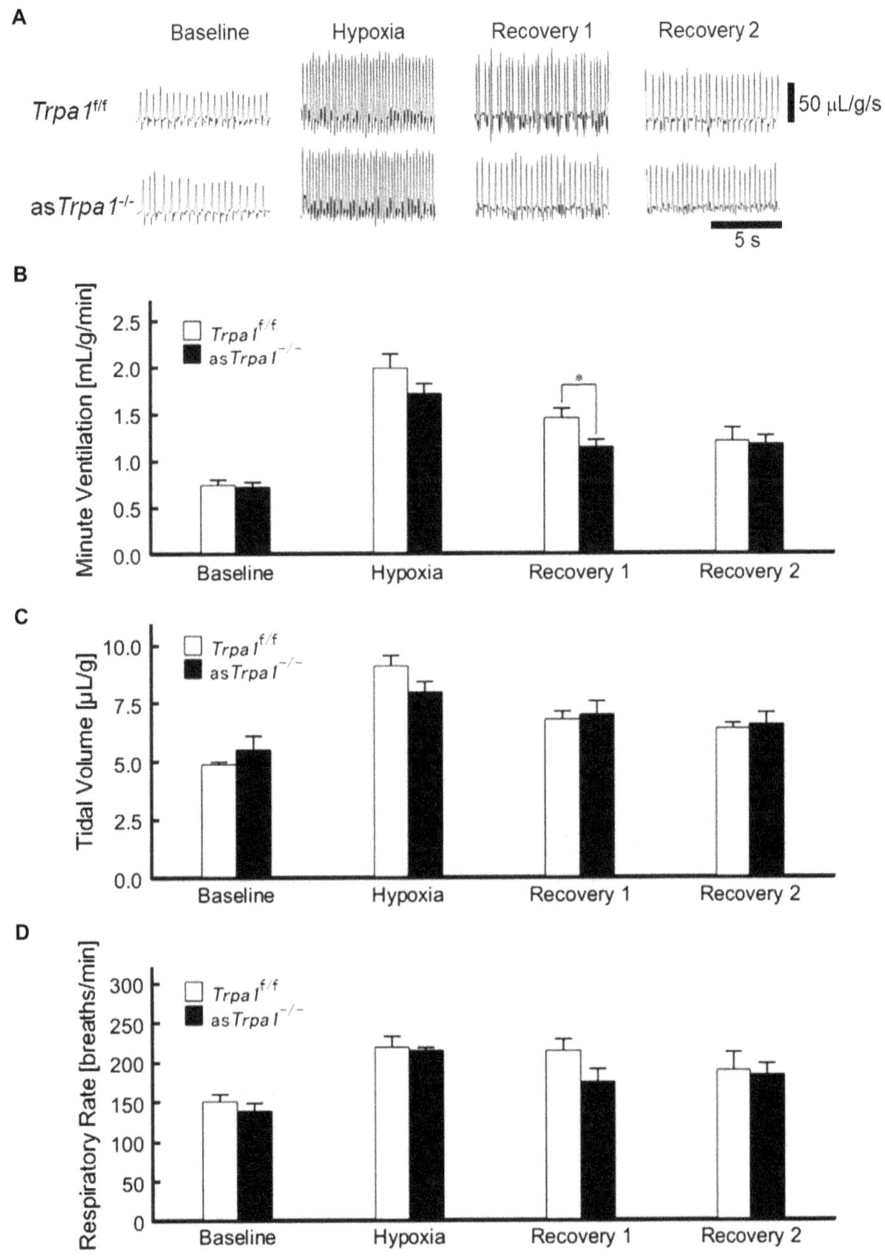

FIGURE 4 | Hypoxic ventilatory responses in as*Trpa1*$^{-/-}$ and *Trpa1*$^{f/f}$ mice. **(A)** Representative recordings of respiratory flow (inspiration upward) in room air (baseline), 7% hypoxia, Recovery 1 (first 5 min), and Recovery 2 (second 5 min). In both as*Trpa1*$^{-/-}$ and *Trpa1*$^{f/f}$ mice, minute ventilation (V_E) increased during hypoxia and then decreased in Recovery 1, remaining significantly elevated over the baseline level throughout both recovery phases. In Recovery 1, V_E was smaller in as*Trpa1*$^{-/-}$ than *Trpa1*$^{f/f}$ mice **(B)** Minute ventilation (V_E) in *Trpa1*$^{f/f}$ ($n = 12$) and as*Trpa1*$^{-/-}$ ($n = 6$) mice in successive ventilatory phases. Of note, V_E was significantly smaller in as*Trpa1*$^{-/-}$ than *Trpa1*$^{f/f}$ in Recovery 1 ($p = 0.034$). **(C)** Tidal volume (V_T) in successive ventilatory phases. There was a significant interaction between transient receptor potential ankyrin 1 (TRPA1) conditions (as*Trpa1*$^{-/-}$ and *Trpa1*$^{f/f}$) × ventilatory response phases ($F_{3,48}$ in as*Trpa1*$^{-/-}$ and *Trpa1*$^{f/f}$ mice = 3.318, $\varepsilon_{GG} = 0.658$, $p < 0.05$) but not between TRPA1 condition and V_T in any of the ventilatory phases. Pairwise comparisons in as*Trpa1*$^{-/-}$: Baseline vs. Hypoxia ($p < 0.001$), Baseline vs. Recovery 1 and Baseline vs. Recovery 2 (both $p < 0.01$), and Hypoxia vs. Recovery 2 ($p < 0.05$) and in *Trpa1*$^{f/f}$ Baseline vs. Hypoxia ($p < 0.001$), Baseline vs. Recovery 1, Baseline vs. Recovery 2, Hypoxia vs. Recovery 1, and Hypoxia vs. Recovery 2 (all $p < 0.01$). **(D)** RR in successive ventilatory phases. There was a significant main effect on RR of the ventilatory response phases ($F_{3,48} = 17.967$, $p < 0.001$) but no significant interaction between RR and TRPA1 conditions ($F_{3,48} = 1.396$, $p = 0.08$). There were no significant pairwise differences between ventilatory response phases in either as*Trpa1*$^{-/-}$ or *Trpa1*$^{f/f}$. Data are means ± SE. $^{*}p < 0.05$; Bonferroni corrected.

involved in the central control of sympathetic activity and cardiovascular function, including systemic hypertension (Marina et al., 2016b), which are enhanced by acute and particularly repeat hypoxia episodes sensed by carotid chemoreceptors (Prabhakar et al., 2015). There is a biological plausibility that medullary astrocytes, respiratory neurons, and peripheral

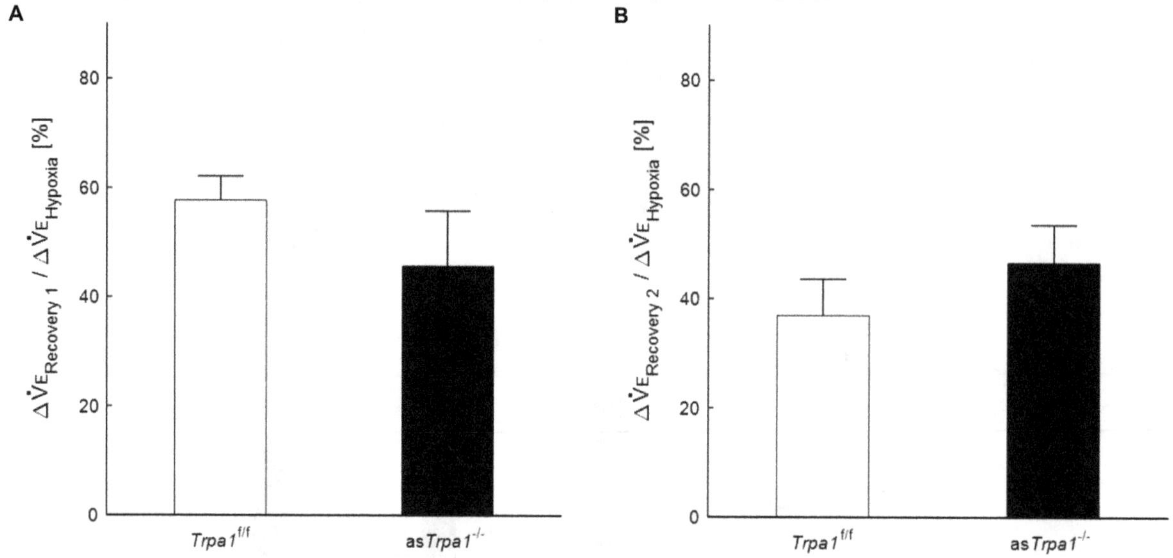

FIGURE 5 | Post-hypoxic persistent respiratory augmentation in astrocyte-specific *Trpa1* knockout mice. The $\Delta V_{ERecovery}/\Delta V_{EHypoxia}$, denoting PHRA, were not significantly different between as*Trpa1*$^{-/-}$ and *Trpa1*$^{f/f}$ in either Recovery 1 **(A)** or Recovery 2 **(B)**. Data are means ± SE.

chemosensing intertwine with each other in shaping PHRA. Alternative study designs are needed to further explore this issue.

In the present study, AA failed to affect V_E, although RR was increased in mice receiving a high dose of AA in room air. This phenomenon suggests that AA can affect breathing, i.e., inhibition of astrocyte activation may alter breathing patterns. In line with this notion, we showed that HVR was attenuated by a high dose of AA. However, AA blunted PHRA much more, suggesting that PHRA is activity-dependent plasticity.

There may be a concern over the time-dependent stability of minute ventilation on the background of a high dose of AA. Our additional investigation revealed that minute ventilation was stable over 240 min in this condition (**Supplementary Figure 1**). Likewise, another set of control investigations showed that hypoxia loadings repeated three times provide close reproducibility (**Supplementary Figure 2**).

One potential limitation of this study could be a lack of the animal's temperature control. In the classical "closed chamber" whole-body plethysmography, tidal volume is calculated by measuring the chamber pressure based on the combined gas law stating that the ratio of the product of gas pressure and volume to the absolute gas temperature is equal to a constant (Drorbaugh and Fenn, 1955). The chamber pressure is recorded while the chamber is sealed, and the body temperature weighs in on the result (Mayer et al., 2014; Rourke et al., 2016; Baby et al., 2018). In practice, however, the body temperature changes are so small during the hypoxic challenges of a couple of minutes that they are usually neglected for the sake of simplicity (Onodera et al., 1997). In the present study, we adopted the "open flow" plethysmography in which the chamber gas is continuously suctioned at a constant flow rate during the continuous recording. We calculated the tidal volume by integrating the airflow whose changes are proportional to those in the chamber pressure (Lundblad et al., 2002). In this case, tidal volume is expressed at ambient temperature (25°C), which obviates the need for taking the animal's body temperature. Another limitation of this study was that we failed to examine metabolic rate in knock-out mice or its potential alterations by AA, which could influence respiration. Metabolic aspects require further exploration using alternative study designs.

The ultimate purpose of this research was to refer to the mechanism of post-hypoxic short-term respiratory plasticity in unanesthetized humans, which is essential to get insights into the pathophysiology of and preventive measures for periodic breathing, e.g., sleep apnea. This purpose stemmed from the studies showing that PHRA is involved in the mitigation of periodic breathing in sleep apnea (Georgopoulus et al., 1992; Mahamed and Mitchell, 2007; Mateika and Syed, 2013; Mateika and Komnenov, 2017) and heart failure (Ahmed et al., 1994); the notion supported in a computer simulation study (Eldridge, 1996). Our results showed that astrocytes, but not the astrocytic TRPA1 channel, were involved in the development of PHRA, suggesting that the TRPA1 is engaged in shaping HVR but not PHRA. The TRPA1 channel likely plays a (patho)physiological role in acute hypoxic conditions such as an attack of bronchial asthma (Shen et al., 2012). In diseases with periodic breathing such as sleep apnea, astrocytes may contribute to its prevention by exerting PHRA. Additionally, the observation that $\Delta V_{ERecovery1}/\Delta V_{EHypoxia}$ tended to be smaller in the female as*Trpa1*$^{-/-}$ mice raises the implication of a greater role of astrocytic TRPA1 in the female gender, which requires further exploration.

In conclusion, we have provided novel aspects of PHRA's role linking it to astrocyte activation and suggesting that this tandem arrangement contributes to respiratory stability and potentially might be influential in the prevention of periodic breathing. However, caution should be exercised in the translation of animal findings to human settings before further exploratory research. We conclude that astrocytes mediate the post-hypoxic persisting respiratory augmentation by mechanisms other than the hitherto recognized role of TRPA1 channels in hypoxia sensing.

ETHICS STATEMENT

The animal study was reviewed and approved by Ethics Committee for Animal Experiments of the Murayama Medical Center.

AUTHOR CONTRIBUTIONS

IF conceived and designed the study, performed the animal experiments, analyzed the data, and drafted the manuscript. KT performed the statistical analysis and drafted the manuscript. MP edited and revised the manuscript. YK, MY, and YH participated in the design of the study. AN and YM provided the animals and revised the manuscript. HO supervised the experiments and revised the manuscript. YO conceived and designed the study, analyzed the data, and revised the manuscript. All authors contributed to the article and approved the submitted version.

REFERENCES

Agulhon, C., Sun, M. Y., Murphy, T., Myers, T., Lauderdale, K., and Fiacco, T. A. (2012). Calcium signaling and gliotransmission in normal vs. reactive astrocytes. *Front. Pharmacol.* 3:139. doi: 10.3389/fphar.2012.00139

Ahmed, M., Serrette, C., Kryger, M. H., and Anthonisen, N. R. (1994). Ventilatory instability in patients with congestive heart failure and nocturnal Cheyne-stokes breathing. *Sleep* 17, 527–534. doi: 10.1093/sleep/17.6.527

Angelova, P. R., Kasymov, V., Christie, I., Sheikhbahaei, S., Turovsky, E., Marina, N., et al. (2015). Functional oxygen sensitivity of astrocytes. *J. Neurosci.* 35, 10460–10473. doi: 10.1523/JNEUROSCI.0045-15.2015

Asano, T., Mori, T., Shimoda, T., Shinagawa, R., Satoh, S., Yada, N., et al. (2005). Arundic acid (ONO-2506) ameliorates delayed ischemic brain damage by preventing astrocytic overproduction of S100B. *Curr. Drug Targets CNS Neurol. Disord.* 4, 127–142. doi: 10.2174/1568007053544084

Baby, S. M., Gruber, R. B., Young, A. P., MacFarlane, P. M., Teppema, L. J., and Lewis, S. J. (2018). Bilateral carotid sinus nerve transection exacerbates morphine-induced respiratory depression. *Eur. J. Pharmacol.* 834, 17–29. doi: 10.1016/j.ejphar.2018.07.018

Beltrán-Castillo, S., Olivares, M. J., Contreras, R. A., Zúñiga, G., Llona, I., von Bernhardi, R., et al. (2017). D-serine released by astrocytes in brainstem regulates breathing response to CO_2 levels. *Nat. Commun.* 8:838. doi: 10.1038/s41467-017-00960-3

Charles, K. J., Deuchars, J., Davies, C. H., and Pangalos, M. N. (2003). GABAB receptor subunit expression in glia. *Mol. Cell. Neurosci.* 24, 214–223. doi: 10.1016/S1044-7431(03)00162-3

Croft, W., Dobson, K. L., and Bellamy, T. C. (2015). Plasticity of neuron-glial transmission: equipping glia for long-term integration of network activity. *Neural Plast.* 2015:765792. doi: 10.1155/2015/765792

Dahan, A., Berkenbosch, A., DeGoede, J., van den Elsen, M., Olievier, I., and van Kleef, J. (1995). Influence of hypoxic duration and post-hypoxic inspired O_2 concentration on short term potentiation of breathing in humans. *J. Physiol.* 488, 803–813. doi: 10.1113/jphysiol.1995.sp021012

De Pittà, M., Brunel, N., and Volterra, A. (2016). Astrocytes: orchestrating synaptic plasticity? *Neuroscience* 323, 43–61. doi: 10.1016/j.neuroscience.2015.04.001

Devinney, M. J., Huxtable, A. G., Nichols, N. L., and Mitchell, G. S. (2013). Hypoxia-induced phrenic long-term facilitation: emergent properties. *Ann. N. Y. Acad. Sci.* 1279, 143–153. doi: 10.1111/nyas.12085

Drorbaugh, J. E., and Fenn, W. O. (1955). A barometric method for measuring ventilation in newborn infants. *Pediatrics* 16, 81–87.

Eldridge, F. L. (1973). Posthyperventilation breathing: different effects of active and passive hyperventilation. *J. Appl. Physiol.* 34, 422–430. doi: 10.1152/jappl.1973.34.4.422

Eldridge, F. L. (1976). Central neural stimulation of respiration in unanesthetized decerebrate cats. *J. Appl. Physiol.* 40, 23–28. doi: 10.1152/jappl.1976.40.1.23

Eldridge, F. L. (1996). "The North Carolina respiratory model," in *Bioengineering Approaches to Pulmonary Physiology and Medicine.* ed. M. C. K. Khoo (Boston, MA: Springer).

Eldridge, F. L., and Gill-Kumar, P. (1980). Central neural respiratory drive and afterdischarge. *Respir. Physiol.* 40, 49–63. doi: 10.1016/0034-5687(80)90004-3

Eldridge, F. L., and Millhorn, D. E. (1986). "Oscillation, gating, and memory in the respiratory control system," in *Handbook of Physiology, Section 3: The Respiratory System: Control of Breathing, Part 1. Vol. 2.* eds. N. S. Cherniack and J. G. Widdicombe (Washington, DC: American Physiological Society), 93–114.

Feldman, J. L., Mitchell, G. S., and Nattie, E. E. (2003). Breathing: rhythmicity, plasticity, chemosensitivity. *Annu. Rev. Neurosci.* 26, 239–266. doi: 10.1146/annurev.neuro.26.041002.131103

Fukushi, I., Takeda, K., Uchiyama, M., Kurita, Y., Pokorski, M., Yokota, S., et al. (2020). Blockade of astrocytic activation delays the occurrence of severe hypoxia-induced seizure and respiratory arrest in mice. *J. Comp. Neurol.* 528, 1257–1264. doi: 10.1002/cne.24828

Fukushi, I., Takeda, K., Yokota, S., Hasebe, Y., Sato, Y., Pokorski, M., et al. (2016). Effects of arundic acid, an astrocytic modulator, on the cerebral and respiratory functions in severe hypoxia. *Respir. Physiol. Neurobiol.* 226, 24–29. doi: 10.1016/j.resp.2015.11.011

Fuller, D. D., and Mitchell, G. S. (2017). Respiratory neuroplasticity - overview, significance and future directions. *Exp. Neurol.* 287, 144–152. doi: 10.1016/j.expneurol.2016.05.022

Funk, G. D., and Gourine, A. V. (2018). CrossTalk proposal: a central hypoxia sensor contributes to the excitatory hypoxic ventilatory response. *J. Physiol.* 596, 2935–2938. doi: 10.1113/JP275707

Funk, G. D., Rajani, V., Alvares, T. S., Revill, A. L., Zhang, Y., Chu, N. Y., et al. (2015). Neuroglia and their roles in central respiratory control; an overview. *Comp. Biochem. Physiol. A Mol. Integr. Physiol.* 186, 83–95. doi: 10.1016/j.cbpa.2015.01.010

Georgopoulus, D., Giannouli, E., Tsara, V., Argiropoulou, P., Patakas, D., and Anthonisen, N. R. (1992). Respiratory short-term poststimulus potentiation (after-discharge) in patients with obstructive sleep apnea. *Am. Rev. Respir. Dis.* 146, 1250–1255. doi: 10.1164/ajrccm/146.5_Pt_1.1250

Gourine, A. V., and Funk, G. D. (2017). On the existence of a central respiratory oxygen sensor. *J. Appl. Physiol. (1985)* 123, 1344–1349. doi: 10.1152/japplphysiol.00194.2017

Gourine, A. V., Kasymov, V., Marina, N., Tang, F., Figueiredo, M. F., Lane, S., et al. (2010). Astrocytes control breathing through pH-dependent release of ATP. *Science* 329, 571–575. doi: 10.1126/science.1190721

Gourine, A. V., Llaudet, E., Dale, N., and Spyer, K. M. (2005). Release of ATP in the ventral medulla during hypoxia in rats: role in hypoxic ventilatory response. *J. Neurosci.* 25, 1211–1218. doi: 10.1523/JNEUROSCI.3763-04.2005

Gregorian, C., Nakashima, J., Le Belle, J., Ohab, J., Kim, R., Liu, A., et al. (2009). Pten deletion in adult neural stem/progenitor cells enhances constitutive neurogenesis. *J. Neurosci.* 29, 1874–1886. doi: 10.1523/JNEUROSCI.3095-08.2009

Guyenet, P. G. (2014). Regulation of breathing and autonomic outflows by chemoreceptors. *Comp. Physiol.* 4, 1511–1562. doi: 10.1002/cphy.c140004

Guyenet, P. G., Stornetta, R. L., Souza, G. M. P. R., Abbott, S. B. G., Shi, Y., and Bayliss, D. A. (2019). The retrotrapezoid nucleus: central chemoreceptor and regulator of breathing automaticity. *Trends Neurosci.* 42, 807–824. doi: 10.1016/j.tins.2019.09.002

Haydon, P. G. (2001). GLIA: listening and talking to the synapse. *Nat. Rev. Neurosci.* 2, 185–193. doi: 10.1038/35058528

Henneberger, C., Papouin, T., Oliet, S. H., and Rusakov, D. A. (2010). Long-term potentiation depends on release of D-serine from astrocytes. *Nature* 463, 232–236. doi: 10.1038/nature08673

Higashino, H., Niwa, A., Satou, T., Ohta, Y., Hashimoto, S., Tabuchi, M., et al. (2009). Immunohistochemical analysis of brain lesions using S100B and glial fibrillary acidic protein antibodies in arundic acid- (ONO-2506) treated stroke-prone spontaneously hypertensive rats. *J. Neural Transm.* 116, 1209–1219. doi: 10.1007/s00702-009-0278-x

Huxtable, A. G., Zwicker, J. D., Alvares, T. S., Ruangkittisakul, A., Fang, X., Hahn, L. B., et al. (2010). Glia contribute to the purinergic modulation of inspiratory rhythm-generating networks. *J. Neurosci.* 30, 3947–3958. doi: 10.1523/JNEUROSCI.6027-09.2010

Jourdain, P., Bergersen, L. H., Bhaukaurally, K., Bezzi, P., Santello, M., Domercq, M., et al. (2007). Glutamate exocytosis from astrocytes controls synaptic strength. *Nat. Neurosci.* 10, 331–339. doi: 10.1038/nn1849

Kang, N., Peng, H., Yu, Y., Stanton, P. K., Guilarte, T. R., and Kang, J. (2013). Astrocytes release D-serine by a large vesicle. *Neuroscience* 240, 243–257. doi: 10.1016/j.neuroscience.2013.02.029

Lahiri, S., Smatresk, N., Pokorski, M., Barnard, P., and Mokashi, A. (1983). Efferent inhibition of carotid body chemoreception in chronically hypoxic cats. *Am. J. Phys.* 245, R678–R683. doi: 10.1152/ajpregu.1983.245.5.R678

Lorier, A. R., Huxtable, A. G., Robinson, D. M., Lipski, J., Housley, G. D., and Funk, G. D. (2007). P2Y1 receptor modulation of the pre-Bötzinger complex inspiratory rhythm generating network *in vitro*. *J. Neurosci.* 27, 993–1005. doi: 10.1523/JNEUROSCI.3948-06.2007

Lundblad, L. K., Irvin, C. G., Adler, A., and Bates, J. H. (2002). A reevaluation of the validity of unrestrained plethysmography in mice. *J. Appl. Physiol.* 93, 1198–1207. doi: 10.1152/japplphysiol.00080.2002

Magistretti, P. J. (2006). Neuron-glia metabolic coupling and plasticity. *J. Exp. Biol.* 209, 2304–2311. doi: 10.1242/jeb.02208

Mahamed, S., and Mitchell, G. S. (2007). Is there a link between intermittent hypoxia-induced respiratory plasticity and obstructive sleep apnoea? *Exp. Physiol.* 92, 27–37. doi: 10.1113/expphysiol.2006.033720

Marina, N., Ang, R., Machhada, A., Kasymov, V., Karagiannis, A., Hosford, P. S., et al. (2015). Brainstem hypoxia contributes to the development of hypertension in the spontaneously hypertensive rat. *Hypertension* 65, 775–783. doi: 10.1161/HYPERTENSIONAHA.114.04683

Marina, N., Kasymov, V., Ackland, G. L., Kasparov, S., and Gourine, A. V. (2016a). Astrocytes and brain hypoxia. *Adv. Exp. Med. Biol.* 903, 201–207. doi: 10.1007/978-1-4899-7678-9_14

Marina, N., Teschemacher, A. G., Kasparov, S., and Gourine, A. V. (2016b). Glia, sympathetic activity and cardiovascular disease. *Exp. Physiol.* 101, 565–576. doi: 10.1113/EP085713

Mateika, J. H., and Komnenov, D. (2017). Intermittent hypoxia initiated plasticity in humans: a multipronged therapeutic approach to treat sleep apnea and overlapping co-morbidities. *Exp. Neurol.* 287, 113–129. doi: 10.1016/j.expneurol.2016.05.011

Mateika, J. H., and Syed, Z. (2013). Intermittent hypoxia, respiratory plasticity and sleep apnea in humans: present knowledge and future investigations. *Respir. Physiol. Neurobiol.* 188, 289–300. doi: 10.1016/j.resp.2013.04.010

Mayer, C. A., Di Fiore, J. M., Martin, R. J., and Macfarlane, P. M. (2014). Vulnerability of neonatal respiratory neural control to sustained hypoxia during a uniquely sensitive window of development. *J. Appl. Physiol.* 116, 514–521. doi: 10.1152/japplphysiol.00976.2013

Mitchell, G. S., and Johnson, S. M. (2003). Neuroplasticity in respiratory motor control. *J. Appl. Physiol.* 94, 358–374. doi: 10.1152/japplphysiol.00523.2002

Mori, T., Tateishi, N., Kagamiishi, Y., Shimoda, T., Satoh, S., Ono, S., et al. (2004). Attenuation of a delayed increase in the extracellular glutamate level in the peri-infarct area following focal cerebral ischemia by a novel agent ONO-2506. *Neurochem. Int.* 45, 381–387. doi: 10.1016/j.neuint.2003.06.001

Navarrete, M., Perea, G., Fernandez de Sevilla, D., Gómez-Gonzalo, M., Núñez, A., Martín, E. D., et al. (2012). Astrocytes mediate *in vivo* cholinergic-induced synaptic plasticity. *PLoS Biol.* 10:e1001259. doi: 10.1371/journal.pbio.1001259

Okada, Y., Sasaki, T., Oku, Y., Takahashi, N., Seki, M., Ujita, S., et al. (2012). Preinspiratory calcium rise in putative pre-Bötzinger complex astrocytes. *J. Physiol.* 590, 4933–4944. doi: 10.1113/jphysiol.2012.231464

Onimaru, H., Yazawa, I., Takeda, K., Fukushi, I., and Okada, Y. (2021). Calcium imaging analysis of cellular responses to hypercapnia and hypoxia in the NTS of newborn rat brainstem preparation. *Front. Physiol.* 12:645904. doi: 10.3389/fphys.2021.645904

Onodera, M., Kuwaki, T., Kumada, M., and Masuda, Y. (1997). Determination of ventilatory volume in mice by whole body plethysmography. *Jpn. J. Physiol.* 47, 317–326. doi: 10.2170/jjphysiol.47.317

Ota, Y., Zanetti, A. T., and Hallock, R. M. (2013). The role of astrocytes in the regulation of synaptic plasticity and memory formation. *Neural Plast.* 2013:185463. doi: 10.1155/2013/185463

Oyamada, Y., Murai, M., Harada, N., Ishizaka, A., and Okada, Y. (2008). Age-dependent involvement of ATP-sensitive potassium channel Kir6.2 in hypoxic ventilatory depression of mouse. *Respir. Physiol. Neurobiol.* 162, 80–84. doi: 10.1016/j.resp.2008.04.003

Pamenter, M. E., and Powell, F. L. (2016). Time domains of the hypoxic ventilatory response and their molecular basis. *Compr. Physiol.* 6, 1345–1385. doi: 10.1002/cphy.c150026

Pokorski, M., Masuda, A., Paulev, P. E., Sakakibara, Y., Ahn, B., Takaishi, S., et al. (1990). Ventilatory and cardiovascular responses to hypoxic and hyperoxic static handgrip exercise in man. *Respir. Physiol.* 81, 189–202. doi: 10.1016/0034-5687(90)90045-Z

Pokorski, M., Takeda, K., and Okada, Y. (2016). Oxygen sensing mechanisms: a physiological penumbra. *Adv. Exp. Med. Biol.* 952, 1–8. doi: 10.1007/5584_2016_67

Pokorski, M., Takeda, K., Sato, Y., and Okada, Y. (2014). The hypoxic ventilatory response and TRPA1 antagonism in conscious mice. *Acta Physiol.* 210, 928–938. doi: 10.1111/apha.12202

Porter, J. T., and McCarthy, K. D. (1997). Astrocytic neurotransmitter receptors in situ and *in vivo*. *Prog. Neurobiol.* 51, 439–455. doi: 10.1016/S0301-0082(96)00068-8

Powell, F. L., Milsom, W. K., and Mitchell, G. S. (1998). Time domains of the hypoxic ventilatory response. *Respir. Physiol.* 112, 123–134. doi: 10.1016/S0034-5687(98)00026-7

Prabhakar, N. R. (2016). Carotid body chemoreflex: a driver of autonomic abnormalities in sleep apnoea. *Exp. Physiol.* 101, 975–985. doi: 10.1113/EP085624

Prabhakar, N. R., Peng, Y. J., Kumar, G. K., and Nanduri, J. (2015). Peripheral chemoreception and arterial pressure responses to intermittent hypoxia. *Comp. Physiol.* 5, 561–577. doi: 10.1002/cphy.c140039

Rajani, V., Zhang, Y., Jalubula, V., Rancic, V., SheikhBahaei, S., Zwicker, J. D., et al. (2018). Release of ATP by pre-Bötzinger complex astrocytes contributes to the hypoxic ventilatory response via a Ca^{2+} –dependent P2Y1 receptor mechanism. *J. Physiol.* 596, 3245–3269. doi: 10.1113/JP274727

Receno, C. N., Glausen, T. G., and DeRuisseau, L. R. (2018). Saline as a vehicle control does not alter ventilation in male CD-1 mice. *Physiol. Rep.* 6:e13702. doi: 10.14814/phy2.13702

Rourke, K. S., Mayer, C. A., and MacFarlane, P. M. (2016). A critical postnatal period of heightened vulnerability to lipopolysaccharide. *Respir. Physiol. Neurobiol.* 232, 26–34. doi: 10.1016/j.resp.2016.06.003

Santello, M., Toni, N., and Volterra, A. (2019). Astrocyte function from information processing to cognition and cognitive impairment. *Nat. Neurosci.* 22, 154–166. doi: 10.1038/s41593-018-0325-8

Schiera, G., Di Liegro, C. M., and Di Liegro, I. (2020). Cell-to-cell communication in learning and memory: from neuro- and glio-transmission to information exchange mediated by extracellular vesicles. *Int. J. Mol. Sci.* 21:266. doi: 10.3390/ijms21010266

Sheikhbahaei, S., Turovsky, E. A., Hosford, P. S., Hadjihambi, A., Theparambil, S. M., Liu, B., et al. (2018). Astrocytes modulate brainstem respiratory rhythm-generating circuits and determine exercise capacity. *Nat. Commun.* 9:370. doi: 10.1038/s41467-017-02723-6

Shen, M. Y., Luo, Y. L., Yang, C. H., Ruan, T., and Lai, C. J. (2012). Hypersensitivity of lung vagal C fibers induced by acute intermittent hypoxia in rats: role of reactive oxygen species and TRPA1. *Am. J. Phys. Regul. Integr. Comp. Phys.* 303, R1175–R1185. doi: 10.1152/ajpregu.00227.2012

Shigetomi, E., Jackson-Weaver, O., Huckstepp, R. T., O'Dell, T. J., and Khakh, B. S. (2013). TRPA1 channels are regulators of astrocyte basal calcium levels and long-term potentiation via constitutive D-serine release. *J. Neurosci.* 33, 10143–10153. doi: 10.1523/JNEUROSCI.5779-12.2013

Sims, R. E., Butcher, J. B., Parri, H. R., and Glazewski, S. (2015). Astrocyte and neuronal plasticity in the somatosensory system. *Neural Plast.* 2015:732014. doi: 10.1155/2015/732014

Tadmouri, A., Champagnat, J., and Morin-Surun, M. P. (2014). Activation of microglia and astrocytes in the nucleus tractus solitarius during ventilatory acclimatization to 10% hypoxia in unanesthetized mice. *J. Neurosci. Res.* 92, 627–633. doi: 10.1002/jnr.23336

Takahashi, N., Kuwaki, T., Kiyonaka, S., Numata, T., Kozai, D., Mizuno, Y., et al. (2011). TRPA1 underlies a sensing mechanism for O_2. *Nat. Chem. Biol.* 7, 701–711. doi: 10.1038/nchembio.640

Takata, N., Mishima, T., Hisatsune, C., Nagai, T., Ebisui, E., Mikoshiba, K., et al. (2011). Astrocyte calcium signaling transforms cholinergic modulation to cortical plasticity *in vivo*. *J. Neurosci.* 31, 18155–18165. doi: 10.1523/JNEUROSCI.5289-11.2011

Takeda, K., Pokorski, M., Sato, Y., Oyamada, Y., and Okada, Y. (2016). Respiratory toxicity of dimethyl sulfoxide. *Adv. Exp. Med. Biol.* 885, 89–96. doi: 10.1007/5584_2015_187

Tateishi, N., Mori, T., Kagamiishi, Y., Satoh, S., Katsube, N., Morikawa, E., et al. (2002). Astrocytic activation and delayed infarct expansion after permanent focal ischemia in rats. Part II: suppression of astrocytic activation by a novel agent (R)-(−)-2-propyloctanoic acid (ONO-2506) leads to mitigation of delayed infarct expansion and early improvement of neurologic deficits. *J. Cereb. Blood Flow Metab.* 22, 723–734. doi: 10.1097/00004647-200206000-00011

Tawadrous, F. D., and Eldridge, F. L. (1974). Posthyperventilation breathing patterns after active hyperventilation in man. *J. Appl. Physiol.* 37, 353–356. doi: 10.1152/jappl.1974.37.3.353

Uchiyama, M., Nakao, A., Kurita, Y., Fukushi, I., Takeda, K., Numata, T., et al. (2020). O_2-dependent protein internalization underlies astrocytic sensing of acute hypoxia by restricting multimodal TRPA1 channel responses. *Curr. Biol.* 30, 3378.e7–3396.e7. doi: 10.1016/j.cub.2020.06.047

Verkhratsky, A., Matteoli, M., Parpura, V., Mothet, J. P., and Zorec, R. (2016). Astrocytes as secretory cells of the central nervous system: idiosyncrasies of vesicular secretion. *EMBO J.* 35, 239–257. doi: 10.15252/embj.201592705

Wagner, P. G., and Eldridge, F. L. (1991). Development of short-term potentiation of respiration. *Respir. Physiol.* 83, 129–139. doi: 10.1016/0034-5687(91)90098-4

Wajima, D., Nakagawa, I., Nakase, H., and Yonezawa, T. (2013). Neuroprotective effect of suppression of astrocytic activation by arundic acid on brain injuries in rats with acute subdural hematomas. *Brain Res.* 1519, 127–135. doi: 10.1016/j.brainres.2013.05.002

Yamamura, S., Hoshikawa, M., Dai, K., Saito, H., Suzuki, N., Niwa, O., et al. (2013). ONO-2506 inhibits spike-wave discharges in a genetic animal model without affecting traditional convulsive tests via gliotransmission regulation. *Br. J. Pharmacol.* 168, 1088–1100. doi: 10.1111/j.1476-5381.2012.02132.x

Yanagisawa, M., Aida, T., Takeda, T., Namekata, K., Harada, T., Shinagawa, R., et al. (2015). Arundic acid attenuates retinal ganglion cell death by increasing glutamate/aspartate transporter expression in a model of normal tension glaucoma. *Cell Death Dis.* 6:e1693. doi: 10.1038/cddis.2015.45

Zappia, K. J., O'Hara, C. L., Moehring, F., Kwan, K. Y., and Stucky, C. L. (2017). Sensory neuron-specific deletion of TRPA1 results in mechanical cutaneous sensory deficits. *eNeuro* 4:ENEURO.0069-16.2017. doi: 10.1523/ENEURO.0069-16.2017

Zorec, R., Parpura, V., and Verkhratsky, A. (2018). Astroglial vesicular network: evolutionary trends, physiology and pathophysiology. *Acta Physiol.* 222:e12915. doi: 10.1111/apha.12915

Permissions

All chapters in this book were first published by Frontiers; hereby published with permission under the Creative Commons Attribution License or equivalent. Every chapter published in this book has been scrutinized by our experts. Their significance has been extensively debated. The topics covered herein carry significant findings which will fuel the growth of the discipline. They may even be implemented as practical applications or may be referred to as a beginning point for another development.

The contributors of this book come from diverse backgrounds, making this book a truly international effort. This book will bring forth new frontiers with its revolutionizing research information and detailed analysis of the nascent developments around the world.

We would like to thank all the contributing authors for lending their expertise to make the book truly unique. They have played a crucial role in the development of this book. Without their invaluable contributions this book wouldn't have been possible. They have made vital efforts to compile up to date information on the varied aspects of this subject to make this book a valuable addition to the collection of many professionals and students.

This book was conceptualized with the vision of imparting up-to-date information and advanced data in this field. To ensure the same, a matchless editorial board was set up. Every individual on the board went through rigorous rounds of assessment to prove their worth. After which they invested a large part of their time researching and compiling the most relevant data for our readers.

The editorial board has been involved in producing this book since its inception. They have spent rigorous hours researching and exploring the diverse topics which have resulted in the successful publishing of this book. They have passed on their knowledge of decades through this book. To expedite this challenging task, the publisher supported the team at every step. A small team of assistant editors was also appointed to further simplify the editing procedure and attain best results for the readers.

Apart from the editorial board, the designing team has also invested a significant amount of their time in understanding the subject and creating the most relevant covers. They scrutinized every image to scout for the most suitable representation of the subject and create an appropriate cover for the book.

The publishing team has been an ardent support to the editorial, designing and production team. Their endless efforts to recruit the best for this project, has resulted in the accomplishment of this book. They are a veteran in the field of academics and their pool of knowledge is as vast as their experience in printing. Their expertise and guidance has proved useful at every step. Their uncompromising quality standards have made this book an exceptional effort. Their encouragement from time to time has been an inspiration for everyone.

The publisher and the editorial board hope that this book will prove to be a valuable piece of knowledge for researchers, students, practitioners and scholars across the globe.

List of Contributors

Valérian Tanner
Medicine School, Faculty of Biology and Medicine, University of Lausanne, Lausanne, Switzerland

Raphael Faiss and Jonas Saugy
Institute of Sport Sciences, University of Lausanne, Lausanne, Switzerland
REDs, Research and Expertise in Anti-Doping Sciences, University of Lausanne, Lausanne, Switzerland

Nicolas Bourdillon and Grégoire P. Millet
Institute of Sport Sciences, University of Lausanne, Lausanne, Switzerland

Laurent Schmitt
National Centre of Nordic-Ski, Research and Performance, Prémanon, France

Christian Arias-Reyes, Jorge Soliz and Vincent Joseph
Centre de Recherche de l'Institute Universitaire de Cardiologie et de Pneumologie de Québec, Université Laval, Québec, QC, Canada

Ning Wang, Ying-Jie Peng, Xiaoyu Su, Nanduri R. Prabhakar and Jayasri Nanduri
Institute for Integrative Physiology, Center for Systems Biology of O2 Sensing, The University of Chicago, Chicago, IL, United States

Vittore Verratti
Department of Psychological, Health and Territorial Sciences, University "G. d'Annunzio" of Chieti-Pescara, Chieti, Italy

Alessandro Tonacci
Institute of Clinical Physiology, National Research Council of Italy, Pisa, Italy

Danilo Bondi
Department of Neuroscience, Imaging and Clinical Sciences, University "G. d'Annunzio" of Chieti-Pescara, Chieti, Italy

Annalisa Chiavaroli, Claudio Ferrante and Luigi Brunetti
Department of Pharmacy, University "G. d'Annunzio" of Chieti-Pescara, Chieti, Italy

Antonio Crisafulli
Department of Medical Science and Public Health, University of Cagliari, Cagliari, Italy

Paolo Cerretelli
Institute of Bioimaging and Molecular Physiology, National Research Council of Italy, Segrate, Italy

Akylbek Sydykov
Department of Internal Medicine, Excellence Cluster Cardio-Pulmonary Institute (CPI), Member of the German Center for Lung Research (DZL), Justus Liebig University of Giessen, Giessen, Germany
Department of Mountain and Sleep Medicine and Pulmonary Hypertension, National Center of Cardiology and Internal Medicine, Bishkek, Kyrgyzstan

Argen Mamazhakypov
Department of Internal Medicine, Excellence Cluster Cardio-Pulmonary Institute (CPI), Member of the German Center for Lung Research (DZL), Justus Liebig University of Giessen, Giessen, Germany

Meerim Sartmyrzaeva, Nadira Kushubakova, Melis Duishobaev, Abdirashit Maripov and Akpay Sarybaev
Department of Mountain and Sleep Medicine and Pulmonary Hypertension, National Center of Cardiology and Internal Medicine, Bishkek, Kyrgyzstan
Kyrgyz Indian Mountain Biomedical Research Center, Bishkek, Kyrgyzstan

Sebastián Castillo-Galán and Bárbara Riquelme
Laboratorio de Neurobiología, Facultad de Ciencias Biológicas, Pontificia Universidad Católica de Chile, Santiago, Chile

Rodrigo Iturriaga
Laboratorio de Neurobiología, Facultad de Ciencias Biológicas, Pontificia Universidad Católica de Chile, Santiago, Chile
Centro de Excelencia en Biomedicina de Magallanes (CEBIMA), Universidad de Magallanes, Punta Arenas, Chile

Jinyan Lin, Lele Fan, Yuming Han, Juanjuan Guo, Zhiqiang Hao, Lingna Cao, Jiamin Kang, Xiaoqin Wang, Jianping He and Jingang Li
National Engineering Laboratory for Resource Development of Endangered Crude Drugs in Northwest China, Key Laboratory of the Ministry of Education for Medicinal Resources and Natural Pharmaceutical Chemistry, College of Life Science, Shaanxi Normal University, Xi'an, China

Garoa Santocildes, Ginés Viscor, Teresa Pagès and Joan Ramon Torrella
Secció de Fisiologia, Departament de Biologia Cel. lular, Fisiologia i Immunologia, Facultat de Biologia, Universitat de Barcelona, Barcelona, Spain

Josep Lluís Torres
Departament de Química Biològica, Institut de Química Avançada de Catalunya (IQAC-CSIC), Barcelona, Spain

Sara Ramos-Romero
Secció de Fisiologia, Departament de Biologia Cel. lular, Fisiologia i Immunologia, Facultat de Biologia, Universitat de Barcelona, Barcelona, Spain
Departament de Química Biològica, Institut de Química Avançada de Catalunya (IQAC-CSIC), Barcelona, Spain

Daniela Parrau and Ismael Hernández
Unidad de Fisiología y Fisiopatología Perinatal, Programa de Fisiopatología, Facultad de Medicina, Instituto de Ciencias Biomédicas, Universidad de Chile, Santiago, Chile

Sebastián Quezada
School of Health and Biomedical Sciences, RMIT University, Bundoora, VIC, Australia

Marcela Díaz
Departamento de Promoción de la Salud de la Mujer y el Recién Nacido, Facultad de Medicina, Universidad de Chile, Santiago, Chile

Germán Ebensperger, Emilio A. Herrera, Aníbal J. Llanos and Roberto V. Reyes
Unidad de Fisiología y Fisiopatología Perinatal, Programa de Fisiopatología, Facultad de Medicina, Instituto de Ciencias Biomédicas, Universidad de Chile, Santiago, Chile
International Center for Andean Studies, Universidad de Chile, Santiago, Chile

Rodrigo Calderon-Jofre and Fernando A. Moraga
Laboratorio de Fisiología, Hipoxia y Función Vascular, Departamento de Ciencias Biomédicas, Facultad de Medicina, Universidad Católica del Norte, Coquimbo, Chile

Daniel Moraga
Departamento de Medicina, Facultad de Ciencias de la Salud, Universidad de Tarapacá, Arica, Chile

Elena Stocco, Maria Martina Sfriso, Martina Contran, Silvia Barbon, Veronica Macchi, Diego Guidolin, Raffaele De Caro and Andrea Porzionato
Department of Neuroscience, Institute of Human Anatomy, University of Padova, Padua, Italy

Giulia Borile and Filippo Romanato
Department of Physics and Astronomy "G. Galilei," University of Padova, Padua, Italy
Institute of Pediatric Research Città della Speranza, Padua, Italy

Mona Lichtblau, Tsogyal D. Latshang, Sayaka S. Aeschbacher, Fabienne Huber, Philipp M. Scheiwiller, Stefanie Ulrich, Simon R. Schneider, Elisabeth D. Hasler, Michael Furian, Konrad E. Bloch, Stéphanie Saxer and Silvia Ulrich
Department of Pulmonology, University Hospital Zurich, Zurich, Switzerland

Michele Dei Cas, Camillo Morano and Rita Paroni
Department of Health Sciences, Università degli Studi di Milano, Milan, Italy

Sara Ottolenghi
Department of Health Sciences, Università degli Studi di Milano, Milan, Italy
Department of Medicine and Surgery, Università degli Studi di Milano-Bicocca, Milan, Italy

Roberto Dicasillati
Department of General Surgery, ASST Santi Paolo e Carlo, San Paolo Hospital, Milan, Italy

Gabriella Roda
Department of Pharmaceutical Sciences, Università degli Studi di Milano, Milan, Italy

Michele Samaja
Department of Health Sciences, Università degli Studi di Milano, Milan, Italy
MAGI Group, Brescia, Italy

Valentina V. Gultyaeva, Dmitriy Y. Uryumtsev, Margarita I. Zinchenko, Vladimir N. Melnikov, Natalia V. Balioz and Sergey G. Krivoschekov
Laboratory of Functional Reserves of Human Organism, Scientific Research Institute of Neurosciences and Medicine, Novosibirsk, Russia

Juliane Hannemann
Institute of Clinical Pharmacology and Toxicology, University Medical Center Hamburg-Eppendorf, Hamburg, Germany
Institute DECIPHER, German-Chilean Institute for Research on Pulmonary Hypoxia and Its Health Sequelae, Hamburg, Germany

Kathrin Cordts and Lena Schmidt-Hutten
Institute of Clinical Pharmacology and Toxicology, University Medical Center Hamburg-Eppendorf, Hamburg, Germany

Rainer Böger
Institute of Clinical Pharmacology and Toxicology, University Medical Center Hamburg-Eppendorf, Hamburg, Germany
Institute DECIPHER, German-Chilean Institute for Research on Pulmonary Hypoxia and Its Health Sequelae, Hamburg, Germany
German Centre for Cardiovascular Research (DZHK), Partner Site Hamburg/Kiel/Lübeck, Hamburg, Germany

Edzard Schwedhelm
Institute of Clinical Pharmacology and Toxicology, University Medical Center Hamburg-Eppendorf, Hamburg, Germany
German Centre for Cardiovascular Research (DZHK), Partner Site Hamburg/Kiel/Lübeck, Hamburg, Germany

Anika Seniuk
German Centre for Cardiovascular Research (DZHK), Partner Site Hamburg/Kiel/Lübeck, Hamburg, Germany
Institute of Cellular and Integrative Physiology, University Medical Center Hamburg, Hamburg, Germany

Chi-un Choe
Department of Neurology, University Medical Center Hamburg-Eppendorf, Hamburg, Germany

Jorge Duque Escobar
German Centre for Cardiovascular Research (DZHK), Partner Site Hamburg/Kiel/Lübeck, Hamburg, Germany
Department of Cardiology, University Heart and Vascular Center, Hamburg, Germany

Florian Weinberger
Insitute of Experimental Pharmacology and Toxicology, University Medical Center Hamburg-Eppendorf, Hamburg, Germany

Jihang Zhang
Institute of Cardiovascular Diseases of PLA, The Second Affiliated Hospital, Third Military Medical University (Army Medical University), Chongqing, China

Fangzhengyuan Yuan, Chuan Liu, Shiyong Yu, Shizhu Bian, Jie Yang, Hu Tan, Jingbin Ke, Yuanqi Yang, Chunyan He, Chen Zhang and Lan Huang
Institute of Cardiovascular Diseases of PLA, The Second Affiliated Hospital, Third Military Medical University (Army Medical University), Chongqing, China
Department of Cardiology, The Second Affiliated Hospital, Third Military Medical University (Army Medical University), Chongqing, China

Xiaohan Ding
Department of Geriatric Cardiology, Chinese PLA General Hospital, Beijing, China

Rongsheng Rao, Zhaojun Liu and Jun Yang
Department of Medical Ultrasonics, The Second Affiliated Hospital, Third Military Medical University (Army Medical University), Chongqing, China

Ivan Lopez, Reinaldo Aravena, Daniel Soza and Alicia Morales
Atacama Large Millimeter/Submillimeter Array, San Pedro de Atacama, Chile

Silvia Riquelme
Departamento de Medicina, Facultad de Ciencias de la Salud, Universidad de Tarapacá, Arica, Chile

Huifang Liu and Noryung Tenzing
Research Center for High Altitude Medicine, Qinghai University, Xining, China
Key Laboratory for Application of High-Altitude Medicine, Qinghai University, Xining, China
Affiliated Hospital of Qinghai University, Xining, China

Martha Tissot van Patot
Retired, Fort Collins, CO, United States

Muge Qile, Ri-li Ge and Tana Wuren
Research Center for High Altitude Medicine, Qinghai University, Xining, China
Key Laboratory for Application of High-Altitude Medicine, Qinghai University, Xining, China

Chaohong Li, Chenlu Zhao, Lu Huang and Yuzhen Liu
Henan Key Laboratory of Neural Regeneration and Repairment, Life Science Research Center, The First Affiliated Hospital of Xinxiang Medical University, Weihui, China

Baosheng Zhao
Department of Thoracic Surgery, The First Affiliated Hospital of Xinxiang Medical University, Weihui, China

Fang Fan, Jinxiao He, Hao Wang, Minghua Zeng and Xin Sun
Department of Pediatrics, Xijing Hospital, Fourth Military Medical University, Xi'an, China

Hui Su
Department of Geratology, Xijing Hospital, Fourth Military Medical University, Xi'an, China

Haifeng Zhang
Teaching Experiment Center, Fourth Military Medical University, Xi'an, China

Qianqian Dong
Department of Natural Medicine, School of Pharmacy, Fourth Military Medical University, Xi'an, China

Wenjuan Xing
School of Aerospace Medicine, Fourth Military Medical University, Xi'an, China
State Key Laboratory of Space Medicine Fundamentals and Application, China Astronaut Research and Training Center, Beijing, China

Isato Fukushi
Faculty of Health Sciences, Uekusa Gakuen University, Chiba, Japan
Clinical Research Center, Murayama Medical Center, Musashimurayama, Japan

Yasumasa Okada
Clinical Research Center, Murayama Medical Center, Musashimurayama, Japan

Kotaro Takeda
Clinical Research Center, Murayama Medical Center, Musashimurayama, Japan
Faculty of Rehabilitation, School of Healthcare, Fujita Health University, Toyoake, Japan

Mieczyslaw Pokorski
Institute of Health Sciences, University of Opole, Opole, Poland
Faculty of Health Sciences, The Jan Dlugosz University in Czestochowa, Czestochowa, Poland

Yosuke Kono, Masashi Yoshizawa and Yohei Hasebe
Clinical Research Center, Murayama Medical Center, Musashimurayama, Japan
Department of Pediatrics, Faculty of Medicine, University of Yamanashi, Yamanashi, Japan

Akito Nakao and Yasuo Mori
Laboratory of Molecular Biology, Department of Synthetic Chemistry and Biological Chemistry, Graduate School of Engineering, Kyoto University, Kyoto, Japan

Hiroshi Onimaru
Department of Physiology, Showa University School of Medicine, Tokyo, Japan

Index